MENTAL ILLNESS AND SOCIAL POLICY

THE AMERICAN EXPERIENCE

MENTAL ILLNESS AND SOCIAL POLICY

THE AMERICAN EXPERIENCE

The
NEW YORK HOSPITAL

By WILLIAM LOGIE RUSSELL

ARNO PRESS
A NEW YORK TIMES COMPANY
New York • 1973

Reprint Edition 1973 by Arno Press Inc.

Reprinted from a copy in
The Medical Library Center of New York

MENTAL ILLNESS AND SOCIAL POLICY:
The American Experience
ISBN for complete set: 0-405-05190-5
See last pages of this volume for titles.

Manufactured in the United States of America

Library of Congress Cataloging in Publication Data

Russell, William Logie, 1863-1951.
The New York Hospital: a history of the psychiatric service, 1771-1936.

(Mental illness and social policty: the American experience)
Reprint of the ed. published by Columbia University Press, New York.
1. Mentally iss--Care and treatment--New York (City)
2. Psychiatric hospitals--New York (City)
3. New York hospital. I. Series. [DNLM: WX28 AN7 H8R 1945F]
RC445.N7N57 1973 362.2'1'097471 73-2414
ISBN 0-405-05224-3

THE NEW YORK HOSPITAL

A History of the Psychiatric Service

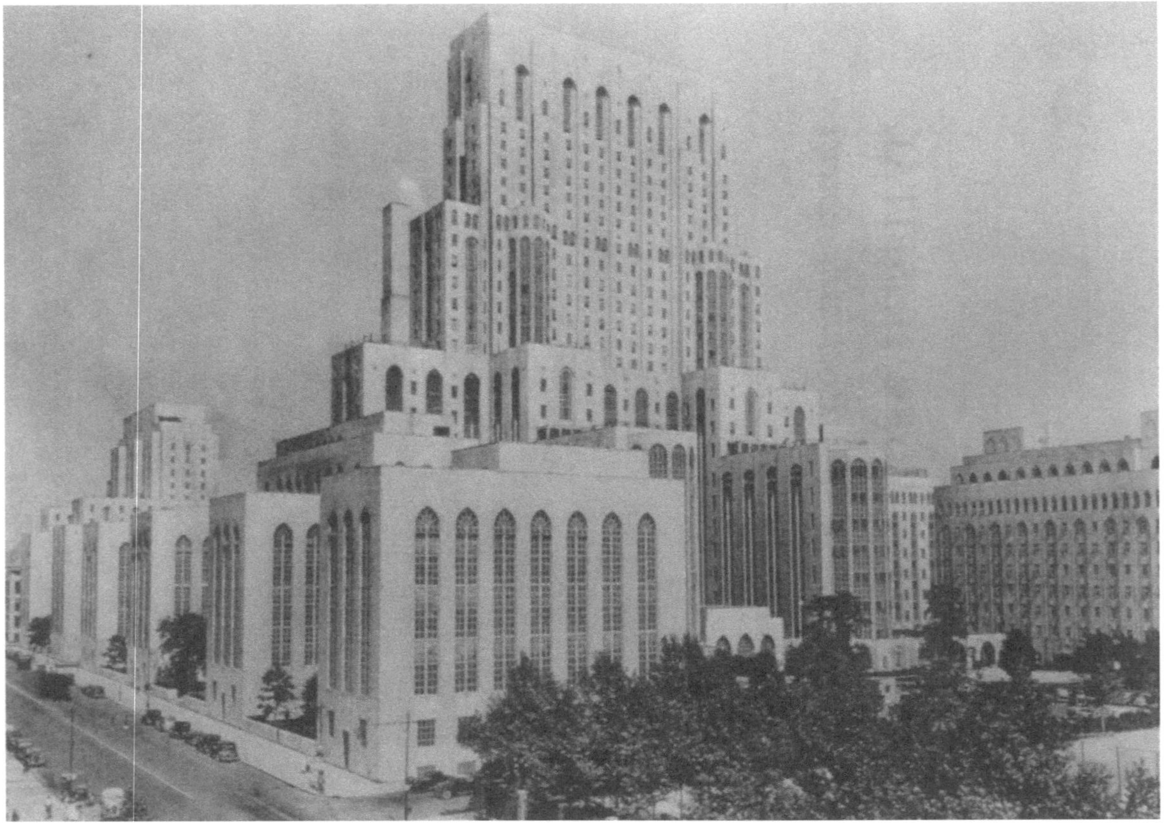

NEW YORK HOSPITAL AND CORNELL UNIVERSITY MEDICAL COLLEGE

The NEW YORK HOSPITAL

A History of the Psychiatric Service 1771-1936

By WILLIAM LOGIE RUSSELL

PROFESSOR OF PSYCHIATRY, EMERITUS, CORNELL UNIVERSITY MEDICAL COLLEGE

CONSULTING PSYCHIATRIST, NEW YORK HOSPITAL

New York · COLUMBIA UNIVERSITY PRESS · 1945

A WARTIME BOOK: THIS COMPLETE EDITION IS PRODUCED IN FULL COMPLIANCE WITH THE GOVERNMENT'S REGULATIONS FOR CONSERVING PAPER AND OTHER ESSENTIAL MATERIALS

FOREIGN AGENT: OXFORD UNIVERSITY PRESS, HUMPHREY MILFORD, AMEN HOUSE, LONDON, E.C. 4, ENGLAND, AND B. I. BUILDING, NICOL ROAD, BOMBAY, INDIA

MANUFACTURED IN THE UNITED STATES OF AMERICA

DEDICATED

TO THE GOVERNORS OF THE SOCIETY OF THE NEW YORK HOSPITAL
WHO ESTABLISHED THE FIRST CURATIVE SERVICE
FOR THE MENTALLY ILL IN NEW YORK
AND BROUGHT IT TO ITS PRESENT EMINENT POSITION
IN PSYCHIATRIC PRACTICE, EDUCATION,
AND RESEARCH

FOREWORD

When the New York Hospital was established in 1771, chains, flogging, and other severe measures were still considered necessary in the treatment of the mentally ill. The hospital was the first and for years the only one in New York, and the second in British America. Provision for the mentally ill was in its earliest policy and plans. The history of its psychiatric service covers, therefore, the whole period during which humane and scientific considerations have been replacing the former severity and neglect.

Contrary to contemporary belief, the governors of the hospital considered mental illness to be curable, and they proceeded to provide a service which should be devoted mainly to curative treatment. This has been the leading aim of the service ever since. Now that it has been in operation for about a century and a half, it seems appropriate to present an account of it, with the hope that this may be a means of quickening interest in the treatment of the mentally ill by the use of facilities and organization which only a liberally supported hospital can supply. This seems to be particularly advisable at the present time when, happily, individualistic treatment has become the major interest in psychiatric thought and practice.

Until well towards the close of the nineteenth century, effort in behalf of the mentally ill in America was devoted almost exclusively to procuring facilities and to forming organizations for using them effectively. For many years little individualistic treatment, psychiatric education, or scientific investigation could be undertaken. This was exemplified at the New York Hospital, and a large part of this account of its psychiatric service was necessarily determined by these considerations. Something of value may, however, be learned from the objects aimed at and the manner and extent of their accomplishment. In retrospect, progress seems to have been remarkably slow. It was, of course, governed considerably by contemporary medical, psychiatric, and social progress. Long delay, even of years, in making advances the need of which was clearly recognized, was sometimes due to lack of funds. Notable advances, however, which occurred at intervals, seem to have been determined by the force and vision of some leading spirit or militant committee of the Board of Governors, or by the understanding and ability of a physician of the service. It can now be seen that progress would have been sounder and more rapid if the recommendations of the physicians had been followed more frequently and more promptly. Progress was undoubtedly retarded by adherence, after it had been generally discarded, to a form of organization in which medical direction of administration was unduly limited. The manner in which the lessons of experience removed this impediment may prove instructive to those who, even yet, especially in the public psychiatric hospitals, propose reverting to this discredited form of organization.

The influence of the psychiatric service of the New York Hospital, established and operated by a group of public-spirited citizens, with state aid and participation in the beginning and for a number of years, contributed to the awakening of the interest and understanding which brought about public provision for the hospital treatment of the mentally ill in New York. The introduction from Europe of a new principle and system of treatment by "management of the mind" or "moral treatment," undertaken by the governors in 1815, and for the practice of which they established Bloomingdale Asylum,[1] influenced all future provision for the treatment of mental illness in America.

Since the advent of the twentieth century the resources of the service have been enriched by means of remarkable advances in medicine, psychiatry, and arts and crafts, and also in social and economic standards. The most advanced facilities and services of medicine, surgery, and the specialties are now intensively utilized in the study and treatment of the mentally ill. The number of physicians, nurses, technicians, and others in the personal-service organization has been more than doubled. The introduction of medical and nursing education has had a large part in advancing the character of the service. It is hoped that the experience met with in endeavoring to conduct a school of nursing may be of some value in furthering this means of providing adequate nursing in the treatment and prevention of mental illness.

Of special interest is the extent to which it has been possible to develop occupational, recreational, and social measures of treatment. These were considered the principal resources in the "new system of treatment" for which Bloomingdale Asylum was established, but their development long baffled the earnest, persistent efforts of the governors and physicians. Now, with other organized forms of treatment, they have such a large place in the service that it is considered that they constitute

[1] Now called New York Hospital–Westchester Division.

"a complete therapeutic organization." The intensive utilization of organized measures of treatment is outstanding in the New York Hospital psychiatric service. Equal advances have, however, been made in the individual study and treatment indispensable to the understanding and "management of the mind."

The spirit of the service has also from its establishment been disposed to scientific investigation and contributions to the advancement of knowledge of mental illness. Previous to the twentieth century only a few studies, some of which were, however, of considerable value, were undertaken. It was not until the laboratory was established and system and precision were introduced in the clinical work that scientific studies and contributions to psychiatric literature became, with increasing volume, an established practice in the service.

Extension of the service beyond attention to patients admitted to the hospital began with the establishment of short courses of psychiatric instruction and practice for student nurses of general hospital schools, and of psychiatric outpatient and ward consultation service in connection with the other departments of the New York Hospital. Individual physicians of the service have also engaged in mental hygiene activities and in teaching. Finally, the resumption of the original close relations with the other departments of the hospital, which were discontinued in 1821 by the removal to Bloomingdale, has been accomplished by the establishment of the Payne Whitney Psychiatric Clinic in 1932. This provision rounds out the service and enlarges its capacity for usefulness in clinical practice, mental health and preventive work, psychiatric education and scientific investigation. Now psychiatric service is as available as any other form of medical service to all the patients of the New York Hospital. The governors built better than they knew when in September, 1792, they admitted, by resolution of the board, the first mentally ill patient, provided he was "considered by the Physicians of the Hospital as curable." They exhibited a sense of values and of service for all their successors to follow.

This account of the service comes far short of revealing the relief from anxiety, despair, weakness, and incapacity accomplished since then in the treatment of more than twenty-five thousand patients. This has been, however, the real work and the true measure of its value. It has been directed to the restoration of mentally ill persons of more than ordinary education and usefulness. To furnish treatment for such persons of moderate means or, by reason of their illness, temporarily dependent is the main purpose for which the service is operated. The results obtained seem to suggest that the essentials of the intensive type of organization and treatment which the New York Hospital has been enabled to develop during the many years of its operation should be available to every mentally ill person in need of active hospital treatment whatever his circumstances.

Most of the material used in the preparation of this book was obtained from the records and archives of the New York Hospital. Much, however, as well as courteous and valuable aid, was obtained from the library of the New York Academy of Medicine, the New York Historical Society, the New York Society Library, the New York Public Library, and the Cornell–New York Hospital Medical Library, all of which is gratefully acknowledged. The material relating to the early history of the service collected by the late Dr. Mortimer W. Raynor has been an incentive as well as a source of information. All or parts of the manuscript were read by Professor Oskar Diethelm and Dr. James H. Wall of the New York Hospital–Cornell Medical College staff, by Dr. Archibald Malloch, Librarian of the New York Academy of Medicine, and by Dr. Emma Peters Smith, historian. Their helpful advice and encouragement are deeply appreciated. Acknowledgment is made to the American Foundation for Mental Hygiene for permission to quote from Albert Deutsch, *The Mentally Ill in America* (1937).

Mrs. Robert S. Hutchins and Miss Lois Thurston have had a large part in the preparation of the manuscript. Mrs. Hutchins was especially helpful in obtaining the material relating to old New York and to the establishment and early operation of the service. Miss Thurston has contributed greatly to the extent and accuracy of the references and to the preparation of the manuscript for publication.

W. L. R.

New York
October 14, 1944

CONTENTS

PART FIVE

Planning for Classification and Removal—State Supervision and Laws, 1852–1877

PART SIX

A Medically Directed Private Charity, 1877–1894

PART SEVEN

The Dawn of Modern Scientific Psychiatry at Bloomingdale, 1894–1911

PART EIGHT

Fulfillment of Some Long-cherished Aspirations, 1911–1926

PART NINE

A Complete Organization for Service, Education, and Research, 1926–1936

APPENDICES

ILLUSTRATIONS

It is the future
which must prevail over the past,
and from it we take our orders
regarding our attitude
towards what has been.

—GASSET

PART ONE

Introduction: The Close of the Eighteenth Century

I: PSYCHIATRIC THOUGHT

THE New York Hospital was established at a time when a new day was dawning for the mentally ill. It was near the close of the eighteenth century and the intellectual and spiritual awakening which characterized that prolific century was about to be transformed into practical accomplishments. Advancing knowledge was taking the form of scientific disciplines. The dignity of the common man and his rights as an individual were assuming an importance far beyond what had previously been acknowledged. It was recognized that there were rights and privileges that could not properly be denied him, however humble or unfortunate he might be. Social responsibility for the weak and dependent, for the welfare and treatment of the physically and mentally sick, and for the rational and humane treatment of offenders against public peace and safety, was recognized. It was a period of prison reform and of the establishment of almshouses, asylums, and educational institutions. In medicine, knowledge of anatomy and physiology, and clinical observation and experience were commencing to supplant authority and poorly controlled theoretical considerations as a guide to practice. Pinel considered that

> the principles of free enquiry which the revolution has incorporated with our national politics, have opened a wide field to the energies of medical philosophy. But it is chiefly in great hospitals and asylums, that those advantages will be immediately felt, from the opportunities which are there afforded of making a great number of observations, experiments, and comparisons.[1]

Medical thinking and practice still lacked precision, however, and specialization was seldom undertaken. Personality deviations (called madness or lunacy), neuroses or nervous disorders, and idiotism were considered much as other diseases, in general medical teaching, writing, and practice. Belief in possession, magic, and witchcraft, which for ages

[1] Philippe Pinel, *A Treatise on Insanity*, trans. D. D. Davis (Sheffield, 1806), p. 46.

had been accepted as an explanation of mental illness, had at this period been practically given up by physicians. The supposed influence of the heavenly bodies, especially the moon, was, however, still discussed with respect, though not without considerable doubt, by eminent medical writers and teachers.[2]

Throughout the history of medicine, in every period, there have not been lacking writers and practitioners who have ventured to advocate and to endeavor to practice rational and humane conceptions and methods in the consideration and treatment of the mentally ill. Their views and example had, however, never been widely enough accepted by their contemporaries to accomplish a general advance. At the close of the eighteenth century a widespread enlightenment had been awakened, and only an attention-compelling demonstration was needed to set in motion the advancement that was to grow and extend, with increasing momentum, through the nineteenth century and on to the present day. Such a demonstration was furnished in 1792—the same year in which the first mentally ill patient was admitted to the New York Hospital—when Dr. Philippe Pinel at a Paris hospital created a sensation by releasing a large number of patients from chains and fetters and replacing the severe repressions and drastic medical practices, that were then universally employed, with a system of "moral treatment." In England also, in the same year, William Tuke, a Quaker merchant, was establishing at York a "Retreat," at which the treatment was characterized by kindly, intelligent consideration, freedom from gross restraints and repressions, and by measures directed to physical and mental rehabilitation and exercise in wholesome interests and activities. In America, at the Pennsylvania Hospital in Philadelphia, Dr. Benjamin Rush, like a voice in the wilderness, was calling for more rational, humane, and effective treatment for the mentally ill patients than was at that time furnished anywhere. As will be noted later, these developments in Europe and at the only hospital then in British America, influenced greatly the establishment and the character of the provision for mental illness made by the Society of the New York Hospital.

In the English colonies in America, and, after the Revolution, in the new states, social organization and provision for public health and for the treatment of the sick, had made little progress. Sanitary and public health and welfare measures were grossly inadequate. Epidemics of infectious diseases were frequent and devastating. In the whole country

[2] Thomas Arnold, *Observations on the Nature, Kinds, Causes and Prevention of Insanity* ('ed ed., London, 1806), I, 251.

there was only one organized hospital [3] and there were few physicians. Almshouses had been established in a few places. Wretched, poorly organized, and meagerly supported, they received dependents from any cause, and were also houses of detention for delinquents as well as the sole refuge for the dependent physically and mentally ill. At Williamsburg, Virginia, an institution solely for the mentally ill was established in 1773. It was called a hospital although not medically organized, and was the first attempt at separate provision for the mentally ill in the Colonies, setting an example that was widely followed throughout the country in the following century. It was not until nearly the close of the colonial period that any provision was made for medical education. This could scarcely be adequately accomplished until hospitals became available. Even in Philadelphia, however, where there was a hospital, and where a medical school was established in 1765, the difficulties in organization were so great that little headway was made for several years. The experience in New York, where there was no hospital, was even more difficult. A medical school was, however, established by King's College and three students were granted diplomas in 1769. It was at the graduation exercises that year that Dr. Samuel Bard delivered the memorable address which accomplished the first steps in the campaign for the establishment of "the Hospital in the City of New York."

There were at that time no laws or regulations for governing medical practice, and many of the practitioners had received no formal medical instruction and training, except possibly that obtainable by a sort of apprenticeship with a practicing physician. In order to obtain an adequate medical education and experience in hospital practice, it was necessary to resort to European medical schools and hospitals, and the leading physicians in New York were those who had been given that advantage. It was natural that the British schools would ordinarily be chosen, and it was in these schools that Dr. Samuel Bard, Dr. Peter Middleton, and Dr. John Jones, who were the petitioners for the charter of the New York Hospital, as well as most of the other physicians who were members of the medical staff of the hospital in the first few years of its operation, received the principal part of their medical education. They were thus indoctrinated with the views and practices that were followed in the European colleges and hospitals to which students repaired. Unfortunately, neither the hospital records nor publications by members of the medical staff reveal their views in regard to mental illness and its treatment, nor the considerations that led to its inclusion

[3] The Pennsylvania Hospital.

in the hospital provisions. A review of the medical doctrines and practices that were followed in the schools and hospitals in which the first physicians of the New York Hospital received their medical education may, therefore, be the best and perhaps the only means available for obtaining information relating to these questions.

In considering mental illness as understood by the medical profession at the time the New York Hospital was established, it is necessary to realize that, at that time, differentiation of forms of disease and morbid reactions such as can now be made was not possible. The eighteenth century physician had a different conception of the nature of man and of his illnesses than prevails today, and total reactions had a more exclusive place in his considerations. The medical doctrines and practices that were followed in the study and treatment of disease, generally, were considered to be fully adequate for the understanding and treatment of mental illness. The prevailing view was that this form of illness was invariably occasioned by morbid disturbances in the brain and nervous system, and that measures directed to these were the only medical treatment that would be effective. Theoretical considerations dominated medical thought and practice, and, with modifications and combinations, the medical teachers, writers, and practitioners of the period adhered to one or another of the many prevailing doctrines. Among these doctrines the following appear to have been the most important:[4] 1) Irritability or Neurosism; 2) Organicism; 3) Vitalism; 4) Naturalism; 5) Humorism. Of these, Irritability or Neurosism seems to have been of the greatest significance and importance in the development of knowledge of the nervous system and its functioning. By this doctrine all phenomena observed in the human organism were considered explainable by the quality of irritability of its tissues. This quality was manifested by contraction of the tissue on stimulation, or by transmission of impressions to the brain by the nerves. It was noted that irritability was, of itself, sufficient for the performance of such vital natural actions as circulation, secretion, digestion, absorption, and elimination, and that these could be performed without perception, volition, or even sensation, which were considered to be mental powers.[5] This seems to have been an early approach to an understanding of the vegetative nervous system.

Those who followed the doctrine of Organicism held to a mechanical

[4] C. G. Cumston, *An Introduction to the History of Medicine* (New York, 1926). This account of the medical doctrines of the 18th century was for the most part obtained from this work.

[5] Arnold, *op. cit.*, II, 41.

view of the organism, which was regarded as a group of organs. Life was considered to be the sum total of the life of the separate organs, and sickness was due to the failure of one or several of them. Inadequate functioning of the organs was the cause of "a bad mixture of the humors." [6] Sickness and death were the result of deterioration of the heart, lungs, or brain; death being due to cessation of all movement.[7] The condition of the blood and movement of the solids were viewed as mechanical causes of disease. Importance was attached to firmness or looseness of the particles which compose the solids of the body, to pressures and obstructions, to balance or equilibrium between the solids and fluids, and to density, viscosity, thinness, or "depravity" of the fluid.[8] Pressure on the medullary substance of the nerves was believed to produce an uneasiness which might result in "delusive sensation." "Sufficient . . . pressure upon the medullary substance . . . may be the remoter cause of consequential madness." A feeling of anxiety might be produced by pressure from "the nervous integuments or neighboring membranes" that were "praeternaturally compacted and of too close a texture." [9] The brain was considered to be the seat of "delusive sensation," but it was not the only one; as "sanguinary or serous obstructions are capable of exciting false ideas. . . . Thus, the stomach, intestines, and uterus are frequently the real seats of madness, occasioned by . . . these viscera being obstructed in such a manner as to compress the many nervous filaments which here communicate with one another by the mesenteric ganglia." [10] Notwithstanding this mechanical view of the human organism, it was found necessary to resort to the conception of "sympathy" or "consent." Every sensitive part of the body was considered to be in sympathy with the whole, and disturbances in the digestive tract or elsewhere might by this process affect the brain and cause mental disorder.

Vitalism taught that the organism was controlled as a whole by some central force or principle.[11] This doctrine attached much importance to movement. Three movements were referred to: circulatory, secretory, and excretory. The more extreme Vitalists held to the doctrine of a living soul that presided over the organism in health and disease.[12] Reference was also made to a central "inciter" or "impeller," the Ενορμων or Ὁρμην

6 Bordeu, quoted by Cumston, *op. cit.*, p. 351.
7 Lancisii, quoted in *ibid.*, p. 319.
8 Baglivi, quoted in *ibid.*, p. 327.
9 William Battie, *A Treatise on Madness* (London, 1758), pp. 39, 46.
10 William D. Perfect, *Annals of Insanity* (2d ed., London, 1801).
11 Barthez, *Les Nouveaux Elements de la science de l'homme* (1774). See Cumston, *op. cit.*, p. 356.
12 Stahl. See Cumston, p. 374.

conceived by Hippocrates as the spring from which all action flowed.[13]

The doctrine of Humoralism was of ancient lineage. The humors were blood, black bile, yellow bile, and phlegm. Illness was attributed to changes in the quantity, consistency, or constituents of one or more humors. The effect on the fluid conveyed by the nerves was believed to be a cause of mental illness.

The doctrine of Naturalism was concerned principally with disease as a natural history problem. It was considered that "Nature alone preserves health in the greater number of men and cures their diseases. . . . It is to scrupulous observation of Nature and the attempts to imitate her that medical art owes its origin." [14] The naturalists proposed to classify mental disorders along the lines that had been introduced in the study of botany and other sciences. In fact, Linnaeus, the botanist, who was also a physician, undertook such a classification.

Near the close of the century, Bichat (1771–1802), who has been called the link between the eighteenth and nineteenth centuries, drew attention to the importance of considering that, though the entire organism is made up of particular organs, these organs, in turn, consist of tissues and of the functions of these tissues, which must be taken into account in explaining the nature and reactions of the organism. He drew attention to the operation, not only of the vital principles of sensibility and contractility, but also of non-vital principles such as gravity, chemical action, and elasticity. He advocated consideration not only of the physiological sciences and medicine, but also of the physical sciences such as astronomy, physics, and chemistry.[15] This understanding had a wholesome effect on medical thought, teaching, and practice.

The way by which impressions were transmitted to and from the brain by the nerves, and by which thought and volition were determined in health and disease, was a knotty problem that was long a subject of much speculation. A prevalent conception was that the nerves were filled with a soft milky cellular substance ("like a Rush with its Pith") which conveyed to the brain "Vibrations, Undulations and Tremors," and that by the same process impressions were conveyed from the brain to the organs of sense and the muscles.[16] Another conception was that the nerves conveyed a fluid "inconceivably fine . . . secreted in the brain . . . and serving as a medium of communication between the mind

[13] H. D. Gaubius, *On the Passions*, trans., J. Taprell (London, c. 1780), p. 38.

[14] *Ibid.*, p. 336.

[15] Bichat. See Cumston, *op. cit.*, p. 361.

[16] George Cheyne, *The Natural Method of Curing the Diseases of the Body and the Disorders of the Mind Depending on the Body* (5th ed., London, 1753), p. 94.

and the body." The transmission of "vitiated" impressions to the brain was considered to be the basis of delusional thinking. "A certain morbid or *irritating* principle or quality of that fluid [nervous fluid . . . or electric aura] acting upon the brain is the *primary* cause of Insanity . . . but what the *specific* nature of that morbid quality or principle is, it is impossible to conceive, and it will, no doubt, for ever remain a secret." [17] Those who held to a mechanical view of the organism believed that the nerves were solid, and that impressions were conveyed by variations in the firmness or looseness of juxtaposition of the particles of which they were composed. They also considered that obstructions, pressure, tension, and relaxation in the brain and other parts of the nervous system might affect the sensibility and contractility of the delicate fibres and produce such disturbances in both the fluids and solids that mental disorder would result.

The mind was conceived to be a concrete entity, or a mysterious force lodged in or connected with the human organism, especially the brain. William Cullen, an eminent clinician and teacher at Edinburgh University when Dr. Samuel Bard and others who later became members of the medical staff of the New York Hospital were students there, considered the nervous system to be "the connecting medium between the soul and the body, the organ of sensation, intellect, memory, judgment, voluntary, involuntary, mixed and sympathetic motions of the animal economy, the basis of the doctrine of excitability and collapse, and of the effect of custom on our corporeal and mental functions." [18] Some believed that the "nervous fluid" was entirely under the control of the soul.[19] Others were, however, commencing to think that the relations between the soul and the body were too mysterious to be understood, and that it would be advisable to confine consideration to the "laws of union."

Although the conception of mental illness and its treatment as exclusively a disease of the brain and nervous system continued to hold first place in medical thought and practice, the systematic observation and study of mental manifestations and of mental factors in etiology were, at the close of the eighteenth century, receiving much attention. It was in this period that modern psychiatry began to take on its present form. To this advance many contributed, and Pinel was the leading spirit. He was much more than a humane reformer. In fact, Vincenzo

[17] William Pargeter, *Observations on Maniacal Disorders* (Reading, England, 1792), p. 15.
[18] William Cullen, *Treatise on Materia Medica* (Dublin, 1789).
[19] Georg Ernst Stahl, quoted in Cumston, *op. cit.*, p. 374.

Chiarugi in Florence, Joseph Daquin in France, and others had preceded him in introducing humane, rational measures in the treatment of the mentally ill, and Tuke was proceeding at York without knowledge of Pinel's accomplishment. Pinel had, however, that clearness of perception of the significant and essential in matters directed to human welfare that is engendered by a kindly feeling for others, and he was an independent thinker who was imbued with the scientific spirit. He found that the theories, classifications, and treatment of the writers he consulted were of little advantage in his efforts to understand and treat his patients.

I, therefore [he wrote], resolved to adopt that method of investigation which has invariably succeeded in all the departments of natural history, viz. to notice successively every fact, without any other object than that of collecting materials for future use; and to endeavour, as far as possible, to divest myself of the influence both of my own prepossessions and the authority of others. With this view, I first of all took a general statement of the symptoms of my patients. To ascertain their characteristic peculiarities, the above survey was followed by cautious and repeated examinations into the condition of individuals. All our new cases were entered at great length upon the journals of the house.[20]

This was a first lesson in modern psychiatric practice. The hospital work of Pinel and his publications mark the beginning of a movement for better study and treatment of the mentally ill which made a striking advance during the nineteenth century and has not yet reached its full fruition.

As the eighteenth century advanced, contributions to psychiatry in medical literature steadily increased in number and magnitude, and psychological considerations became more frequent and extensive. By the close of the century most of the general treatises on mental disorders contained much relating to the nature of the mind and to the role of mental factors in the production of symptoms. Classifications of mental disorders in accordance with psychological conceptions were presented. It was proposed that Insanity should be considered as a single Genus with two varieties, "Ideal Insanity" and "Notional Insanity." The former term embraced disorders in which objects perceived were unreal or not correctly recognized, as in delirium; the latter embraced disorders in which objects were perceived as objects of sense, but the patient "conceives such notions of the powers, properties, designs, state, destination, importance, manner of existence, or the like, of things and per-

[20] Pinel, *op. cit.*, pp. 2–3.

sons, of himself and others, as appear obviously, and often grossly, erroneous, or unreasonable, to the sober and judicious parts of mankind." [21] Much importance was attached to the production of mental and nervous manifestations as the result of the retention or suppression of any customary evacuation, or of "metastases, or translations to the brain, as in repelled gout, . . . cutaneous eruptions," and so on. Ideas of this kind were accepted by many until late in the nineteenth century. Changes in the "nervous fluid" were, however, considered to be the principal cause of mental disorder. Extreme excitement was agreed by all to be due to great activity of the circulation of the small vessels of the brain, and the physical and mental symptoms of melancholia, it was thought, would appear "when the brain is compressed by a gradual accumulation of blood in the veins, and sinuses, without any increase in the activity of the small arteries." The physical reactions to the emotions were distinguished from those of the "animal desires or aversions" in which corporeal feelings were felt only "in parts of the body where uneasy sensation arouses the desire." Feelings in the praecordium and uneasy feelings in the abdomen were considered to be of etiological as well as of symptomatic significance. Some believed that the cardiac region and the abdomen were the real seats of mental disease. Pinel considered that the seat of periodical mania was in the epigastric region.[22] The growing interest in psychological and social considerations in the study and treatment of mental illness met with much opposition from those who considered that disease of the mind was a fantastic notion. The objectors pointed to what they regarded as characteristic postmortem observations, though in many instances no anatomical abnormalities were discovered. Changes in the pulse, the skin, the eyes, the muscular system, the hair, the blood, the bile, the digestive system, and numerous physical signs and symptoms were cited as proof of the physical character of the illness.[23] And, though personality and its reactions and all the conditions by which they are affected, whether physical or mental, have gradually become the center of interest in the study and treatment of mental illness, many physicians still find it difficult to accept as a real medical activity the study of the personality and intensive attention to the personal, domestic, and social problems of a patient, such as is required in the practice of psychiatry.

That the emotions, especially the strong emotions or passions, had

[21] Arnold, *op. cit.*, I, ix.

[22] Pinel, *op. cit.*, p. 17.

[23] Thomas Mayo, *Remarks on Insanity; Founded on the Practice of John Mayo, M.D.* (London, 1817), pp. 20 *et seq.*

a large place in the production of mental illness was generally accepted. H. D. Gaubius (1705–1780), of the University of Leyden, had the title of "Professor of the Passions." Too intense application to study or to business affairs, and too great activity of the imagination were also considered important. The role of the emotions in the causation and cure of physical symptoms was recognized, as was the powerful influence of sex problems in the etiology of neurotic and psychotic disorders. In regard to nervous conditions in young patients, one writer states that when they occur "about a certain Time in their Lives (as they often do) then they generally proceed from some Disorder in that great Affair, which ought, if possible, to be set to Rights." [24] It was believed, however, that mental factors operated entirely by effects on the physical organism, and it was to these that effective study and treatment must be directed. It was considered that "delusive sensation," "delirious pressure," and disturbances in the irritability of the brain and nervous system were fundamental in the causation of mental disease. The lungs, heart, liver and all the viscera subservient to digestion, as well as the kidneys, uterus, and bladder, were considered to have an "innate sympathy" with the emotions.[25] Attention was directed to "Caenesthesis or Self-feeling" as the sensations that arise in the internal organs and other parts of the body, and to symptoms occasioned by its disturbance.[26] Quite full and fairly accurate descriptions were given of the physical reactions that accompany strong emotions, such as fear, anxiety, anger, grief, sudden surprise, joy, and the like. Although modern historians are disposed to regard the Wesleyan religious movement of the late eighteenth century as "a sorely needed stimulus to the dulled conscience of the time," [27] the medical authors of the period considered that the intense emotional excitement and the sense of guilt and fear aroused by this and other strongly emotional religious appeals were productive of mental illness. Domestic misfortunes, obstructions to matrimony, effects of the Revolution, and religious fanaticism were considered important; also "suppressed exertion of the passions," and "severe restriction upon the sexual propensity."

The importance of constitutional factors was clearly recognized. The hypersensitive state sometimes observed even in nursing babies was

24 George Cheyne, *The English Malady, or, A Treatise of Nervous Diseases of All Kinds* (Dublin, 1733), p. 153.

25 Thomas Trotter, *A View of the Nervous Temperament* (London, 1807), p. 31.

26 Alexander Crichton, *An Inquiry into the Nature and Origin of Mental Derangement* (London, 1798), I, 110.

27 R. Hingston Fox, *John Fothergill and His Friends* (London, 1919).

considered to be evidence of a susceptible constitution. A writer on "the nervous temperament" refers to it as "a disposition of the mind." He believed, however, that "deranged sensations and inverted sympathies of the Great Sympathetic Nerve" were produced and that "causes . . . whether moral or physical exert their influence on this portion of the nervous system whose office directs the most important operations in the animal economy . . . so all violent emotions, in their turn, induce affections of the chylopoietic viscera." [28] It was observed that fear occasioned diarrhoea and incontinence of urine, anger affected the liver, grief the stomach, and terror produced complete palsy. Hope, on the other hand, affected the respiration and caused "quick and powerful distribution of the blood." [29] It was also noted that mental pleasures and pains "are not felt in the mind but in the body; they undulate about the heart, and breast, producing great and remarkable physical changes there; the influence of which is often extended throughout the vascular and nervous parts of our whole frame." [30] The remote effects of emotional influences in infancy and childhood were recognized. The number of women who were unable to nurse their babies was deplored and attention was directed to the advantage of "a mild and serene condition of mind" in wet nurses.[31] It was considered that the milk of a nurse of "profligate morals" might corrupt a well-bred child. It was suggested that stammering might sometimes be attributed to harshness of parents when the child was learning to speak.[32] The methods of education were criticized:

> Does it not happen that a boy is kept for many years together to the irksome task of loading his memory with a vocabulary of mere words; and that the active faculties of his soul for the want of proper exercise become inert, and are at last incapable of being exerted on subjects of abstract thought without pain? . . . A boy frequently becomes learned at the expense of common sense, and now and then at that of his judgment.[33]

Reference is made to precipitating a delirious episode by mentioning the word "earthquake," or "the Lisbon earthquake," to a man who had survived the catastrophe. It is also stated that Boileau-Despréaux, French poet and critic, was emasculated when a child, by a turkey cock, and that this accounted for his hatred of women, and also of the Jesuits, who were said to have first introduced the turkey into Europe.[34]

[28] Trotter, *op. cit.*, p. 234.
[29] Crichton, *op. cit.*, II, 137, 119.
[30] *Ibid.*
[31] Trotter, *op. cit.*, p. 96.
[32] Crichton, *op. cit.*, II, 80–81.
[33] *Ibid.*, I, 267.
[34] *Ibid.*, I, 383.

Even at this early stage of the development of modern psychiatry, it was observed that there were types of personalities in which traits were present that had psychopathological significance. "The serious and thoughtful boy has less sensibility in the nerves of his organs of external sense, than force of mind. . . . He is silent, absent, and often solitary; and if this state be not corrected by the most judicious management, he becomes unfit for every active commerce with the world." Of the "opposite type" it is said: "The mind of the other is too much exalted at the expense of the external senses, and, therefore, the foundation is laid for a predisposition to singular illusions." [35] This seems to indicate recognition of the introvert and the contrasting extrovert. A person of "Melancholic Temperament" is described as of "serious thoughtful disposition and disposed to fear and caution," less moved by impressions, ready to be engaged in constant application to one subject, "one particular object or train of thinking . . . remarkably tenacious of whatever emotions [he] happens to be affected with . . . readily seized with an anxious fear . . . may easily grow to partial insanity." This was considered to be due to "torpor in the motion of the nervous power both with reference to sensation and volition," and to "general rigidity of the simple solids . . . balance of the sanguiferous system . . . upon the side of the veins." The condition of the sanguine was the opposite.[36]

In clinical practice the time-honored terms "mania" and "melancholia" were universally employed, and many accurate descriptions of the symptoms of these forms of reaction are recorded. In the early records of the New York Hospital, the mentally ill patients as a class are designated "maniacs," and the recorded diagnosis in nearly all admissions is "mania." The term "dementia" was also used in the literature, but the distinction between failure in mental development and deterioration in mental disease was not always clearly made, and both were frequently designated "idiotism." The frequency of alternating states of mania and melancholia was noted, and attention was directed to the recognition of this by authors of previous periods back to Greek and Roman times. It was also noted that, in these alternating cases, "the physical constitution of the patient ought always to be taken into account and it is, perhaps, of all causes, the one which has the most influence in producing one or the other of these events." Hysteria, hypochondriasis, and many other ailments were commencing to receive attention and were desig-

[35] Crichton, *op. cit.*, I, 312.

[36] William Cullen, *First Lines of the Practice of Physic* (Worcester, Mass., 1790), III, 212–216.

nated neuroses or nervous disorders. They were defined as nervous disturbances, hitherto reckoned witchcraft, enchantment, sorcery, and possession. It was also considered that "they are so far to be classed among mental disorders that a *disposition of the mind,* not easily defined, attends every degree and stage of them." [37] They were said to be most prevalent among the more prosperous classes. It was stated that a third of the complaints of the "people of condition" in England were of this character.[38] They were regarded as "the Diseases of the Wealthy, the Voluptuous, and the Lazy (tho' perhaps not always an absolute and outrageous Intemperance.)" Cheyne, writing as early as 1733, entitled his book "The English Malady." It was said also that suicide was more prevalent in England than in other countries. Tea, "a beverage suited to the taste of an indolent and voluptuous age, particularly hurtful to the female constitution," coffee, tobacco ("the Indian Leaf") which "powerfully acts on the nervous system," alcohol, and opium came in for a share in responsibility for "the nervous temperament." The drama of the period was referred to as "another hotbed of this diseased sensibility"; also some of the works of fiction, "love sick trash," three quarters written by women, "some of whom are known to have drunk deep of the fountains of pleasure and adversity." [39] Blame was also laid on the excessive bleeding, purging, and vomiting practiced by some physicians, and the administration to "dyspeptic and hysterical females" of "mercurial courses till their very teeth have been in hazard of dropping from their sockets." [40] Morbid matter in the blood (scorbutic), flatulent improper aliments, and other causes affecting the gastrointestinal tract were thought to account for certain sensations that were peculiar but not painful and might be considered nervous. Trotter found in nervous disorders "all the signs that are said to mark *angina pectoris.*" All writers of the period attached much importance to the effects of the emotions. The role of alcohol in the etiology of both the extreme mental disorders and of the neuroses was considered of great importance.

In the light of present knowledge, the medical doctrines of the late eighteenth century seem so crude and so remote from those of the twentieth that the value of the foregoing brief review might be considered doubtful were it not that, in the establishment of the New York Hospital, these doctrines and the methods derived from them had a large place in determining the measures employed in the treatment of the mentally ill.

[37] Trotter, *op. cit.*, p. 200.
[38] Cheyne, quoted, in *ibid.*, p. xvii.
[39] Trotter, *op. cit.*, p. 91.
[40] *Ibid.*, p. 119.

II

PSYCHIATRIC PRACTICE

THE medical treatment of the mentally ill, at the close of the eighteenth century, consisted principally of measures that were routine practice in every form of illness. About the middle of the century, a writer on mental disorders had described as follows the "Medicines and Methods by which a lasting Cure might be obtained":

1. Proper evacuations of the several proper Kinds; 2. Attenuating and deobstruent Medicines of which I find the mild ponderose to be generally the best; 3. The gentle Astringents and Strengtheners of the Solids; 4. A proper and specific Diet, with Air and Exercise. "Whatever exceeds this," he adds, "is calculated either for the easy Death, or to keep up the Courage and Hopes, of the Patient." [1]

The objects of this plan of treatment were:

1. to thin, dilute, and sweeten the whole Mass of the Fluids, . . . 2. to divide, break, and dissolve the saline, acrid, and hard Concretions generated in the small Vessels, and to destroy all Sharpness and Acrimony lodged in the Habit, and to make the juices soft, sweet, and balsamick, . . . 3. to restore the tone and elastick Force, to crisp, wind up and contract the Fibres of the whole system.[2]

Dr. Rush of the Pennsylvania Hospital followed a similar plan of treatment and, "after reducing the action of the bloodvessels to a par of debility with the nervous system," [3] by means of bleeding, blisters, issues, salivation, emetics, purges, and reduced diet, he proceeded to build up the patient by stimulating aliment, drinks, and medicines.

The "several proper kinds of evacuations" were bleeding, purging, and vomiting. Bleeding was by venesection, arteriotomy, cupping, and leeches. It was a nearly universal practice. It was also used as a preventive measure and people went to the barber for bleeding as they did for hair trimming. In clinical practice it was the essential remedy in states of mental excitement, which all agreed were invariably caused by increased activity of the circulation in the small arteries of the brain. In melancholia also it was thought that there was congestion of the veins and sinuses of the brain which could be relieved by bleeding. The dis-

[1] George Cheyne, *The Natural Method of Curing the Diseases of the Body and the Disorders of the Mind Depending on the Body* (5th ed., London, 1753), p. A3.

[2] Cheyne, *The English Malady, or, A Treatise of Nervous Diseases of All Kinds* (Dublin, 1733), pp. 78–79.

[3] Benjamin Rush, *Medical Inquiries and Observations upon the Diseases of the Mind* (Philadelphia, 1812), p. 98.

covery of the circulation of the blood had given rise to an idea that in this would be found the key to the understanding and treatment of disease, and it was even said that "in every case, insanity does not occur without its being accompanied by marks of a diseased action of the bloodvessels." [4] This furnished sufficient reason for bleeding in every case. There had, however, always been those who counseled against indiscriminate and excessive bloodletting, and at the close of the century their number was increasing. Its use began to be restricted to the early stages of mental illness, and to young, robust patients of sanguine temperament, with a hard full pulse and with definite signs of increased activity of the circulation of the brain. Local bleeding from a small artery of the head or foot, and cupping or leeches were more frequently used instead of venesection. Blisters, setons, and issues were used to draw off "morbid serum" from the blood and to operate as revulsives. Foot baths, fomentations, sinapisms, friction of the scalp, and the application of irritating substances, or an ice bag or clay cap were used to divert blood from the brain. The excessive bleeding and other drastic measures employed in the treatment of the mentally ill were considered, by Pinel and others, to account for the rapid and irretrievable deterioration observed in some of the cases admitted to the hospitals. Bloodletting, however, in one or another form and degree, continued to be employed as a remedy well into the nineteenth century.

Purgatives and emetics were given not only to relieve gastrointestinal disturbances but also as a means of depleting the blood vessels, of relieving the organism of acrid humors, and of correcting morbid conditions in the solids and fluids of the body. Emetics were considered to be especially effective. One author wrote: "I know not in Nature a more universal and effectual Remedy." [5] Others, however, were finding that emetics were "in general very hurtful in madness," and that they should be used only when "the disease has its source in the stomach, . . . or when it may present some humoral engorgement in the viscera of the lower belly." [6] There were "rough" and "gentle," "lenient" or "cooling" purgatives and emetics, and the general tendency at the close of the century was to rely more and more on the milder ones.

Errhines or stenutatories were medical snuffs. They were used to "promote excretion of mucid lymph secreted in the glandular pituitary

[4] Alexander Crichton, *An Inquiry into the Nature and Origin of Mental Derangement* (London, 1798), II, 333.

[5] Cheyne, *The English Malady*, p. 142.

[6] M. Joseph Daquin, *La Philosophie de la folie*, quoted by John M. Galt, *The Treatment of Insanity* (New York, 1846), p. 15.

membrane which lines the cavity of the nostrils and the sinuses of the brain; . . . absterge redundant stagnated lymph from the . . . head. . . . In melancholia and mania tranquilla," they were recommended for "agitating the body, and rousing the torpor of the nervous system, . . . encouraging a more brisk circulation, and conveying energy and vigour to the animal functions." [7] The general purpose in the use of all evacuants was said to be "the grinding, breaking, and dissolving the Cohesion, Viscidity and Sharpness of the Fluids, and throwing them off by the fastest and most patent outlets." [8] In this way "delirious pressure," which caused hallucinations and delusions, was supposedly relieved or prevented. The mechanical effect of "rough" purges, and especially of emetics and stenutatories, was also considered to be beneficial, as "by agitating the whole frame, they excite a general commotion in the nervous system—promote an uniform circulation—produce a determination to the surface of the body . . . remove obstructions in the sanguiferous system." [9]

These effects provided artificial physical exercise for patients who were too indolent to exercise voluntarily; it was said that they

> not only discharge or dislodge the delirious load of stagnating fluids, but also by their convulsive influence upon the muscles of the abdomen and indeed upon every animal fibre of the agitated body crowd as it were a great deal of exercise in a small portion of time, and that without the consent of the patient, or even the trouble of contradicting his lazy inclinations.

The author adds that it is "no easy task to persuade or even to force any person, whether a Lunatic or not, who has long indulged in idleness, to put his body in motion." [10]

The purpose served by "attenuating and deobstruent Medicines" was to remove

> indolent obstructions [which] have their seat either in the secretory tubes of the glands, or in other vessels smaller than those which carry red blood, in the glandular follicles, or in the spaces of the *tela cellulosa,* in which there is deposited, by the exhaling arteries, a fluid which soon becomes too thick to be taken up by the absorbent veins.[11]

While water was considered a good dissolvent, it did not have "activity and agility enough to get into the small vessels," and required the assistance of medicines of active volatile character.

[7] William Pargeter, *Observations on Maniacal Disorders* (Reading, England, 1792), p. 91–93.

[8] Cheyne, *The English Malady,* p. 159.

[9] Pargeter, *op. cit.,* p. 73.

[10] William Battie, *A Treatise on Madness* (London, 1758), pp. 86–87.

[11] Robert Whytt, *Observations on the Nature, Causes, and Cure of Those Disorders . . . Called Nervous . . .* (3d ed., Edinburgh, 1767), p. 406.

Astringents and bitters which "have the experienced though unaccountable efficacy of contracting the material particles which constitute an animal body," [12] were given for the purpose of strengthening the solids and promoting the juxtaposition of particles of which they were composed and which had become loosened. Preparations of iron, mineral waters, and Jesuit bark (Cinchona) were given for this purpose.

Antispasmodics were used in states of tension, spasm, and convulsions. Musk, castor, valerian, hyoscyamus, and camphor were most frequently employed. "The gums," especially asafoetida, were also considered useful. Opium, "this noble medicine, which has been happily called 'the medicine of the mind,'" [13] was used to procure sleep and to relieve tension, restlessness, and mental distress, but the danger of increasing the dose was realized. The administration of mercury to the point of producing salivation was frequently resorted to. Dr. Rush considered this of advantage "to abstract morbid excitement from the brain to the mouth," and to remove visceral obstruction and fix complaints on the mouth. Others, however, were opposed to extreme salivation, and restricted the administration of mercury to syphilitic subjects. Digitalis was, at one time, thought to be a useful remedy in mental excitement. Wines and cordials were frequently prescribed as part of a supporting or stimulating plan of treatment, but distilled liquors were, by most observers, considered inadvisable, and total abstinence from alcoholic beverages in depressions and neurotic disorders was advocated by some.[14]

The use of water in the form of general baths or applied locally had always been regarded as a valuable therapeutic measure. The warm bath was, at the close of the eighteenth century, used in the treatment of melancholia but only in cases with "rigidity and dryness of the fibre," which could be readily "discovered by hardness, crispature, and dark colour of the hair." [15] Not all observers were in favor of it in manic excitement. Cold baths were used as tub baths and showers for the tonic effect, and, in hospital practice, sometimes as means of punishment. Sea bathing was frequently prescribed, especially in the treatment of neurotic disorders. Douche to the head, foot baths, and hand baths were recommended in cases in which the blood vessels of the brain were considered to be over active. Friction and massage were practiced with a view to diverting blood from the brain and to removing obstructions in the glands, small vessels, and intercellular spaces. Physical exercise by walk-

12 Battie, *op. cit.*, p. 86.

13 Rush, *op. cit.*, p. 103.

14 See Thomas Trotter, *A View of the Nervous Temperament* (London, 1807); Battie, *op. cit.*; Daquin, in Galt, *op. cit.*

15 Pargeter, *op. cit.*, p. 97.

ing, gymnastics, games and sports, dancing, horseback riding, and manual labor, was universally commended. Electricity in the form of "sparks, shocks, and fluid" was, to a limited extent, coming into use as a treatment measure. In some instances the head was covered with flannel and "shocks through the cranium" were given.[16] It was observed that "an intermittent fever coming upon a madness of long standing, had cured it,"[17] but many years passed before fever therapy was considered to be an effectual form of treatment.

Although the importance of diet was fully recognized, the recommendations relating to it were quite general in character and fail to indicate that it was a subject of precise study. So important was diet considered, however, that one writer declared that "Manias, real Lunacy, Madness, and a disordered Brain . . . can possibly be accounted for, from no other natural Cause but a Mal-regimen of Diet."[18] A "low diet," sometimes to the point of fasting, was invariably prescribed during the depleting period in the treatment of acute excitement. A liberal diet was, however, considered necessary in the convalescent period, and in depressed states. A mild and vegetable diet was frequently recommended in the treatment of nervous disorders. "Rich dishes" with fats and heavy sauces were considered objectionable. For constipation it was advised that the diet should be of a character that would reduce the faecal mass, in order to diminish the load on peristalsis (contrary to the present prescribing of "roughage"). Some increase in the fluid intake, slow mastication, the free use of fruit, and avoidance of much bread, flour puddings, and pastry were recommended. To reduce weight, "low living and exercise" seemed to be the main reliance; tea and coffee were frequently prohibited, as were alcoholic beverages, with the occasional exception of a light wine. For patients who would not eat voluntarily, the "spouting pot" was sometimes used as a means of forcible feeding, but was said to be "painfully unpleasant."

The psychiatric writers of the eighteenth century devoted much attention to the nature and operation of the mind in health and disease. They recognized the role of the emotions in the causation and cure of physical symptoms, and the powerful influence of sex problems in the etiology of neurotic and psychotic disorders. It was not, however, until near the close of the century that treatment by mental measures began to approach a systematic form. Before 1780 Gaubius of Leyden had taught that the physician,

16 William Perfect, *Annals of Insanity* (2d ed., London, 1801), pp. 406–409.

17 Pargeter, *op. cit.*, p. 115.

18 Cheyne, *The Natural Method*, p. 90.

in the execution of his office, when he has to do with the whole man, being a compound of body and mind, if he directs all his assistance to the body only, without any regard to the mind, he, in reality, will often do little towards curing his patient, and will either miss his aim, or at least omit some important part of the things necessary for that purpose. . . . The mind frequently brings disorders on a sound body, or mends a diseased one; and the body in its turn not rarely discomposes a quiet mind and quiets a disturbed one.[19]

Notwithstanding this evident comprehension of the need of treatment for the mind as well as the body, there was apparently little system or precision in the measures employed. Patience, and "great mildness in our demeanor and manner," was recommended, together with an effort to gain the confidence of the patient and to discover any moral means that might, perhaps, avail in his treatment. It was advised that no deception be practiced, except "pious frauds" such as a fake operation or procedure for the purpose of dispelling a particular delusion. Removal from home and freedom from visitors were considered essential in the more profound types of mental illness. When coöperation and orderly behavior were resisted, "catching the eye" of the patient immediately upon coming into his presence was considered to be effective. To inspire him with "awe and dread" was an accepted plan of procedure. Firmness, harsh threats—even of death—seclusion in darkness, restricted diet, stripes and blows, sudden ducking in cold water almost to the point of drowning, the strait waistcoat, chains, cords, manacles and other means of producing fear were, by the most eminent medical practitioners and teachers, regarded as legitimate and necessary measures. On the principle that "no two different perceptions can subsist at the same time," the pain and acute discomfort produced by blisters, caustics, vomits, rough cathartics, and stenutatories were considered to be therapeutic.[20] The psychological value of recreations, occupation, and social relations was clearly recognized, but their utilization by means of systematic organization has been acccomplished only in our own times. By the close of the century, however, the movement for more rational and effective "management of the mind" or "moral treatment," as it was variously designated, was clearly going forward. About this time also, Dr. Franz Anton Mesmer (1734–1814), notwithstanding the disapproval which his ideas, practices and ethical standards received from his contemporary colleagues, was bringing into medicine, however imperfectly, ideas and techniques for the understanding and treatment of mental

[19] H. D. Gaubius, *On the Passions,* trans. J. Taprell (London, 1780[?]), pp. 51–52.
[20] Battie, *op. cit.,* p. 85.

illness that have gradually assumed a large place in psychiatric thought and practice.[21]

Although the importance of alcoholism was at this period undoubtedly recognized, its study and treatment had apparently not yet been undertaken by physicians as a definite problem. At least, Dr. Thomas Trotter, who published an essay on drunkenness, stated in his introduction: [22] "I have not any precursor in my labours, nor example in the records of physic." He commented on the neglect of the effects of alcohol by physicians and by society, and mentioned a number of bodily and mental disorders which he attributed to this cause. It was generally recognized, he stated, that "the drunkard appears to act the part of a man of deranged intellect," and he added: "In medical language, I consider drunkenness, strictly speaking, to be a disease; produced by a remote cause, and giving birth to actions and movements in the living body, that disorder the functions of health." Trotter believed that temperament as well as physical condition, had a large part in determining the reaction of an individual to alcohol. He referred to a statement of Captain Bligh of the *Bounty* that the men who had been set adrift by the mutineers and who were on a very small allowance of food and water were inebriated by a teaspoonful of rum.[23] He noted that head injuries increased susceptibility. He did not consider intoxication necessary for the production of ill effects. There were also "sober drunkards." Treatment consisted in the usual depletion measures for acute conditions with immediate abstinence from alcohol. This was followed by treatment directed to physical rehabilitation. Drunkenness was, however, "a disease of the mind," and the patient should be treated kindly and patiently. It was useless to upbraid him, and it might drive him to suicide. It was important to gain his confidence and thereby "bring him under our control." He should be studied, and the particular cause, time, and place of his love of the bottle should be ascertained. Something should be "proposed that will effectually wean his affections from it, and strenuously engage his attention." Total abstinence was essential. Trotter noted that one rarely met with a reformed drunkard—a proof "that little had been done hitherto with success."

The number of drugs employed in the treatment of disease in the eighteenth century was enormous. Most of them have been long since discarded and are no longer found in the pharmacopoeias. The drastic

21 Margaret Goldsmith, *Franz Anton Mesmer: the History of an Idea* (London, 1934).
22 Thomas Trotter, *An Essay . . . on Drunkenness* (London, 1804), p. 2.
23 *Ibid.*, pp. 29–30.

character of some of the treatment measures seems also, in retrospect, to be remarkable. The physicians of this period were, however, as conscientious and zealous for the welfare and cure of their patients as the physicians of any other period, including the present. Nor were they lacking in ability to observe and think, and they were regretfully aware of the painful character of some of the measures they considered necessary. It has been said of them that "their prognosis was generally sound, and it is probable also that their success in treatment was not so far behind our own as was their knowledge of pathology." [24] Is it not possible that our successors may view with equal perplexity some of the practices of the present day in the treatment of the mentally ill?

Nor, at the close of the century, were the prevailing practices free from contemporary criticism. Something may, perhaps, be learned from the advice of a physician of the period to his colleagues, who, he said, "might as well dissect the top of the osophagus [*sic*] for the cause of globus hystericus, as attempt to fix the pathology of these versatile movements in the secreting or other organs; or inspect the brain of a hypochondriac for the picture of his blue devils." [25] Pinel, also, was endeavoring to persuade his colleagues that "in diseases of the mind, as well as in all other ailments, it is an art of no little importance to administer medicines properly, but it is an art of much greater and more difficult acquisition to know when to suspend or altogether to omit them." [26] Nor was the outlook of these physicians on the field of mental illness altogether narrow.

Following the lead of Pinel and others, it was beginning to be realized that "treatment requires that the full life history be considered." Like all physicians who earnestly study and treat their patients, they were optimistic.

> We have, therefore, as Men, the pleasure to find that Madness is, contrary to the opinion of some unthinking person, as manageable as many other distempers, which are equally dreadful and obstinate, and yet are not looked upon as incurable: and that such unhappy objects ought by no means to be abandoned, much less shut up in loathsome prisons as criminals or nuisances.[27]

Dr. Benjamin Rush, at the close of one of his chapters,[28] stated: "After the history that has been given of the distress, despair, and voluntary

[24] R. Hingston Fox, *Dr. John Fothergill and His Friends* (London, 1919).
[25] Trotter, *A View of the Nervous Temperament*, p. 221.
[26] Pinel, *A Treatise on Insanity*, trans. D. D. Davis (Sheffield, 1806), p. 10.
[27] Battie, *op. cit.*, p. 93.
[28] Rush, *op. cit.*, p. 97.

death, which are induced by that partial derangement which has been described, I should lay down my pen, and bedew my paper with my tears, did I not know that the science of medicine has furnished a remedy for it." They were thoroughly convinced of the medical character of mental illness, and sought the interest of all physicians in the problem. Gaubius remarked in a lecture at the University of Leyden,

This care of the human mind belongs to us. It is the most noble branch of our office; and by how much the more diligently any one of us cultivates it, with so much the more propriety, as Hippocrates says, will he be worthy of the title of a Philosophic Physician, and to be esteemed *"Isotheos"* or Godlike. . . . Our art will not be consummately perfect, till it can render men, not only as robust, but also as ingenious and as good as possible. . . . Rouze [*sic*] yourselves therefore all you who have abilities, and by your joint observations, experiments and endeavours, and if there be any other sort of promising or useful attempts, by them improve, polish, and render compleat, this medicinal philosophy.[29]

Although, as in our own time, the majority of physicians did not concern themselves to any great extent with the study and treatment of mental illness, the subject received attention in the medical colleges, and eminent medical teachers were among those who lectured and wrote on the subject. Few physicians, however, specialized in psychiatric practice.

In the latter part of the eighteenth century medical thought and interest began to have a distinct trend toward prevention. It was commencing to be realized that heredity might be a factor, and constitutional predisposition or the "nervous temperament" was clearly recognized.[30] The significance of influences operating in infancy and early childhood was noted. "Even children at an early age are not beyond the reach of moral causes," writes Trotter. Other references to this subject were given in the preceding chapter. A general scheme of living, for the maintenance of mental health is given by Arnold, as follows: [31]

1. Temperance. . . ; 2. Exercise; 3. the due Regulation of the Passions; 4. Attention to the operation of the imagination. . . ; 5. Improvement of the reasoning faculties; 6 . . . Avoidance of too long-continued uniform thinking, and of excessive watching; 7. Avoidance of the other occasional causes of insanity. . . ; 8. Rational views of God and religion.

The menace to mental health of the unregulated sale of opium and of spirituous liquors was considered to be serious. In regard to the

29 Gaubius, *op. cit.*, pp. 113–114.

30 Trotter, *Nervous Temperament*, pp. 169 *et seq.*

31 Thomas Arnold, *Observations on the Nature, Kinds, Causes and Prevention of Insanity* (2d ed., London, 1806), II, 320.

latter it was said that wine was introduced into Great Britain in the thirteenth century, and that it was at first "confined to the shop of the apothecary." The writer added that "it would have been well, had it been still confined there . . . spirituous liquors are," he stated, "not mentioned in that period of our history. They were probably unknown until our army went to assist the Dutch in obtaining their independency." [32] Prohibition of the sale of these liquors was advocated by some writers. "Prevention, at least with regard to vinous spirits, is entirely within our power. For which reason it deserved the serious consideration of our governors, how far it is their duty by a total prohibition of the cause to prevent those frequent effects of temporary but real Lunacy." [33] The danger of resorting to alcohol for relief from anxiety and "tediousness of life" was pointed out.

Some of the medical writers of the period, as in our own times, directed their literary productions to lay as well as medical readers. One author stated that his book was designed "principally for common intelligent Readers, and those who suffer under Nervous Distempers, though not regularly bred to the Practice of Physick," and that therefore "Lunacy and Madness" were omitted.[34]

At the time of the establishment of the New York Hospital, access to hospital treatment, or even to the protection and sustenance provided by the asylums, was available to an exceedingly small proportion of the mentally ill. In the year 1792 there were in England only fifteen institutions for this class of sick persons,[35] three of which were departments of general hospitals. In the United States there were two, which together had accommodations for perhaps one hundred patients. The population at this time was approximately four million people (in 1790 it was 3,929,214). Consequently, a large number of mentally ill persons constituted a problem in the various communities. The belief in witchcraft and possession, and in the depravity of mentally ill persons, still lingered in the emotional attitude toward them, even though it was no longer openly declared. It was generally believed also, even by physicians, that many of the mentally ill were insensitive to cold and deprivations and that they were extraordinarily strong. Consequently, they were frequently confined, even while at their own homes, in attics or cellars or specially constructed receptacles, with little light and no heat, without proper clothing, bedding, or toilet facilities. Cords and

[32] Trotter, *On Drunkenness*, p. 150.
[33] Battie, *op. cit.*, p. 83.
[34] Cheyne, *The English Malady*, p. 175.
[35] D. H. Tuke, *Chapters in the History of the Insane in the British Isles* (London, 1882), p. 514.

chains were used to restrain them, and the attention given to their physical health, food, cleanliness, and exercise was scarcely that given to domestic animals. Many wandered homeless about the country, dependent for food and shelter on what they could obtain by begging. If they became troublesome, the public authorities confined them with criminals in lockups and houses of detention, where they were subjected to the same treatment as criminals, being whipped, fastened in the stocks, and roughly handled by brutal keepers.

Those who were sufficiently controllable to be suitable for private homes were, if they were without friends to provide for them, auctioned off to the lowest bidder who would board them; or they were placed, with other paupers, in almshouses, in which no adequate provision was made for their proper treatment.[36] In the hospitals and asylums, the relatively few patients who were accommodated were attended by physicians and treated medically in the manner already described in this chapter. It is necessary to realize that all hospitals, and the treatment administered by them, were, at that time, extremely crude. Sanitary construction and plumbing, central heating and lighting, elevators, and facilities for transportation, nursing, and medical procedures, were lacking. Anaesthetics had not yet been discovered, nor the role of bacteria in surgery and medicine. There were no training schools for nurses, and no dietitians. If judgment is made on the basis of the prevailing hospital standards of the respective periods, the early institutions for the mentally ill were relatively perhaps no poorer than some of those of the present day.

The report of a committee of the British House of Commons made in 1815 on institutions for the mentally ill reveals in great detail the standards of the period.[37] Those of the two institutions in our own country may be learned from Deutsch's history, Morton's *History of the Pennsylvania Hospital,* and Rush's treatise on insanity. Some of the drastic measures employed in medical treatment were routine for a large proportion of the patients. At the Bethlehem Hospital in London it was the custom to bleed all of the patients about the end of May. This was followed by emetics once a week for several weeks, and after this purgatives were given. "That," said the physician, "has been the practice invariably for years, long before my time . . . and I do not know any

[36] Albert Deutsch, *The Mentally Ill in America* (New York, 1937).

[37] House of Commons, *Report together with the Minutes of the Evidence and an Appendix of Papers from the Committee Appointed to Consider Provision Being Made for the Better Regulation of Madhouses in England* (London, 1815).

better practice." [38] At the Pennsylvania Hospital bleeding was a constant practice. Patients were bled to syncope, and purged until the alimentary canal failed to yield anything but mucus.[39] In most of the institutions disturbed patients were confined in "cells," which were usually located in the basement. In some instances the windows were so high that patients could not see out, and they were not always glazed. The rooms were not warmed, and there was no lighting at night. Beds were of straw; the attendants were so few in number, and frequently so indifferent, that the straw was sometimes not changed for weeks, even after it had become filthy. Chains and manacles were an approved form of restraint; by some of the physicians who testified before the English Committee, they were said to be preferable to other forms. Patients were fastened to the wall or to the bed by a chain attached to the waist, the ankle, or the arm. In addition they might also wear leg locks and wristlets. At one of the British hospitals 70 of 400 patients were chained; in another, 10 of 122 were in chains and 8 to 10 were fastened to tables and were quite naked. In a private asylum only one of 14 patients was without fetters or handcuffs. Attendants or keepers usually carried a whip, and it was considered proper to subdue a patient by blows. The advance towards treatment by management and by more considerate and rational methods was indeed by the close of the eighteenth century gradually going forward. Progress was slow, however, and though the principles and practices then advocated have been generally adopted, a few years ago a survey of the public hospitals for the mentally ill revealed that handcuffs and chains had not yet been entirely discarded. Restraint by means of chains or the strait waistcoat was considered to be a means of punishment, as were also cold shower baths, plunges into cold water by surprise, cold water poured into the sleeves, confinement in darkened cells, deprivation of food and other means of control by fear. A tranquilizing chair and a whirling apparatus or gyrator were employed at some and condemned at other hospitals.

The time had, however, arrived for the introduction of better conditions and methods. Pinel was endeavoring to reorganize the Paris hospitals. He urged the importance of administration as a treatment measure: "to place first in point of consequence, the duties of a humane and enlightened superintendency, and the maintenance of order, in the services of the hospitals," [40] to employ only capable and humane at-

[38] House of Commons, *Committee Report*, p. 110.
[39] Thomas G. Morton, *History of the Pennsylvania Hospital* (Philadelphia, 1895), p. 125.
[40] Pinel, *op. cit.*, p. 222.

tendants, and to prohibit violence in the management of the patients, to establish a night service, to provide for occupation and amusement, to classify the patients so that they might not prove detrimental to one another, and to make provision for an adequate dietary. He observed that many patients showed greater improvement when left to nature and the kindly intelligent ministrations of the exceptionally capable lay superintendent of the hospital and his staff of well-governed attendants than when they were subjected to the drastic medical treatment which was routine practice. He concluded that in the treatment of mental illness blind routine diverted attention from "the more important management of the mind," and from the study of the illness, the "history of its symptoms, of its progress, of its varieties, and of its treatment in and out of hospitals." He saw, "with wonder, the resources of nature when left to herself, or skilfully assisted in her efforts. My faith in pharmaceutic preparations was gradually lessened, and my scepticism went at length so far, as to induce me never to have recourse to them, until moral measures had completely failed." [41]

Management instead of medicines and repression was finding many advocates. "If insanity is purely a mental alienation," wrote Trotter,[42] "the method of cure must turn chiefly on a mode of discipline addressed to the weakened powers of intellect. . . . A physician . . . must live among them [patients] that he may learn the genius of every individual case, if his discipline is to conduce to their recovery." Dr. Rush at the Pennsylvania Hospital, by means of communications to the board of managers, was endeavoring to provide better conditions for the mentally ill patients. In 1789 he advised them that the cells of the hospital were damp in winter, too warm in summer, offensive to smell, and "Dishonorable to the Science and Humanity of Philadelphia." He asked for bath rooms and for means of occupation for the patients, for separate buildings for the mentally ill with separate floors for each sex, for intelligent men and women to direct amusements and recreations, for better furniture, for close stools for the cells.[43] Not all of his proposals were accepted by the managers, but, as means were provided, progress there and elsewhere was gradually achieved.

[41] *Ibid.,* p. 109.

[42] Trotter, *A View of the Nervous Temperament,* p. 279.

[43] Memorial addressed by Rush to the Managers of the hospital, 1810. See Francis R. Packard, *History of Medicine in the United States* (new ed., New York, 1931), I, p. 215.

PART TWO

The First Hospital in New York and Its Department of Psychiatry 1771-1821

III: "THE HOSPITAL IN THE CITY OF NEW YORK"

IN 1771 "The Society of the Hospital in the City of New York" received its charter. In 1810 the title was changed, by act of the legislature, to the Society of the New York Hospital. The first building, situated on Broadway at Worth Street, was partially destroyed by fire in 1775, and it had scarcely been restored when the Revolutionary War broke out and New York was occupied by British troops. With the exception of a short period before the arrival of the British, during which a few soldiers of the Revolutionary Army were received for treatment, the building during the war was used as a barracks for Hessian soldiers and was left in a bad state of dilapidation. After peace was declared and the city was evacuated, municipal and state affairs, as well as those of the populace, were so disorganized that it was not until January, 1791, that the governors were enabled to open the hospital for the reception of patients. The building had, in the meantime, been occasionally used, first for a meeting of the State Legislature,[1] and later, at times, to house newly arrived immigrants. Dr. Richard Bayley conducted at the hospital the anatomical studies and lectures that precipitated the "Doctor's Riot" in 1788, in which several persons were killed.

The city which the hospital was designed to serve was already the largest in the country and its population—then about 35,000—was growing rapidly. New York was said by the newspapers to be "everyday growing into symmetry, elegance, and beauty," and was called "The Naples of America." [2] A considerable proportion of the population were Negro slaves. New York was an active seaport in which, during the year 1791, over 1,800 vessels were docked.[3] Sailors and constantly arriving nonresidents helped, therefore, to swell the population and add to the

[1] Jan. 12, 1786; also on Jan. 13, 1790.
[2] *N.Y. Daily Advertiser,* Nov. 23, 1790, and July 11, 1791.
[3] I. N. P. Stokes, *Iconography of Manhattan Island* (New York, 1926), V, 1276.

social and sanitary problems. Many conditions existed which were prejudicial to satisfactory social, ethical, political, economic, and sanitary standards. Scarcely anywhere else could the need for hospital service for both the mentally and physically sick have been more pressing.

The city limits embraced the entire island of Manhattan, though only the area below Canal Street was divided into city lots. Most of the streets were still unpaved. Some were so narrow that there was no space for sidewalks. Many of the more wealthy inhabitants escaped the inconveniences of the city by living in Bloomingdale and other sections of Manhattan Island that had previously been separate villages. There was no sewer system. There was a brick covered drain in Broad Street; other drains were open. In spite of the fact that negro boys were employed to sweep the streets, and garbage was collected daily, refuse was thrown into the open, cattle roamed freely, and filth abounded. The water supply, drawn from wells, was inadequate and a menace to health. The year 1791 was marked by pestilence and fires: after a long period of immunity, there was a violent outbreak of yellow fever, and two disastrous fires occurred. Fire protection and control were achieved by means of buckets and hose supplied by householders. Heating was altogether by means of wood-burning fireplaces—coal was practically unknown. Candles and oil lamps furnished light indoors, while in the streets, lamps were placed on poles or attached to the houses, at intervals of 114 feet.[4] Transportation was slow and laborious. A stage journey to Philadelphia took two days, broken by an overnight stop at Princeton or Trenton. There were regulations governing carts and hackney coaches, and horses and carriages were taxed for the maintenance of the streets.

Finance and business were poorly organized. Funds for public purposes were sometimes raised by lottery. There were no public schools. Advertisements of private schools are found in the newspapers of the period, and charity schools, at which, besides tuition, clothing, fuel, books, and paper were furnished, were conducted by the churches. A school was also conducted by the commissioners of the almshouse. Advertisements for teachers called, in some instances, for masters who were capable of teaching both Dutch and English, the languages in general use. King's College, established in 1754, was suspended during the war. In 1784 it was revived by the Regents of the University of the state, which in 1787 granted a charter for the establishment of Columbia College. The New York Society Library was established in 1754; in 1791 it was the only one in the city. In 1791 four daily and two weekly news-

[4] New York city, *Minutes of Common Council, 1784–1831*, I, 633. (Order of March 29, 1791.)

papers were published,[5] and five magazines, of which the principal were the *Columbian, American,* and *American Museum.*

There were twenty churches, the oldest of which were the Dutch Reformed, founded in 1626, and Trinity, founded in 1697. It was in the latter that, at the first graduation exercises of King's College Medical School in 1769, Dr. Samuel Bard delivered the address which determined the establishment of the New York Hospital. There were also a Jewish Synagogue and a Friends' Meeting House. Under the colonial government, Roman Catholic worship was forbidden, and it was not until 1785 that the first Catholic church was erected.

Social and political activities centered chiefly in the taverns, some of which were provided with large halls for dinners, dancing parties, public meetings, and other gatherings. Dancing schools were advertised in the newspapers. An influential group called "The Moot" used to meet at King's Arms Tavern. Another and larger group was known as "The Social Club." Dr. Samuel Bard belonged to the latter and was considered, according to the club's roster, "Loyal, tho' in 1775 doubtful, remained at N. York—A good man." [6]

Governor's Island was laid out in groves and gardens with a house and pavilions and was used as a pleasure resort. There were also "pleasure gardens," named "Vauxhall" and "Ranelagh," after similar resorts in London. "Ranelagh," founded in 1765, was located on the Anthony Rutgers estate, which was afterwards the site of the New York Hospital. The hospital was sometimes referred to as "the hospital at Ranelagh." As the one theater, located on John Street, aroused great opposition, no other was established until 1798 when the John Street Theatre was closed and the Park Theatre was opened. There were panoramas and galleries of paintings to be visited, as well as the American Museum of Antiquities, established by the Tammany Society in 1790. Athletic sports and games were popular; also yacht racing off Sandy Hook, horse racing, fox hunting, cock fighting, sailing, skating, cards, and dancing.

Following the Revolution, lawlessness was rampant. There was an increase in cursing and vile language, the existence of God was denied, and men seldom went to church. Bowling Green, the haunt of dissolute characters, was frequently the scene of disorder and crime. "Bawdy houses" flourished, with over a thousand known prostitutes—nearly one in thirty-five of the stationary population. Liquor was sold in about 1,400

[5] *Bibliography of American Newspapers 1690–1820,* Part VIII, New York City, comp. Clarence S. Brigham (published in *Proceedings of the American Antiquarian Society,* XXVII, 1917, New Series, Part 2).

[6] M. Harrison Bayles, *Old Taverns of New York* (New York, 1915), p. 248.

places; licenses were issued by the mayor, with no limit on the number, and the mayor and treasurer were paid by a percentage of the license fee. "Incredible quantities" of liquor were sold to individual customers and drunkenness and gambling were common, even among the clergy.[7] A person was not considered drunk as long as he could stand up and drink more. The myth of the masterful way in which our ancestors carried their liquor, soberly explained by some present-day writers as due to the vitamins in their food, is not sustained by the annals of this period in New York. In an article in the *Medical Repository* in 1802, the following example of the drinking habits of a laboring man is given: As he went to work in the morning he would take a small glass (half a gill) of bitters or gin and perhaps a second. As he returned home for breakfast he would take two or three more such glasses. This before eight o'clock. On the way back to work he would have a large glass (a gill), in the midforenoon another, and a third as he returned home to dinner. On his way back after dinner he would have another, also two more in midafternoon, and still another as he returned home after work. Thus, a quart was consumed in the day, with more to follow, probably, in the evening. The expenditure was about four shillings, or a half dollar a day.[8]

Pauperism was common. Vagrants were arrested and returned to their place of legal residence or confined in the bridewell.[9] Among them were many feeble-minded and insane persons. The prisons were "miserable and filthy holes." They served for the confinement of all disorderly persons, the mentally ill as well as others. Imprisonment for

[7] *Medical Repository*, I (1804), 2d Hexade, pp. 90–91.

[8] *Ibid.*, VI (1803), 333. The light-hearted attitude toward excessive drinking is illustrated by the following verses, which appeared in the *New York Daily Advertiser* on Sept. 20, 1791:

What care I, if my wife should scold?
When drunk I cannot hear her:
When warmed with liquor I'm so bold,
Egad, I never fear her.

If Susan furious then should rave,
I manfully abuse her:
Or, if she should a favour crave,
I scornfully refuse her.

I know if I
Should once comply,
Her tongue would run the quicker:
What can subdue
So curs'd a shrew?
Why, liquor, liquor, liquor.

[9] Bridewell, a prison for debtors and others accused of minor crimes.

debt was still the law, and many respectable persons were held in houses of detention and prisons. In 1808 the number of persons imprisoned for debt was 1,317, of whom 591 were women; 697 owed less than $10. By 1791, however, this state of lawlessness and disorganization was giving place to more orderly conditions. Groups of citizens had formed organizations for promoting improvements. Among these was a "Society for the Relief of Indigent and Distressed Debtors in Prison." There was also a "Manufacturing Society for furnishing Employment to the Honest and Industrious Poor." This society conducted a workshop in which one hundred and thirty spinners and fourteen weavers were given employment.[10] The commissioners of the almshouse distributed firewood, money, and relief for sickness in the homes, considering that this was "less expensive in the long run, to the public," than supporting them in the almshouse. Destitute children were "bound out" with families, after a trial period in order to determine whether the children and "masters" would be satisfactory to one another. Inspections were made and complaints investigated. Other benevolent organizations were the Humane Society, the Chamber of Commerce, St. Andrews Society, and the Masonic Order; the General Society of Mechanics and Tradesmen, and the Manumission Society for Negro Slaves, which was supported chiefly by the Friends.[11]

Provision for the treatment of the sick was, at the time the New York Hospital was established, extremely inadequate, not only in New York but everywhere else in America. The first directory of the city in 1786 contained the names of 27 men who were either "doctors" (23) or "surgeons" (4). The directory of 1791 contained the names of 59 medical men, listed as 49 physicians and 10 surgeons, 6 of whom were "Drs.," and 4 "M.D." Of the last mentioned, two, Dr. Samuel Bard and Dr. Samuel Borrowe, were connected with the hospital; names of later appointees—Drs. E. H. Smith, Valentine Seaman, David Hosack, S. L. Mitchill, and John Charlton—also appeared in this directory. Of the ten surgeons, two were also listed as druggists, one as a barber, and two as dentists. A law, known as "An Act to regulate the practice of Physick & Surgery in the City of New York," passed on June 10, 1760, provided that

> no person whatsoever shall practice as a Physician or Surgeon in the said City of New York before he shall first have been examined in Physick or Surgery and approved of and admitted by one of his Majesty's Council, and the Mayor of the City of New York for the time being, or by any three or

10 Stokes, *op. cit.*, V, 1276. (March 16, 1790.)

11 Benson J. Lossing, *History of New York City* (New York, 1885), I, 49.

more of them, taking to their assistance for such examination such proper person or persons as they in their discretion shall think fit.

Anyone practicing without this testimonial was subject to a fine of five pounds. This law, however, probably became obsolete after the Revolution and it was not until 1792 that the State Legislature passed an Act to regulate practice in the city. Many practitioners were, therefore, without proper qualifications: it was said that quacks were as "thick as locusts in Egypt." [12] At the opening of the Revolution in 1776, in the whole country not many more than 350 physicians—among a total of some 3,500 practitioners—had received medical degrees.[13] Apothecaries were, as in England, considered experts in the use of medicines and did much prescribing.

A few outstanding physicians, most of whom had received their medical education in European colleges and hospitals, were active in the promotion of standards and facilities in medical practice and education. It was they who brought about the establishment of the King's College Medical School in 1767, the Hospital in 1771, and the New York Dispensary in 1790. The most prominent practitioner in New York in 1791 was John Bard, father of Samuel. He was described as a striking figure in his red coat, cocked hat, and gold-headed cane, as he rode about the city in a low pony phaeton driven by a faithful Negro, almost as venerable as himself. He was the only physician who used a vehicle; all others walked, or hired a "chair." Dr. Bard was as ardent as his distinguished son in the advancement of medicine. He encouraged the latter in his endeavors to establish a hospital. He had been instrumental in the establishment of the college; in 1788 he was one of the organizers of the Medical Society of the City of New York, and was a leading spirit in founding the New York Dispensary in 1790.

Before the New York Hospital was established, hospital treatment was not available in New York City for the rich or poor.[14] The almshouse (also called the "Publick Workhouse and House of Correction") was opened in 1736 on the site of the present City Hall; it had a six bed infirmary, 25 by 23 feet, on the second floor. The first physician to the almshouse was Dr. John Van Beuren; he was succeeded in 1765 by his son Beekman, who served until the Revolution. The almshouse was a two-story build-

[12] Joseph M. Toner, *Contributions to the Annals of Medical Progress and Medical Education in the United States, before and during the War of Independence* (Washington, D.C., 1874), p. 37.

[13] *Ibid.*, p. 105.

[14] In 1658 under the Dutch regime "a clean and suitable house" was established as a hospital. It was still operated in 1680.

ing, 56 by 24 feet. "In the cellar . . . on the west a strong room or cage for the refractory" [15] was located, and no doubt served in the treatment of many mentally ill persons. The daily paper published an order authorizing five or six English sailors to go unarmed to convey "a crazy woman" to the almshouse. Some provision for "lunatic and Mad Persons" was also made in the bridewell. In 1785 the Common Council authorized that not more than five rooms be partitioned off in the attic story there for the confinement of such persons. A new almshouse was erected in 1796, but it was not until 1816, when the institution was removed to "Belle Vue Place" on Kip's Bay, that buildings for hospital purposes were provided. Although mentally ill patients in increasing numbers were accommodated, service for them was inadequately supplied; and separate provision was not made by the city until 1839, when the New York City Lunatic Asylum was established on Blackwell's (now Welfare) Island. In the meantime, as will be related in succeeding chapters, the New York Hospital was, at first in the hospital itself and later in a special institution, providing the only properly organized facilities available for the treatment of the mentally ill in the whole state. Nor were the other states, except two, any better off.

The State Hospital at Williamsburg, Virginia, which had been opened in 1773, was a small institution without medical organization. The building was of two stories, and 100 by 32 feet in dimensions. It contained 24 rooms and cells, and accommodated 20 to 30 patients. The admission records of 1775 to 1778 are defective or missing; omitting these years, the records from October 12, 1773, to November 3, 1779, show the admission of only 36 patients. At the end of that period 18 remained in the hospital. There was no resident physician. A "Keeper" was in charge, and a physician of the vicinity was appointed to examine and give any necessary immediate treatment to patients on admission, and "at such other times as may be necessary." [16]

By contrast, the Pennsylvania Hospital was, in origin, organization, relations, and purposes, quite similar to the hospital in New York. The charter of the Pennsylvania Hospital was granted in 1751. Both the petition, which was written by Benjamin Franklin, and the charter reveal that the "principal motive which inspired the founders of the Pennsylvania Hospital as well as the main argument expressed in the Petition was the care and treatment of lunaticks . . . that they may

[15] R. J. Carlisle, *An Account of Bellevue Hospital* (New York, 1893), p. 5.

[16] Henry M. Hurd, *Institutional Care of the Insane in the United States and Canada* (Baltimore, 1916), III, 708–709.

be restored in reason and become useful members of the community." The hospital was opened in "Judge Kinsey's Mansion" for the reception of patients in February, 1752, and, of the first two patients admitted, one was a "lunatick." It was not until December, 1756, that the new hospital building was ready for occupation. The first floor was especially constructed for the accommodation of the mental patients; in 1841 a special department was established at some distance from the rest of the hospital.[17] The character and work of the Pennsylvania Hospital were, undoubtedly, well known to the founders of the hospital in New York. Dr. Benjamin Rush, attending physician at the Pennsylvania Hospital, had a wide reputation not only as a practitioner, but as a medical author and as a public-spirited citizen. He was greatly interested in mental disease, and did much to advance the treatment of the mentally ill in the hospital.

Dr. John Bard, who was living in Philadelphia when the Pennsylvania Hospital was established, was the physician and friend of Franklin. His son Samuel became acquainted with Franklin in London, and was introduced by him into the most influential circles. Samuel also made the acquaintance of Dr. John Fothergill, the Quaker physician of London who did much to obtain funds for both the Pennsylvania and the New York hospitals. Samuel Bard's teachers in Edinburgh, especially William Cullen, John Brown, Robert Whytt, and Alexander Monro II, were actively interested in mental disorders, and in the mental aspects of disease in general. There can be no doubt, therefore, that Bard and others among the physicians concerned with the establishment of the hospital, who had been students of medicine in Europe and had been there exposed to the influence of the movement for more humane and intelligent treatment of the mentally ill, were aware of the importance of making hospital provision for them. The leading citizens of New York, who were supporters and, in some instances, governors of the hospital, were also, no doubt, well acquainted with corresponding groups in Philadelphia and could hardly have failed to obtain considerable knowledge of the character and work of the Pennsylvania Hospital. The example set by this hospital in giving the needs of the mentally ill such a leading place in their purposes and plans, and the demonstration of the practicability and advantages of hospital treatment, must surely have influenced the founders of the hospital in New York in determining the principles, policies, and plans to be followed.

The charter of the New York Hospital does not contain any specific

[17] Thomas G. Morton, *History of the Pennsylvania Hospital* (Philadelphia, 1895).

reference to the mentally ill or "lunatics." The petition has, unfortunately, disappeared; it may have been destroyed by a fire in the State Library at Albany several years ago. It is evident, however, from various references, that it was the deliberate intention of the governors of the hospital to make provision for the mentally ill. In October, 1774, the following resolution was adopted by the board:

That the Committee for superintending the Building of the Hospital be Authorized to appropriate the cellar part of the North Wing or such part of it as they may judge necessary into wards or cells for the reception of Lunatics.

As has already been mentioned, fifteen years elapsed after the hospital building had been completed, before it was officially opened for the reception of patients. In the meantime, as the population of the city increased there was much sickness from contagious and other diseases, and the need of facilities for medical teaching became more pressing. Queries concerning the unused hospital became acute. In October, 1790, the Medical Society of the State of New York, which was especially interested in the establishment of a dispensary for outpatient service, placed on its minutes the following:

Might not the New York Hospital, now empty and useless, be advantageously converted into an Alms House, with cells for lunatics, the present Alms House into a Dispensary, the garden into a Botanic Garden, and the funds of the Hospital appropriated for their support? [18]

In November the Common Council of the city followed this proposal with an application to the governors for the use of their building as an almshouse.[19] This was disapproved by the governors in December, as "foreign to the object of their charter," but a committee was appointed to consider maintaining a dispensary. Soon afterwards the advice of Dr. Samuel Bard and Dr. Malachi Treat was requested in regard to arrangements for the admission of patients into the hospital. Evidently the question of opening had been under consideration for several months, as on January 3, 1791, James Murray, William Edgar, Jacob Watson, and Theophylact Bache were mentioned as "the Committee appointed on the 22d Day of April last," and were ordered to "forthwith, procure the means necessary for the reception of eighteen Patients in the Hospital, and admit that number, as soon as Convenient." [20] The committee was also ordered to "inform the Corporation of the City, that they can

18 Stokes, *op. cit.*, V, 1276 f. (Note for Oct. 14, 1790.)
19 New York city, *Minutes of Common Council, 1784–1831.* (Nov. 26, 1790.)
20 New York Hospital, *Minutes of the Governors,* Jan. 3, 1791.

be accommodated with one or two wards, in the Hospital, for the reception of such sick in the Alms House as they may think proper to send and support there." It is interesting that, although it later became a constant practice for the commissioners of the almshouse to send patients to the New York Hospital, the offer just mentioned was declined by the Common Council "as it would tend to increase the expences of the Alms House." [21] On January 21 the governors added Aaron Burr and William Maxwell to the "Committee appointed to open the Hospital," and ordered "that the Powers of the Committee be continued; and that they give public notice in such a way as they shall think best, that the Hospital is open for the reception of patients." [22] A week later, on January 28, 1791, the following notice appeared in the *New York Daily Advertiser:*

NEW YORK HOSPITAL
By order of the GOVERNORS *of the Hospital*
Public notice is hereby given

that they have made preparations for the reception and entertainment of patients and that on Tuesday the first of February, the physicians and surgeons will attend for the administration of the sick. Tuesdays and Fridays between the hours of one and two are appointed, taking in days; notwithstanding, however, one physician and surgeon will attend every day, at the same hours; and the apothecary all day; that in cases of accident and emergency, no unnecessary delay may happen. Such as wish to be admitted must apply to some one of the Governors who are Isaac Roos [Roosevelt]; Theophylact Bache; Henry Haydock; John Keefe; Aaron Burr; William Edgar; Alexander McComb; John Murray; William Denning; Thomas Pearsall; Samuel Franklin; John Murray, jun; George Bowne; Lawrence Embree; Jacob Watson; Sampson Fleming; Gerard Walton; Thomas Buchanan; Alexander Robertson; Hugh Gaine; William Backhouse; William Maxwell; Robert Bowne; Richard Morris; John Lawrence; and Robert R. Livingston, and who will in all proper cases, give letters of recommendation.

JOHN MURRAY, *chairman of the Committee/appointed for that purpose. Jan. 28.*

The hospital was located on a plot of three and a third acres between Barley and Catherine Streets (now Duane and Worth) on the west side of Broadway. This was virtually the limit of Broadway at that time, and there were few houses in the vicinity. The site was elevated above the surrounding country, and the land sloped gently to the Hudson River, of which there was an attractive view. The building was of stone, simple in design but dignified. Until other hospitals were established it was

21 New York city, *Minutes of Common Council, 1784–1831.* (Jan. 17, 1791.)
22 *Minutes of the Governors.*

popularly referred to as "The Hospital." Its opening was an event of considerable significance to the social organization of the city, and to the advancement of medical practice and medical education in New York, and was not without influence and practical helpfulness in other parts of the country. It quickened and mobilized the philanthropic spirit of the people, and furnished a concrete object for their interest and attention. With the Pennsylvania Hospital it led off in the splendid hospital development by private benevolent organizations which is such a distinctive feature of hospital provision in America. It is remarkable that, in the establishment of these two pioneer hospitals, one of the "principal motives" was the care and cure of the mentally ill; and it is unfortunate that this was not accepted as a standard to be followed by all succeeding hospital organizations. Had this occurred, the understanding, treatment, and prevention of mental illness in America would probably have been far in advance of what has been reached today.

IV

FACILITIES AND ORGANIZATION, 1791-1808

THE hospital building had been much damaged during its occupancy by Hessian soldiers, and was neglected during the years that immediately followed. Full occupancy could not be undertaken, and the committee to attend to the opening were authorized to admit only eighteen patients. No record of the total number admitted during the first year has been found. A committee appointed to estimate the sum necessary to support the hospital, however, reported in February, 1792, that the expenditures during eleven months had been £580, or 2 *s.*, 5½*d.* per day for each patient treated. This implies an average daily total of about fourteen patients. The total capacity of the building is not stated. In estimating the sum needed, however, the committee reported that £1,370 would be required for a year's support of 60 patients—probably close to the maximum that the governors felt prepared to accommodate. The annual reports of successive years show that at the close of 1795 this number had been exceeded; there were then 73 patients, and at the close of 1802—the last year before the enlargement of the building—the number was 147. After another story had been added in 1803, the number of patients increased, and at the close of 1807 there were 207 under treatment.

The only available means of depicting the interior construction and the equipment and furnishings of the New York Hospital in the period from 1791 to 1808 is to present the meager references in official records [1] and in publications designed for other purposes.[2] No detailed descriptions have been found. The interior construction was principally of wood, with plastered walls which were whitewashed from time to time. In 1805 Dr. Hosack recommended that they be painted. The floor plans shown on page 39 are apparently the only ones that have been preserved. There were, it will be noted, four wards on the main floor, besides the offices of the steward, the matron, and the apothecary. The library, 27 feet by 19 feet 6 inches, was also on this floor. There was a second floor and, after the building was enlarged in 1803, a third, but plans of these have not been found. The total number of wards in the enlarged hospital was 16. The lying-in ward was on the second floor, the surgical amphitheater on the third, and there were 23 other rooms.

1 New York Hospital, *Minutes of the Governors, Minutes of Visiting Committee, Superintendent's Expenses.* In the pages that follow, much of the detail has been derived from these official records.

2 *A Brief Account of the New-York Hospital* (New York, 1804, 1811).

The plan of the basement floor shows two wards in the north section, which were "fitted up for the temporary accommodation of patients whose particular disease renders it necessary to remove them from intercourse with others." [3] No description of these "wards or cells" has been found, but that this was the space provided for the "Maniacs" seems

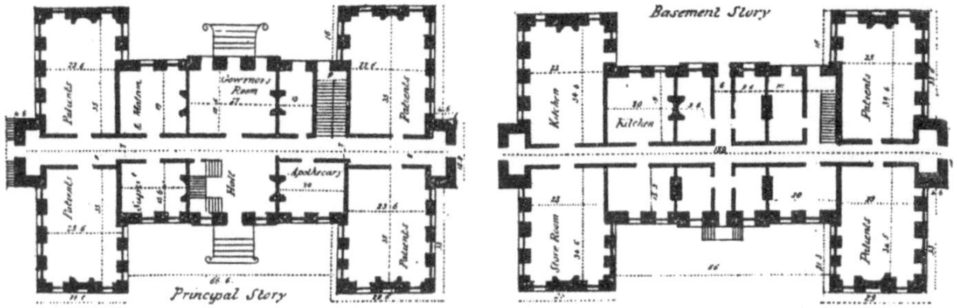

THE NEW YORK HOSPITAL, 1776: FLOOR PLANS

probable. There were several rooms on this floor the purpose of which is not in all instances indicated on the plan. The storeroom and kitchen are shown in the south section of the plan, and in the central section is a smaller kitchen. The wards of the hospital were described as "spacious, and susceptible of complete ventilation," and it was added that "the sick enjoy a fine atmosphere, in a situation that cannot be encroached upon by the neighboring buildings." [4]

There was no water distribution system in the building. There was a well, the water of which was said to be excellent and "like other water drawn from equal depths in this latitude, of the temperature of 54 degrees of Fahrenheit's scale." [5] The carrying of water was, however, an onerous and time-consuming task. The toilet facilities were quite primitive; a "privy," probably more than one, accessible from the wards.[6] This was evidently a dry-earth closet, as it was recommended that lye or ashes should be thrown in every week, especially in the warm months. The proposal was made that a door, closed by a spring or a pulley, be placed at the entrance of the passage from the hospital in order to exclude as much as possible of the bad air and smell. Commode chairs were used on the wards, and the physicians mentioned the necessity of emptying them promptly after use. In one instance, it was recommended

[3] *Ibid.* (1811), p. 11. [4] S. L. Mitchill, *Traveller's Guide* (New York, 1807).
[5] Mitchill, *op. cit.*
[6] New York Hospital, *Minutes of the Governors,* April 2 and June 4, 1805.

that the single chair, evidently kept in the ward for general use, be kept out of sight in a closet and cleaned carefully by the nurses. The advantages of water closets and sewers were mentioned and the governors were advised to "recommend and urge to the magistracy of the city, such a measure."

Bathing facilities were apparently in a "bathing house" separate from the wards; attention was directed to "the state of the air in going to and returning from them, as well as their not being heated as often as they ought to be." The physicians considered that tin bathing tubs, of which there was only one, could be used with great advantage on the wards. The patients suffered much from cold every winter in the north and west wards, and in all the wards the windows were either loose or in such an open state as to admit much cold air. Double casements or sashes were suggested for the windows with a northern and western exposure. At that time the only means of heating the wards and corridors was by means of fireplaces in which wood was burnt. Coal stoves were recommended by the physicians, and also the use of coal in the fireplaces. Open stoves for burning coal were actually introduced in December, 1806. This was, at first, considered to be an experiment, and the Visiting Committee were instructed to purchase a type of stove that could not be used by the patients for cooking purposes. It was added, however, that other means of warming drinks might be easily provided by the superintendent. Stoves were deemed unnecessary in wards with a southern or eastern exposure. The suggestion was made that in cold weather some of the patients might be moved to the southern wards. Since, at that time, "maniacs" were generally believed to be insensitive to cold, it is unlikely that the cells were provided with heat. If these cells were located in the basement shown in the plan, some heat might, however, have been derived from the kitchen and laundry. The hospital was lighted by candles, oil lamps and lanterns. The odor of the wards and the need of better ventilation were frequently mentioned. In the wards for venereal cases, the odor was sometimes so offensive that the physicians found it difficult to remain long enough to attend to the patients.

The bedsteads were of wood, but, on recommendation of the physicians, these were gradually discarded and replaced with iron ones. "Sacking" was proposed in place of boards for bed bottoms because it would "add so much to the comfort of the sick that the advantages in their recovery far outweigh all considerations of expense," and "particularly in the surgical ward, pillows of different kinds are wanted, not only of the ordinary sort to raise the head, but very soft and easy ones to support wounded limbs, and to rest diseased parts on." Blankets were imported from England. The physicians asked for a larger supply of sheets and other articles of bedding in order that changes could be made more frequently and recommended that, when patients were admitted, filthy or infected clothing should be destroyed and, if necessary, new clothing supplied. White flannel shirts and worsted stockings were considered "indispensably necessary," because colored articles did not show so readily that they were dirty.

In occupying new wards, the separation of convalescent, venereal, and postoperative patients was suggested, as well as of "those who are phthisical and require an uniform temperature." All these reports of the physicians were referred by the governors to a committee which recommended that most of the suggestions should be adopted and carried into effect. The committee considered, however, that instead of outside sashes for the windows, it would be sufficient if they were well caulked during the winter. They also proposed white linen or tow cloth shirts for the summer season.

It is necessary to keep in mind that, if the hospital was lacking in comfort and conveniences, the homes of even the most affluent citizens were also without them. If the equipment and furnishings, and the domestic and nursing service, were crude, it was because no better were obtainable and the funds of the hospital were insufficient. The hospital was for the poor who, at best, were obliged to bear such hardships and deprivations as are only exceptionally met with today. Of what modern hospital could it be reported, as occurred at the New York Hospital in June, 1799, that "the Patients were generally well satisfied" with the following dietary?

BREAKFAST

Sunday & Tuesday—Rye Coffee sweetned with Molasses, & Bread.
Thursday & Saturday—Cocoa, sweetned with Molasses, & Bread.
Monday Wednesday & Friday—Mush & Molasses.

DINNER

Sunday & Tuesday, Ox head & Meat Soup with Indian Dumplins (sic).
Thursday & Saturday, Ox head & Meat Soup with Bread & Vegetables in their Season—
Monday Wednesday & Friday—Rice & Molasses—

SUPPER

Monday Tuesday Thursday & Saturday—Mush & Molasses—
Wednesday & Friday, Rye Coffee or Cocoa with Bread—

4 quarts of Milk pr. Day—Bread to be of Rye & Wheat flour.
1 quart of Molasses for 24 Persons [7]

This dietary was for patients "whose diseases in the opinion of the Physicians and surgeons do not require particular food." In 1806, on the recommendation of the physicians and surgeons, it was changed to:

Breakfast: (every day) Rye Coffee with half a gill of Milk sweetened with Sugar; or Indian gruel with Molasses or Sugar. N.B. The difference between gruel or mush has only reference to its consistence.

Dinner: (4 days) Rice with Molasses or Milk and an ounce of Butter to each patient.
(3 days) Meat and Soup with Vegetable.

Supper: (4 days) The same as for breakfast.
(3 days) Common tea sweetened with Sugar and half a Gill of Milk.

Roasted and Broiled Meats as well as Liquors are only to be served at the particular desire of the Physicians.[8]

The nursing service was a source of constant concern to both the governors and the physicians. There were, apparently, more than a few Sairy Gamps, and many years were to elapse before nurse training was established and nursing became a fine art in the hands of women of education and refinement. Nurses were frequently recruited from former patients in the hospital. The maximum number employed at any time before 1808 was, as far as can be ascertained from the payrolls, never more than thirteen. This was at a time when the number of patients was about 178, a proportion of 13.7 patients to each nurse. The physicians wanted one nurse to every ten patients, and, in addition, a head nurse and an "orderly man" to every two wards. The governors, however, found that only one head nurse and one orderly could be added at that time. The only position listed especially in connection with the mentally ill was that of "maniac keeper" or "cell keeper." This position was occupied for at least six years by James Williams. The letters "B.M." after his name were then used throughout the records to designate a Negro. They are attached to the names of several of the female nurses also, and in one instance the nurse, who was Williams' wife, is named "Phillis Blk Nurse." The records show that from an early period Negroes, some of them slaves, were admitted as patients, and there were two "black wards."

[7] *Minutes of the Governors*, May 7, 1799.
[8] *Minutes of the Visiting Committee*, Nov. 14, 1806.

No lists of positions, no payroll, and no descriptive references to the various positions in the hospital organization prior to 1795 have been found in the records examined. The position of steward was established in June, 1791, at a salary of forty shillings a month, but it was not filled until June, 1792, when John Reay was appointed at a salary of forty pounds a year. The steward was virtually superintendent of the hospital and was, eventually, given that title. He purchased current supplies and kept records of patients admitted and discharged, entering their names in the "Book of Admission." It was also his duty to visit the wards every morning and evening; to attach to each bed a card showing the name of the patient and of his physician; to have the names of the patients called; note absentees; and aid the nurses in maintaining order and discipline. It was a lawless period: many of the patients were sailors or other transients; drunkenness was rampant; and the records show that "going over the wall" was a frequent occurrence. Many patients were discharged for disorderly behavior. Of 1,094 patients discharged in 1806, 58 were "disorderly," and 64 "eloped." A minute of the Visiting Committee of January 15, 1808, states:

> It appears that many of the Pauper Patients are in the practice of going over the Wall, & by means of the excesses they run into during their absence from the House, their cure is render'd tedious & expensive to this Institution. The Superintendent is directed to report all such to the Committee that they may be order'd discharged—or if they are not in a situation to be discharged that orders may be given to chain them in their respective Wards.

At the same meeting it was noted that:

> Isaac Palmer a Pauper in No. 9 having in direct violation of the order of the Visiting Committee (of which he was particularly informed) gone over the Wall. The Committee called in said Palmer, informed him he must either leave the House, or submit to be chained . . . & he agreed to be chained.

Other employees listed in 1795 are a matron, five nurses, one orderly man, one gardener, one porter, two washerwomen, one assistant cook, and one housemaid. During these early formative years, the governors, especially the Visiting Committee, participated actively in many details of administration. The Visiting Committee visited the hospital twice a week, and the Inspecting Committee once a week. All committees were held to a strict accounting by the board, and failure to report was repeated in the minutes of each meeting of the governors until the report was submitted or the committee discharged.

When the hospital was opened, the medical organization consisted of Dr. Samuel Bard and Dr. Malachi Treat, who had been appointed as

"Physicians in Ordinary" in 1774. Dr. Peter Middleton and Dr. John Jones, who had been appointed at the same time, were no longer available, as the former had died and the latter had moved to Philadelphia. In January, 1791, Dr. John Charlton and Dr. Thomas Jones were appointed to replace them. No other medical appointments were made until May, 1792, when Dr. William P. Smith, and Dr. Samuel Nicholl were elected physicians and Drs. Richard Bayley, James Tillary, Wright Post, and Richard Kissam were elected surgeons. In July of the same year the governors made a distinct separation between the surgical and medical departments. Changes occurred from time to time during the next few years, when Drs. John R. B. Rodgers, Samuel Borrowe, David Hosack, Valentine Seaman, Samuel L. Mitchill, Elihu H. Smith, William Hammersley, Edward Miller, James S. Stringham, and others were added to the list of those who belong to the early history of the hospital, and who brought into the medical service the quality and distinction which have always characterized it.

In January, 1792, William Dickson, Jr., who occupied the position of Apothecary, was appointed Resident Assistant to the Surgical Department. He was the first house surgeon. The apothecary was at that time considered a sort of semimedical person. It was necessary for him to have considerable knowledge not only of medicines but of therapeutics, and he was subjected to examination by the physicians before he was appointed. He shared with the house surgeon the responsibility of reporting to the attending physicians and surgeons the condition of their patients, and of prescribing for the sick "in ordinary cases" during the absence of the physician. He was required to report to the board the patients received and discharged, and to keep an account of them in a book. The Rules of the Hospital adopted by the governors in September, 1801, required the apothecary to alternate with the house surgeon in attending women at childbirth, "that is to say, one time the Apothecary and the next time the House Surgeon where the labour is natural."

On account of the significance to the development of the resources of the hospital for the treatment of the mentally ill, it seems proper to mention here that Thomas Eddy was elected a member of the Society in May, 1793, and in June a member of the Board of Governors, of which in May, 1794, he was elected Secretary. He was always zealous in advancing the facilities and organization for the treatment of the mentally ill.

V

TREATMENT OF THE MENTALLY ILL IN THE GENERAL MEDICAL SERVICE, 1792–1808

Although the mentally ill are not specifically mentioned in the charter of the Society of the New York Hospital, there is ample evidence that active treatment of them was a well-considered part of the policy and purpose of the governors. In an *Address to the Citizens of New York* published in 1794, the governors referred to their disappointment in the loss of their first building in 1775, which "was so far completed, as to afford hope that, in a few weeks, an asylum would be opened for the poor sick, and maimed, languishing under the various diseases of body and *mind.*" [1] The address goes on to say,

> Among the many maladies to which mankind is liable, none are more to be lamented than insanity. For this class of patients, *convenient wards are provided* [1] and several of that description have been cured, and others much relieved. . . . Religion and Humanity strongly plead in favor of a fellow creature, deprived of the means of subsistence joined to . . . a disordered mind.

In the previous year the governors had, by resolution, exempted the mentally ill, or "lunatics," from the rule that curable patients, only, could be admitted to the hospital. In 1797 an announcement of policy contained in the annual report of the governors to the State Legislature stated that "Persons labouring under incurable decrepitude or long continued Ailments of any kind, are considered as fitter Objects for an Alms House than for this Hospital, which is properly an Infirmary for 1st. Medical Treatment, 2d. Chirurgical Treatment, 3d. Maniacs." Thus, soon after the opening of the hospital the particular interest in the mentally ill which has always animated the governors, commenced to assume a place of growing importance in their considerations.

The "wards or cells" for which, in October, 1774, the Building Committee were instructed by the board to make provision in the "cellar part of the North Wing," seem to have been the only special accommodation made for the mentally ill patients or "maniacs." The hospital site was elevated and the cellar in the back of the building may have been sufficiently exposed to provide space for windows. The governors had in 1773, during the planning of the building, ordered that the lower floors of the wings should be raised for the purpose of giving light to the cel-

[1] No italics in original.

lars,[2] and an estimate of one of the contractors contains twelve windows for the basement. Evidently, however, the cells in the cellar were used only in the treatment of extremely difficult cases.

Mentally ill patients were in other parts of the hospital also. Alexander Anderson, a medical student [3] who kept a diary, recorded that, in May, 1794, he "went to the Hospital and took a walk through the garden and saw Eccles, a maniac." In June he recorded that, when he was at the hospital, "Cockle, the lunatic gave a jargon really ridiculous, and concluded with showing that he was in a 'continual whirlwind of reprobation and not of reformation.' " The rather curious name of this patient as well as that of Eccles are in the admission book. Again in February, 1796, the diarist records that he

> went to the Hospital. Dr. Bard attended there and visited the patients. Talcott, an insane person introduced himself among us and read over a curious jargon which he had written. As he is quite harmless, he has liberty to walk about the Hospital. His appearance is that of a decent quaker and his language pretty good.

As the subject of Anderson's graduation thesis was "Chronic Mania," and as he mentions several mentally ill patients under treatment in their homes, it may be assumed that his interest in patients of this type was more than ordinary. Only once, however, does he record a visit to "the rooms fitted up in the cellar" where he saw "a distracted woman," and he adds, "This sight affected me with very dismal reflections." That patients were not transferred to these cells without consideration for attention to them is indicated by the following from the *Minutes of the Governors*, September 3, 1797:

> The President reports that the situation of Philip C. (a Maniac) is such as very much disturbs the quiet of the House. Therefore, Resolved that the Visiting Committee be requested to inform his family that the board thinks it necessary he be immediately removed to one of the Cells, and that it will be proper to make an additional charge for someone to attend him.

Evidently the treatment of the mentally ill was, until the special department was established in 1808, considered to belong to the general medical service of the hospital, and the first enlargement of the hospital was occasioned by the desire of the governors to make more extensive

[2] New York Hospital, *Minutes of the Governors:* "At Hulls on Tuesday the 10th Augst 1773."

[3] Later a well-known doctor and engraver, he was a student receiving instruction at the hospital in 1793–1796. A copy of the diary is at the library of the New York Historical Society; original at the Low Library, Columbia University.

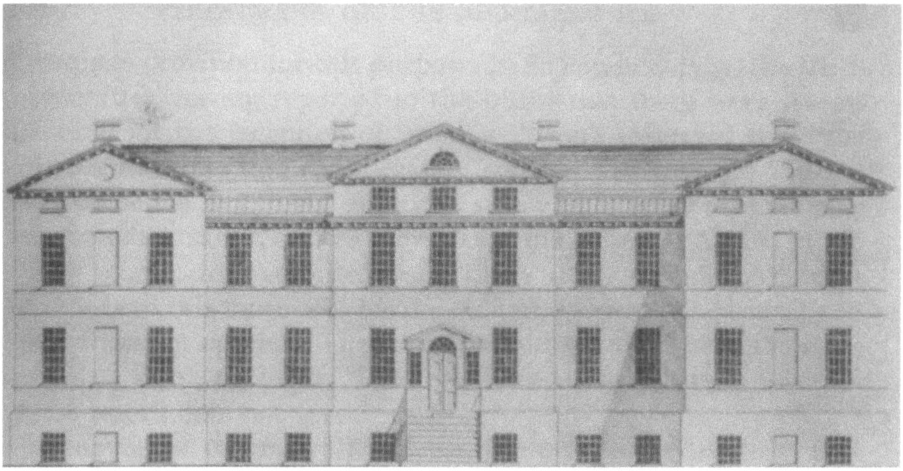

A FRONT VIEW OF THE NEW YORK HOSPITAL, 1776

IN THE "CELLAR PART OF THE NORTH WING . . . CELLS FOR THE LUNATICS" WERE CONSTRUCTED.

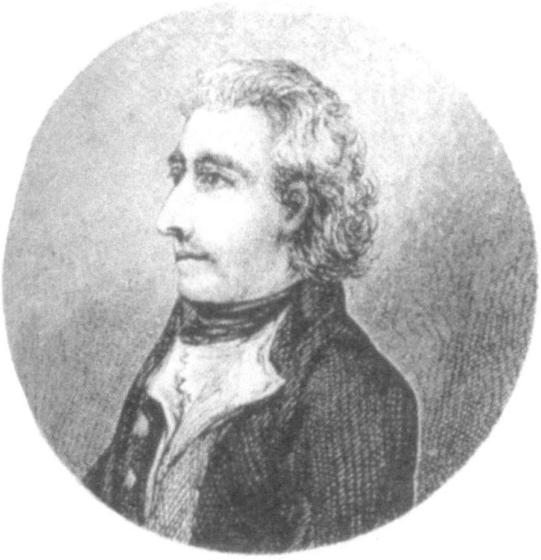

ALEXANDER ANDERSON

MEDICAL STUDENT, 1793-1796

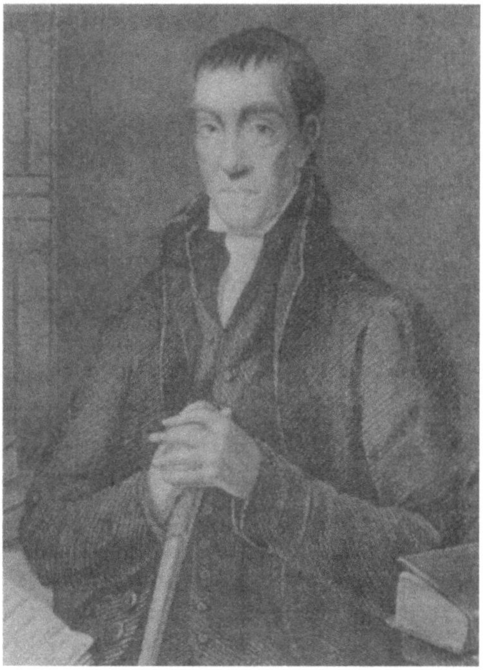

THOMAS EDDY

HIS COMMUNICATION ON "MORAL TREATMENT," PRESENTED TO THE BOARD OF GOVERNORS IN 1815, LED TO THE ESTABLISHMENT OF BLOOMINGDALE ASYLUM. ONE OF THE GOVERNORS OF THE HOSPITAL, 1793-1827

and adequate provision for this purpose. In September, 1797, the Visiting Committee, having reported to the board that there were several applications for the reception of "maniacs," were informed that "the Board took the same into consideration and resolved that the Visiting Committee be left at Liberty to receive such and as many as there may be accommodations for, and as they may think proper." Again, in the following month, it is recorded that "the Visiting Committee report in favour of erecting more cells for the Maniacs, which being considered the Board were of opinion 'That the Committee should have the same done if they think necessary.' " Where these additional cells were located the record does not reveal.

The number of mentally ill patients, however, increased from that time on, and by June, 1802, the need of additional facilities was so pressing that a committee was appointed "to consider if some plan of arrangement can be made, by an addition to this building, or otherwise, for the accommodation of Lunatics." In August this committee reported that they had consulted an architect, and were ready to submit a plan. After much consideration had been given to the relative advantages of an additional story on the building or a wing, it was, in March, 1803, decided that construction of the former would be undertaken during the ensuing summer. In their annual report to the legislature, the governors stated that

> they have long lamented, that an Hospital, otherwise so well adapted for the alleviation of human misery, should not furnish an Asylum convenient and inviting for the reception of that class of our fellow Creatures, who are deprived of the use of their Reason . . . and perhaps none are more entitled to pity and compassion, or have a more powerful claim on us as professors of christianity.

They hoped to be able to finance the proposed construction but, if their funds proved to be inadequate, they would "trust to the goodness of providence and to the benevolence of the Legislature and their fellow citizens." In their next annual report, for 1803, the governors were able to announce that the additional story had been completed, furnishing "convenient and airy accommodations for one hundred and twenty more patients," and that it was now possible "to provide suitable apartments for Maniacs, a description of patients that imperiously demand our sympathy and our most sedulous care and attention." The new story greatly improved the appearance of the hospital, which is described in a publication of the period as follows:

The grounds of the hospital were in 1801 inclosed with a handsome brick wall. The roof has been covered with slate, and adorned with a cupola. A third storey has also been added to it. Within the inclosure are fine and healthy walks, and rests, for the convalescent patients. The approach to the hospital is between beautiful rows of elms.[4]

In April, 1804, the governors appointed a committee to meet with the physicians and surgeons to "take a view of the Hospital," and report on the best plan for making suitable accommodations for the "Maniacs," the governors "being desirous to have this description of Patients provided for in the best possible manner." The committee advised that "the north east Ward and the west middle Ward on the upper story should be divided into convenient cells and that the cells already provided in the two north tower wards should be continued to be appropriated as heretofore."[5] No description of the north tower wards is available, and whether the "cellar part of the North Wing" was so designated, or where cells which had been provided in some other part of the hospital were located, cannot be stated with certainty. The committee further advised that the women should be kept in one apartment entirely separate from the men and attended to by female nurses. They also recommended "grates" for the windows; that the cells should be painted and "in every respect made comfortable, and convenient"; and that the corridor leading to the cells in the lower part of the building be floored, and the whole ceiled and finished. The board, in adopting the report, substituted for the northeast ward the ward opposite the west ward and the north room adjoining. No further description and no floor plan are available. The elimination of male attendants from the management of difficult female patients may seem commonplace now but at that time it was a real step forward. The practice of allowing females to be attended by males was then generally prevalent; a remnant still remains in some states where the transfer of mentally sick women by constables and deputy sheriffs is the custom.

The deep satisfaction of the governors in the improved facilities for the treatment of the mentally ill is feelingly expressed in their annual report to the legislature for the year 1804:

Of all the Evils which afflict the Human Race, the deprivation of Reason is the most awful and deplorable; and it has been an object of anxious solicitude on the part of the Governors to extend more fully the benefits of this institution to persons suffering under so great a calamity. It is with much

[4] S. L. Mitchill, *Traveller's Guide* (New York, 1807).
[5] *Minutes of the Governors*, April 3 and 11, 1804.

satisfaction they are enabled to state, that convenient apartments are prepared, where all suitable means are provided for the relief and recovery of all such maniacs as may be sent from different parts of the State, to the Hospital.

In the whole state there was still no other hospital in which a mentally ill person could obtain protection and treatment, and the applications for admission kept increasing. One year later, 1805, the governors were again appealing to the legislature for aid to enable them to increase their accommodations. They proposed to erect two wings to the hospital building, one of which was to be "exclusively appropriated for the reception of Maniacs who would then have ample accommodations, adapted to the different forms and degrees of insanity, to the relative situations of the patients, and their various connexions in life." Already the necessity of classification was becoming apparent, and, while at that time no person suffering from any form of illness who could afford the expense of treatment at home went to a hospital, in the case of the mentally ill the alternatives for the affluent and poor alike were frequently prison or neglect and brutality in private as well as public care. The governors, therefore, drew the attention of the legislature to the position of the hospital as the only "public institution in this State for maniacs," and asked that "this part of the establishment should be placed on an adequate and respectable foundation." They felt that the humanity and honor of the state demanded this, as "with the uniform increase of patients in general, and the size of the edifice, it is not possible to afford those advantages to this afflicted class of persons which they require, and which the feelings and wishes of the Governors would induce them to impart." [6] In response to this appeal, the legislature extended to 1857 the annual appropriation of $12,500 that had been previously granted.[7] Thus supported, the governors proceeded to make plans for a separate building for the mentally ill, instead of a wing to the existing building as first proposed. This will be described, with an account of its organization and operation, in the next chapter.

The total number of mentally ill patients treated in the general medical service of the hospital, previous to the establishment of the separate department, was quite small. The first recorded admission of a patient of this character was authorized by resolution of the Board of Governors, indicating that such admissions had previously been considered

[6] *Minutes of the Governors,* Jan. 20, 1806.

[7] In 1810 the Legislature also granted an annuity of $3,500 for 10 years to help pay for the new building. This was discontinued in 1817.

inadvisable. On September 18, 1792, the following resolution was adopted:

It having been represented to the Board, that John Alner, an Inhabitant of this City is deranged in his senses: and that his Family are desirous he should be admitted to this Hospital: Resolved that if said John Alner shall be considered by the Physicians of the Hospital as curable and therefore a proper object of this Institution that he be admitted on paying all the necessary expenses during his continuance in the Hospital.

It is noteworthy that one of the conditions for admission was that he should be curable. No record of the actual date of admission has been found, but in January, 1793, the rate to be charged Alner was fixed by the board at twenty shillings a week.

Until 1795 no classification by diagnosis was made in the statistical tables in the minutes and the annual reports. In the report for 1795, the table records one case of mania remaining in the hospital from the previous year, and 14 discharged during the year. There is no record of any admissions. The report for 1796 gives no record of any admissions nor of any remaining from the previous year. Eleven cases of mania and one of melancholia were, however, recorded as discharged, and 4 cases of mania and 1 of melancholia were in the hospital at the close of that year. The statistics of admissions and discharges from 1797 to 1807 are complete except for those of 1799, which are missing. All available figures on mania and melancholia from the opening of the hospital until the establishment of the separate department in 1808 are contained in Table 1 on page 51.

The total number of admissions of mentally ill patients that can be accurately determined was 410, and by adding admissions in 1795 and 1796, the number of which is estimated from numbers recorded as discharged or remaining over from the previous year, this may be increased to 429. The years 1793, 1794, and 1799 must be entirely omitted. Of the total number considered to be accurate, mania was the diagnosis in 394 cases, and melancholia in 16 cases. This was the classification that prevailed in America at that time. Idiots were, however, placed in a separate class. It is noticeable that the number of yearly admissions increased after the new story was added in 1803. Among the cases treated during the years 1795–1807, there were also recorded, besides the "maniacs," 33 cases of epilepsy, 16 of hysteria, and 15 of hypochondriasis. The medical designations under which these patients were listed are among those employed at the present time, but no doubt a large proportion of the cases would now be differently classified. The discharge

TABLE 1

CASES OF MANIA AND MELANCHOLIA TREATED IN THE NEW YORK HOSPITAL, 1792–1807

Year	Remaining from Previous Year	Admitted during Year	Total Treated	Discharged						Remaining at End of Year
				Cured	Relieved	Disorderly or Eloped	To Alms House	Died	By Request	
1792	..	1[a]	..	..	..	..	..	..	..	..
1793[b]	..	1	..	..	..	..	..	..	1	..
1794[b]	..	3	..	1	..	..	..	..	1	..
1795[c]	1	14[?]	15[?]	5	3	2	1[d]	2	1	..
1796	1[?]	15[?]	16[?]	3	3	2	..	2	2	5
1797	5	18	23	4	6	1	..	2	1	9
1798	9	20	29	15	..	2	..	1	2	9
1799[e]	..	..	..	..	..	..	..	..	..	..
1800	4	37	41	27	4	4	3	1	..	2
1801	2	38	40	13	16	..	..	4	..	7
1802	7	43	50	20	7	5	4	2	..	12
1803	12	33	45	19	7	3	1	4	..	11
1804	11	46	57	22	5	5	2	3	5	15
1805	15	60	75	30	4	3	3	8	7	20
1806	20	68	88	29	..	10	..	7	21	21
1807	21	47	68	18	3	2	..	4	17	24

a From a note to that effect in the *Minutes of the Governors*, Sept. 18, 1792. No doubt there were others.

b From lists of admissions in Admission Book of Aug. 21, 1793–March 26, 1799, apparently incomplete. No entries in the Admission Book subsequent to this.

c All figures from here on obtained from Annual Reports of the Governors.

d Discharged Incurable, not to Alms House.

e No records.

Patients when discharged signed a certificate such as the following:

> This is to Certify that I *Jas. C.*—— was admitted on the 6th Day of Feby 1795 a Patient into the New York Hospital, afflicted with Lunacy and am now discharged; by my own desire. Witness my Hand, at the New York Hospital, this 20th Day of Feby 1795.
>
> James C.——

of 14 of the 33 epileptics, 12 of the 16 cases of hysteria, and 12 of the 15 hypochondriacs as "cured," and the death of 5 of the cases of hysteria seem to indicate this. Thirty-eight percent of the cases designated mania or melancholia were discharged "cured" and 7 percent died; the number of patients so designated who were admitted from the opening of the hospital until 1808 constituted 4½ percent of all patients admitted.

These figures are probably an understatement of the total psychiatric cases treated.

The conception of mental illness and the methods employed in the study and treatment of the patients were probably no different from those which prevailed everywhere and which have been described in preceding chapters. Although none of the physicians of the hospital during this period appear to have specialized in mental disease, a few of them can, by means of publications available, and otherwise, be shown to have had considerable interest in the subject. The "wards or cells in the cellar part of the building" were, until additional and more adequate accommodations were provided in 1803, the only special structural provision for "maniacs." The character of these cells is, in some measure, indicated by the following extract from a report made to the governors by Dr. Hosack in 1805:

> The lower apartments at present occupied by the Maniacs are in a state that renders them very unfit for their accommodation—in consequence of having never been painted the Cells have become so imbued with filth that they are extremely offensive and unwholesome especially in the summer season—these apartments should be immediately painted both inside and outside—the floors should be washed and sanded every week. . . . The beds of the Maniacs are not as frequently changed as is necessary considering the propensity to filthiness attending this description of the sick.[8]

The "maniac keeper" was probably not distinguished for his gentleness, and as in other places a whip was probably one of his resources in difficult situations. In the superintendent's account of October 1, 1799, is an item for the purchase of a "cat & nine tales for Sel Keeper . . . 4 s." Violence was controlled by chains, which were also used as punishment for refractory cases. Altogether, there were no doubt ample grounds for Alexander Anderson's entry in his diary, after a visit to the cellar in 1793, that "this sight affected me with very dismal reflections." The cells into which the space appropriated for the mentally ill in the story added in 1803 was divided, were probably much more suitable than those in the cellar, and possibly the latter were afterwards seldom or never used. At least, the reports of the Visiting Committee after 1805, wherein the distribution of the patients in different wards was sometimes stated, mentioned only "upper cells," and the number of patients in these was never more than three and usually only one or two. Most of the "maniacs" seem to have been accommodated on Ward 2, the number recorded in the reports being from ten to fifteen. Judging from the

[8] *Minutes of the Governors*, June 4, 1805.

entries found in the *Minutes of the Visiting Committee* from March 1, 1805, to the opening of the Asylum, only men were admitted to Ward 2. Women patients were admitted directly to the "upper cells"; men also were apparently treated there. Prior to the opening of the Asylum, the last admission to Ward 2 occurred in May, 1808, and the last discharge, on June 16 of that year. Occasionally, however, mentally ill patients were evidently admitted to other wards. The maximum daily number in the service during 1807 was 20. It will be recalled that Alexander Anderson mentioned in his diary meeting mentally ill patients in the garden and in the general wards as he made rounds with the physicians, several years before accommodations for "maniacs" had been provided above the "cellar part of the North Wing." The disposition of these patients throughout the hospital and the manner in which they were treated, cannot, however, because of the lack of adequate information, be accurately described.

So scanty is this information that it seems appropriate to present an abstract of the only account of a case of mental illness treated at the New York Hospital during this period which was found in the medical literature. This contains some of the views relating to mental illness which were prevalent at the time. It appeared in the *Medical Repository,* a journal which was established in 1797 by two physicians of the Hospital, Dr. Samuel L. Mitchill and Dr. Elihu H. Smith, in association with Dr. Edward Miller, later a member of the hospital staff. It was the first medical periodical to be published in America. The communication was by Dr. Smith and was entitled "Case of Mania Successfully Treated By Mercury." [9]

Abstract

Mary Mathews—admitted to N.Y. Hospital, Aug. 16, 1796. Age 17. England—U.S. few weeks.

Always feeble—subject to "something like hysteria"—though never in form of fit or convulsion. "Wind rising from her stomach, struggling for breath, a sensation like swelling of her tongue, heat in all her body, and an universal uneasiness."

About a week before admission, as she was walking in a field some miles from town, "was suddenly taken insane." Symptoms increased to admission. No nourishment for a week. "Efforts so violent that it was necessary to cause her to be confined in a cell, and to be strait-waistcoated." No passage of bowels for week before admission. Rejected medicine and food. 16th and 17th, "Completely tore off and rent apart three strait-waistcoats; neither of which, probably, could have been rent by the utmost combined effort of

[9] *Medical Repository,* I (1797), 181.

two strong men." Forced grating of cells, drank dirty suds in wash room—first thing known to swallow since her disease commenced. "Five or six persons were, with difficulty, able to force her back to her cell." Went naked—indifferent, "Disposed herself in various and scarcely conceivable attitudes, and continued for hours in postures which well persons could not have assumed, much less have rested in." Noticed no persons, divided time in singing "methodistic hymns" and putting up short prayer. "That her disease did not proceed from any insane religious impression is evident from her never having expressed any anxiety before, during, or after her illness: nor did she seem to suffer from apprehension of any kind." Uniform exertion was to escape when door opened—no uneasiness to effect this when it was shut. Made no endeavor to hurt attendants and visitors.

Aug. 18, 8 or 9 days without food or movement of bowels. No sleep nor repose—violence not diminished. "As the vital energy seemed principally determined to the external muscles, leaving the stomach and intestinal canal, in particular, in a state of apparent torpidity, it occurred to me that, notwithstanding her long inanition and violent exertions, any thing which would considerably diminish the muscular force would tend to equalize the distribution of that energy, and would promote a cure."

Desired to bleed her, but was impossible to use the lancet. No force could open bent arm. Cupping-glasses used—occiput, temples, and forehead—6 oz.—of "black blood" taken away. More calm after. Took broth and gruel. Relapsed into violence. Drank water and vomited. Cupping repeated on 22d. Patient fainted. No other effect. 23d—No food, no sleep, strength diminished. "I resolved to try the effect of salivation; hoping that if I could succeed in exciting a powerful action in the absorbent system, it would divert a part of the vital energy from the muscles, and awaken the torpid power of the brain, stomach and bowels. Three drachms of strong mercurial ointment were accordingly rubbed in." 24th—Gums slightly affected. Grew calm and rational; took food, purging powders, given an injection. Clothed, removed to a clean bed "in the nurses' room."

In a few hours again violent: "broke every frangible article in the nurses' apartment; and again tore off her clothes." "Reconducted to the cell." Cathartics operated freely. Mercury renewed—gentle salivation—restored reason. 26th, removed into "the principal ward for women, and proper medicines and regimen were directed for the restoration of her health. "Occasional turns of anxiety and distress." "These were particularly troublesome about two o'clock in the afternoon, when there was increase in heat, and in the frequency of the pulse." Returned to family 7th of September.

Dr. Smith commented on the case as follows:

[She] attributed [her] conduct to witchcraft, or something of the kind, which made the wind in the stomach, that she used to complain of, to ascend to her head; and the said heat of her body was so intolerable that she could not endure the least covering. Her skin was never remarkably hot during her insanity; but after the return of her reason, her feet were affected with such a burning heat, that she could only be relieved by placing them in cold water; and she was troubled with irregular flushes, over her whole body, for several days. With respect to the disease of Mary Mathews, which I have called *mania,* it may perhaps be questionable whether it has been denominated so with propriety. It deserves to be remembered that the whole duration of her illness, as near as we can determine, was fourteen or fifteen days. Is it possible that this was its period, that it then ceased, from having completed its course, or that it was more easily inclined to stop at that time than at another? Is it possible that this is a variety of hysteria? of intermitting fever, which sometimes assumes the shape of mania, and to which quotidian exacerbation, after the insanity was removed, may be supposed to correspond? Or is it possible that the cause of Yellow Fever, whatever it may be, which, in different persons, affects different parts of the system, and appears under almost every form of disease, to whose operation foreigners seem peculiarly liable, and were so this year, could have excited the mania of this girl, whose period is that of many fevers, and whose cure, supposing it to have been effected by the salivation, is not hostile to this supposition?

The reason must determine which, or whether any of these conjectures deserve consideration.

It may have some significance that in his graduation thesis on "Chronic Mania," Alexander Anderson stated, in discussing treatment, that restraint should be avoided as long as possible, "lest the strait jackets, and chains and cells should induce a depression of spirits seldom surmounted." He also expressed doubts of the propriety of "unexpected plunging into cold water," or of "two to six hours in spring water or still colder," as well as the "refrigerant plan" of bleeding, purging, vomiting, streams of cold water on the head, blisters, pressure on the carotids which, he said, belonged more properly to the treatment of phrenitis. Quite likely Anderson reflected the views of his teachers and of the practices he had observed at the New York Hospital. That much tender consideration was given the patients of the hospital, including and even particularly the mentally ill, is revealed in the expressions of the governors in their minutes and in their communications to the legislature and the public, and in the spirit and character of their decisions, as well as in the reports of the physicians on the state of the hospital, and in the scanty glimpses obtainable of the treatment of individual patients.

What attention was given by the physicians to the mentally ill patients in the hospital cannot be fully ascertained. Dr. Hosack was perhaps more interested than the others. He alone reported the condition of the cells of the "maniacs" to the governors and recommended improvements. Notes of his lectures [10] made by a medical student show that he discussed

[10] Notes by Robert Hathaway on Lectures delivered at Rutgers College, 1829 and 1830.

"idiosyncracys" (principally phobias), hypochondriasis, sleep, the role of the passions (emotions) in the production and cure of physical ailments, phrenitis, and neuroses. His views of the effect of the emotions on bodily states were perhaps rather extreme. Grief, he considered, affected the abdominal viscera, produced obstruction of the liver and particularly injured the stomach, "that very sensible organ which with its numerous ganglions may be styled a second brain." Anger, he said, caused a certain excitement of the sanguineous system, producing hemorrhage from the liver, apoplexy, and epilepsy. A manuscript of Hosack, in the New York Academy of Medicine Library, is entitled "Observations on Mania." In this he stated that there was "in the whole range of medical science no subject more interesting or less satisfactory . . . a subject involving the most refined consideration both of medical and philosophical nature, and in this inquiry we feel the imperfection of both sciences in their utmost extent." He considered that "there is no reason to think that the disease is purely mental . . . some material disease of the brain [had been considered] as a universal cause." He referred to Pinel, Arnold, Crichton, Morgagni, Haslam, Chiaruggi, and other writers in mental disease; also to Locke, Hume, and Tooker, showing that he was a student of the subject. He used as illustrations cases that he had observed in the hospital. He leaned rather heavily on his authorities and expressed few opinions of his own. In treatment, he advised that the same principles should be followed as in the treatment of bodily diseases: "We act upon the sound parts to change the condition of those that are diseased." He described the "moral treatment of Pinel" as consisting in part of "employment of mind and body." There is also in the Academy of Medicine Library a manuscript of Hosack on "Occupation and Employment of Maniacs." His remarks therein do not indicate that they were based on actual experience and observation at the New York Hospital. In the same library there are notes by Hosack on Samuel Tuke's letter to Thomas Eddy in 1815, in which Tuke expressed his views on the importance of moral treatment; and notes on Tuke's "Practical Hints," which was another communication to Thomas Eddy when the governors were considering the question of an institution for moral treatment in the country. In a proposed classification of diseases, Hosack included those of the mind, employing the general term "Vesaniae," with Mania, Melancholia, Oneirodynia, and Amentia as varieties.

When the new department for the mentally ill was established in 1808, Hosack was one of the candidates considered for the position of Attending Physician. In 1819, after Dr. Handy resigned, Hosack was appointed to give "suitable medical assistance to the Lunatics, until a Physician is regularly appointed," and served for three months.[11]

In an interesting letter of March 6, 1796, to Alexander Anderson, then a student of his, Dr. Mitchill, another physician of the hospital, gave an account of his views on "Illusions of human Senses," which revealed considerable thought and interest in the subject. As this letter discloses views on mental illness held by a leading physician and adds a little to the scanty material relating to psychiatry in the New York Hospital at this early period, it seems valuable enough to present in full.

Dear Sir;

I regret that I cannot find for you a Copy of my Pamphlet published at Albany in 1789 on the *Illusions of human Senses.* I must therefore endeavour to give you an Abstract of it from my notes and from memory together with such ideas on the Subject as have occurred to me upon deeper Reflection, since that time.

The Principle which I endeavoured to establish was this; "That conditions of body occur, in which the Organs of Sense do, from *internal causes* and *without the aid of external agents,* take upon themselves a configuration or impression, similar to that which is usually induced by the action of material Objects & Occurrences from without."

1. This sometimes happens when the Person whose Sensations are thus perverted is *himself quite conscious of the deception,* and can then counteract in a good degree the influence of these false suggestions upon the mind, by the effects of will and the exercise of Judgment. Now and then this singuular state of one or more of the Senses comes on in a Person who is in other Respects well in Health; and in such cases the change wrought is generally feeble and fugitive. The Spectra left upon the Retina after looking at the Sun or any other bright or high-coloured body are of this sort; and the Case of our late Professor Nicoll, as he related it to me, was a very remarkable one, wherein the Ears as well as the Eyes were strangely affected while he was perfectly aware of the imposition. High-wrought Imagination and ardent Poetic fancy seem to belong to this Head.

2. Another memorable instance of such illusions is, when beside this affection of the Sensorial Organs *there is a belief wrought, at least for the time being, of the Reality of what appears.* The whole of the phenomena of *dreaming,* Incubus and of *delirium* are of this kind— In dreaming, the shapes and colours of things seen, the distinctness of notes and voices, and even in some instances the pleasureable and painful perceptions referable to the Sense of Feeling, oftentimes surpass any thing that can be Impressed upon the Eye, Ear or Touch, even by real Objects, in a State of Wakefulness. A belief of their *actual existence* is from the Senses so operated upon, impressed upon the mind; but this belief instantly vanishes on waking; and the whole Series of events that just before seemed with so much distinctness to be present, is confessed to be an Illusion.—

[11] *Minutes of the Governors,* Nov. 3, 1818, and Jan. 5, 1819.

In Nightmare and Delirium too, the person who roves, tho' firm in the persuasion for the present, that things are truly as he fancies them, acknowledges his Error and stands self convicted as soon as the fit is over. The false suggestions in these Ailments, are as in dreaming, founded in morbid conditions of the organs of Sense induced without the customary operation of external Bodies.

3. A third case is where the images presented to the Sensorium by morbid Sensation are not only *"not" present, but where they are wholly different from any thing which exists; and have consequently no prototype in Nature.* Wicked Persons & such as are highly superstitious and enthusiastic, whose minds are under deep concern; or are violently agitated, and whose organs of Sense are irritable, are very often the Subjects of this illusion. Hence Devils in all imaginable forms, Angels in every possible variety of Shape, Spectres, ghosts and apparitions, are frequently seen by persons suffering this form of Dissease, and Visions, Revelations and extraordinary Communications made to them. They see invisible things; they hear Sounds not audible. The irritable condition of the Eyes suggests to them *inward light* beaming with celestial influence upon them, and giving a foretaste of Heaven; or impresses them with the notion of *fire* and *flames* threatening them with infernal torture and anticipating the pains of Hell. There is nothing hideous, deformed or monstrous which may not thus be presented to the Mind originating in *distempered Sense,* and giving rise to *fallacious Experience.*

4. There is yet another example of morbid Sensation wherein *the impressions made upon the Senses from "inward Causes" are stronger than those occasioned by external occurrences.* And this condition of the organs is so permanent & obstinate that it continues during the time of wakefulness and is not to be dispelled by any effort of the will. When this happens in a single point or in a few respects, it constitutes *partial Insanity.* When false perceptions ensue on many objects they constitute *general or total Mania.*— The *fury* of such Madness will depend upon the avidity or force of the distempered sensation.— Its *duration* will be proportionate to the permanent or indelible nature of the impression.— And here there is generally the strongest Conviction of the truth of the false Perception. From this erroneous principle proceed an endless variety of odd deductions and applications, flowing however in many instances, logically enough from the premises.

I consider the State of Body to which Mania belongs as a *morbid Sensation,* wherein without correspondent Exerting *powers from without,* a condition of some or other of the Organs of Sense is induced *from inward causes* similar to what usually happens from the *opperation of external agents* and which probably would be brought on by these.—Let the causes of this be what they may whether they be imagined to be in *the Brain,* in the *Arterial System,* or in the *Organs of Sense,* such is the Law of the Animal Economy that *false Sensations* suggest *unreal perceptions,* and these give rise to *groundless Notions;* and thus a belief, persuasion or conviction is produced, and *upon the evidence of the Senses too,* of the Existence of Non-entities & all manner of unreal representations.—

As to the *Seat* of Madness, I have strong doubts of its being in the Brain.

The disorder of the thinking powers is *secondary* and I believe always *subsequent to vitiated Sensations.* The Organs of Sense then, or *Sentient Extremities of the Nerves,* which have been considered by Darwin with great appearance of Truth, to be the Seats of Thought, are I apprehend, *particularly and primarily diseased in Madness.* Dissections of the Brain in Maniacs have thrown little or no light upon this Malady; and the Brain has been found excessively deranged in its Structure by Disseases, as Distention, Suppuration Concussion &c in other Ailments, without producing any corresponding Disorder of Mind; and I consider it vain and fruitless to search the Brain for the cause of Mania. *As it is grounded in false Sensation, the Organs of Sense must be examined with a view to detect the mischief there.* The principal internal Stimulus acting upon the Sentient Extremities of the Nerves is *the Blood;* and if an irregular distribution of blood, its Circulation with too great or too little force, in Quantity too large or too small, &c. are capable of inducing Disorders or morbid changes in the Organs of Sense, then a large share of Maniacal Affections is inherent in the *Sanguiferous System.*

I am, dear Sir, with much esteem & regard yours

SAM. L. MITCHILL.[12]

Anderson relates in his diary that he discussed his thesis on Chronic Mania with Dr. Mitchill several times, and on one occasion, he was "given such a view of the metaphysical ideas which such a Discussion will involve as almost intimidated me from undertaking the subject." [13] He mentions that he had similar talks with Dr. Bard and Dr. Hosack. Among the lectures attended by Anderson as a student, "The Passions" and "The Power of Habit" by Dr. William Hammersley are the only ones that indicate that mental diseases may have had a place in the course. Significant of the persistence of discarded conceptions were, perhaps, the lectures delivered to the students on "The Moon," "The Stars" and other astronomical subjects. Anderson was, himself, emotionally susceptible to the idea of the influence of the moon, as he noted that "it is somewhat singular that my asthmatic complaint is contemporary with her [mother's] hysteric affections and both occur at the changes of the moon," though he added that "this may be call'd old womanish—but such is the fact, and such occasions I find no relief from the use of stimulants." [14] Lectures were also given on the medical theories widely held in the eighteenth century (see Chapter I). Anderson's attendance at clinical lectures at the hospital were frequently noted in the diary, though the forms of illness presented were omitted. The title ("Chronic Mania") of his graduation thesis is evidence that instruction in mental

[12] Courtesy of the New York Historical Society.
[13] Anderson's diary, Feb. 17, 1796.
[14] *Ibid.*, June 16, 1798.

illness was included in the medical course. As a public defense of the thesis, in the presence of an audience which included the governor of the state, was part of the examination, a presentation that would be creditable both to examiners and student would naturally be anticipated.

The comparatively few mentally ill persons who were treated at the New York Hospital during the sixteen years under consideration, were a small proportion of the total of such persons in the city and state who were in need of hospital treatment. Many still languished in cells, cages, and other secure receptacles in almshouses, lockups, and in homes. Several mentally ill patients seen at their homes and in the streets were mentioned in Anderson's diary, some of them quite seriously ill. In one instance he took his violin with him on a visit to a patient, but the playing seemed to be without effect. One young man traveled to Philadelphia with Anderson, and on the trip was so overactive and eccentric as to occasion much comment. At times this patient was considered to be a menace to his family. Another lad who was in "a state of stupidity" at home, suddenly regained his reason when his father was temporarily ill, and became an attentive nurse, day and night. A few weeks later it was noted that as soon as the father recovered the son relapsed into his previous condition. Suicides in the community were also mentioned in the diary. Many cases of mental illness must have received attention from the private medical practitioners.

There were few publications on any medical subjects. The only medical periodical published in New York was *The Medical Repository,* and it was the first in America. Reference to a few of the communications in the numbers issued during the period under consideration may, perhaps, in some measure reveal the prevailing views and practice relating to the mentally ill. An abstract of Dr. Smith's report of a case of mania treated with mercury has already been presented. All of the communications were reports of cases. One entitled "The Efficacy of Cold in Madness" [15] referred especially to the "good effects of cold in apoplexia mentalis or delirium sine febre," which was perhaps another term for acute mania. It was reported that five cases had been successfully treated, two of which had been "abandoned by two eminent physicians." The method consisted merely of intensive application of cold water to the head until the patient shivered, at which point the treatment was discontinued for an hour and then resumed. One advantage in this treatment was, at least, that the patient escaped the more drastic measures

[15] *Medical Repository,* IV (1801), 209.

usually employed. The cure of "madness" by the administration of digitalis was reported in one communication,[16] and the use and action of this drug were discussed in a number of articles in this journal.

"A Case of Lunacy with a new Argument in favour of the Vitality of the Blood" was reported by a "Student of Medicine in Virginia." [17] The argument is not clearly presented, but the case illustrated the hard lot of the mentally ill at this time. The patient was a man of thirty-five. probably an epileptic, who had no home and suffered much privation. He was easily affected by alcohol, and when he ate much or drank ardent spirits in excess he had convulsions. He gradually "lost his ordinary understanding," and there was increasing "idiocy." He died in the night on a public road. An autopsy revealed "gastro-intestinal disease with stricture of the duodenum and hypertrophy of the stomach walls." The brain was not examined.

Another communication related that a patient, who was under the care of an attendant, swallowed a full-size teaspoon, while the attendant was gone, at the patient's request, to bring water from the opposite side of the room. Eighteen days later the spoon was located by palpation in the ilium and was removed by operation. The wound healed by first intention, and two months later the patient was well enough to be removed to Nantucket for convalescence.[18]

Still another case was that of a man of twenty-five who, when emotionally excited, was subject to "violent spasmodic affections, resembling painful epilepsy, alternating with insanity of a very singular kind." In the attack described, the patient during a heated argument became "more and more incoherent" and was finally seized with convulsions. "As soon as the muscular exertions ceased, his countenance assumed the lineament of deepest sorrow, his voice changed to most solemn tragedy; no actor ever surpassed him. Family and friends were undertaker, sexton, pall-bearers and mourners at the funeral of lost relatives." He attended to nothing said to him. "His eyes were open, but his sense was shut." This patient was relieved by extremely strong pressure on his abdomen and the case was designated "Convulsions alternating with temporary Insanity." [19]

Not infrequently the cases reported as tetanus, hydrophobia, and other forms of illness were apparently psycho-neurotic. A case in point was reported as "A Case of Tetanus Cured by the Cold Bath." [20] The patient was a man of thirty who was

[16] *Ibid.*, p. 313.
[17] *Ibid.*, II, 2d Hexade (1805), 135.
[18] *Ibid.*, IV, 2d Hexade (1807), 369.
[19] *Ibid.*, V, 2d Hexade (1808), 146.
[20] *Ibid.*, IV (1801), 76.

suddenly seized, while in bed, with spasms of his lower extremities, which shortly after affected his whole system, but particularly his stomach, which was drawn in a hard lump, and protruded to a considerable distance. His pains were excrutiating. He had violent vomiting and purging, which came on an hour after the seizure and continued about two hours. At one time he had emprosthotonos, at another opisthotonos,[21] to the greatest degree, and sometimes complete tetanus. The muscles of his face were drawn in every direction and deglutition was entirely impeded.

He was bled, placed in a warm bath and "all the remedies laid down by medical writers" were administered. No relief resulted, and "the cold sweat of death appeared to be upon him, his tongue had refused its office, his eyes sunk, having a glassy appearance and his exit was every moment expected." It then occurred to the physician that a cold bath might have a good effect, and he was "carried in a blanket to a forge dam that was near at hand, and plunged in. He was then insensible. His spasms immediately abated and, in twenty minutes, totally ceased." He remained feeble for a few days, after which he rapidly recovered and remained well. "This," said the report, "was a complete tetanus, and, I think, a tetanus from wounds &c would yield to the same mode of treatment."

A girl of fifteen who claimed to have been bitten by a spider was reported as "A Case of very Singular Nervous Affections supposed to have been occasioned by the Bite of a Tarantula." [22] (This was in Rhode Island.) The symptoms were that the same afternoon in which she was bitten she felt the hand and arm of the side bitten twitch several times. That night she had a pain in this arm and hand, which shifted into her stomach and increased till the morning of the third day, when "she went into fits." These fits were reported as resembling hysteria but more nearly "hysteric paroxysms combined with St. Vitus' Dance." It was noticed that in her fits she moved her hands and fingers as though she was keeping time to music. When music was introduced she beat her hands and fingers upon her breast in imitation of dancing so hard that the attendants felt it necessary to interpose their hands to protect her. She was best pleased when her father's hand was placed for this purpose, but later, when she had improved somewhat, this partiality changed to extreme aversion. Music now became the remedy, and was the only thing that moderated the spasms. It was noticed that she was able to distinguish colors and objects while her eyes were closed and she was

21 Emprosthotonos: the body bent forward. Opisthotonos: the body bent backward.
22 *Medical Repository,* I, 2d Hexade (1804), Art. I.

"partly in a fit." She could detect her father's presence even when the room was dark. People flocked to see her and her "ability to distinguish colors &c was vulgarly attributed by some to witchcraft." The physician was evidently impressed by these manifestations and questioned whether "holding a substance in one's hand made a slight alteration in its surface which her extreme sensibility could discover, and having before held that hand, could she perceive the similarity? I was led so to conclude, or leave the phenomena unaccounted for." As the case progressed, the patient began to make dancing movements with her feet while still in bed. When she "lay in a motionless state upon the bed, every nerve and muscle being contracted" music of a violin close to her ear aroused her. This patient developed many other symptoms. After she left her bed, she would dance when music was played until she was exhausted, "jumping a considerable distance from the floor." The physician considered that "her dancing was nothing more nor less than a modification of those spasms, one terminating in the other, and vice versa." In some of her paroxysms she "threw up" pins and needles which, the physician considered, she had unwittingly put in her mouth "in the agony attending her fits." Ten months after the supposed bite by a spider, the spot became painful, red, and "mortified." The discharge from it was "as green and almost as thick as inspissated beef gall." The fits abated when the discharge began, and four months later there had been no return. The case was considered by the physician to be "a real tarantismus," and in support of his opinion he stated that "the spider of Italy [tarantula] produces a disorder which, as their physicians say, is cured by music." "A case so replete with the wonderful," he adds, "is not, perhaps, easily to be found in the annals of medicine. If my theory be right, may we not expect much benefit from music in hysteria?"

A monograph entitled "Observations on the Influence of the Moon &c" was reviewed in the *Repository* in 1801,[23] the writer of which, the reviewer stated, was a firm believer in lunar influences. The following is a quotation from the monograph:

> On the mind it [full moon] produces the most powerful effects; as an equanimity of temper, a disposition to cheerfulness, and an aversion to anger in people of irascible dispositions. Perhaps there may be discovered in the atmosphere a mixture of airs, at the periods, favorable to the intellectual faculties. In this state of mind, physicians visit their patients and relations; their friends labouring under contagious diseases, and are not so liable to receive infection.

[23] *Ibid.*, IV (1801), 285.

In Philadelphia at this time Dr. Benjamin Rush was actively engaged in the study and treatment of the mentally ill, and the medical students who received instruction from him and attended his lectures and demonstrations at the Pennsylvania Hospital, entered into practice with some knowledge of the nature and problems of mental disease. It was not until 1812, however, that Dr. Rush's treatise entitled *Medical Inquiries and Observations upon the Diseases of the Mind* was published, and many years elapsed before another work of similarly comprehensive character was published in America. Dr. Hosack was, apparently, the only physician of the New York Hospital at this period whose interest in the subject might, if greater opportunity had been presented to him, have resulted in contributions that would have revealed more fully than is now possible the character of the cases and the methods of study and practice then current in the hospital.

VI

A NEW DEPARTMENT AND ITS "MEDICAL ASYLUM," 1808

THE word "asylum" means simply a place of refuge in which one may feel safe from some imminent harm. When institutions for the mentally ill were first established, the title "Asylum" was considered peculiarly appropriate because it was generally assumed that the primary object was to provide a refuge or asylum for sorely afflicted persons, who were at that time treated in the community with neglect, cruelty, and abhorrence. In conformity with custom, therefore, the new building at the New York Hospital, provision for which was mentioned in the preceding chapter, was given the official title of "Lunatic Asylum." Usually, it was called simply "The Asylum," and sometimes the whole institution was referred to as "The New York Hospital and Lunatic Asylum." The term "asylum," however, fails to convey the conception of a medical institution and of active curative measures of treatment. Many persons, even at the present time, associate with the term "asylum for the insane" only gross and hopelessly incurable forms of mental disorder, and, notwithstanding the change of the title of the institutions from "asylum" to "hospital," the persistence of this conception has been and still is a serious obstacle to adequate hospital and medical treatment of the mentally ill. The governors of the Society of the New York Hospital, feeling perhaps some intimation of the inadequacy of the title, and in order to indicate that they considered the asylum to be as truly medical as any other part of the hospital, referred to it in their annual report for 1808 as "a medical asylum." They had learned from their own observation and experience that the mentally ill were sick persons who were in need of active hospital treatment, and were in many instances curable. As early as 1794 they had observed that "several of that description have been cured and others much relieved." [1] Their further experience seemed to them to confirm this observation, as is explicitly stated or implied in the minutes of their meetings, in their reports and appeals to the legislature, in their public announcements, and in the policies and plans pursued by them. Their views were illustrated in their response to an order of the Secretary of the Treasury of the United States that "no Seamen afflicted with Mania, or any other kind of incurable disorders, be allowed the benefit of the Hospital for any period however short." [2]

[1] New York Hospital, *Minutes of the Governors,* June 6, 1794. [2] *Ibid.,* May, 1821.

The governors had, soon after the hospital was opened, made an agreement with the Government to furnish hospital treatment to sick seamen at a stipulated rate, to be paid from a sickness insurance fund which was maintained by the collection of twenty cents a month from the wages of all seamen in the merchant marine. An arbitrary limit was placed upon the number of seamen who could at any time be in the hospital, and a time limit of payment for four months was set, "be his situation, at the time, what it may." [8] Foreigners employed on American ships, and even native seamen if they had not been on more than one or two deep sea voyages, were, notwithstanding their payment to the fund, declared to be ineligible for support in the hospital. Venereal cases were also refused support, and finally cases of mania. The governors, who knew that adequate service could not be furnished if these arbitrary procedures were complied with, felt obliged to admit seamen as they did other patients, without regard to any particular number, form of illness, or duration necessary for their cure. They listed the "super-numerary" seamen separately, and they sent bills regularly to the government and insisted upon payment. A committee was appointed to study the situation and report. This committee learned from the Secretary of the Treasury that the arbitrary time limit was because, owing to certain "impositions," the fund had become inadequate. It seemed to the committee that it was remarkable that, while the Congress had evidently contemplated that the sick sailor should, if curable, be treated until he was cured, the Treasury Department were of the opinion that "under a diminished or augmented fund" treatment for "two or six months would as well answer the intention of the Law." It seemed to them that, because of "impositions," the government considered it proper "to retaliate, by imposition on the poor sick Sailor, and refuse him admission, because their own agents have defrauded them or neglected their duty." Thus, they reported, "now another disease, which more than any other excites our Sympathy and has stronger claims upon our Charity, must also be totally excluded, because the Secretary chooses to say that *Mania* is incurable." Several cases illustrating the jeopardy to recovery and even to life that would be entailed by compliance with the arbitrary orders of the Treasury Department, were described in the report, and characterized by the committee as "shocking to humanity, and the principle that dictates them an outrage upon justice and common sense." This experiment in compulsory sickness insurance, more than a century ago, not only reveals the humane principles and standards

[8] *Ibid.*, Nov. 6, 1821.

observed in the administration of the New York Hospital, but it may now serve as a warning of what may be expected if any similar long distance, bureaucratic system of management of the treatment of the sick is again undertaken.[4]

In establishing a special service for the mentally ill, the governors, animated by the idea of curability, endeavored to provide facilities for the best form of active treatment of which they had knowledge. They were not physicians, and there was apparently no physician available to them who was sufficiently versed in mental illness and its hospital treatment to provide them with medical guidance and leadership. They were obliged, therefore, in planning the new building and its organization, to follow prevailing standards and to depend upon their own judgment and on the experience they had obtained during the sixteen years in which the mentally ill had been treated in the general medical service. The building, now ready for the reception of patients, had, under the direction of a committee consisting of Thomas Franklin, Gilbert Aspinwall, John R. Murray, William Johnson, and Samuel Mansfield, been planned and constructed with careful attention to the purpose it was designed to serve. An architect, whose name was unfortunately not recorded, was employed, and as much information as possible was obtained in regard to other institutions. For this purpose a subcommittee visited the hospital in Philadelphia, at which mentally ill patients had been treated for more than half a century. The following description of the new building is taken from an account of the New York Hospital which was prepared by William Johnson, a member of the building committee; it was published by the governors in 1811.

The building denominated *the Lunatic Asylum,* is also of grey stone. It is situated on the southerly side of the ground, at a short distance from the principal building, and corresponding with it, in its exterior appearance and style of architecture. Being separate from the other house, the sick are not incommoded by the lunatics, who have separate yards inclosed, one for males, and the other for females, where such as can be trusted at large, are permitted to walk in the open air.

This building, on account of the declivity of the ground, has a sub-basement, besides a basement and two principal stories. Its length is 90 feet; it is 40 feet deep in the centre, and 65 feet at the wings, which project 12½ feet on each side. The sub-basement contains 10 rooms, 11 feet long and 8½ feet wide and 9 feet high; 3 rooms, 16½ feet long and 11½ feet

[4] *Minutes of the Governors,* Nov. 6, 1821.

From 1806 to 1819 the number of "supernumerary" seamen treated was 1649, none of whom had been paid for. The governors eventually memorialized Congress. (*An Account of the New-York Hospital,* New York, 1820.)

wide, and a kitchen, 23½ feet long and 16½ feet wide. There is a hall running through the centre, from one end to the other, into which the doors of the rooms or cells open, opposite to the windows. This hall is paved with marble, and in it are fixed seven circular iron stoves, communicating with iron pipes fixed in brick flues, reaching to the top of the building; each flue passes through the corners of the rooms, so as, by means of iron doors and valves, to communicate heat to two rooms, in each story. All the rooms or cells, except the four largest, and those in the upper story, are arched with brick, and the walls are also brick, whitewashed; so that there is no wood, and the floors being filled in with brick, the building is completely fire-proof; and the patients, while they have sufficient heat, in the winter season, cannot possibly set fire to any part of the building, or injure themselves. The basement story contains the same number of rooms, and of the same size with those in the sub-basement. In each of the two principal stories, are also 10 rooms, 11 feet long and 8½ feet wide; two rooms, 17 feet long and 11½ feet wide, and two rooms, 24 feet long and 17 feet wide, which open into a hall 11 feet wide. The height of the principal story is 14½, and of the upper story, 12½ feet.

There is a yard inclosed, 75 feet in length and 65 feet in breadth, and another between the house and the street-wall, on the southerly side, about 200 feet long and 50 broad, in which the patients take the air, and amuse themselves.

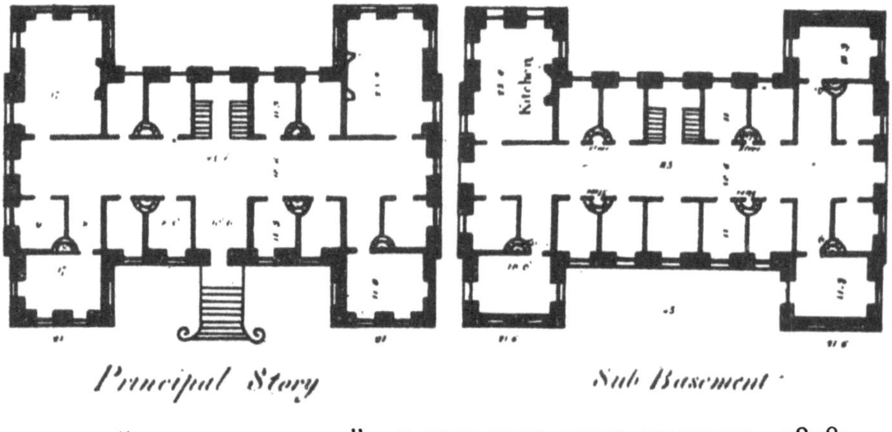

THE "MEDICAL ASYLUM" OF THE NEW YORK HOSPITAL, 1808: FLOOR PLANS

The height of the building, from the ground, in front, is about 46 feet. It contains 60 rooms of different dimensions, which will contain about eighty patients. The apartments are adapted for persons of every condition, the rich and the poor, equally subject to this worst of human miseries, who may be here accommodated according to their various circumstances in life.

This description and the accompanying illustrations show that, notwithstanding the lack of features and facilities that are now considered essential, the building was far in advance of any previous provision for the mentally ill in New York, and perhaps in America. The governors had already learned that classification of the patients was essential and that separate provision for outdoor activities should be made. The basement rooms with walls and ceilings of brick were fireproof, secure, and not easily damaged, though they must have been rather cheerless. Those in the upper stories were, however, of different character. The rooms were commodious and had ample windows. The heating arrangements, though superior to those in the rest of the hospital, were crude though ingenious. Significantly, the erroneous belief that the mentally ill were insensitive to cold and hardship no longer determined the conditions of their treatment. The toilet facilities were imperfect, as circulating water and plumbing had not yet been introduced into the hospital. There was a special kitchen, but the lack of designated space for dining rooms, service and treatment rooms, and for other facilities illustrates the gap between present conditions and those of that period. The building was designed to accommodate 80 patients. It was frequently overcrowded and, in March, 1815, the governors decided that 75 were as many as could be properly accommodated, and thereafter that number was seldom exceeded. The cost of the building was $53,600.

A contemporary medical evaluation of this "new hospital for the relief of insane persons" may be gathered from the following, which appeared in the *Medical Repository:*[5]

In the course of our work, frequent and respectful mention has been made of that excellent and useful institution, the New-York Hospital. . . .

The governors of the Hospital have . . . been enabled to execute a work which had been long in meditation. This is a house expressly for the reception and accommodation of maniacs. . . . The best information was sought, and the most instructive precedents examined. And in the summer of 1806 the foundation of the new hospital for the relief of insane persons was laid. It has since been carried on with a steady hand, under the direction of Thomas Franklin, Gilbert Aspinwall, John R. Murray, William Johnson and Samuel Mansfield, Esqrs., the committee for superintending the building. It is now nearly finished and will soon be opened for the reception of patients.

Persons of all conditions whether affluent or indigent, may be accommodated, according to their respective situations in life. The cells are made strong, and the confinement rigorous, in proportion to the violence of men-

[5] V, 2d Hexade (1808), 416–418.

tal derangement, and the corresponding bodily disorder. Care is taken also to sever the servants of the house who attend the kitchen and laundry from all communication with the patients. None are to be admitted to them but the needful and proper attendants. It is intended to place the maniacs who are received into this asylum under the care of a special physician. It will be expected of him that he should study the various forms of insanity with the strictest attention: and by a steady perseverance in that pursuit, it may be reasonably hoped he will acquire more than usual knowledge of mental diseases. Where consultations shall be necessary, the consulting physicians of the New-York Hospital will also be medical counsellors of the Lunatic Asylum. On the 6th of June, 1808, ARCHIBALD BRUCE, M.D. was appointed the physician.

This building was erected at an expense of at least fifty thousand dollars. Its architecture is well suited to the intended purpose, both as to design and execution. Its object is to relieve mankind from one of the heaviest afflictions of life. And it may be affirmed with truth, that the Lunatic Asylum of New York does honour to the city in which it stands, and the country to which it belongs. The eye is not offended in this institution with the sight of padlocks and bolts, nor the ear by the rattling of fetters and chains. And it is believed that the discipline can be established among the maniacs without the use of the whip.

The gratification of the governors for this addition to their resources was expressed in their annual report to the legislature for the year 1808:

The completion of this usefull and necessary edifice affords an acquisition to the Institution, which does honour to the State, in providing a medical Asylum for this most unfortunate portion of the human race, and the Governors trust that they have not only fulfilled their engagements with the Legislature, and gratified the wishes and expectations of the public, but that the House has been constructed on such a plan and the work executed in such a manner, as reflects credit on the Institution.

In anticipation of the organization of the service, a committee consisting of Gilbert Aspinwall, Thomas Eddy, John R. Murray, Thomas Franklin, and William Johnson, were appointed in February, 1808, to prepare a system of rules and regulations for the government of the "Asylum for Maniacs." This committee evidently found the task somewhat disconcerting, and in May they reported that they had sought diligently for some result from the experience of others upon which they might form rules for their government, and had decided that, until they could be assisted by some months' experience, they would be incompetent, and recommended that another committee be appointed. They nevertheless made some suggestions, one of which was especially significant and important. For the organization of the service they reported that from the particular nature of this Institution your Committee are of the opinion, (and that opinion has been formed upon mature reflection) that one Physician only, be appointed to the Asylum, during the pleasure of the Governors. That he shall be required to visit the Asylum every day, and keep a register of patients, and until Rules are formed, he is to conform to such regulations as the Committee shall direct.[6]

This proposal apparently originated in the minds of the committee as a result of the service for the mentally ill that had thus far been engaged in by the hospital. It was not in accordance with the views of the physicians of the hospital, who in August, 1817, recommended that the medical service of the Asylum be "conducted on the same principles" as the other services.[7] The committee also recommended that an "overseer" be appointed to have charge of the Asylum, with a woman, preferably his wife, as assistant.

The committee were continued and were authorized to carry their recommendations into effect. A month later they were reappointed and designated the "Asylum Committee," with instructions to report monthly to the board. At the same meeting, Dr. Archibald Bruce was appointed Physician to the Asylum. Other candidates were Dr. William Handy, who nine years later succeeded Dr. Bruce, and Dr. David Hosack. The committee were independent of the Visiting Committee (the Executive Committee of the Board) and of all other committees. They were responsible for the admission of patients to the asylum and for the rates charged. They employed and discharged all persons engaged in the service, and were responsible for the manner in which it was conducted and for all transactions. It was arranged that supplies would be furnished by the superintendent and apothecary of the hospital. This marked the establishment of the present department of psychiatry of the New York Hospital, and the form of organization on the foundation thus laid has stood the test of time and experience; its essentials have ever since been adhered to and developed in the service for the mentally ill of the hospital.

To what extent the policies and plans pursued by the governors in this service were influenced or guided by any of the physicians of the hospital is not disclosed in the records. Occasionally, it is recorded that the advice of the asylum physician was requested in regard to a particular matter. Nevertheless, what is found in the records indicates that, for many years, the policies and plans of development and administration

[6] *Minutes of the Governors,* May 3, 1808.

[7] *Ibid.,* Aug. 5, 1817, p. 307. (Report of committee to confer with the physicians and surgeons.)

were originated and executed by the governors, and that this continued for years until, under the direction of full-time resident physicians, the administration gradually became more and more fully medical.

Little ceremony attended the opening of the asylum for the reception of patients. There were no formal exercises, and no such announcement to the public as appeared in 1803 when the new story was added. On July 14, 1808, the Asylum Committee held their first meeting, and adopted the following simple resolution:

It appearing that the present accommodations of the Lunatics in the Hospital are extremely inconvenient & the Asylum being thought in a sufficient state of preparation to receive them, Resolved that the superintendent be directed to remove the Lunatics from the Hospital to the Asylum; that before their removal they be thoroughly cleansed, their hair cut, and heads washed, and furnished new Clothes, and new beds and bedsteads, as soon as may be.[8]

On the following day, nineteen patients were transferred from two wards of the hospital, and one other was admitted from the almshouse.[9] On July 17 it was noted that three applications "on account of the unprepared state of the House have been put off for a few days." At the September meeting of the Board, the committee reported that "the General State of the patients have [*sic*] been much improved since their admission into the Asylum."

The population of the City of New York was, in 1808, approximately 80,000, and that of the state about 900,000. For this large population, the little asylum of 80 beds was the only place where anything approaching hospital treatment could be obtained for the mentally ill, and the New York Hospital was the only hospital of any kind in the state.[10] Nor was any separate provision for the mentally ill undertaken by the city until 1839, when the New York City Lunatic Asylum was established; nor by the state until 1843, when the first state asylum was opened at

8 Asylum Committee Minutes, the first entry.

9 In other accounts of the New York Hospital, it is stated that when the Lunatic Asylum was opened on July 15, 1808, 19 patients were transferred and 48 others were admitted, making a total of 67. This mistake was probably first made by misreading the governors' annual report for 1808, in which it is stated that 19 patients were transferred on July 15, and that "since then" 48 others had been admitted—meaning clearly that 67 was the total number admitted during that year. The actual facts are that the records contain the names of 22 patients who were transferred to the asylum from Wards 1 and 2 of the Hospital on July 15, of one other admitted from the almshouse on the same day, and of 44 others who were admitted by the close of the year, making the total of 67 as in the annual report.

10 Although provision of a sort was made for the dependent sick in the Almshouse, the first specially designed general hospital buildings at Bellevue were not erected until 1816, and it was not until 1825 that an organized hospital service was established. R. J. Carlisle, *Account of Bellevue Hospital* (New York, 1893).

Utica. In the meantime, and for many years, hundreds of mentally ill persons were confined, with practically no consideration for their proper treatment, in prisons, in strong rooms in almshouses, or in their homes, while others wandered as vagrants, sometimes perishing from starvation and exposure. Is it surprising that not even yet has public and private provision caught up with the long-neglected need for the proper study, treatment, and prevention of mental illness?

The only law relating to mental illness at the time the Asylum was established, was Chapter 31 of the Laws of New York of 1788:

> Whereas, There are sometimes persons who by lunacy or otherwise, are furiously mad, or are so far disordered in their senses that they may be dangerous to be permitted to go abroad; therefore,
>
> Be it enacted That it shall and may be lawful for any two or more justices of the peace to cause such person to be apprehended and kept safely locked up in some secure place, and, if such justices shall find it necessary, to be there chained.

This law, it may be noted, contains not the slightest sign of recognition of the medical needs of a mentally ill person. In March, 1809, however, the legislature, at the suggestion of the governors of the hospital,[11] passed an act which authorized

> the Overseers of the Poor of any city or town, by and with the consent of the Common Council of such city, or of two justices of the peace of the county in which such town shall be, whenever any poor person legally settled in such city or town (and maintained at the public charge), and who was, or shall become, lunatic or insane, to contract with the governors of the New York Hospital for the maintenance and care of such lunatic, on such terms as they may deem meet; and transport such lunatics to the Hospital, and the sums agreed on are to be paid to the Hospital by the overseers of such city or town.[12]

This law marked the first movement of the state towards making provision for the hospital treatment of the mentally ill, the culmination of which is the present (1944) great state system of twenty hospitals for civilians, two for criminals, and nine schools for the feeble-minded and epileptic.

The governors had already on July 18, 1808, adopted the following:

> Resolved that no patient be admitted into the Asylum only as pay patients, and that untill the first day of May next, when Maniacs who are paupers supported by the Towns are offered from the several Towns in the State, they shall be received, the Overseers of the poor for the Town to which they

11 New York Hospital, Annual Report for 1808.

12 New York State, Laws of 1809, Chapter 90.

belong—*Paying* or Securing payment for the same at not less than *Two Dollars* per week which shall include boarding and cloathing.

This rate was the same as that charged for pauper patients from New York City, and was said scarcely to cover the cost. With reference to support, the patients in the asylum, as well as those in the hospital, were classified as "Paupers," "Pays," and "Seamen." There was also the list of "Supernumerary Seamen," and, pursuant to a law passed in April, 1818, which authorized the inspectors of the State Prison to transfer insane prisoners "to the Lunatic Hospital at New York, the directors of which are required to receive such persons, and to confine them according to the rules of that Institution," two such prisoners were admitted. The reference to "moral treatment" in the medical certificate relating to these cases is not without significance:

The Board of Surgeons and Physicians are of opinion, that Jerome S. is a case of confirmed Insanity, and that Mary R. is also Insane, but that she would probably be restored to her reason by morral treatment in some Asylum.[13]

The proportion of patients from other places than New York City was exceedingly small, only 35 during the thirteen years of operation of the Asylum at the New York Hospital, 12 of whom were from Albany.[14] Apparently the town and county officials found that maintenance in the almshouses and prisons was less expensive.

Residents of New York were admitted as pay patients for as little as three dollars a week; those from other states were charged not less than five dollars a week. The maximum rate received from any patient during the period was thirteen dollars a week, and few paid more than the minimum. Evidently, the policy, still pursued, of considering the economic situation of the patient with reference to his treatment and the needs of his family was inaugurated at this early period. Typical examples of the action of the board are the following:

September 27, 1808. Mary A.—in consequence of her Husband Philip A. having a large family and in reduced circumstances have concluded to admit her at $2 per week.

October 24, 1815. It being represented that Gad D. is not in a situation to pay three dollars a week for the board of his Son. The Superintendent is therefore directed to reduce the price to Two Dollars per week from the time of the last payment.[15]

[13] *Minutes of the Governors,* June 2, 1818.

[14] Admission Book, Westchester Division.

[15] *Minutes of the Asylum Committee.*

Promissory notes were frequently accepted in lieu of immediate payment, in one instance at least from the patient. Rates of those admitted as private patients were sometimes reduced by the committee to a point below reimbursement. In the case of those who were entirely dependent when admitted, charges were rendered to the poor law authorities of their place of residence. Colored patients were admitted; some who were slaves were paid for by the owners at the rate of five dollars per week.

Probably because of the peculiar difficulties attending the control and treatment of mentally ill persons at home, the proportion of patients of the more opulent and cultured class was apparently larger in the asylum than in the hospital. Among those admitted were physicians, lawyers, clergymen, teachers, students, chemists, merchants, bankers, mill owners, and planters from Georgia, as well as some who were designated "lady" and "gentleman." As there were 60 rooms in the building, of which 45 were "single rooms," the facilities for classification were apparently ample. The relative income from "pays" was larger in the asylum than in the hospital. The income from this source was, in 1820, in the asylum, $2,664.17; in the hospital, with far more patients, it was $497.91.[16]

Averse to the admission of "idiots," the governors ruled in 1810 that they were "improper objects for the House" and that none would be admitted unless dangerous to society. In April, 1816, they recorded that they considered it necessary "to have all Idiot Patients removed, and particularly such as belong to the city, and under the charge of the Almshouse—as the new accommodations at Bellvieu [*sic*] can now accommodate such." [17]

16 *Minutes of the Governors*, Feb. 1821.

17 *Minutes of the Asylum Committee*, April 4, 1816. This was when the first "Bellevue Hospital" was erected.

VII

GENERAL ADMINISTRATION OF THE FIRST ASYLUM

PENDING the "some months' experience" which the committee felt to be necessary to render them competent to prepare a set of rules and regulations for the government of the asylum, various general orders were issued relating to some immediate need or situation. It is noteworthy that the first of these orders, which was issued three days after the service was established, was directed to the protection of the patients from prejudicial experiences. The public have always been curious concerning the behavior occasioned by mental disorder, and the governors were no doubt aware that in some places in Europe and also in America a visit to the "Lunatic Asylum" was considered a means of entertainment, and an admission fee was sometimes charged.[1] For the purpose of regulating visiting, therefore, on July 18, 1808, they ordered that no person was to be admitted as a visitor except by permission of a governor, physician, or surgeon, or when accompanied by the superintendent, and visiting hours were established. They also ordered that "in future, patients of this house shall not be permitted to go into the other house to remove dead bodies—or anything pertaining to this business." The clerk was instructed to present a list of the patients to the committee at each meeting and the physician was requested to report on the condition of the patients, particularly any who were no longer entitled to the benefits of the institution. It was also ordered that no patient should be admitted without a written order of one of the committee.

The detention of patients against their will must, at this time, have given the governors some concern. There was no statutory provision to give them the necessary authority. The law of 1788 provided that a mentally ill person might be "kept safely locked up in some secure place," [2] and the law of 1809 authorized overseers of the poor to contract with the governors of the New York Hospital for the care and maintenance of mentally ill paupers. It may have been considered that these provisions and the terms on which appropriations of funds for the Society were made by the legislature, "particularly to provide suitable apartments for maniacs," and other similar specifications, carried with

[1] At the Pennsylvania Hospital the fee was, in 1822, increased from 12½¢ to 25¢. Thomas G. Morton, *History of Pennsylvania Hospital* (Philadelphia, 1895), p. 153.

[2] See p. 73.

them adequate authority. Among the private patients, there were some from states other than New York and others who were apparently admitted without any legal formalities and whose detention was not warranted by any statutory provision. That the governors found it necessary to assume authority to detain patients has already been related.[3] Nor, after the asylum was established, did they hesitate to transfer to it, for disciplinary purposes, patients in the hospital service who were merely disorderly. On November 9, 1813, the nurse on Ward 5 complained to the Inspecting Committee of the bad conduct and language of the patients. The committee reported that "if the same cause again occurs, we directed the offending ones to be removed to the Asylum." The superintendent of the hospital evidently considered this to be sufficient authority, as it was further recorded that on November 20 he removed Ann T. to the asylum, and that the committee conferred with her and thought it proper that she should be continued on light diet till she seemed disposed to better conduct. On December 6, Ann made acknowledgment of her bad conduct, and was released from the asylum and discharged from the hospital "cured."[4] The few available histories of patients who were treated in this early asylum reveal that patients not infrequently protested against their detention, and occasionally ran away. There is, however, nothing in the records to indicate that the governors were ever called upon to defend their acts.

It was not until May, 1809, that the Asylum Committee felt enabled to propose to the governors a few "Rules for the government of the Asylum." Their understanding and interest in the importance of "a certificate with the state of the patient's case from a physician of the town from which the patient is sent," is revealed in Rule 3. Their appreciation of the necessity of medical control of visits to the patients is evident in Rule 6. And that they were proceeding systematically to build a plan of administration based on careful observation and experience can be gathered from Rule 7. These rules were presented to the governors on May 2, but the record does not indicate that any action in regard to them was taken at that time. They were as follows:

First. That no patient be received unless payment or Security for their maintenance, Cloathing &c, be first obtained, the price to be regulated by the circumstances of the Case.

Second. That when a patient is received from the Alms House of this City, the Superintendent of the Alms House shall send a written request

[3] See p. 43.

[4] New York Hospital, *Minutes of the Inspecting Committee,* Dec. 6, 1813.

for his admission—and when such are discharged, They shall in all cases be returned to the Alms House with a certificate from the Attending Physician of the state of the patient at the time of discharge.

Third. That when a patient is sent from other Towns in this state the overseers of the poor shall send a certificate with the state of the patients case from a physician of the town from which the patient is sent—and on the requisite security being given he shall be received, and when such patient is discharged he must be delivered to the overseers of such town, at the expence of said Town, with a certificate from the attending physician of the case of such patient when discharged—the security received from the overseers of the poor is to embrace the expence of removal.

Fourth. That a regester expressing all the necessary descriptions be kept of the Admission, death and discharge of patients.

Fifth. To prevent too frequent visiting of patients it shall be requisite for every Visitor to obtain a written permission from a Governor or the attending physician—or they may visit by permission of the Superintendent, the hours of Visiting shall be only from Ten to Twelve in the morning and from Three to Five in the afternoon.

Sixth. When the attending physician shall deem it proper to prevent a patient from being visited by friends or acquaintance he must [give] Orders to the keeper to that effect, and it shall be the duty of the keeper to obey such Orders.

Seventh. As cleanliness and regularity are of the first consequence in an institution of this kind, the Inspecting and Asylum committee are enjoined to be vigilent in the execution of their duties, and for the purpose of collecting information on the subject of proper rules, and regulations for the government of the Asylum, they will note in their minutes whatever may appear important or usefull.[5]

There is no further reference to rules for the asylum in the records until June, 1811, when a more complete set appeared in a revised copy of the by-laws of the hospital. It will be noted in these, that the physician was required to attend only three times a week, instead of daily as was recommended by the committee first appointed to prepare rules.[6] Later experience was to show that this was unfortunate. It is also unfortunate that the complete histories contemplated in Rule XV of the 1811 rules are available only in 75 cases recorded by Dr. Handy in 1817 and 1818. The term "pay patients" in Rule VIII does not imply privately supported patients only. It also relates to patients who were supported by the various poor authorities. The section from the 1811 by-laws is as follows:

I. The building erected for the benefit of lunatics, shall be denominated the "Lunatic Asylum," and appropriated solely for the reception of lunatics.

[5] *Minutes of the Governors,* May 2, 1809.

[6] See p. 71.

II. The physician of the asylum shall attend the same, at least, three times every week, and oftener, if necessary.

III. The asylum committee shall have the same powers, and perform the same duties, with relation to the asylum, as those of the visiting committee with relation to the hospital; except that all purchases for the use of both houses are to be made by the superintendent, or visiting committee.

IV. The asylum committee shall appoint a proper person to be keeper of the asylum, and also a female keeper.

V. The keeper shall perform the duties of the superintendent, and under his direction, so far as relates to the asylum.

VI. The servants employed in the asylum, shall be appointed and discharged by the asylum committee.

VII. Medicines shall be sent from the apothecary's shop to the asylum, in like manner as they are sent to the wards, under the direction of the physician to the asylum.

VIII. None but pay-patients are to be received into the asylum.

IX. The asylum committee may admit patients into the asylum, without any recommendation, upon such terms as they shall think reasonable; but before the patient is received, the committee shall take security, or payment in advance, for the expenses of maintenance of such patient, the charges of burial, in case of death, and of removal, in case the patient is sent back to his or her friends; and whenever a patient is sent to the asylum, it is recommended that a statement of his case, drawn up by a physician, or some of his friends, should be sent with him, for the information of the physician of the asylum.

X. No patient shall be received from the almshouse, without a written request to admit him from the superintendent thereof. Any such patient, when discharged, shall be returned to the almshouse, and a certificate, by the physician of the asylum, of the state of his case shall be sent with him.

XI. Lunatics sent by the overseers of the poor of any town in this state, may be received on the same terms as those sent by the city and county of New-York. But the asylum committee shall take security for the payment, and for the expenses, of sending the patient back to the town, when discharged.

XII. Every such patient when discharged, shall be sent back to the town from which he was received, and a certificate like that mentioned in the tenth section shall be sent with him.

XIII. A register shall be kept by the keeper, under the direction of the asylum committee, in which he shall record the admission and discharge of all patients, with such other matters as the committee may think proper.

XIV. No visitor shall be admitted into the asylum without permission from a governor, physician, or surgeon of the hospital, or from the superintendent; nor at any other than at such stated hours, as shall be from time to time appointed for that purpose, by the asylum committee. And the physician of the asylum may absolutely prohibit all visitors from such patients as he thinks proper, or allow them, under such restriction as he shall judge necessary.

XV. The physician of the asylum shall cause to be kept a register, in which shall be entered every case under his care, the name, age, place of residence, and occupation of the patient, the probable cause and history of his disorder, the remedies used, the termination of his disease; and such other circumstances as may tend to elucidate the case, and the nature of the disease—which register shall be kept in the asylum, under the care of the committee, who shall provide a proper book for that purpose; and they shall cause all special and remarkable cases to be entered, at the end of every three months, by the clerk of the hospital, in a book, to be kept in the library and in all cases where it may be thought proper, the names of the patients or parties may be omitted.

In the absence of any precise account of the organization of the asylum, or any roster of the persons employed, it is impossible to state the number and character of the positions, or the distribution of responsibilities and duties. The order in which nurse positions were listed in the superintendent's accounts for the years 1809 to 1816 suggests, however, that from two to six men and from six to ten women were employed in the nursing service. Names that appear in the superintendent's accounts seem to indicate that some of those on the payroll of the asylum had previously been patients there. In a few instances, a charge for a private nurse or "servant" appeared in the accounts. The wages were the same as at the hospital, ranging from $7 to $10 a month for both men and women, with two or three exceptions for those apparently holding superior positions.

When the patients were transferred from the hospital to the asylum on July 15, 1808, the "cell keeper," James Williams (B.M.), and his wife Phyllis, "who have charge of the Lunatics, at present," were continued in their positions, to be, however, "under the superintendant or such person as may be appointed keeper of the asylum." [7] The Asylum Committee apparently had some misgivings in regard to Williams's capability in the enlarged and improved service. On March 7, 1809, they reported to the governors that he had "behaved improperly," and had been excused because it was found that "his improper conduct was the result of passion, and that passion caused by anxiety for the institution." The committee, however, evidently felt that some change should be made in order to improve the attention given to the patients: on April 4 they reported that "some of the patients being of respectable standing in Society, your committee have deemed it proper to place them under the care of respectable keepers," and that to this end they had (on March 21) appointed James Cowan and his wife who were "well recommended

[7] *Minutes of the Asylum Committee*, July 14, 1808.

and are without children." In this same report, they said that "James the keeper of the Asylum having . . . behaved very improperly, it has been deemed expedient to discharge him." The departure of James—with, it may be hoped, his "cat and nine tales—" coupled with the avowed intention of the committee to employ "respectable keepers," seems to mark an advance in the standards of the service in keeping with the improved facilities.

James Cowan and his wife remained until November 1, and were succeeded by "a young man and elderly woman." At the same time Lewis Sandford was appointed "caretaker of the Asylum," at a salary of $300 a year, which by February, 1816, was increased to $600. The dignity and importance of this position assumed greater proportions with advance in the character of the service. Eventually it was frequently referred to in the records as "superintendent of the asylum" and was so designated in some of the annual reports. The salary continued gradually to be increased, and in 1820 it had reached $720. From time to time vacancies and appointments in the positions of keeper, assistant, and servant were noted in the minutes. Some of those employed were designated "blk." The terms "nurse" and "nursing" were sometimes employed in references to the care of individual patients. Notwithstanding, however, the trend of progress and the earnest purpose of the governors to provide humane, rational, curative treatment, it was long before the established idea of confinement, restraint, repression, and punishment by "keepers" ceased to determine the phraseology and the measures employed in the consideration and treatment of the "maniacs."

The Asylum Committee entered upon their duties with great interest and zeal. They met regularly once a week, and occasionally held special meetings. Individual members visited the service more frequently. Thomas Franklin, especially, sometimes made as many as 28 visits during a month. The duties of the committee were similar to those of the Visiting Committee of the hospital. No patient was officially admitted without the approval of at least one member of the committee. They fixed the rates; considered many questions relating to patients; filled vacancies in the various positions; and exercised disciplinary powers.

In order that the Visiting and Asylum Committees might devote themselves more exclusively to executive duties, in 1809 the governors found it advisable to add a committee whose duty it would be "to discover conditions that need attention," both in the hospital and the asylum. The new body was called the "Inspecting Committee." Their valuable reports relate to the physical condition and the order, cleanliness, and ventilation of the rooms, halls, and "cells"; to the bedding, clothing, furniture, and equipment; to sanitation in general; to their observations of the patients and of their management by the attendants; and to the attendance of the physician as required by the by-laws. These reports are straightforward and sometimes sharply critical. It is noteworthy that the committee apparently found less to criticize in the asylum than in the hospital. Especially remarkable is it that no adverse comments in regard to the character and qualifications of the attendants were made. Comments such as the following appear with great frequency:

Inspected the Lunatic Asylum, the halls and cells of which are kept in the best condition and all other matters in relation to this institution appear to be well regulated. The Patients are treated with humanity and care by the manager and are daily visited by the Physician.

Note with satisfaction the attention of Wilson to the care of the Lunatics, particularly exemplified in his obtaining chairs for the Patients who require continued confinement, which adds much to their comfort.

Found them in excellent order, particularly the Asylum.

Adverse criticism was, however, not entirely lacking.

In the Asylum three patients entirely naked two of them chained to the floor showed how much would be gained to humanity by an establishment which would admit of milder treatment and one that would produce moral effects without the use of severity.[8]

Man entirely naked. Hope that some mode might be found of keeping him clothed.

Less order and regularity among the patients than formerly.

Privies in the yard are in very filthy condition, men and women frequently go at the same time; each sex should have a separate place.

Other committees of the governors occasionally reported observations of some significance to the treatment of the mentally ill. In April, 1812, the Committee on Repairs was instructed to have the height of the brick wall around the yard raised so as to "prevent escape of Lunatics & patients." This distinction recalls the persistence of established conceptions relating to the mentally ill, notwithstanding that in practice it was accepted that they were really patients. The Visiting Committee, in reporting the "irregularity and infamous behavior of the girls on No. 5," stated that "improper connections frequently occur with men

[8] This report was made in November, 1816, after Thomas Eddy had in April, 1815, presented his address in which he advocated the erection of an asylum in the country for "moral treatment."

in and about the Hospital, and the situation of the Lunatics are frequently rendered very bad by their infamous conduct." [9]

Some reluctance in providing facilities is apparent in the delay in installing water closets in the hospital. An experimental installation was declared to be a failure because the water in the pipe froze. In October, 1818, the Visiting Committee expressed their approval of water closets, but, in consequence of the lateness of the season and the great number of patients, they advised postponement of the project "until a future day." In January, 1819, the "Committee on Water Closets" reported against their introduction on the grounds that they would freeze in the proposed location, and that in private houses in which they had been tried they had "been generally abandoned."

Items in the superintendent's accounts occasionally furnish a little information in regard to the service, and in view of the lack of any contemporary detailed description, every scrap or glimpse is valuable. Typical entries in these accounts include: "making and mending straight jackets"; "three straight jackets $9 (sold one for $4.00)"; "mending irons"; "snuff for Asylum"; "bladder of snuff $4.25"; "ice for patient .18 [cents]"; "for fetching a Crazy man Back .88"; and "Paid for Mending windows broke by an assylum patient $3.15." [10] Much clothing was purchased for the patients, as was required by contracts with the poor law authorities. Various articles such as tubs, mats, brushes, and tables were purchased from the State Prison, indicating that the disposal of such articles by sale to public institutions has been practiced in New York from a very early period.

The character of the nursing service continued to be of concern to the governors until the establishment of the school of nursing in 1877. As early as 1821 a committee reported to the governors [11] that the number of "nurses" in the general hospital service in January of that year was sixteen. Of these one was appointed in 1801, one in 1815, one in 1816, one in 1818, two in 1819, and two in 1820. Three were rated "Good"; four, "tolerable Good"; four, "Inferior or Not Competent"; and five, "Bad." Of six men, one was rated "Good"; three, "Bad"; and two, "Inferior." Apparently the asylum service was not included; no precise record of the number employed there at any time has been discovered.

A former state "Commissioner in Lunacy" wrote in 1886, in reference

9 *Minutes of Visiting Committee,* July 24, 1818.
10 Superintendent's Daily Expenses, 1810–1818, and General Expenses, 1808–1821.
11 *Minutes of the Governors,* Feb. 6, 1821.

to the treatment of the mentally ill in the New York Hospital prior to the establishment of the asylum, that "the attendants were but little above the common order of poor-house keepers, or jailers," but that "in the Asylum of the Hospital, the patients were treated in the most humane manner, by the best class of officers and attendants." [12] The absence of adverse criticism by the Inspecting Committee, already noted, may indicate that, in some way, a better class of employee may have been secured for the asylum than for the hospital. The committee whose report on the hospital nursing service has been cited recommended the adoption of a progressive wage schedule including a 50 percent increase after five years, an additional 33⅓ percent after another five years, an annuity of $25 at the end of twenty years' service, and the further provision that "in case of disability to obtain decent support, and the want of means adequate thereto, the same shall be comfortably supported through life in the Hospital."

The consideration given by the governors to the interests of the patients was again shown by the issuing, in 1811, of an order that no patient was to be permitted to sign any "Instrument of Writing without being first inspected by the Asylum Committee or one of them and the consent of the same obtained." [13] Their treatment of a request from Ezra Stiles Ely, who asked "the concurrence of the Committee in his publishing an Acct. of the Lives of certain patients in the asylum and the probable causes of their Lunacy," had similar significance. It was

> Resolved that the means used by Ezra Stiles Ely to obtain the necessary information to enable him to write the acct. of patients in the assylum was improper, as being without the consent of the Committee—and the Committee feel themselves bound not only to withold their consent to the publishing, but to retain the Manuscript handed them as they feel a conviction that making public the names and conduct of the unfortunate people admitted as patients in the assylum would militate against the prosperity of the institution and injure the feelings of relatives and Friends—and the chairman is requested to furnish Ezra Stiles Ely with a Copy of this resolution as an answer to his application.[14]

A proposal to have the asylum visited weekly by "a number of respectable matrons residing in the city" was similarly discouraged,[15] after having been referred to the physician of the asylum. A month later "further consideration of the subject [was] dispensed with."

[12] Stephen Smith, "The Care of the Insane in the State of New York Historically Considered," *Am. J. Insanity*, XLIII (1886), 59–65

[13] *Minutes of the Asylum Committee*, Sept. 3, 1811.

[14] *Ibid.*, Feb. 4, 1812.

[15] *Minutes of the Governors*, Jan. 2, 1816.

The records show little evidence that the physician of the asylum was consulted in regard to the administration. There can be no doubt, however, that reports and recommendations made by him received respectful consideration. In December, 1812, one such suggestion in regard to "some new Arrangements in the Asylum yard for the greater seclusion of the Patients" was immediately "referred to the Asylum Committee and the Committee on Repairs to make such alterations as in their discretion may appear most advisable." Dr. William Handy's report to the governors in June, 1818, was read at their August meeting, and "so much of said Report as relates to the construction of Lunatic Asylums [was] referred to the Building Committee of the new Asylum" (Bloomingdale), and in September a printing of five hundred copies was ordered. Another report, by Dr. John Neilson who had been recently appointed, was received in January, 1820. These are the only medical reports relating to the general state of the asylum service that have been found in the records.

What has been learned in regard to the asylum physicians of this period has not disclosed any particular previous training or experience in the hospital treatment of the mentally ill. The physicians were general practitioners. This may, perhaps, account for the neglect of the governors to refer to them more frequently matters in which professional knowledge and judgment would have been helpful. For example, in October, 1815, a committee of governors was appointed "to prepare a sett of Questions to be asked on the admission of each patient." The committee must have found the task too difficult, for in January, 1816, they were "discharged from further consideration of the subject." In July, 1815, the Inspecting Committee remarked in their report that "Mary *C.* & —— *H.* two assylum patients are not proper objects for further detention." Apparently nothing was done about this. The committee, in February, 1816, reported that in inspecting the asylum they had

> met with several cases which in their opinion cannot be considered entitled to further claim on the benevolence of that institution . . . one case in particular, that of Miss H. which is considered not a desided [*sic*] case of insanity—or if so in any degree, is so faintly marked (from all the Committee have been able to assertain) as to create a doubt in their minds as to the propriety of detaining her any longer.

The record does not indicate that these cases were referred to the physician or that any action was taken. It is frequently noted that, to persons ill informed concerning the character of the several varieties of mental illness, many patients appear to be quite well, especially in the protecting environment of a hospital.

The understanding and zeal of the governors in regard to the medical, scientific, and educational purposes of the hospital and the asylum, were shown in many ways. The Inspecting Committee reported any neglect of medical service discovered by them, and the negligent were called to account by the governors. The physicians and the medical schools were encouraged and assisted in utilizing the facilities of the hospital and its library in the teaching of medical students. On several occasions resolutions were adopted for the purpose of encouraging scientific studies and the collection of histories of particular cases.

VIII

THE ASYLUM MEDICAL SERVICE

During the thirteen years in which the asylum was operated at the New York Hospital, the position of asylum physician was held by three doctors in turn. All engaged in private practice also, and nothing has been found in the records to indicate that they were paid for their service to the asylum. The first to occupy the post was Dr. Archibald Bruce, who was appointed on July 14, 1808. He had not previously been connected with the hospital, nor, as far as can be learned from various sources, was he particularly qualified in mental disease. A graduate of Columbia College, he studied medicine with Dr. Nicholas Romayne and Dr. David Hosack, and obtained his M.D. degree from Edinburgh University in 1800. The following three years were spent in European travel and in making a valuable collection of minerals. In 1803, Dr. Bruce entered into private practice in New York. With Dr. Romayne he was instrumental in obtaining the passage of the enabling act under which the state and county medical societies were organized, and in establishing the state and New York county societies. He aided in securing a charter for the College of Physicians and Surgeons in 1807, and was appointed registrar and professor of materia medica and mineralogy. In 1811 he was one of those who left the College to establish a medical school at Rutgers (then Queens) College. Bruce's only contribution to medical literature was his graduation thesis, *De Variola Vaccina.* He is best known for his work in mineralogy—his name survives in "Brucite," a native magnesia which he discovered and analyzed. He was the founder and first editor of the *American Journal of Mineralogy,* "our earliest *purely scientific* Journal, supported by *original American communications.*" [1] Dr. Bruce resigned from the asylum in September, 1817, and died of apoplexy on February 22, 1818, at the age of forty-one.

His successor, Dr. William Handy, was appointed in September, 1817, but on November 3, 1818, resigned because of ill health. A fuller account of Dr. Handy and of his service at the asylum is given in Chapter IX. After his resignation there was a period in which it was considered necessary "to provide suitable medical Assistance for the Asylum until a Physician is regularly appointed." It was not until January 5, 1819, that Dr. David Hosack was "regularly appointed." He had been an attending physician at the New York Hospital since 1797, and, as we have seen,

1 Silliman's *Journal of Science and Arts* I (1818), 3.

his writings and lectures display considerable knowledge and interest in mental disease. His assignment at the asylum was probably a temporary one, as on May 4 nominations were again considered, the names presented being Dr. Hosack, Dr. Handy, Dr. John Neilson, and Dr. J. R. B. Rodgers. Dr. Neilson was elected. At the time he also was an attending physician of the hospital. He remained physician of the asylum until it was removed to Bloomingdale and he was appointed physician there. He was evidently much respected as a citizen and as a physician and was invariably attentive to his duties. Neilson was described at the time of his death as having had "in his profession, large observation and experience," and being "prompt, skillful, faithful, successful, eminent." [2] Little information relating to him, however, has been found, and there seem to be no histories of his patients at the "medical asylum" or publications by him, except an article on dispensaries published in 1836.

The records do not reveal the extent to which other physicians may have assisted in the service. The reports of the Inspecting Committee, however, mention that Dr. Bibby sometimes made visits in behalf of Dr. Bruce, and, in his report to the governors in 1818, Dr. Handy acknowledged his indebtedness to Dr. Joshua Fisher for faithful attendance and to Dr. Campbell, the house physician, for "able assistance and polite friendly aid." For the purpose, perhaps, of providing officially for assistance by a house physician, the governors in August, 1820, by resolution placed the physician of the asylum "upon an equal footing with the Physicians of the Hospital . . . respecting the nomination of House Physician." There is, however, no record of an appointment in this position until after the removal to Bloomingdale in the following year.

Notwithstanding the frequent requests and resolutions of the governors in regard to case histories, few have been found. In fact, Dr. Handy in one of his histories in 1818 mentioned that "as there exists no record of . . . cases of long standing in the Asylum, much pains have been taken to procure some authentic history of them." [3] The good resolutions were not always productive. For example, in November, 1809, the governors adopted the following:

> The Governors being informed that the Physician of the Asylum has opened a regester for the purpose of entering therein the names of all the patients, who are now in the building or may be hereafter admitted, and

[2] John Knox, *The Character and End of the Perfect and Upright: a Discourse . . . on the Occasion of the Death of John Neilson, M.D., June 28, 1857* (New York).

[3] Dr. Handy's case history No. 23.

also of those who have been received since the erection of the asylum, and stating the practice pursued for the cure with its termination.

Resolved that the plan adopted by the Physician meets with the approbation of this Board, and he is requested to add the History of each patient so far as relates to the cause, that most probably produced the insanity and the Volume Neat and strongly bound, be deposited in the Library.

In June, 1811, a by-law was adopted by which the physician was again required to keep a register of this description including, in addition to the information called for above, "other Circumstances, as may tend to elucidate the case, and the Nature of the disease." In November, 1812, the Inspecting Committee reported that the register of the keeper was regularly kept but they had not seen the register of lunatics kept by the physician, and were informed that it was at his house. In October, 1815, the governors requested the Asylum Committee to call on Dr. Bruce and inquire of him respecting the Register of Cases. The following month the chairman reported that he had called on the physician, who had promised "to attend to the subject." A motion was thereupon passed directing him to report at the next meeting. His report, received at the December meeting, was merely that "when appointed Physician to the Asylum, he could not have supposed it to have been the intention of the Governors that he should, Independent of his situation of Physician, act as Apothecary and Registering Clerk." This was naturally unsatisfactory to the governors, and a formal charge of neglect of duty was made. After a hearing which did not improve the situation, Dr. Bruce, on January 2, 1816, presented to the board the following communication, which is produced in full because very little information has been obtained in regard to this physician and his service:

The undersigned respectfully begs leave to submit to the President and Governors of the New York Hospital the following grounds of defence relative to a resolution of the Governors passed at a Meeting on the 19th ultmo.

The undersigned has ever since he received the Appointment of Physician to the Lunatic Asylum expressed himself as averse to any aggravation of the situation of Patients committed to his care by rendering them the subjects of public record and to that effect begs leave respectfully to refer to a report presented by him to the President & Governors in the hope that what was therein contained might have the effect of mitigating this worst of Maladies. As it is the object of the Governors of the New York Hospital to contribute everything in their power towards alleviating human distress and Misery, it has always been considered by the undersigned his duty to afford them every reasonable assistance. He has with this view ever since his appointment visited the Asylum agreably to the regulation at least three times a week, has always held himself subject to such extra attendance as might be deemed necessary and has not unfrequently where the situation of a Patient has required it, visited three times a day.

In addition to the above attendance as Physician to the Asylum the undersigned has been constantly subject to visits of enquiry by the Friends of Patients, many of which visits are attended with very considerable loss of time.

It frequently happens that previous to a Patient being Admitted into the Asylum the undersigned has been requested, and could not from motives of Humanity refuse, to visit.

The undersigned is often consulted by Letter from different parts of this State and the United States respecting Paupers which he has always considered it incumbent on him to answer.

The undersigned takes the Liberty of stating these circumstances in order that it may be understood how much of his time is occupied independent of his immediate duties at the Asylum, he therefore respectfully represents to the President and Governors of the New York Hospital in regard to keeping a register of Cases the necessity of the assistance of some person whose business it may be to attend to the collection of such Facts as may lead to the development of the history of the Case.

Very respectfully submitted

ARCHIBALD BRUCE, M.D.[4]

This was considered satisfactory and the Asylum Committee was requested "to confer with the physician on the proposition made by him, in order to carry the same into effect."

The only other communication by Dr. Bruce relating to the service was a report requested by the governors on cases "attributed to the immoderate Use of ardent Spirits," which was presented in June, 1814. He reported that, of 572 patients admitted to the asylum since it was opened, 65, of whom 16 were females, were cases of this character. There were also 17 others whose intemperance he considered to be an effect of mental illness already present. He gave a brief account of a few cases to illustrate the difficulties and failure attending treatment, and of one case in which total abstinence had been accomplished. As preventive measures "of this Cause of Mania," he recommended: 1. That intoxication be considered a punishable offense, and that "Persons who are in the habit of using ardent Spirits to excess, so as to render themselves Nuisances to Society, . . . be subjected to Confinement for a longer or shorter period . . . in an Establishment expressly for the purpose. . . . to be occupied in some useful pursuit, & when discharged to find Security for good behavior;" 2. "Discouraging the Consumption of Ar-

[4] New York Hospital, *Minutes of the Governors*, Jan. 2, 1816. The Register of Patients contains the names of patients admitted from the date of the opening. No medical observations recorded during Dr. Bruce's period of service have been found.

dent Spirits by substituting the use of light Wines,—Cider, Malt liquors—&c." The duties on wines were to be "in proportion to the quantity of Ardent Spirit which they contain, and this in a ratio that would render the price of Ardent Spirit too expensive for the laboring Class of the Community." The license for small shops, "particularly for those who retail Ardent Spirits under the form of Drams," should be heavy; that for vending wines, malt liquors, etc., should be proportionately low. 3. "No debt contracted for Drams, to be recoverable by Law." [5] This was apparently the contribution mentioned by Dr. Bruce in his answer to the charge of neglect of duty, and was evidently based on records which were, as reported by the Committee, "kept at his own home."

The effect of alcoholic beverages in the production of mental illness was already a subject of concern, as it still is, to those engaged in the treatment and prevention of this illness. Thomas Eddy, one of the governors of the hospital, was, with others, endeavoring "to prevent the increase of taverns and dram shops in this city, and to lessen the number of those which already exist." He considered that to destroy "this wide spreading mischief," an entire prohibition of home distillation and a heavy import and excise on foreign spirits" would be necessary; but he adds, "No legislature would dare pass such a law, and no administration could carry it into execution. . . . It is painful to reflect that it is only in our power to attempt partial remedies, and to endeavour to regulate what we cannot prevent." [6] Mr. Eddy's views and attitude in regard to this serious problem may with advantage receive the careful consideration of those to whom it is a subject of concern at the present time. Following Dr. Bruce's communication, the monthly reports of the Asylum Committee gave the number of patients admitted whose illness was attributed to the intemperate use of alcoholic beverages.

Among the motives which animated the governors of the New York Hospital, the spirit of the Christian religion had a large place. They considered that this spirit should pervade the whole organization, and that, in the treatment of the patients, provision should be made for furnishing access to the consolation of religion. From an early period chapters were read from the Bible every Sunday at ten in the morning and at three in the afternoon in each ward, by the "most sober patient" there, who was appointed for that purpose by the superintendent.[7] It was, however,

[5] For full text see Appendix, p. 489.

[6] Samuel L. Knapp, *The Life of Thomas Eddy* (New York, 1834), p. 206.

[7] Rules and Orders for the Government of the New-York Hospital, 1804 and 1811.

not until 1813 that a chaplain was engaged. This was the Reverend John Stanford,[8] who for several years had given his services freely to the State Prison, the Almshouse, the Orphan Asylum, the hospital and several other charitable institutions in the city. He visited the wards once or twice a week, and besides conversing and praying with individual patients he conducted informal services. Moreover, "with one of the governors of the Hospital" he formed a plan for giving some education to the lame children in the institution. "This system produced the happy effect, not only of teaching them to read, but it kept them still, and thus facilitated their cure." His first sermon as "regularly appointed chaplain in the City Hospital" was preached on July 1, 1814. It was, however, not until August 31, 1819, that "by request of the governors and physicians, he performed divine service in the lunatic department." The service was attended by about forty of the patients and by several of the governors, the physicians, and the superintendent.

The text was "Comfort the Feeble-Minded." The new chaplain discussed what he understood to be causes "by which a feeble mind is produced." "Some persons," he said, "are naturally feeble minded." Other "causes" were excessive use of ardent spirits, financial loss, death of relatives, disappointment in love, "consciousness of sin against God," or having committed "the unpardonable sin." For all of these he proposed the solace and healing power that were to be found in religion. In a report to the governors of January 4, 1820, Mr. Stanford stated that he would request one of the children in the Orphan Asylum to write a copy of his address to be presented to the Board. A nicely bound, hand-written copy of this remarkable sermon is preserved at the Westchester Division of the hospital.[9] A note appended to it is as follows:

> In future services in the Asylum, I shall think it most prudent to avoid particular reference to their mental derangement, as like unfortunates of other classes they shrink at being told of their unhappy situation. Still, I considered myself justified in describing their case, and offering them consolation in this plain introductory discourse.

In November, 1819, Mr. Stanford was elected a member of the Society of the New York Hospital. "This," his biographer states, "furnishes another evidence of the high estimation entertained of his private and public character."

With the transfer of the department for the mentally ill to Bloomingdale in June, 1821, the "medical asylum" at the New York Hospital

[8] C. G. Sommers, *Memoir of the Rev. John Stanford* (New York, 1835).

[9] Published in *Am. J. Insanity*, IV (1848), 39.

was discontinued. No medical histories of patients treated after Dr. Handy resigned have been found. Nor have any publications by the asylum physicians been noted in the medical journals of the period. Theodore Romeyn Beck, a medical student who presented at his graduation from the College of Physicians and Surgeons an "Inaugural Dissertation on Insanity," [10] may have received instruction at the asylum. The medical literature of that period in America contained very few articles relating to mental illness. A pamphlet with the title "An arrangement of those parts of the phenomena of the human mind, which belong to the function of *Somnium*, a state which is intermediate between waking and sleeping," by Samuel L. Mitchill, attending physician of the hospital, published in 1815, was found in the library of the New York Historical Society. In this he discusses various abnormal mental states. Dr. Mitchill's interest in mental disorder has already been referred to.[11] Cases of hysteria, epilepsy, hypochondriasis, and an occasional case of "mania" were admitted into the medical service of the hospital, and there is no reference in his article to the asylum.

The number of patients admitted to the "medical asylum" of the New York Hospital during the thirteen years of its operation was 1,148. The largest number treated in any one year was 179, in 1812. After the governors had limited the number to be accommodated to 75, the largest in any year was 151, in 1820. Of the patients discharged, 503, about 44 percent, were recorded as "cured," and 174, about 15 percent, as relieved. One hundred and eleven died. This was nearly 10 percent, and is probably indicative of a large proportion of very acute forms of illness. Apparently some patients were retained for long periods. The reason for this is not clear, but the deplorable conditions in almshouses as places for the mentally ill may have had an influence. The asylum was, however, much more than a custodial institution. There is considerable evidence that much intelligence and kindly consideration were shown. A patient who had returned to his home and business addressed the physician as "My dear friend," and, after giving an account of his present condition, added:

When I reflect upon what was probably the state of my mind the last summer, and upon the uncommon number of cases of insanity, many of which resulted in violent deaths, I have a reason to be extremely grateful that I was preserved—that I was attended by and received the benefits of friendship and affection, skill and benevolence. How vastly ameliorated must be

10 *Am. Med. and Philosophical J.*, II (1812), 349.
11 See p. 57.

the condition of the human family from the improvements in the healing art and the many conveniences afforded by benevolent institutions! And, Sir, how different must be the reflections of the man, who, by attention and skill, has restored to his family and friends, a fellow creature, from those of the duellist, who has blasted the prospects and agonised hearts, perhaps in a single instant, of father and mother, brother and sister, and wife and children!!

This patient had been sufficiently disturbed to be placed in a strait-jacket. Another, while at the asylum, wrote to his parents:

The excellent accommodations, and the kind treatment I have experienced, make me extremely ashamed that I am not able to acknowledge that I owe a debt of gratitude to the Doctor and Mr. Wilson which I am totally unable to repay by any act of mine. During the time I have been here, I have had at the first, one or two fits of insanity which rendered it necessary to chain me; but otherwise I have experienced as much care and attention as I could have done at home, or anywhere else.

The history of this patient relates that he was chained because he was attempting to break a door. Further evidence of the character of the nursing attention is contained in a report to the governors by Dr. Neilson in January, 1820:

I am happy to have it in my power Gentlemen, to testify to the diligence and attention, with which the different attendants apply themselves in promoting the comfort of the patients. . . .

The services of Mr. Willson the principal keeper are highly valuable, his indefatigable judicious and affectionate attention to the unfortunate beings, who are committed to his care, merits your warmest approbation."

The chaplain, in a report to the governors on January 4, 1820, stated:

It is pleasing to myself and must be gratifying to you, to be informed that for the several years I have attended this Hospital, and the familiar intercourse with which I have indulged the patients, I have never yet had a single instance of complaint of inattention or ill treatment from those who have charge of them.

What Williams (B.M.), the first "keeper" at the asylum may have been guilty of when he "behaved very improperly" and was discharged, was not explained.[12] Perhaps he used his "cat and nine tales" too heavily, or was otherwise brutal to the patients. Only one specific act of violence was found in the records of treatment. A patient in an alcoholic delirium, during a "furious paroxysm" endeavored to commit violence on the superintendent. "The latter, in self defence, as he informs, by a blow

[12] See p. 81.

with his fist knocked him down on his bed, and afterwards exposed him to the shower bath." Soon afterwards the patient was found "in a convulsive fit," and after repeated convulsions for four days he died.

In most of the accounts of the development of hospital treatment of the mentally ill in New York and America, the little "medical asylum" of the New York Hospital seems to be pretty completely eclipsed by its much larger offspring at Bloomingdale. In its relations with the other services of the hospital, the asylum was, with due consideration of the change in circumstances, somewhat like the present Payne Whitney Clinic. In the first few decades of the nineteenth century, medical practitioners were far from ignorant or indifferent in regard to mental illness. Whether the asylum service had any part in promoting this interest, and whether the service was utilized as the other services of the hospital were, in the teaching of medical students, cannot be stated with certainty, though it seems highly probable. That it had a part in awakening and shaping the public interest that led eventually to legislation and public hospital provision for the treatment of the mentally ill, is generally conceded. In regard to this, the testimony of Dr. Stephen Smith in his article in 1886 on the history of the care of the insane in New York [13] is of interest.

Dr. Smith was born in 1823, and may have been acquainted with some of the physicians, governors, and others who had personal knowledge of the asylum and its affairs when it was operated at the New York Hospital. He was well informed concerning the provision made for the treatment of the mentally ill and was an active and earnest State Commissioner in Lunacy from 1882 to 1889, the year before the passage of the State Care Act, of which he was a strong promoter. In the article referred to, he quoted from the act of the legislature providing the appropriation which enabled the New York Hospital to erect its asylum in 1808, that the appropriation was "particularly to provide suitable apartments for the maniacs, adapted to the various forms and degrees of insanity." This, Dr. Smith wrote, was "the first public recognition in this State of the fact that there are various forms and degrees of insanity which require the classification of the insane, in suitable apartments." In further reference to the asylum he wrote: "There are many evidences of the value of the experience gained in this institution, and of the influence which its management exerted upon the public mind. It led to the first effort of the State to make special provision for the insane poor, hitherto confined in poorhouses." After describing the deplorable

13 Smith, "The Care of the Insane . . ."; see p. 84, above.

condition of mentally ill persons in the jails and poor houses through the state, he added: "In the asylum of the New York Hospital, they were treated in the most humane manner, by the best class of officers and attendants." He quoted much of Dr. Handy's 1818 report to the governors,[14] and commented that the report showed

that there were in New York, at that early day, men who had the most thoroughly correct views of the care and treatment of the insane, and of the proper qualifications of attendants. It cannot be doubted that these opinions had a wide dissemination among the leading citizens, many of whom were governors of the hospital.

Similar evidence is contained in an article on "Insanity in the State of New York" which says of the New York Hospital:

The Governors having been among the first in this country to recognize insanity as a disease amenable to medical and moral treatment . . . identified their Board intimately with the lunacy history of the State. To the successful administration of their trust is to be attributed the earlier interest excited in behalf of a class of the insane, whose claim for care rested in the public recognition of their helpless situation.[15]

That the asylum as well as the hospital were objects of public interest is attested by a visit from the President of the United States (James Monroe) in 1817, at which he "visited both Houses, and expressed himself much pleased with the general arrangement and good order of the establishment."[16]

Twelve of the governors were members of the Asylum Committee for varying periods during the thirteen years of the service of the department at the New York Hospital. To these men are due honor and gratitude for the sound foundation on which the service has since been built.[17]

[14] See Chapter IX.

[15] *Am. J. Insanity*, XIII (1856), 41.

[16] *Minutes of the Governors*, July 1, 1817.

[17] For list and periods of service see Appendix, p. 532.

IX

PRINCIPLES AND PRACTICE OF DR. WILLIAM HANDY: PHYSICIAN OF THE ASYLUM, 1817-1818

ALTHOUGH Dr. William Handy was physician of the asylum for only fourteen months, he made a contribution to the advancement of the service, and to this account of it, which is outstanding. Previous to his appointment he had been in private practice in New York City for ten years. He was born in Newport, Rhode Island, on September 21, 1766, and was, therefore, 51 years of age when appointed to the asylum. He received his medical degree from the University of Edinburgh in 1788 and spent the following two years in travel, in the course of which he visited India. Upon his return to America he entered private practice in Charleston, South Carolina. In 1794, the death of his father necessitated Dr. Handy's retirement from medical practice until 1808, when he resumed it in New York.

The records are silent as to whether Handy had received any particular training or experience in the treatment of the mentally ill previous to his appointment as physician of the asylum in September, 1817. Apparently, however, he had at least been a student of the subject and was deeply interested. His clinical histories of 75 patients together with his report to the governors in May, 1818, constitute a graphic description of the medical treatment in the asylum service, and of, perhaps, what was best in psychiatric principles and practice in America at that time. That his work was known and appreciated by his medical colleagues is revealed in an obituary in *The New York Medical and Physical Journal* upon his death in 1828:

> It was his custom during this period to record the most interesting cases that occurred in that institution; and had his connection with it continued, it was his intention to have pursued this object with the same fidelity and accuracy with which he began it. His conduct here claimed the decided approbation of the Governors of this charity. . . . His judgment was clear and discriminating, his duties were fulfilled with conscientious rectitude.

Dr. Handy's report [1] to the governors in May, 1818, gives such a full account of his principles and methods of practice that it seems to be sufficiently important as a psychiatric document of the period, as well as of the asylum of the New York Hospital, to be incorporated in this

1 Handy, *Report of the Physician of the New-York Lunatic Asylum; Addressed to a Committee of Its Governors and Published at their Request* (New York, 1818). Signed by William Handy, May 15, 1818.

account of the service. His references to construction and organization relate to the planning and operation of a new asylum which was then under consideration.

To *Thomas Franklin, Jacob Sherred, and Cornelius Dubois, Esquires, chairman, and members of the committee of the New-York Lunatic Asylum.*

GENTLEMEN;

As your monthly records exhibit regular returns of the patients, and you have by long and assiduous attention become familiar with the management of the asylum and its dependencies, it can hardly be expected, that under a more general view of the institution, I shall be able to add to your knowledge of its important interests. But as with the privilege of your example, and of co-operating with you in your benevolent design, there cannot, it is hoped be any misconception of the motives which govern me, I beg leave to lay before you in the form of tables a statement of the cases admitted from the 13th of September last to this date (a period of eight months) with their results, and of others received prior to that month, and within the same time discharged; referring to you for a more particular account, to the accompanying volume,[2] which contains their histories, in so far as it has been practicable to obtain them, and their medical treatment. I shall take the liberty to add some general observations on lunatic asylums, and on the treatment of insanity, having exclusive reference to the comfort, convenience, and cure of the unfortunate persons labouring under that most awful malady.

The number of admissions in the period refered to, is thirty-eight, of which twenty-eight were males, and ten females. Of the former, there have been discharged cured, thirteen, improved three; two by request, and two have died. Of the eight remaining in the house, four are much improved, three have been recently admitted, and one is a man sixty-eight years of age, labouring under that species of insanity, which sometimes occurs in advanced life, from a diminution of perception and memory, and is termed amentia senilis. It is to be observed, that T. H. who, on the 25th of October, was entered on the minutes of the committee as relieved only, was discharged cured. Of the ten female patients, one has been discharged cured, one an improper object, three by request, and one had died. Of the remaining four, one was admitted the 18th, one the 27th of March, one the 24th of April, one the 12th instant; and they are all nearly in the state in which they came in. During the time stated, of patients who were in the house previous to the first of September, there have been cured one male, and one female; four males and one female have died, three males and two females have been discharged by request, and one male as an improper object; the (three) females and two of the males, improved. The cases which ended fatally were of long standing, connected with palsy, epilepsy, consumption and dropsy.

The whole number cured since the 13th of September, is fourteen, twelve of whom were males, and two females. In the same time, there have been

[2] Preserved at the Westchester Division. The tables referred to are missing.

relieved, and much improved, five; discharged by request, twelve; as improper objects, two; and eight have died.

The number of patients now in the house is seventy-seven, of whom forty-nine are males, and twenty-eight females. Fourteen males,[3] and nine females are variously and usefully employed in such occupations as appear to be the best adapted to their several cases, deriving in this manner, more benefit perhaps, than the establishment, under its present arrangements, could otherwise afford them.

It is desirable that early measures should be taken to discharge C. H. whose case you are acquainted with, and to enable him to return to his connections in Scotland, who, I am informed, are respectable people. His confinement appears to have a tendency to revive, and it may perpetuate the disorder from which he is fast recovering. And which, for its entire cure, may require nothing but his enlargement. Should he from his present restraint unfortunately relapse into the dreadful state in which he was admitted, it is not difficult to foretel[l] to what a series of painful reflections so deplorable an event would give rise.

W. M. a custom house patient, as he is called, labouring under palsy, is an improper object of our attention. The means adapted to his cure, would be more advantageously applied in the hospital.

There are several old cases of both sexes in the house, of whose recovery there exists but a faint probability; and there are others in a course of improvement.

Accompanying the tables of cases, is a list of names, showing annexed to each, as nearly perhaps as the difficulty and obscurity of the subject admits, their supposed causes.[4] How far such an exposition may or may not be useful, it is not pretended to determine. I shall hazard one remark on the occasion, that religious terror, arising from erroneous perceptions, is much more frequently the effect than a cause of mental derangement.

It will be evident to you, that from any pharmaceutical course that has been pursued in the treatment of our patients, there is but little to boast. Medicine indeed, has been rarely given, except when strongly indicated by such symptoms of bodily disease, as were supposed instrumental in exciting, or had been connected with the disorder of the mind. Under such circumstances chiefly, do we rely on its efficacy: but we do not believe in the specific power of any drug in curing madness. Although mercury has been given to a number of our patients, there is but one instance in which it was considered that the recovery was the result of its use, and that was the case of J. L. G. discharged the 31st of March.

Mild cathartics, and warm bathing, have long appeared to me of more general utility than any other means employed as physical agents in the treatment of insanity, and the latter, in an especial manner, in melancholic cases. Drastic purges, unless when particularly demanded, have been of far less benefit.

[3] The number of men employed is noteworthy.
[4] This table has not been found.

Blood-letting, judiciously used, in violent paroxysms, has on many occasions been of great efficacy, but is of far less general application than is often supposed; and, without the most accurate discrimination, will be productive of great mischief. So far as I have been able to judge, local bleeding, as it is termed, has not that general advantage over the general operation, as to justify the trouble of performing it; and I am almost led to pronounce it a more than useless resort in cases of mental disorder. Very ample experience does not dispose me to think more favourably of setons in the neck.

Blistering the head, the back of the neck, or between the shoulders, has also been of doubtful effect; and more dependence has been placed on the same operation on remoter parts.

In three old cases, the actual cautery has been applied in its fullest extent, to the head, in the manner proposed and practised by Monsieur Valentin, a French surgeon, of reputation, as I am told; and although succeeded by exfoliations of the outer table of the scull, the result has not justified a repetition of so severe a remedy.

As a means of temporary mitigation, under a furious paroxysm, accompanied by strong arterial action and increased heat, the shower bath has been usefully applied. Though it is not to be supposed that any case of madness is to be removed by its operation, as has often occurred in certain states of febrile disease, much advantage may be derived from its proper application.

The means of safe keeping by bars and bolts, and cords and chains, are abundant, and easily obtained; but it should be the supreme object of those who have assumed the supreme responsibility of governing the insane, to restore to their reason and to society the greatest possible number of these afflicted beings; and we have no hesitation in believing, that this will be most certainly accomplished by strict attention to a moral regimen. The greatest improvements in the treatment of madness have been of this nature; and the most approved physical agents of modern times were familiar to our remotest ancestors. With such views, the recovery of the deranged is not to be forgotten in the mazes of abstract research, nor in those wild speculations on the nature of the reasoning faculty, under the influence of which it is often difficult to determine where the greatest alienation exists, whether in the patient, or in him who has the care of him.

The order and internal economy and government of the New York Lunatic Asylum have justly placed it in the highest rank among the best institutions of our country; and the most improved establishments of the kind in Europe, do not afford a source of higher congratulation on the benefits they have afforded to the most afflicted of our race. The period is not remote, when a variety of circumstances conspired to render the very name of a madhouse a subject of terror and dismay. The prevailing opinion of the friends of its unhappy tenants was, that they were placed within its walls, not as in a situation, where they might by lenity and kind treatment, be restored to the blessings of health and reason, but as in a place of safe keeping; disabled from injuring themselves and others; where, from the supposed nature of their disorder, they neither deserved nor would receive the compassion of their keepers, and where they would inevitably languish and die. Thanks to the wisdom and humanity of the times in which we live, lunatic asylums have not only excited the attention of the benevolent everywhere, but have also been the subject of legislative investigation in one of the most enlightened countries of Europe. It was on inquiry discovered in England, that the contributions which had been made with a liberal hand towards their support, both in town and county, where [were] shamefully misapplied, and lavished on these, who, by neglect and cruelty, had merited and received the severest reprehensions of an abused people. Under their former structure, everything that met the view of the exiled sufferer, about to enter them, was suited to convey the idea of confinement and restraint and that he was immured in, and subject to the hardship of a prison; an impression of lasting and pernicious tendency. He was indeed, there shut up from the world, separated from his friends, and covered from the light of day; and, amidst the aggravated horrors of a dungeon, the chains which rivetted his ghastly figure to the ground, bound also in everlasting night, the distinguishing attributes of his being. In such a situation, without an effort to revive the suspended energies of his mind, with nothing to awaken him to a sense of his human nature, without a ray of consolation, of affection, or of sympathy to beam upon him, he remained a neglected, forgotten and abandoned prisoner. Thus forlorn, the whole plan and system of his custody, were of a nature to drive him to despair, and to the hopeless, the awful condition of irremediable madness. Asylums for the insane ought no longer to be viewed as places of personal security merely, but the temporary abode of a class of fellow beings, having the strongest claims to our sympathy and regard; furnished with the means of comfort, amusement, and employment adapted to the circumstances of their condition and the nature of their disease.

In the supervision and general superintendence of such an institution, I would take the liberty to recommend for the most obvious reasons, permanency of appointment, when justified by the qualifications of the elected. The appointed should be reasonable, humane, moral and religious, possessing stability and dignity of character, mild and gentle in their temper and deportment, but resolute in their purposes, and of great self command; never attempting by ill directed efforts and superior strength, to subdue the unconscious violence of their charge; of just and sagacious observation, and endued with clear and unclouded minds; so compassionate, and of such intelligence, as not only to take an interest in the unhappy lot of the objects of their trust, but to be able to assist them in the recovery of their reason. In their ordinary visits, they should approach the insane with an air of gentleness and kindness, expressive of concern for their unhappy condition, a deportment, which will not fail to augment their respect and confidence, on occasions requiring a more stern and distant intercourse. They should watch, with discriminating and unwearied attention, those favorable moments of drawing them from their hallucinations, their fantasies and wanderings, which frequently occur in the intermissions of many cases, both of madness and melancholy. The blunders of the ignorant and unskilful in the treatment of bodily disease, are generally of rapid effect, and may soon end in the death of their victim; but in the management of the insane, they are of slow, deep, and lasting consequence.

In the arrangement and structure of the asylum now erecting, whether as connected with this house, or as a separate establishment, I beg leave to suggest, that while it is of much importance that it be so constructed as to convey no idea but that of comfort, it may also admit of a classification of the patients during the day, according to their sexes, condition of life, and various states of derangement, in separate apartments of convenient dimensions. This is an object of such moment that although requiring an additional number of attendants, appears to be deserving of serious consideration; and it is confidently believed, that its advantages would amply repay any additional expence which might arise from a variation of form. It is also recommended that a distinct building be provided for the most raving and noisy, who should be constantly under the inspection of a faithful, humane and discreet attendant.

A convalescent should at all times be separated from the most insane. While permitted to see in the countenances and conduct of those around him, multiplied examples of the deplorable state from which he is emerging, what can be more adapted to overthrow his feeble and yet tottering intellect?

The furious maniac; who from occasional, but remote acts of violence, may have required the most rigid restraint, ought at times to be released from his chain and his cell, to be led forth to the refreshing influence of an untainted air, and the liberty of such exercise as may promote so free and equal a circulation, as shall counteract that morbid structure and disorganization, whatever their nature, which confirm and prolong his disease, and finally render it incurable. When released, it is advised that he should not associate with the deranged, but continue under the eye of an attendant, both capable and willing to improve every advantage of his ameliorated condition. It is only by thus extending the freedom of the violent that we can ascertain the changes their malady may have undergone. Neglect in performing so imperious a duty is a negative act of unpardonable cruelty which there are strong reasons to believe, has often doomed to immeasurable suffering many a wretched inmate of a lunatic asylum. What must be the feelings of that being, who, month after month, and year after year, fettered with chains, and shut up in darkness, yet possessing the powers of intellect, is incapable of rousing the sympathy of his keepers, and can contemplate in the grave only, the termination of his suffering? With what an aggravated sense of horror must we view his forsaken condition, if at the same time, he is cut off from the cheering light and consolations of the Gospel, the blessed refuge of the afflicted? It is stated, that at the house of correction at Kendal in England, a maniac, who had lucid intervals of nine to ten months duration, was confined in a solitary cell for ten whole years, without occupation, and without seeing a human being but those who brought him food.

In the arrangements of the new asylum, it is presumed that considerable advantage would be derived from an exclusive appropriation of two large apartments for the sick of the two sexes, having allowed to each an attendant, who should remain with them during the night as well as the day. With such a provision, the sufferer, in whose mind the light of reason has been long extinguished, might, during that gleam of intellect, which frequently attends the closing scene of life, be made to know that he is a human being meriting and receiving the compassion and kind offices of his fellows. Without such accommodation, many do, and must unavoidably die unseen.

There is perhaps nothing of more real importance to the comfort and recovery of the sick and insane, as respects the internal provisions of the house, than a plentiful supply of water. At this establishment, some difficulty and delay have attended the prescriptions for tepid bathing, an application not only of great utility in many cases of mental disorder, but essential also for washing and purifying the skin, and promoting that cleanliness which is so necessary to health, as well as comfort, in every situation. Where the quantity of this most necessary article is most abundant, conveniences under the usual calls of nature, may be so constructed and arranged in some of the apartments, and especially in those of the sick, as that their contents may be removed by a stream of water, conveyed by pipes in the walls of the building, passing constantly through them.

It appears to me that the marble floor of the hall of the basement of this house, without possessing any particular advantage from its material, produces a degree of dampness, not only uncomfortable, but hurtful to the persons who daily occupy it in our colder seasons.

The expediency, propriety, and utility of public worship, cannot be too strongly inculcated, under proper regulations and restrictions, in every building appropriated to the reception of persons labouring under mental disease.

With respect to the amusements and various occupations of the deranged, as a means of arresting their wanderings, and thereby contributing to their recovery, many useful remarks may be found in some of the publications on insanity. I would recommend that in all their recreations, whether of labor, or skill, or amusement, they should be separated from each other, and classed, as far as circumstances will admit, with the sane, engaged in similar amusements and pursuits. It has been found that such employments and recreations as require the most bodily exertion, have been the most beneficial.

It is submitted to the committee, if a full supply of the succulent vegetables of the season, would not be a reasonable, as it is considered a proper and salutary indulgence, to the patients of this institution.

I cannot, Gentlemen, close this long report, without an apology for so great a trespass on your time, and expressing to you my high sense of the support afforded me in the arduous duties of my appointment, as well as by your example, as by a prompt acquiescence in the means which have been occasionally proposed for the benefit and comfort of the patients of the asylum. For your uniform tokens of personal respect and kindness, I beg you to receive my warmest acknowledgments.

To Mr. Wilson, the superintendent, I am much indebted for his faithful attendance, and ready co-operation with me under the various circumstances in which his services have been required. To Doctor Joshua Fisher, for his able assistance in every department of duty claiming my attention, we are under the highest obligations; and for the polite and friendly aid on various emergencies, of Doctor Campbell, the house physician, I cannot adequately express my thankfulness; and it is with no ordinary emotions that I acknowledge the respectful civilities of the superior and subordinate officers, generally, of the New-York Hospital.

I am with much respect
GENTLEMEN, your obliged
and obedient servant
WILLIAM HANDY

Asylum 15th May, 1818

Although the by-laws required the physician to visit the asylum regularly three times a week, the record of attendance shows that Dr. Handy seldom failed to make a visit every day. His 75 clinical histories furnish the only detailed descriptions of the patients and their treatment in the asylum that have been found. All except eight relate to patients who were admitted during the years 1817 and 1818. The total number admitted during these years was, however, 124. Some of the cases which had been in the asylum for a longer period were also reviewed, and special measures of treatment were undertaken with a view to improving their condition. Of a man of thirty who had been in the asylum since 1812, it was recorded that he had been confined to bed since his admission, and was found in October, 1817, to be sullen and silent. Treatment was instituted by the use of actual cautery and scarification of his scalp. In January, 1818, it was recorded that no benefit had resulted. The patient was then taken from his cell into the yard every day and encouraged to work. In a few days he became more tractable, offered his hand to the physician for the first time, and accepted work. On July 25 he was considered sufficiently well to be transferred to the almshouse. A woman of thirty-eight who had been admitted in 1808 was, in June, 1818, noted to be sullen, reticent, and so violent that she was in a strait jacket. She was released from confinement and permitted to walk with a nurse in the hall and later in the city. She became mild, orderly, and submissive, the change being attributed to the liberty granted. In August it was recorded that she was "tranquil and inoffensive."

Although Dr. Handy's histories relate only to a little more than half of the total number admitted during the years 1817 and 1818, they were probably fairly representative of the general run of admissions to the asylum. Fifty-one of the 75 patients were men, and 24 were women. A similar preponderance of men prevailed through the whole period of operation of the first asylum, though later, as will be related, there were far more women than men. Eleven of the patients had received previous treatment at the asylum. The majority were comparatively young, more than half being not more than 30, and 4 were under 20. Only 11 were over 40, and only one over 60. In a number of instances, the age was stated to be "about" that given. Among their occupations the men included one banker, 5 merchants, 5 mechanics, 3 manufacturers, 3 coachmen, 7 seamen, 2 farmers, one chemist, one domestic (male), one tavern keeper, one law student, and one "gentleman." One woman was a washerwoman, and one a sailor's wife. With these exceptions the occupations of the women, or those of their husbands, were not mentioned. Twenty-five of the patients were residents of New York City. The residence of 26 others was not given, and it seems probable that they also resided in the city. Two were from the state prison. The others, except one from Boston, were residents of 21 towns and cities of New York State, one from each except Albany, from which 2 were received.

Considerable effort was made to obtain histories of the patient's illness previous to admission, and when this was unsuccessful, it was, Dr. Handy wrote, "much to be regretted on all occasions." In about a third of the cases no previous history was recorded. In others, the history was too meager to be of much value. In quite a large proportion, however, the information obtained was, considering the times and circumstances, remarkably full and pertinent. A tendency to attribute the illness to some definite single "cause" was frequently noticeable. Mental causes were such as death of a relative, loss of property or position, domestic infelicity ("excited by a scolding wife," "some connubial jealousies"), religious "impressions" ("quarrel with wife over joining the Baptist Church," "Certain religious impressions and imagery of damnation for her and her whole family"). Physical causes were such as brain disease, fevers, childbirth, sudden suppression of uterine hemorrhage produced by cold applications, alcoholic indulgence, camphor and mercury fumes. In many instances, however, the complexity of factors in the development of the illness was evidently understood. Evidence of inquiry in regard to heredity is revealed in such entries as, "no insanity in the family," or "disease hereditary," "mother several times in the asylum and now well," "mother in a manic state when patient was born," "father and many relatives had the same trouble." Previous attacks, in which the patient had been treated at home, frequently with restraining apparatus, solitary confinement, and drastic remedies, were recorded in some cases. One woman, apparently a case of dementia praecox, was confined in a dark room at home for two months. She afterwards died of tuberculosis.

The condition of the patients between "attacks" was not always clearly described, and some had been mentally ill for months or years before resorting to hospital treatment. Admission to the asylum was, in nearly all instances, occasioned by manifestations for which restraint and treatment had become imperative.

The description of the cases was evidently not related to any system of classification of mental disorders. All were "maniacs." In only a comparatively few cases can an approximation be made to identifying them in the classifications followed at the present time. Apparently, 21 cases (28 percent of the total) presented some of the characteristics of schizophrenic forms of reaction. The following is an abstract of the history of a case of this kind in which a fairly full account is given of the development of the illness:

CASE 25: Male, age 22. Admitted August 30, 1817. He had already been a patient in the asylum for a short time from July 7 to August 19th. The history previous to his admission was obtained from his physician, and from one of his teachers who had been intimately acquainted with the family for fifteen years. The patient was the only son of fond and indulgent parents. He was educated at the New York Literary Institution, and, from childhood, was remarkable for the correctness of his morals and his application to books. His parents wished him to remain at home and enter his father's business of tanner and currier. This, his teacher believed, "constituted the important crisis of the young man's life." The patient considered that he had been too well educated to waste the prime of his days in mechanical employment, and he was much opposed to the proposal. He was prevailed upon, however, to enter the currying shop. He worked there for six weeks, but complained of a pain in his chest and ill health, and he was then permitted to discontinue. His only employment, thereafter, was occasional attendance at a country store and tavern kept by his father. He took no interest in his father's concerns, and became more and more gloomy, sullen, discontented, and hypochondriacal. He was much under the influence of "religious impressions," reading much in the Bible and attending religious meetings. He disdained the rustic society of the neighborhood, and "his mind appeared to be left a prey to the gloom of solitude." In July, 1815, he went to Charleston, South Carolina, by boat, and returned by land. On the way home he stopped at "the sweet springs in Virginia" and contracted a fever, "which was succeeded by such a state of mental derangement as made it necessary to confine him in a straight jacket." He was brought home, and during the winter of 1816 and 1817, he worked in the store of a physician, and was constantly attending to and prescribing for a variety of ailments with which he considered himself affected, while in the opinion of others he was in good health. About the first of July, "his maniacal symptoms returned and overwhelmed him, he became frantic and has ever since been subject to paroxysms of madness" so violent as to require the use of restraints. His greatest rage was directed to the members of his family. The paroxysms were of short duration, and in the intervals he was rational and agreeable. He was brought to the asylum on July 7th, and was treated with mercury; without benefit. There is no record of this period or that between his discharge on August 19th and his readmission on the 30th. On September 26th, a seton was placed in the back of his neck, and was kept there, discharging freely, until December 13th. No improvement was noted until February 4th, 1818, and few entries were made during the interval from his admission. He was then recorded as "obviously more uniformly consistent in his conduct and conversation." His manner was less restless and hurried, and he was not so irascible. On the 21st it was noted that he was walking in the city, dining with friends, and manifesting to his sisters "at least a partial return of that natural affection for them, the absence of which they have so long and deeply mourned." After spending a couple of days at the house of a friend two miles from town, it was noted on February 24th that "his entire demeanour indeed, during the time mentioned, has been marked with such propriety as to warrant his being pronounced cured of the malady under which he was placed in the Asylum," and he was "accordingly dismissed from the house." On March 21st, he called on the physician, who noted that he had become more corpulent. He was, as formerly, rapid in all his actions, and in his manner of speaking. He was confident of the permanence of his cure. "On its being recommended to him to endeavor to forget that he had ever been an inhabitant of the asylum, he said he thought it would be useful to him in his future career not to forget it, but on the contrary to retain a lively recollection of it, as it might hereafter be a source of amusement as well as instruction to study and contemplate the various aberrations of the human intellect." No further reference to this patient has been found in the records.

The nature of mental illness of this form, and its probable further course, was not, at this period, understood as it is now. Dr. Handy's account of the case, is however, sufficiently accurate to permit of identification. Schizophrenic reactions of the different types are described in a number of the other histories.

Excitement and disorderly behavior of various types and degrees were mentioned in a large proportion of the histories. Sixteen of the cases, about 20 percent, were attributed to "intemperance in the use of ardent spirits." Not all of these cases seemed to present characteristic alcoholic symptoms, but excessive indulgence in alcoholic beverages was so prevalent, at that time, that it was no doubt a factor in the causation of a large number of the cases. Cases of pathological intoxication who were discharged after a few days' treatment; delirium with visions of the devil, tremors, and "furious madness," so severe as "to require to be chained"; hallucinatory states with depression, a feeling of extreme horror, "as if arising from guilt," and attempts to commit suicide; and a paranoic condition in a man of 51, whose wife was reluctant to have him at home even after he appeared to have recovered, seemed to be sufficiently distinguishable.

A considerable number of cases in which excitement and disorderly behavior were inadequately described cannot be positively identified with the forms in the present classifications.

CASE 27: Male, age 25. The record gave a history of 3 previous attacks, none of which was as severe as the present one. The duration of the present illness was, when he was admitted, 3 weeks, during which, it was stated, he had "raved," torn his clothes, and, though he was not vicious or violent, "it was thought necessary to manacle and confine him in a separate apartment." In the asylum, it was recorded that "he raves incessantly," was furious and destructive, and kept in close confinement. He had short periods when he was described as "mild, tranquil, submissive," but it was not until he had been in the asylum for 6 months that improvement seemed to be permanent; and he was allowed to walk in the yard. Soon afterwards it was recorded that he worked about the house with diligence and intelligence, and, after a total period in the asylum of more than 8 months, he was discharged "cured."

CASE 10: A black girl, age 18. On admission she was elated, very talkative, and seized with a delirium or mania "without being outrageous," which was followed by "furious madness requiring the coercion of chains, cords, &c." She had been in the asylum for a year when the first note was made. This stated that she had required the restraint of chains, but for 3 weeks had appeared to be sane and had been admitted to the large apartment with the other female patients. She was described as mild and respectful and was usefully employed in various duties of the house. An interesting observation was that, after it was mentioned to her that she would probably return home soon, she became more talkative and continued "to wear some trifling appendages to her dress, as a substitute, as she thinks for a watch." She relapsed into her previous state of excitement, and was placed in a "cell," and a strait jacket. After a period of treatment by bleeding and tartar emetic, during which she was from time to time allowed to leave the cell on trial, she was recorded as again improving and employed in assisting the attendants with their work. She continued well, and eventually it was stated "that she has voluntarily thrown aside those baubles of which she was once so fond, and her attachment to which marked the continuance of her disease." Three weeks after this note she was discharged "cured."

These two cases seemed to present a manic type of excitement, and there were a few others which could be so considered. Other cases, besides alcoholics, appeared to present delirious types of reaction, a few following childbirth or a fever.

Fourteen were cases in which depression of spirits seemed to be the leading manifestation. Six made desperate attempts to commit suicide. One woman of 47 was reported to have cut her throat several times.

CASE 39: Female, age 45. The history stated that 3 years previous to her admission she had in a period of mental illness, complained of pressure in her head and felt that she "must kill one of her family and must be imprisoned and executed, that the devil reigned and they must pray to him." She also, in this illness, tried to leave the house at night and throw herself into the river, and was described as obstinate, profane, and noisy. She was ill for 8 or 9 months. On admission to the asylum, she was apprehensive of being expelled because of noisy and disorderly behavior, was hopeless of recovery, and feared she would be exposed and become a reproach to her family. She accused her brother of deceiving her in bringing her to the asylum, and was sorry she had not destroyed herself on the passage from Albany. In about 6 weeks she had improved sufficiently to leave the asylum and live with a companion at "The Narrows," Long Island, where the physician of the asylum visited her. She continued to improve and, in a little more than 5 months from her admission, she went home "under the strongest hope and expectation that when once more restored to her family, she would again return to the enjoyment of those intellectual blessings which are above all price."

This was apparently a depression of the anxious, apprehensive type.

CASE 12: Female, 27. Six months previous to admission, she had become depressed after the death of her child. She was described as having been at first thoughtful and melancholy. She then became "completely deranged" and in a "state of great fury," singing day and night. After admission, she was at first talkative, with intervals of silence and melancholy. This patient was admitted about 9 months previous to Dr. Handy's appointment, and little information in regard to her condition during that period appears in the record. Various measures of treatment were noted, including a "shock of electricity through her head; without evident injury." It was also stated that she had been "confined to her cell, under restraint of chains from admission." She was removed from the cell by Dr. Handy and "when disposed to be unruly, the extravagance of her conduct has been overcome by the dread of confinement." Two months later, she was described as no longer mischievous, and as easily governed. She was silent, with occasional answers to questions, and melancholy. She spent the days with the other patients in the large room. She was treated repeatedly by light shocks of electricity through the hypogastrium, and was given a course of mercury until she was salivated. It was not until a year and a half after her admission that she was considered to have recovered and was discharged "cured."

This may have been a case of manic depressive psychosis. Disorderly behavior was, however, at this period, treated with severity, as to rule the patient by fear was considered a proper psychotherapeutic procedure. The confinement of a patient in a cell, the use of a strait jacket, or a chain, and the administration of shower baths, might therefore, in some instances have contributed to the noisy and violent behavior which occasioned the treatment. The treatment of this patient by a "shock of electricity through the head without evident injury," is noteworthy with reference to the electric-shock treatment of today. Another case was apparently one of general paresis, a disease which was not described in medical literature until 1822, four years after this case was recorded.

CASE 23: Male, age not stated. Admitted August 8, 1816. No account of the case was recorded until after Dr. Handy became physician of the asylum in September, 1817. It was stated that great pains had been taken to obtain the history. The cause of the patient's illness had been variously ascribed to loss of property and disappointment in love. Dr. Handy, however, considered that it did not originate from either of these causes. He learned from the patient's brother that the patient, in voyages to tropical countries, had suffered from fever, dysentery, and a pulmonary complaint. In 1813 physicians in New York had stated that his disorder was due either to rheumatism of the head or syphilis. In the winter of 1815–1816 his "mind began to change." He became very talkative, hurried in his actions, manifested angry passions, and his speech was impaired. It was supposed that he must have had a paralytic stroke. "In this state of mental and physical infirmity," he was brought to the asylum. The first observation of his condition in the asylum was noted on October 4, 1817. He was then unable to stand or walk unless supported by another person, and he appeared to be incapable of articulating. On October 17, it was recorded that there were ulcers on his hips and sacral region. On January 12, 1818, he had become very feeble and emaciated, and the ulcers had extended. On the 18th, his countenance was described as "placid and marked with an air of cheerfulness." He had evidently been confined in a strait jacket, as it was directed that it be removed and the "straps of the tranquilizer to be taken from his ankles." It was noted later that the ulcers were healing. On February 17 he was losing strength daily. On March 14 his mind and speech remained as before, and he was growing more feeble. On March 24 he had diarrhoea, and on the 25th he died, "without the smallest previous glimmer of reason."

Six of the 75 patients died, and on one an autopsy was done.

CASE 38: Female, age not stated. The patient had been continuously in the asylum from February 12, 1813, until her death on April 16, 1818. She had been previously admitted on September 12, and discharged "cured" on October 9, 1812. In her earlier asylum residence she was "much more insane," and sometimes required "the usual restraints of the violent." Since September, 1817, her deportment had been generally mild, with no regular combination of ideas, and her conversation was incoherent and desultory. She assisted in various occupations about the house. She had grown feeble and

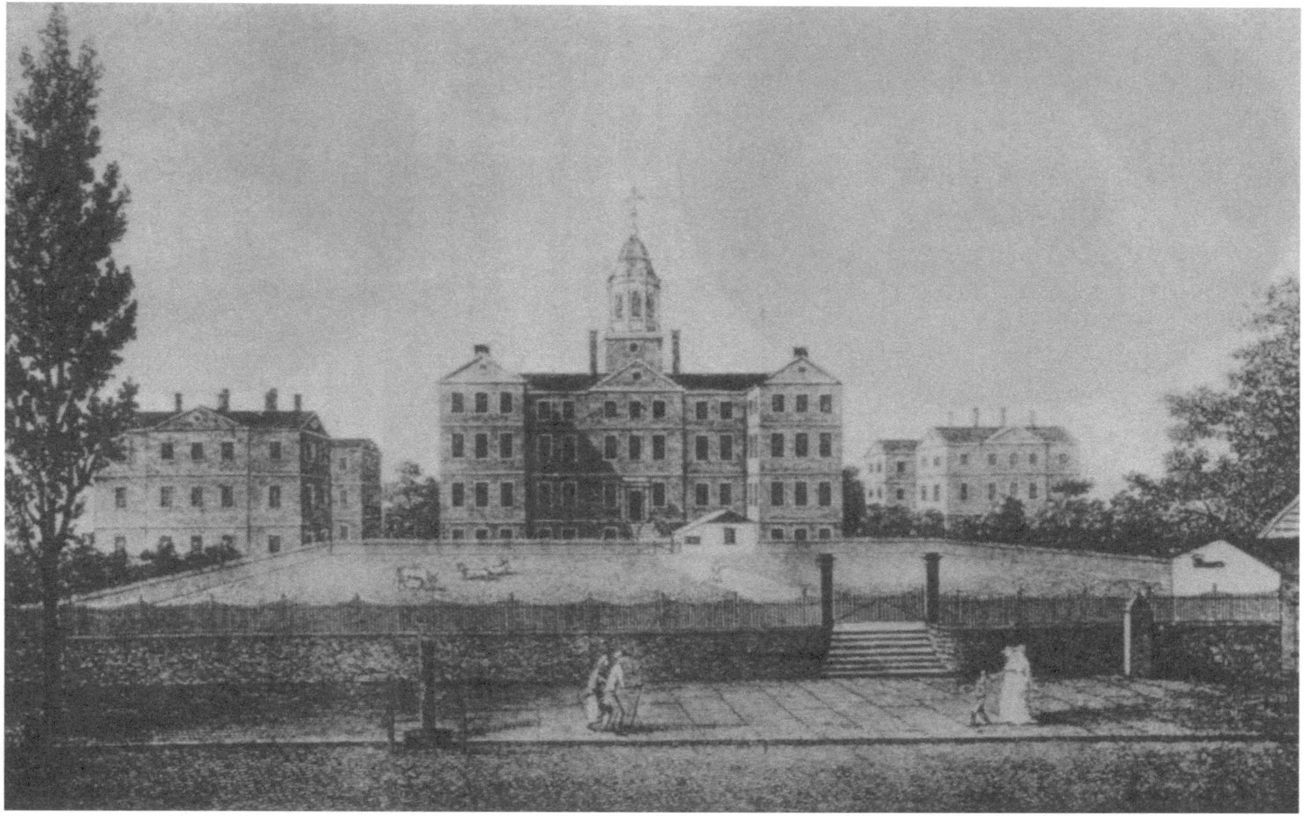

THE NEW YORK HOSPITAL AND "MEDICAL ASYLUM," 1808-1821

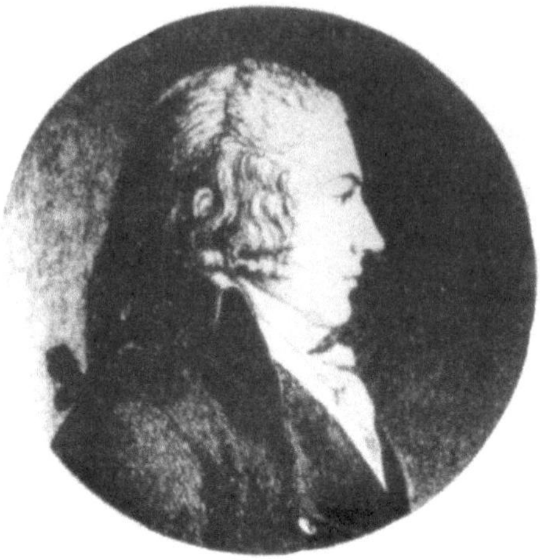

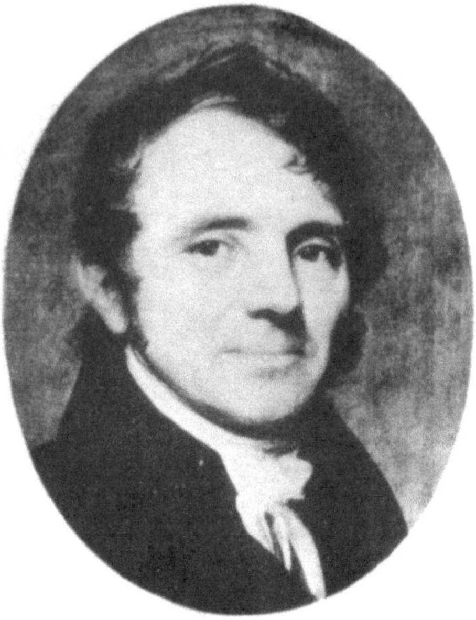

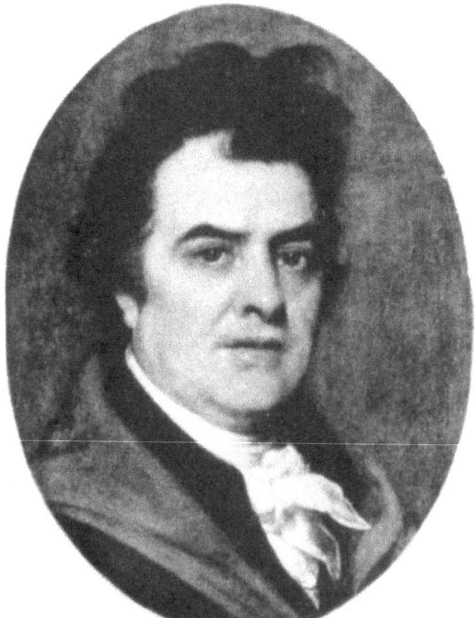

DAVID HOSACK, M.D.
PHYSICIAN OF THE ASYLUM, 1819

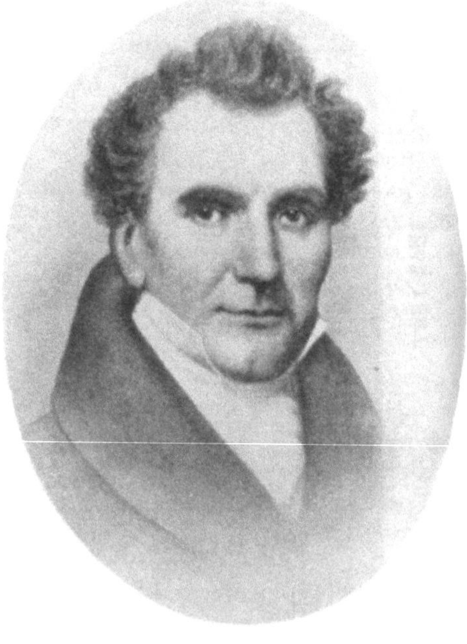

JOHN NEILSON, M.D.
PHYSICIAN OF THE ASYLUM, 1819-1830

emaciated, with frequent weak pulse and dyspnoea. She had "but little cough," and a good appetite. Ten days before death she developed diarrhoea and her lower extremities became "highly oedematous."

The autopsy revealed "evident marks of determination of blood to the brain." An aqueous fluid was discharged from the external surface of the dura mater, and a considerable quantity of a similar fluid was found "in the basis of the scull." The brain on its upper surface, and the interspersed veins "exhibited an extended aspect," and the latter appeared to be much enlarged. Attached to the convex surface of the brain and between the hemispheres was "a firm substance, the fifth of an inch in thickness, of a light buff colour, somewhat resembling fat." The "cineritious substance" was of a paler cast than is generally noticed so soon after death, "say four hours." The corpora striata were of similar paleness. Some water was suffused in the lateral ventricles; the pineal gland contained a gritty matter. In the thorax there were pleuritic adhesions. "Numerous tubercles occupied the lungs themselves, which were also in a state of universal suppuration." The heart was natural in appearance, and the pericardium contained the usual amount of fluid. The abdominal viscera were normal. The uterus was filled and distended with a caseous like substance.

To the physician of the present day, it must seem remarkable that the extensive disease of the lungs discovered by autopsy in this case, was not mentioned in the clinical record. Nothing, however, could better illustrate the progress that has been made in clinical medicine than the character of the physical examinations recorded in these histories. Clinical medicine, as now practiced, was still in its early stages. Precise methods of examination, with instruments of precision, had not yet been introduced into general medical practice. In a large proportion of the histories the admission note contained no reference to the physical condition, and throughout the histories the rate and quality of the pulse, the condition of the tongue, the skin, and the bowels seemed to constitute all that was regularly noted, to which was added, as occasion arose, such gross subjective and objective symptoms as could scarcely escape notice.

In some instances, the general appearance of the patient was noted on admission, with regard perhaps to some lingering respect for the doctrine of humoral pathology and temperament.[5] Such descriptions as "form slender, countenance melancholy, eyes dark and animated expression; Hair and complexion dark," "dark complexion, grey eyes, apparently of sanguineo-melancholic temperament," were frequently recorded. In some instances it was evident that the advantage of knowledge of the personality of the patient previous to the illness was appreciated.

[5] See Chapter I.

Of one patient, it was recorded that "when in health her habit was delicate, modest, intelligent, unassuming, pious." Of another, it was stated that

> in health he was estimable, noble-minded, warm heart, good temper, brave, generous, strong attachments and weak resentments, easily directed by friends, persevering, faithful to purpose however laborious, good and comprehensive talents, first rank as an arithmetician, considerable proficiency in mathematics, particularly such as related to navigation. Temperate, abhorred drunkenness.

It would hardly be proper to assume that Dr. Handy's 75 cases present illustrations of the standards of study and treatment which were followed at the Asylum of the New York Hospital during all of the thirteen years of its operation. However, occasional references in the reports of the Asylum and Inspecting Committees, and other notes made by Dr. Handy relating to a few patients who had been treated at the asylum previous to his appointment, contain the only other information concerning the previous medical treatment and management of patients that has been found. As has already been intimated, it seems highly probable that Dr. Handy made a substantial contribution to the advancement of the standards. He evidently endeavored to adhere to the principles and practices discussed in his report to the governors on May 15, 1818, but he did not discard entirely the prevailing practices. His skepticism of their value, however, led him to exercise moderation and discrimination in their employment. He considered "mild cathartics and warm bathing . . . of more general utility than any other means employed as physical agents in the treatment of insanity." He gave medicines only "when strongly indicated by such symptoms of bodily disease, as were supposed instrumental in exciting, or had been connected with the disorder of the mind."

The medication was apparently fully recorded in the histories. In scarcely a dozen of the cases, were the "rough purges," of jalap, calomel, and gamboge administered. Senna, rhubarb, magnesia, were given in electuaries, and aloes with other substances in pills. Tartar emetic was given in small doses with the purgative in some cases, and, in three or four instances of intense excitement only, in larger doses, when it operated "sursum et dorsum," after which the patient was invariably "tranquil." A course of mercury to produce salivation was administered in ten instances. Dr. Handy stated in his report to the governors that there was "but one instance in which it was considered that the recovery was the result of its use." Digitalis, which was at this time considered by some observers to be a valuable remedy in the treatment of mania, was prescribed in a few cases. The sedatives employed were hyoscyamus, camphor, and, in a very few instances, opium. This form of medication for restlessness, sleeplessness, and excitement was, apparently, resorted to less extensively than it is, by many practitioners, at the present time. Valerian and asafoetida were prescribed in some instances. Bitter tonics, iron, and wine were used in the treatment of feeble patients and convalescents. Medication seemed to be the main reliance in treatment, and the notes consisted principally of the medicines prescribed and their effect. In one case, however, "all medicine at length laid aside" was recorded, as though for the purpose of observing the effect, and it was nearly three months before it was resumed.

Other measures which were, at that period, universally resorted to in the treatment of the mentally ill had a place in the asylum service. For patients who would not eat, "coercion" was sometimes considered necessary. The feeding tube had apparently not yet been adopted. A funnel was, however, used in some way, and in some instances the sight of it was sufficiently persuasive. Dr. Handy approved of bloodletting "in violent paroxysms," and his records mentioned fifteen instances. Venesection was seldom employed, although "copious blood-letting" was recorded in a few instances, and, in one, the patient was bled nine times. The method most frequently used was cupping, and the amount of blood withdrawn was never large. Dr. Handy mentioned in his report to the governors that "in three old cases" he had employed a form of treatment "practised by Monsieur Valentin, a French surgeon." The treatment described in the record of one of his cases consisted of the application of the actual cautery to the scalp, followed by extensive scarification. Blisters were employed with about the same frequency as bleeding. They were usually applied to the ankles, to the back of the neck, and between the shoulder blades. They were sometimes opened and kept discharging for a considerable time, and were then called "issues." A strip of muslin looped through incisions in the skin of the back of the neck was called a "seton," and was used quite frequently.

A warm or tepid bath was mentioned in the record of a few cases. As there was no plumbing and no circulating water in the building, its administration must have been difficult. The shower bath was prescribed much more frequently. It was apparently considered to be refreshing and invigorating, and it was in some instances prescribed for these purposes. More frequently, however, it was evidently a means of discipline and punishment, and was disliked by the patients. Tearing clothing or bedding, removal of all clothing, or soiling the room or cell, was usually followed promptly by exposure to the shower bath. Attempts to escape, or mischievous behavior, such as throwing the hat of one of the patients "into the necessary" in the yard, were punished in the same way. "Restless and mischievous for which he had a shower bath" is another note. Of one patient, it was recorded that "she struck me in the face with the palm of her hand. Directed instantly the shower bath." Three days later it was recorded that she had been "very correct in her conduct since she had the shower bath." This mode of "punishment" was resorted to in the treatment of 15 of the 75 cases. That it was rather futile in some instances is revealed by its use in the treatment of a schizophrenic boy of eighteen, who was reproved for silly behavior and laughing, and, when this was continued, it was ordered that he was "to have a shower bath as a punishment for his disobedience." In another case, a shower bath was given a patient for an attempt to escape from the yard, "to discourage from future attempts." A week later, however, he did escape and went to his home in Albany.

The usual procedure when a patient was excited and disorderly was to place him in solitary confinement in a "cell" or room, presumably one of those in the subbasement. If further measures of control seemed necessary, a strait jacket was used, or he was fastened to the wall by means of a chain. These measures were employed in the treatment of 7 or 8 of the 75 cases. Of one patient it was recorded that he was placed in the "tranquilizer" where he was apparently treated for eight days, and of another, that order was given for the removal of the straps of the "tranquilizer" from his ankles. As the purchase of a chair from the Pennsylvania Hospital at a cost of $28 was noted in the superintendent's accounts,[6] the "tranquilizer" mentioned was no doubt a chair devised by Dr. Rush for the treatment of disturbed patients.

The records show, however, that Dr. Handy was guided by the precepts set forth in his report, and that the patient in confinement was "at times to be released from his chain and his cell, to be led forth to the refreshing influence of an untainted air." Apparently, an effort was made to remove the patients from solitary confinement and restraining apparatus as soon as possible, and a walk in the yard, or a trial visit to the large room where there were other patients was recorded in a number of instances. This course was followed in the treatment of patients who had been in confinement or restraint for a long time, as well as of those recently admitted. Evidently, the plan of treatment of all the patients

[6] Superintendent's General Expenses, July 31, 1811. See p. 234.

was directed to their adjustment to liberty. It was noted of a patient, who was restless and dissatisfied, that she "visited various parts of the house with seeming interest and reasonable satisfaction." Another patient was permitted, from time to time, to visit her children who were in the alms-house. Of other patients, it was noted that they had been in the city with an attendant. One man visited his home "to attend to business." A colored man "went home with an attendant to visit his sick wife." Patients who seemed to be recovering were allowed to "walk out daily and return," and to visit friends in the city. Their liberty was gradually extended to visits, day after day, returning in the evening, and eventually remaining overnight. In some instances, the patient went home "on trial." In one instance, removal of the patient was disapproved, as it was thought inadvisable that he should return to his home in Troy, "until it was fully determined by his remaining a fortnight out of the asylum whether or not he was still in a state of mind to return to his family." This advice was not followed, and it was necessary to return him to the asylum in about two weeks. Although no special provision was made for employment as a measure of treatment, in several instances it was recorded that the patient was usefully employed about the house, or in assisting the attendants. Instructions to this effect were sometimes given by the physician.

After Dr. Handy resigned in November, 1818, the standards of visits to the patients were, as shown by the attendance record, maintained by his successor. No medical histories of this period have, however, been found, and it can only be assumed that the example he had given of intensive study and treatment was, in some measure, followed.

PART THREE

The Founding of Bloomingdale Asylum 1815-1840

X: THOMAS EDDY AND A NEW SYSTEM OF TREATMENT

THE year 1792 is memorable in the annals of psychiatry. The form of provision for the mentally ill that is now found in every well-organized country was derived from a movement which seems to have assumed distinguishable dimensions in that year. Two outstanding events of the year contributed to this; namely, the reforms in the treatment of the mentally ill, dramatically instituted by Dr. Pinel in the hospitals of Paris,[1] and the establishment of the Retreat for the Insane at York, England, by the Society of Friends under the leadership of William Tuke. It is interesting also that in September of the same year the New York Hospital inaugurated its service for the mentally ill by the admission of its first case of that character. The methods of treatment adopted by Pinel, and in the management of the York Retreat, aroused much interest and attention. They became widely known, principally through the publications of Pinel and his followers, and the description of the Retreat published in 1813 by Samuel Tuke, grandson of the founder. A further impetus was given to the movement by the revelations of appalling abuses in the public and private asylums of Great Britain, which were contained in reports of committees of the House of Commons, by which they were investigated.[2]

Progress in making improvements was, however, extremely slow and attended with great difficulty and resistance. In fact, it can scarcely be said, even now, that the movement has everywhere—or, perhaps, any-

[1] Since the above was written it has been noted that, G. Zilboorg, *History of Medical Psychology* (New York, 1941), p. 321, states that Pinel was appointed to Bicêtre Hospital on August 25, 1793. Pinel, in his *Treatise on Insanity* (trans. 1806) p. 53, mentions his nomination as chief physician of Bicêtre "in the second year of the republic." Nevertheless, 1792 is the year usually mentioned in the literature from an early period; e.g., "Eulogy upon Pinel by M. Pariset, Aug. 28, 1828 (trans. *Am. J. Insanity*, II, 211), in which it is stated that "he entered upon his duties at the Bicêtre in the latter part of May 1792." Also in the *Dictionnaire de Médecine* (Paris, 1833), II, 165. Calmeil states: "Bientôt [1792] Pinel détache le premier les chaînes, dans l'hospice Bicêtre."

[2] House of Commons, *Report, together with the Minutes of Evidence, and an Appendix of Papers from the Committee Appointed to Consider Provision Being Made for the Better Regulation of Madhouses in England* (London, 1815).

where—reached its potential fulfillment. The first objective was to abolish a system in which it was considered proper "to detain maniacs in constant seclusion, and to load them with chains; to leave them defenceless to the brutality of underlings, in pretence of danger to be dreaded from their extravagances: in a word to rule them with a rod of iron." [3] Fortunately, it can now be said that such practices have been generally abandoned. The treatment adopted by Pinel and at the York Retreat went, however, much further. It was based on the conception that mentally ill persons were, by no means, deprived entirely of susceptibility to the same influences that determine the behavior of well persons. The motives which actuated both Pinel and Tuke were, indeed, humanitarian. Pinel, however, was a distinguished physician, and he understood the current medical doctrines relating to mental illness, and the measures employed generally in medical practice. He had tried them all, and was dissatisfied with the results. At the Bicêtre Hospital, he had observed that the kindly, tactful, yet just and firm management of the patients by a remarkably able lay superintendent and his staff of well disciplined attendants was apparently accomplishing more for their relief and cure than he was capable of with all his learning and resources as a physician. It seemed to him that he was witnessing a new form of treatment. "Being," he writes, "desirous of better information, I resolved to examine for myself the facts that were presented to my attention; and forgetting the empty honours of my titular distinction as a physician, I viewed the scene that was opened to me with the eye of common sense and unprejudiced observation." His carefully recorded observations revealed to him "that insanity was curable in many instances, by mildness of treatment and attention to the state of the mind exclusively, and when coercion was indispensible, that it might be effectually applied without corporal indignity." [4] Much of what he undertook was directed to the administration of the service. He did not, however, discontinue entirely the medication and other measures that had long been employed in medical practice.

It is interesting that, although Tuke was not a physician and had no knowledge of Pinel, the system of management he adopted at the York Retreat corresponded closely to that of the latter. The conditions at the Retreat were more favorable than those in the public hospitals of Paris. The institution was small, privately supported, and provided for patients who were of a better social grade. Neither chains nor corporal punishment was tolerated. If the strait jacket was used, the patient was

[3] Pinel, *op. cit.*, p. 184. [4] *Ibid.*, p. 108.

allowed to walk about. Instead of manacles and shackles, leather straps were used to restrain the arms and ankles. The arm straps were, in some instances, attached to a belt, which for women was made of green morocco, so as to have the appearance of an "ornament." The main reliance was, however, placed on "moral treatment or management," which was considered to be "of high importance." It was found that "furious mania" was exaggerated by harshness. Tolerance, tact, patient reasoning and persuasion, just, considerate, mild yet firm use of force, when indispensable, were found adequate in difficult situations. As far as possible, patients were treated as though they were normal. An effort was made to interest and employ them in normal activities. They were given the fullest trust and liberty permitted by their condition. Even the most disturbed were not allowed to go unclad, and they were encouraged to adopt orderly habits and to exercise self restraint. Much attention was given to their comfort and social life. Those who were sufficiently orderly and tractable had meals with the superintendent, matron, and other officials. Games, sports, and social entertainments, outdoor and indoor, were provided, and a variety of occupations. The patients entertained their visitors at tea parties and other social gatherings, and visited their own homes and the homes of their friends when possible. Medical treatment was indeed considered indispensable, and a physician was employed to visit the patients "several times a week." The first physician of the Retreat was Dr. Thomas Fowler, whose name is still familiar to physicians who prescribe "Fowler's Solution." After following the accepted forms of medical treatment for a period, Dr. Fowler, like Pinel, observed that medicines were "very inadequate means to relieve the most grievous of human diseases, and that bleeding, blisters, seatons, and evacuants were not of value unless indicated by the general state of the patient's health." He plainly "perceived how much was to be done by moral, and how little by any known medical means." He never forced medicine when the patient objected.[5]

It can scarcely be realized that principles and methods which are now commonplace routine in the operation of practically every properly conducted service for the treatment of the mentally ill, should, when first introduced, have been regarded as a new and specific form of treatment. It was designated "Moral Treatment," or "Management of the Mind," and, by some, it was considered that, as it was directed solely to the mind, it was different from medical treatment and could be administered separately. Pinel was criticized severely by some of his colleagues who ac-

[5] Samuel Tuke, *Description of the Retreat* (Philadelphia, 1813), pp. 71–72.

cused him of believing that the mind could be diseased separately from disease of the body. Much experience was required before the authorities, medical and lay, of hospitals and asylums for the mentally ill, apprehended the extent to which the general organization and administration were involved in this system of treatment of the patients, and that moral and medical treatment could not be separated. Gradually, the physicians, like Pinel, turned their attention to administration as a most effective means of treatment, and the form of organization in which the physician is also chief executive officer came finally to be accepted as the best in the operation of a service for the treatment of the mentally ill. The gradual steps by which this form of organization was adopted in the psychiatric service of the New York Hospital is one of the most interesting and instructive chapters in its history.[6] The hospital physician of today, absorbed in the study and treatment of the individual patients, may, with advantage, consider that the organization and facilities and the form of medical administration which work so effectively with him in the treatment of his patients have been laboriously built up as a means of administering what was at first regarded as "a course of moral treatment," which should be cherished and intelligently used.

It was not long before accounts of the movement in Europe began to appear in America. An abridged edition of Tuke's *Description of the Retreat* was published in Philadelphia in 1813, and the friends of humanity generally, and the Society of Friends particularly, were much impressed by the success which had crowned the benevolent exertions of the Friends at York. The influence of the Retreat was probably responsible for the establishment of the Friends' Asylum, at Frankford, Pennsylvania, in 1817. No one was, perhaps, more impressed than Thomas Eddy, one of the governors of the New York Hospital. Eddy was a Quaker, and, with others of the same faith, he was a tireless worker for the welfare of humanity. He was instrumental in establishing the State Prison, and occupied the position of inspector for seven years, during which time he introduced industries and conducted them so efficiently that during his last year of service, the profits of the prison labor equaled the cost of operation of the prison. Eddy was active in the establishment of the Bible Society, the Free School Society, the Manumission Society, the Savings Bank, the Society for the Reformation of Juvenile Delinquents, and the Humane Society (to provide food and other necessities to the poor, especially to debtors in prison who were required to furnish

[6] W. L. Russell, "A Chapter from the Evolution of Medical Administration," *Am. J. Psychiatry*, IV (1924), 125–133.

their own food). He was also greatly interested in the Indians. He participated actively with Governor Clinton in putting through the Erie Canal. Eddy became a governor of the Society of the New York Hospital in 1793, and his biographer states that new life was given to the board by the plans he proposed. Whatever he undertook he did with all his might, and from the age of thirty-five he devoted most of his life to the public welfare. It was stated by his biographer, however, that

> the claims of Mr. Eddy to a lasting consideration will, I think, rest mainly on the early begun and long continued zeal and abilities which he exhibited on the subject of insanity, and the unfortunate beings afflicted with this calamity. He read much and thought much on the subject of mental derangement, on prison and penitentiary discipline, on the structure and economy of mad-houses, and on the domestic and sanative treatment of the insane.[7]

He was, therefore, as a governor of the hospital, especially interested in improving provision for the mentally ill. He was much respected by the public authorities and was invariably selected by the board to represent them at Albany when legislation affecting the hospital was pending. He was largely instrumental in obtaining funds for the enlargement of the hospital in 1803, and for the establishment of the "Medical Asylum" in 1808. When a separate department for mental illness was established, he was a member of the first Asylum Committee. It is not surprising, therefore, that it was he who proposed to the governors that consideration be given to the new system of treatment of the mentally ill which had been introduced in Europe.

On April 4, 1815, he presented, at a special meeting of the board, a carefully prepared communication on the subject. He explained that it had closely engaged his attention for some years, and that his views had been considerably extended and enlightened by "perusing the writings of Doctors Creighton, Arnold and Rush; but, more particularly the account of the Retreat near York, in England." He had found that "the radical defect in all the different modes of cure that have been pursued, appears to be, that of considering mania a physical or bodily disease," and that "very lately a spirit of inquiry has been excited, which has given birth to a new system of treatment of the insane; and former modes of medical discipline have now given place to that which is generally denominated *moral management.*" He then added:

> Under these impressions I feel extremely desirous of submitting to the consideration of the Governors, a plan to be adopted by them, for introducing a

[7] S. L. Knapp, *Life of Thomas Eddy* (New York, 1834), p. 26.

system of moral treatment for the lunatics in the Asylum, to a greater extent than has hitherto been in use in this country. The great utility of confining ourselves almost exclusively to a course of moral treatment, is plain and simple, and incalculably interesting to the cause of humanity.[8]

He then reviewed the plan of treatment at the York Retreat, as described by Samuel Tuke, and suggested that, in the management of the Asylum of the New York Hospital, the following regulations be adopted: [9]

1st. No patient shall hereafter be confined by chains.

2nd. In the most violent states of mania, the patient should be confined in a room with the windows, etc., closed, so as nearly to exclude the light, and kept confined if necessary, in a straight jacket, so as to walk about the room or lie down on the bed at pleasure; or by strops etc., he may, particularly if there appears in the patient a strong determination to self-destruction, be confined on the bed, and the apparatus so fixed as to allow him to turn and otherwise change his positions.

3rd. The power of judicious kindness to be generally exercised, may often be blessed with good effects, and it is not till after other moral remedies are exercised, that recourse should be had to restraint, or the power of fear on the mind of the patient; yet it may be proper sometimes, by way of punishment, to use the shower bath.

4th. The common attendants shall not apply any extraordinary coercion by way of punishment, or change in any degree the mode of treatment prescribed by the physician; on the contrary, it is considered as their indispensable duty, to seek by acts of kindness the good opinion of the patients, so as to govern them by the influence of esteem rather than of severity.

5th. On the first day of the week, the Superintendent, or the principal keeper of the Asylum, shall collect as many of the patients as may appear to them suitable and read some chapters in the Bible.

6th. When it is deemed necessary to apply the strait jacket, or any other mode of coercion, by way of punishment or restraint, such an ample force should be employed as will preclude the idea of resistance from entering the mind of the patient.

7th. It shall be the duty of the deputy-keeper, immediately on a patient being admitted, to obtain his name, age, where born, what has been his employment or occupation, his general disposition and habits, when first attacked with mania; if it has been violent or otherwise, the cause of his disease, if occasioned by religious melancholy, or a fondness for ardent spirits, if owing to an injury received on any part of the body, or supposed to arise from any other known cause, hereditary or adventitious, and the name of the physician who may have attended him, and his manner of treating the patient while under his direction.

8th. Such of the patients as may be selected by the physician, or the Com-

[8] Thomas Eddy, *Hints for Introducing an Improved Mode of Treating the Insane in the Asylum* (New York, 1815), p. 4.

[9] *Ibid.*, pp. 12–15.

mittee of the Asylum, shall be occasionally taken out to walk or ride under the care of the deputy-keeper; and it shall be also his duty to employ the patients in such manner, and to provide them with such kinds of amusements and books as may be approved and directed by the Committee.

9th. The female keeper shall endeavor to have the female patients Constantly employed at suitable work; to provide proper amusements, books, etc., to take them out to walk as may be directed by the Committee.

10th. It shall be the indispensible duty of the keepers, to have all the patients as clean as possible in their persons, and to preserve great order and decorum when they sit down to their respective meals.

11th. It shall be the duty of the physician to keep a book, in which shall be entered an historical account of each patient, stating his situation, and the medical and moral treatment used; which book shall be laid before the Committee, at their weekly meetings.

Mr. Eddy was, however, not satisfied with proposing the introduction of "moral treatment" into the asylum then operating. He went on to say that

a further and more extensive improvement has occured to my mind, which I conceive, would very considerably conduce towards affecting the cure, and materially ameliorate the condition, and add to the comfort of the insane; at the same time it would afford an ample opportunity of ascertaining how far that disease may be removed by moral management alone, which, it is believed, will, in many instances, be more effectual in controlling the maniac, than medical treatment, especially in those cases where the disease has proceeded from causes operating directly upon the mind. I would propose that a lot, not less than ten acres, should be purchased by the Governors, conveniently situated, within a few miles of the city, and to erect a substantial building, on a plan calculated for the accomodation of fifty lunatic patients; the ground to be improved in such a manner as to serve for agreeable walks, gardens, etc., for the exercise and amusement of the patients; this establishment might be placed under the care and superintendence of the Asylum Committee, and be visited by them once every week: a particular description of patients to remain at this Rural Retreat; and such others as might appear suitable objects might be occasionally removed there from the Asylum.[10]

He closed his comunication with an estimate of cost and a schedule of successful operation and support.

Probably neither Mr. Eddy nor anyone else anticipated, when this communication was presented, the momentous change that was portended in the character of the service for the mentally ill of the New York Hospital. Eddy apparently contemplated such a service both at the hospital in the city and at the "Rural Retreat." What it might have

10 Eddy, *op. cit.*, pp. 15–17.

meant to the development of psychiatry in medical practice, teaching, and scientific investigation if his views and plan had been adopted can scarcely be estimated. The time, however, was not favorable for such a development, and it was not until more than a century had elapsed that social, economic, and scientific advances brought about relationships with the general hospital similar to those he proposed. The communication was referred to a committee, which on July 3 made the following report: [11]

The Committee appointed to consider the Expediency of Erecting another Building for the Accomodation of Insane Persons Report,

That another Building for the Use of those unfortunate persons who have lost the Use of their reason, is not only adviseable, but seems to be absolutely necessary.

That though there are at present more patients in the Asylum by nearly one third, than can with perfect safety, and the best hopes of recovery, be lodged there; many more insane persons, perhaps twenty within a few Months, have by their friends, been soliciting a place in that Building. In speaking of the want of safety, the Committee only mean to express an Opinion, that when two or more insane persons, from the want of room are lodged to-gether in one Cell, the life of the weaker must be somewhat endangered by the stronger, who in a high Paroxysm of insanity might strangle him in his sleep, or otherwise destroy him.

That such additional Building, from the want of room, cannot possibly be erected near the Hospital, in this City.

That there are many reasons for believing, that the recovery from a State of insanity would be greatly promoted, by having a considerable space of ground adjoining the Asylum or Public Building, in which many of the patients might have the privilege of walking, or taking other kinds of exercise.

That considering the various kinds of Insanity, your Committee are clearly of the Opinion, that two Buildings should be erected at the distance of at least One hundred yards from each other—The sedate or melancholy Madman should not have his slumbers broken by living under the same roof with disorderly persons, who by singing, or other Noisy proceedings, will not suffer their Neighbors to sleep.

That for the above, and similar Considerations, it would be advisable to purchase, within a few Miles of this City, at least twenty Acres of land, detached from private Buildings, in a healthy and pleasant situation; where the Water is good, and where Materials for building may be obtained on easy terms; and the portage of Fuel not expensive.

Your Committee are aware that a small lot of ground might suffice for all the Buildings that are now required, or all that this Corporation may, in a short time, be enabled to complete. But they count it advisable to prepare for a period that must certainly come; a period in which such a lot will be

[11] *Minutes of the Governors*, Aug. 1, 1815.

needed, and not easily obtained for it is evident from the topography, and the geographical position of this City, that the time must come, when New York will be not only the greatest City in the United States, or in America; but must rival the most distinguished Citys in the old Continent.

Wherefore it is recommended, that a Committee be appointed, who shall examine the sundry places, corresponding with the above description, that may be purchased. And that they report the means of making the purchase, and of Erecting such Buildings, as seem at this time to be required.

Evidently, the governors, upon consideration, concluded that it would be advisable to build a new asylum for "all the insane." They said so in a memorial to the State Legislature in February, 1816,[12] and gave the following reasons: the increasing number of applications and "the painful necessity of almost daily refusing admittance to new patients," the impracticability of introducing improvements in the treatment of the patients because of inadequate space, and the "indiscriminate mixture . . . of persons of different character, of various and opposite religious sentiments, the serious and profane, the profligate and virtuous." The problem of classification here presented remained for many years a leading issue in the development of the service. It was considered that with more extensive space, the patients might "enjoy more rational and congenial society, a freer and purer air, innocent amusement, agreeable employment, or salutary exercise." The governors realized that further enlargement of the asylum in the city was impracticable. They were, also, fully persuaded of the value of "moral treatment." In the memorial to the legislature they referred to the York Retreat "in which the number of these [insane persons] under its care, restored to society and their friends has far exceeded those afforded by any other establishment," and expressed their intention of "combining a course of moral treatment towards insane persons with the usual medical aid." The records do not show that the regulations proposed by Thomas Eddy for the introduction of "moral treatment" into the service as then conducted were adopted, nor that any particular change occurred in that service. There is, nevertheless, considerable evidence that, following his communication, "moral treatment" had a larger place in the interest of the members of the Asylum Committee and of the physicians.

12 For full text of the Memorial, see Appendix, p. 492.

XI

BUILDING ON THE "SPOT OF LAND" AT BLOOMINGDALE

UPON receiving the report of the committee to which Mr. Eddy's communication had been referred, the governors immediately appointed Thomas Eddy, John R. Murray, and John Aspinwall to "look out for a suitable spot of land and make a purchase." This committee proceeded with great celerity, and on August 1, 1815, reported that they had purchased 38 acres of the estate of Gerard DePeyster at Bloomingdale at $246 per acre.[1]

Bloomingdale, or Bloomendael (Vale of Flowers), was the name applied to part of the upper west side of Manhattan by the early Dutch settlers. (There is a village of the same name near Haarlaem in Holland, from which many of the Dutch settlers came.) Originally, the name was confined to a cluster of about twenty houses and farms in the vicinity of what is now 100th Street; eventually it embraced a large section, the boundaries of which are not accurately known, but which seems to have extended at least as far down as 23d Street and up as far as 120th Street, or farther. It was a beautiful region, described by Washington Irving as "a sweet rural valley, beautiful with many a bright flower, refreshed by many a pure streamlet, and enlivened here and there by a delectable little Dutch Cottage, sheltered under some sloping hill, and almost buried in embowering trees."[2] Many fine homes were built by wealthy New Yorkers among its streams, lakes, and woods. The river was a great attraction and in the summer was dotted with the sails of pleasure boats. The Bloomingdale Road, opened in 1703, started from the Bowery at what is now Union Square and wound diagonally across the city, following roughly the course of Broadway to about 115th Street and Riverside Drive; in 1795 it was extended to 147th Street, where it joined the Kingsbridge Road.

The property purchased for the new asylum was near Bloomingdale Road, about seven miles from Federal Hall on Wall Street. It was an attractive site, with wide views of the river and surrounding country. Most of the governors considered it entirely suitable; some of them,

1 New York Hospital, *Minutes of the Governors*, Aug. 1, 1815.

2 Washington Irving, *Knickerbocker History of New York* (1809).

Most of the information relating to Bloomingdale was obtained from H. S. Mott, *The New York of Yesterday: Bloomingdale* (New York, 1908). I. N. P. Stokes, *Iconography of Manhattan Island* (New York, 1926) and *New York City Guide* (a W.P.A. project, New York, 1939) were also consulted.

however, thought it was too far from the city, and committees were appointed to examine property in other locations. Two years passed before a final decision was reached. Of the other sites proposed, two were strongly recommended by the committees who examined them. One of these was on Barn Island (now Ward's Island). A report in June, 1817, from Frederick DePeyster, Peter Mesier, and Thomas Eddy, who examined this property, advised the board "that it would be wise, prudent, and economical to suspend operations at Bloomingdale; with a view to examine the manifest advantages attending Barn Island." (Thomas Eddy did not sign this report.) Thereupon, the board voted that "all proceedings relative to a new Asylum out of town be suspended." Another committee, consisting of Moses Field, Thomas C. Taylor and Thomas Buckley, was appointed "to confer with the owners of Barn Island, and to look out for a more desireable situation for the contemplated Asylum." They reported on August 5 that they had "had a conference with several of the proprietors [of Barn Island] . . . and have also made a visit to the property" of Richard D. Arden and that of William A. Hardenbrook, but that "neither of these situations will answer the views of the Governors." However, on November 4 this same committee reported that they had purchased 18 acres on the East River, "late the property of Ann Hardenbrook" (apparently the property considered unsuitable on August 5), and had borrowed $4,000 from the Bank of New York in order to make the first payment. This, moreover, was approved by the board at the same meeting. Nevertheless, after due consideration, on December 9, 1817, it was resolved on motion "that the Board do adhere, to the resolution to locate the New Asylum on the grounds at Bloomingdale." Opposition still continued, however, and in February, 1818, Jonathan Little gave notice that at the next regular meeting of the board he would "move to reconsider the location of the New Asylum, in order to fix a site on the ground at the East River." This was the Hardenbrook property. The committee had already been instructed to sell it and did so before the next regular meeting, with a profit to the Society of $2,400.[3]

During the two years in which the location of the new asylum was being considered, the governors were also active in making preparations for its erection and operation. In the memorial to the legislature in February, 1816, a request was made for financial aid "by an annual sum or otherwise." In May, 1816, Thomas Eddy, who had spent much of the

[3] *Minutes of the Governors*, March 3, 1818. A sketch of this property, which was near the present site of the New York Hospital, is in the archives of the Society.

winter in Albany endeavoring to obtain favorable action on the appeal, reported to the board the passage of a bill [4] which granted to the Society an annuity of $10,000 until 1857. The details of this bill were proposed by Mr. Eddy in a letter to Peter A. Jay at Albany, in January, 1816. The letter made clear the intention of the governors to provide an institution in which "all the insane could be accommodated." Eddy estimated that New York City had "one hundred and twenty lunatics," and that it contained one tenth of the inhabitants of the state.[5] On receiving the report, the governors appointed Thomas Eddy, Gilbert Aspinwall, John Murray, Jr., George Newbold, John R. Murray, Thomas Buckley, and Cadwallader D. Colden to "report on a plan for a new Asylum for the maniacs together with the best situation for the same." At the same time a vote of thanks was extended to Mr. Eddy "for his exertions in promoting the views of the Governors, in their late application to the Legislature." This committee, after making a full report in June, were in November discharged from further consideration of the subject, and a Building Committee was named, consisting of the same governors, with Gilbert Aspinwall, John Murray, Jr., and George Newbold omitted, and Peter A. Jay added.

Attention was now given to the preparation of plans and estimates. Mr. Eddy wrote to Lindley Murray of York, England (the celebrated grammarian and the uncle of John Murray, Jr., one of the governors), and enclosed a copy of his communication to the board relating to a new asylum, with a request for information about the York Retreat. Murray replied that he was "putting thy pamphlet and letter into the hands of my benevolent and zealous friend, Samuel Tuke." [6] An interesting and informing letter, dated "7 mo. 17th 1815," was received from Mr. Tuke, and the governors ordered a number of copies to be printed for distribution under the title *A Letter on Pauper Lunatic Asylums.*[7] Mr. Tuke also sent a floor plan of a new asylum at Wakefield, and a pamphlet, entitled *Practical Hints on the Construction and Economy of Pauper Lunatic Asylums,* which he had just published. An eminent physician of New York, Dr. J. W. Francis, visited the York Retreat in November, 1815, and wrote Mr. Eddy "on the success of this important innovation on old prejudices which this institution presented." [8]

[4] *Ibid.*, May, 1816. "An act to enable the Society of the New York Hospital to Erect a New Building for the accommodation of Insane patients passed 17th April 1816."

[5] S. L. Knapp, *Life of Thomas Eddy* (New York, 1834), p. 242.

[6] *Ibid.*, p. 231.

[7] New York, 1815.

[8] J. W. Francis, *Old New York* (New York, 1858), pp. 308–311. It seems possible that Mr. Tuke addressed a previous communication to the governors in 1811. A copy of this com-

The asylum superintendent's accounts contain charges for trips to Philadelphia, assumably to visit the Pennsylvania Hospital, and possibly the Friends' Asylum (opened in 1817), although no records of such visits appear in the Governors' Minutes. In January, 1817, plans were submitted to the governors, and one was approved. In February the Building Committee reported that the estimated cost was about $200,000. They recommended that the necessary funds be obtained by borrowing, and that the annuity from the State be applied to the interest on the loan and to the establishment of a sinking fund. The plan that was approved at this time was evidently quite comprehensive. No copy has been discovered, but it contained five buildings and, in a letter from Mr. Eddy to Patrick Colquhoun, an English philanthropist, in April, 1817, it was stated that the governors intended to erect "separate buildings for men and women patients about 300 feet distant from each other, besides one other building remote from these for noisy patients." [9]

In January, 1818, the committee presented a plan and an estimate of cost amounting to $159,217. Their report was adopted. In February, 1818, this committee appears to have been superseded by the appointment of Thomas C. Taylor, Thomas Eddy, and Thomas Buckley to "be a Committee to be called the Building Committee, whose duty shall be to superintend the erection of said building." From this time on, Thomas C. Taylor appears to have been the active superintendent of construction, devoting all of his time to the project. In some accounts of the asylum, he is credited with having designed the center building.[10] The records do not reveal the appointment of an architect. The superintendent's accounts in July, 1818, however, contain an item for drawing plans, and in October, 1820, a claim of J. O'Donnell for "Architectural service" was rejected by the governors, but it was evidently submitted to arbitration later and was paid in 1821. Mr. Taylor made a number of recommendations in regard to the building, most of which were adopted. In May, 1818, he proposed that instead of blue stone and marble, Newark free stone should be used on all fronts. "This," he said, "may appear extravagant to some of the Governors, but they should remember this building ought to have the appearance of a Palace, rather than of a Goal [jail]." This recommendation was at once adopted.

On March 21, the governors gave the word to commence construc-

munication was very kindly presented to the Society by Dr. Henry Viets of Boston in 1921. See Henry Viets, "A Note from Samuel Tuke to the New York Hospital (1811)," *Am. J. Psychiatry*, I (1844), 425.

[9] Knapp, *op. cit.*, p. 267.

[10] *Minutes of the Governors*, Jan. 2, 1821.

tion, and the following day they met on the property to decide on the position of the building. But before building operations were undertaken, Mr. Taylor reported that the site selected would bring the extension of the building on the northern side too close to the property of Mr. De Peyster; also that it was wet and not easy to drain. As no other part of the property was considered suitable for the main building, an adjoining plot of 21 acres, extending westward to Bloomingdale Road was purchased from Thomas Buckley at $500 per acre. It was on this property that the building was erected, facing south, and at equal distances from Tenth and Eleventh Avenues, which at that time appeared on the city map but were not yet opened. The site was approximately that now occupied by the Low Library of Columbia University, facing 116th Street. It was well elevated and commanded a wide view of the river and the beautiful surrounding country. When the institution was opened in 1821, the asylum owned about 77 acres of land. The property comprised two large irregular pieces; one extending from what is now 107th to 113th Streets, roughly along Tenth (Amsterdam) Avenue and stretching east into the present Morningside Park; the other from 113th to 120th Streets between the west side of Tenth Avenue and the Bloomingdale Road.[11] The cornerstone was laid on May 7, 1818.

In June the governors ordered that "a new set of books be opened for the New Asylum, and all accounts be kept separate from the accounts of the Hospital." This practice has been followed to the present day. Construction of the building apparently proceeded with few noteworthy incidents. There were no labor unions, and no strikes. Mr. Taylor "prepared all the plans," bought the materials, employed journeymen and superintended their work, laid out the grounds, and from November, 1817, to November, 1820, gave to the project his undivided attention. "His knowledge and experience, if not indispensable, was thought of the greatest importance in the execution of the plan." It was estimated that a considerable sum had been saved by means of his services. He had "repelled every suggestion of future compensation for his services, wishing them to be regarded as perfectly gratuitous." The governors, however, considered that this should not be permitted, and in January, 1821, after the building had been completed, voted him a gratuity of $6,000. This, however, he considered too large; he finally accepted $4,000. Reports of the progress of the building and of the ex-

[11] *Atlas of the City of New York* (2d ed., Philadelphia, 1894), Map, Plate 38. (Seen at C. F. Noyes & Co., 225 Broadway, New York.)

penditures were frequently received from Mr. Taylor and minor changes were made from time to time.

In March, 1819, a letter was received from the mayor of the city, in which he suggested "the utillity, and propriety, of prohibiting the workmen at the new building for the accommodation of Insane patients from drinking spirituous Liquors." Whereupon, the following resolution was adopted:

Whereas the custom of supplying workmen, employed in erecting buildings, with spirituous Liquors, has been productive of much evil, and has contributed to encrease the number of patients in this Hospital, as well as of convicts in the Public Prisons, and of paupers in the City Alms House, and it appearing to this Board that it would be improper for this Institution, to countenance so pernicious an example— It is therefore resolved, that the Asylum Building Committee, be directed, and they are hereby directed, to use such measures as they may think proper effectually to prohibit any person from bringing spirituous Liquors upon the Asylum premises, and that they employ no person who shall whilst in their employment, use ardent spirits, and if any person who shall act contrary to the meaning and intention of this Resolution, he shall be promptly discharged.[12]

At the next meeting of the board it was "Resolved, that Thomas Eddy and John R. Murray be a Committee to wait upon the Mayor, in order to solicit him not to grant any License to retail Spirituous Liquors within two hundred yards of our premises at Bloomingdale."

In July, 1819, it is recorded in the Governors' Minutes, that the plants that remained in the hothouse of the Botanical Garden, (established in 1801 by Dr. Hosack and presented to Columbia University by the state), had been presented to the asylum by the university, and that a proper building had been erected to accommodate them. This was the beginning of the greenhouse which has continued to be a means of pleasure and healing for the patients ever since. Some of the palms and other plants then presented survived until a very few years ago.

The progress of construction was noted in the annual report to the legislature each year and in that for 1820 its completion was announced. In the same report the governors stated that they had expended $177,-271.11 for purchasing, enclosing, and improving the land, and in erecting the building and "necessary offices." They had borrowed $137,000 on bond and mortgage and $9,500 from the banks. They anticipated that the rates received for the maintenance and treatment of the patients would be sufficient to defray the ordinary expenses and enable them "to receive paupers sent from different towns in the state, at a very low

[12] *Minutes of the Governors,* March 2, 1819.

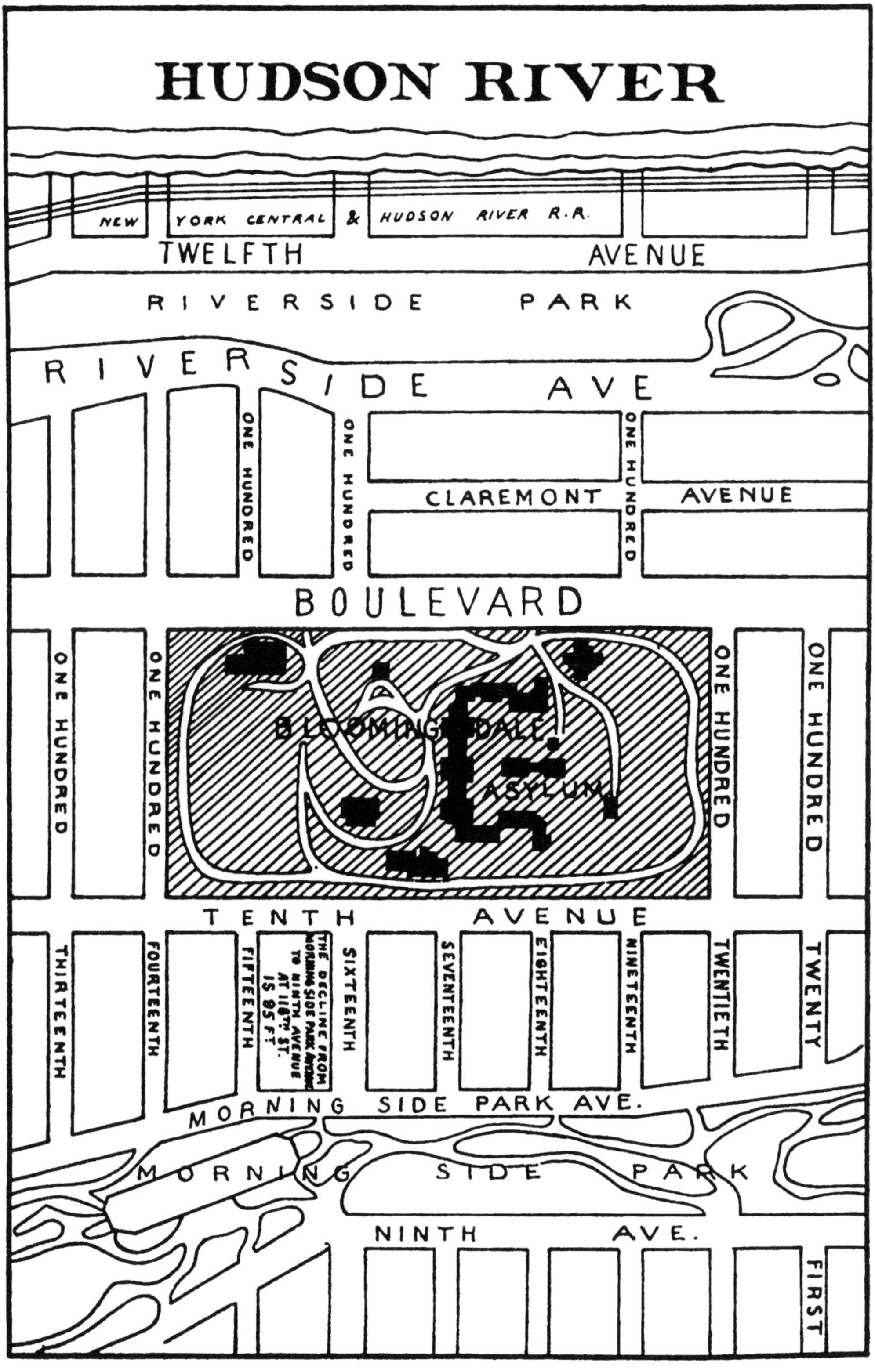

HUDSON RIVER
NEW YORK CENTRAL & HUDSON RIVER R.R.
TWELFTH AVENUE
RIVERSIDE PARK
RIVERSIDE AVE
CLAREMONT AVENUE
BOULEVARD
BLOOMINGDALE ASYLUM
TENTH AVENUE
ONE HUNDRED
ONE HUNDRED
ONE HUNDRED
ONE HUNDRED
ONE HUNDRED
ONE HUNDRED
ONE HUNDRED
ONE HUNDRED
ONE HUNDRED
THIRTEENTH
FOURTEENTH
FIFTEENTH
THE DECLINE FROM MORNING SIDE PARK AVENUE TO NINTH AVENUE AT 116TH ST. IS 95 FT.
SIXTEENTH
SEVENTEENTH
EIGHTEENTH
NINETEENTH
TWENTIETH
TWENTY
MORNING SIDE PARK AVE.
MORNING SIDE PARK
NINTH AVE.
FIRST

rate." A committee was appointed to "look out for a suitable Superintendent and Matron, to take charge of the New Asylum when in readiness to receive patients." The building was considered to be ready for occupancy in November, 1820, and a committee was then appointed to provide furniture. In December another committee was appointed

to inquire into the expense of furnishing the Asylum at Bloomingdale so as to make it ready in every respect for the reception of patients, the cost of all necessary out buildings, and the probable amount of expenditures requisite for the support of the establishment for one year, and also the means which are, or may be within the power of the Governors during the coming year to defray the expenses and to report them particularly to the Governors at a future meeting, with their opinion as to the opening of the Asylum in the next Spring.

The furniture committee, in June, 1821, was authorized to expend an amount not to exceed $6,000; in July they reported that they had procured "a greater part of the furniture necessary for opening at $1683.79." It was ordered that other furniture be sent out from the asylum at the Hospital. May 1 was fixed as the date of opening, and the committee "to look out for a superintendent" were instructed to prepare an address to the public. This address [18] was as follows:

The Governors of the New-York Hospital have the satisfaction to announce to the public, the completion of the Asylum for the insane; and that it will be open for the reception of patients, from any part of the United States, on the first day of June.

This Asylum is situated on the Bloomingdale road, about seven miles from the City Hall of the city of New-York, and about three hundred yards from the Hudson River. The building is of hewn free-stone, 211 feet in length, and sixty feet deep, and is calculated for the accommodation of about two hundred patients. Its sciet [site] is elevated, commanding an extensive and delightful view of the Hudson, the East River, and the Bay and Harbour of New-York, and the adjacent country, and is one of the most beautiful and healthy spots on New-York Island. Attached to the building are about seventy acres of land, a great part of which has been laid out in walks, ornamental grounds, and extensive gardens.

This institution has been established by the bounty of the Legislature of the state of New-York, on the most liberal and enlarged plan, with the express design to carry into effect that system of management of the insane, happily termed *moral treatment*, the superior efficacy of which has been demonstrated in several of the Hospitals of Europe, and especially in that admirable establishment of the Society of Friends, called "THE RETREAT," near York, in England. This mild and humane mode of treatment, when

[18] "Address of the Governors of the New-York Hospital, to the Public, Relative to the Asylum for the Insane at Bloomingdale. New-York, May 10th, 1821."

contrasted with the harsh and cruel usage, and the severe and unnecessary restraint, which have formerly disgraced even the most celebrated lunatic asylums, may be considered as one of the noblest triumphs of pure and enlightened benevolence. But it is by no means the intention of the governors to rely on moral, to the exclusion of medical treatment. It is from a judicious combination of both, that the greatest success is to be expected in every attempt to cure or mitigate the disease of insanity.

In the construction of the edifice and in its interior arrangements, it has been considered important to avoid, as far as practicable, consistently with a due regard to the safety of the patients, whatever might impress their minds with the idea of a prison, or a place of punishment, and to make every thing conduce to their health and to their ease and comfort. The self-respect and complacency which may thus be produced in the insane, must have a salutary influence in restoring the mind to its wonted serenity. In the disposition of the grounds attached to the Asylum, everything has been done with reference to the amusement, agreeable occupation, and salutary exercise of the patients.

Agricultural, horticultural, and mechanical employments, may be resorted to, whenever the inclination of the patient, or their probable beneficial effects may render them desirable. To dispel gloomy images, to break morbid associations, to lead the feelings into their proper current, and to restore the mind to its natural poise, various less active amusements will be provided. Reading, writing, drawing, innocent sports, tending and feeding domestic animals, &c. will be encouraged as they may be found conducive to the recovery of the patients. A large garden has been laid out, orchards have been planted, and yards, containing more than two acres, have been inclosed for the daily walks of those whose disorder will not allow more extended indulgence. The plants of the Elgin Botanic garden, presented to this institution by the Trustees of Columbia College, have been arranged in a handsome green-house, prepared for their reception.

The apartments of the house are adapted to the accommodation of the patients, according to their sex, degree of disease, habits of life, and the wishes of their friends. The male and female apartments are entirely separated, so as to be completely secluded from the view of each other.

Care has been taken to appoint a Superintendent and Matron, of good moral and religious characters, possessing cheerful tempers, and kind dispositions, united with firmness, vigilance and discretion. A Physician will reside in the house, and one or more physicians, of established character and experience, will attend regularly, and afford medical aid in all cases where the general health, or the particular cause of the patient's insanity, may require it. The relations or friends of patients will be at liberty, if they prefer it, to employ their own physicians, who will be allowed to attend patients, subject to the general regulations of the house.

The institution will be regularly visited and inspected by a committee of the Governors of the Hospital, who will, as often as they may think it advantageous, be attended by some of the physicians of the city of high character and respectability.

The charges for board and the other advantages of the institution, will be moderate, and proportioned to the different circumstances of the patients, and the extent of the accommodations desired for them.

Patients at the expense of the different towns of the state, will be received at the lowest rate.

Applications for the admission of patients into the Asylum, must be made, at the New-York Hospital, in Broadway, where temporary accommodation will be provided for such patients as may require it, previously to their being carried to the Asylum out of town. A Committee of the Governors, will, when necessary, attend at the Hospital in Broadway, for the purpose of admitting patients into the Asylum, and to agree on the terms and security for payment to be given.

By order of the board of Governors

MATTHEW CLARKSON, *President*

THOMAS BUCKLEY, *Secretary*
New-York, 10th May, 1821

The building as first constructed consisted only of the central portion of the plan adopted. Its location was the highest point of Manhattan Island, with the exception of Fort Washington. The grounds had been improved as the building was being erected, and much of the property was enclosed by a stone wall. Preparations were made for the reception of patients by the continuation of Dr. John Neilson as Physician of the Asylum and the appointment of Dr. James Eddy as House Physician. Laban Gardiner was appointed Superintendent, and his wife Matron, on March 6. On April 3, 1821, the new institution was, by resolution of the board, named "Bloomingdale Asylum."

XII

THE FIRST TWENTY YEARS, 1821–1840

BLOOMINGDALE ASYLUM was opened officially on June 1, 1821. The transfer of patients from the asylum at the New York Hospital did not, however, commence until June 23, and was not completed until July 27. The number of patients transferred was 52, 31 men and 21 women. Although the first by-laws provided that "part of the Asylum in town shall be reserved for the temporary accommodation of Patients, until they can be conveniently sent to the Bloomingdale Asylum,"[1] the records do not reveal that it was ever used for that purpose. After the patients were removed, service for the mentally ill, which had been conducted at the New York Hospital since 1792, was discontinued there and was not resumed until the Payne Whitney Clinic was established in 1932. It was more than a physical separation. For many years the new asylum received little attention from the other services of the hospital. At first an attempt was made to maintain relations by means of a rule which provided that "as the Physicians and Surgeons are considered by this Committee consulting Physicians to this institution," a physician or surgeon of the hospital staff should visit the asylum once a week for consultation.[2] There is in the records little to indicate that this rule was strictly observed, and eventually such visits were made only when specifically requested. In December, 1823, it was noted in the Governors' Minutes that Dr. Stevens was reprimanded for regulating his visits to the asylum "rather by a virtual compliance with the Spirit of the Bye Laws . . . than by a strict and formal observance of those laws according to their Letter."

During the twenty years immediately following the opening of the new asylum, the interest and efforts of the governors were directed: 1.) to the improvement and extension of the buildings and grounds in order to adapt them more and more adequately to the purpose for which they were designed; 2) to an attempt to introduce "moral treatment" as a system separate from medical treatment; 3) to developing medical capability and authority in the organization, and gradually to delegate to the resident physician the moral as well as the medical treatment; 4) to the classification of the patients with reference to social as well as medical considerations, and towards a well-defined policy of selection. Preparatory to opening the service, the Asylum Committee, which had

1 New York Hospital, *Minutes of the Governors*, Nov. 3, 1821. It was used for sailors, and in 1855 was demolished.

2 *Minutes of the Asylum Committee*, June 28, 1823.

been operating since 1808, was, in May, 1821, reorganized, with Thomas Eddy as chairman and Cadwallader E. Colden, Thomas C. Taylor, John Adams, Thomas Buckley and James Lawrence as the other members. All six were present at the first meeting, which was held on May 5. At this meeting a subcommittee of two to visit the asylum every week was appointed. The appointment was for two months, one member finishing his term each month. This "Weekly Committee" is still a part of the organization. A committee to draft rules for the government of the asylum was also appointed.

In their first report to the governors, in August, 1821, the Bloomingdale committee stated that "on opening the House, many inconveniences and difficulties occurred, that required alterations and improvements in the building, which were found necessary for the security of the patients, and for their comfort and accomodation." Much attention was given to the development of the property and facilities as means of comfort, protection, and healing of the patients. The property was quite irregular in form and, from time to time, small plots were purchased in order to straighten and protect its boundaries. The interest of individual governors was illustrated in the purchase, in October, 1823, of an acre of land adjoining the southeast corner of the property at Tenth Avenue for $219.15, concerning which they noted in their minutes that, if the governors would not accept it, "the members of the Committee have agreed to take it on their own account."

The 38 acres first purchased as a site for the asylum were separated from the property on which the buildings were erected, and it was found advisable to sell them. Twenty-four acres were sold to the Leake and Watts Orphan Asylum in 1834 for $24,755.[3] In 1891 part of this land was sold by the Orphan Asylum to the Cathedral of St. John the Divine for $900,000. In 1835 14 acres, extending from 107th to 109th streets along Ninth Avenue, were sold for $1,500 per acre to Mr. E. L. Williams. In the same year several small plots were purchased. In 1836, an accurate survey of the property was made, and monuments placed to mark its boundaries. In February of that year, the valuation of the property and buildings was reported to be $157,958.13.[4] As soon as the boundaries of the property were fixed, an appeal was made to the City Council to refrain from opening streets through it. The streets were on the city map, however, and a successful application was made to the council and to the State Legislature to have the map changed.

[3] *Minutes of the Governors*, Dec. 2, 1834.

[4] *Ibid.*, Feb., 1837. (Report of Auditing Committee for 1836.)

The property was gradually enclosed, and yards in which shelters were erected were provided for the patients. Yards and apartments occupied by disturbed patients were hidden from curious visitors by fences and shrubbery. The basement of the main building was never considered to be a satisfactory place in which to provide for these patients. The Inspecting Committee in 1827 reported that

the Committee deem it, however, proper to add, that the wards in the Basement stories formed a striking contrast with the airy, cheerful, and comfortable appearance of those in the upper part of the building, and cannot from their sombre and cheerless aspect, but have the most deleterious effect on minds already too much disposed to gloom and melancholy.

It was not until 1836, however, that improvements were made. The committee had again brought to the attention of the governors that the basement was not only cold, dark, and damp, but that it was also infested with rats, "who, as the committee witnessed in the daytime, and were told it was a common occurence, freely traverse the rooms and halls." Thereupon, an area 7 feet wide and 6½ feet deep was constructed along both wings, in front of the basement windows, which were at the same time enlarged; and the brick floor of the halls was replaced with plank.

As only the central portion of the building was erected, references to overcrowding not infrequently appeared in the records, and measures were taken to overcome it. The stairway was extended to the garret, and dormitories and rooms were constructed there for the use of servants. Anticipation of overcrowding may have led the committee, in designating a room to be used as an apothecary shop, to order that "it be occupied by the Resident Physician as a bedroom also, and for a clerk's office." [5] In 1825 the apothecary complained to the Inspecting Committee that he was "much incommoded by being compelled to sleep in his medicine shop." [6]

Complaints were not confined to overcrowding. The problem of classification was soon encountered and inadequate facilities for separating disturbed patients from others not infrequently occasioned comments by visiting governors. The large proportion of "pauper patients," many of whom were incurable as well as extremely offensive in appearance and behavior, was also deplored. As the resident physician gained experience in knowledge and treatment of the patients, his reports to the Asylum Committee presented, with increasing understanding and force, the evil effects of indiscriminate commingling. The "mingling of

[5] *Minutes of the Asylum Committee,* July 21, 1821.
[6] *Minutes of the Inspecting Committee,* March 24, 1825.

the malevolent and harmless, the frantick and melancholick, the convalescent and idiotic, of these capable of rational enjoyment and of those in state of extreme mental deprevation," was termed "highly injudicious." [7] The governors were advised that "in the best asylums patients are classed not only according to sex but also to rank in life and form of disease." The Inspecting Committee also reported, on January 2, 1824, that the

> greater proportion may be stated to be of the pauper class, which from the expensiveness of this establishment was not originally intended. The current expenditures may be covered by the revenue derived from this source, but towards the extinguishment of the great debt but little can be expected. If attention is to be directed to the accomodation of the opulent class of patients, some new mode must be devised preparatory to an event of separating the paupers from this building, which subject, it is supposed, must ere long be introduced by the proper committee.

In April of the same year, when the number of patients was 120, the committee further reported: "This number, according to the present state of the building is probably a full complement. It is hoped that proper arrangements will be made, in due time, to remove those patients who from all appearance are incurable." In August the committee again referred to "the want of a more perfect classification and division," and recommended "separate enclosures or gardens . . . for air, exercise, and amusement." With a hope of affecting some improvement, large rooms in the basement and in the upper story were divided by partitions into smaller rooms to accommodate patients separately.

By 1826, the problem had become so pressing that consideration was given to the erection of two small buildings, one in each yard, for noisy and violent patients. Ezra Weeks, one of the governors, was in fact requested in May to prepare a plan and estimate for a new building. In November, 1827, it was "Resolved, that it is expedient that such alterations or additions be made to the Bloomingdale Asylum, as may effect a complete classification and separation of the Patients." [8] In December, 1829, the first of these buildings, designed for men, was ready for occupancy. It was located back of the northwest wing of the main building at a distance of 117 feet.[9] The walls were of brick, and, to distinguish it from the main building the walls of which were of stone, it was usually designated the "Brick Building" or "Men's Lodge." It was 57 feet long and 32½ feet wide. There were three stories, each with a hall 10 feet

[7] *Minutes of the Asylum Committee.* (Dr. Macdonald's Report, April, 1827.)
[8] *Minutes of the Governors,* Nov. 6, 1827.
[9] Annual Report for 1841.

wide, from which a tier of wards opened on each side. There were 33 wards or rooms, the windows of which were guarded by iron "grates." There was a "bathing-room," a dining room, and a receiving room, the

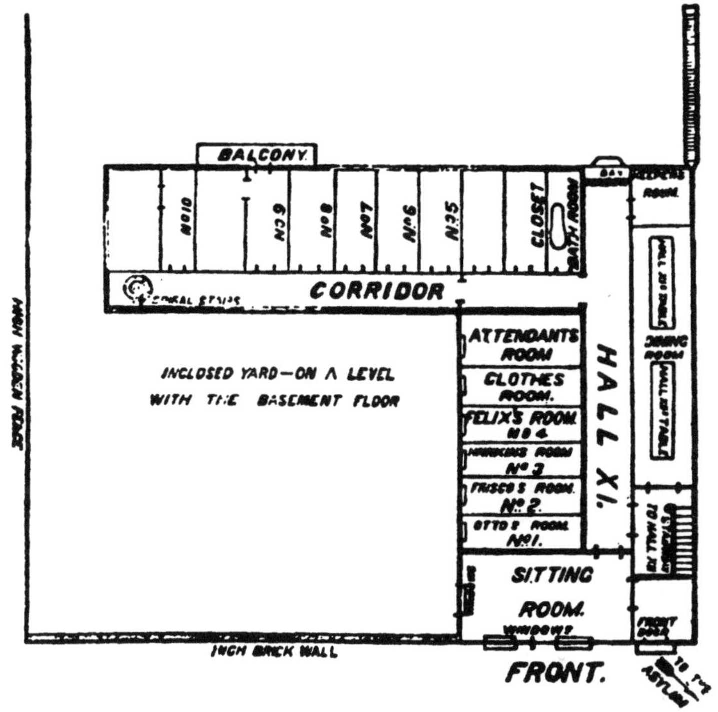

FLOOR PLAN OF THE MEN'S LODGE, BLOOMINGDALE ASYLUM

FROM A SKETCH MADE BY A PATIENT AND PUBLISHED IN CHAMBERS, *A Mad World*, D. APPLETON AND COMPANY, NEW YORK, 1877

two last mentioned being 14 feet long and 10 feet wide. The front windows of the receiving room and of the hall were guarded by strong, iron bars. The bars were an inch thick, and, to prevent the patients from breaking the glass with their hands, were placed so close together that they could only put their fingers through. All the remaining windows were provided with iron sashes, which permitted dispensing with bars. The 16-inch walls contained hollow spaces, which, by means of openings protected by a "piece of iron perforated with small holes," carried off the foul air from the wards. A "Wakefield" stove, which, it was said, did not require "pipes," was installed for heating.

The water supply was from the well in the rear of the main building, and was, by means of a rotary suction and forcing pump, conveyed through a lead pipe to two tubs (tanks), each with a capacity of a hundred gallons, placed in a room adjoining the bathing room. "Inside the Hot Water Tub is placed a cast iron furnace and fed with Fuel from the outside"; in this way the water was heated. A substantial copper bathing tub equipped with brass cocks was supplied with hot and cold water from these "tubs." The water was carried off by a brick drain under the house to an open field.

A yard 139 feet long and 32 feet wide was enclosed by the wall of an adjoining yard, by the end of the building, and by a fence consisting of a stone foundation 3 feet high, into which were built locust posts fastened with strong iron clamps worked into the wall. To these posts were attached upright planks 7 feet long. The cost of the building was $9,103.35 and it was designed to accommodate about 40 patients. The Resident Physician, in his monthly report for December, 1829, contrasted the cleanliness, purity and uniformity of its atmosphere, and the comparative cheerfulness of the patients with the conditions in the basement of the main building. He referred especially to the superiority of the warming apparatus, and of the bathing facilities, the success of which he thought might suggest some improvement in the bathing department of the main building. He reported that "the two most furious maniacs, who were not only confined in their rooms, but kept under severe personal restraint while in the Main Building, have since their removal to the new one, so far improved, as to obtain during the day the unrestrained liberty of the house and yard." [10]

The separation of the disturbed men from the other patients proved so advantageous that the necessity of making similar provision for the women was more and more keenly felt. In August, 1833, when there were 134 patients in residence, thirty of whom had just been transferred from Bellevue, the Resident Physician reported that a separate building for the worst class of female patients was "never more wanting than at this moment." Again in November, 1834, he made a strong plea for "a new building for the accommodation of violent and disorderly Female patients." He dwelt particularly upon the detrimental effects of "the imprecations, the ravings, and the unearthly laugh of the maniac" upon "delicate females in which the predominant feature is fear." The accommodations then available he described as "a dark, dismal, and partly subterranean basement," from which "noise is quite audible in the

[10] *Minutes of the Asylum Committee,* Jan. 2, 1830. How advancing views and standards changed the estimate of the value of this building in regard to treatment may be learned by reference to pp. 214, 250.

upper stories and patients who would otherwise be peaceable, as is frequently observed on a larger scale in mobs without the walls of mad-houses, catch the infuriated spirit and rave in such a manner as to disturb the comfort of all in their neighborhood." He considered that "though the assemblage in the Basement of all such patients as are most offensive be to a certain extent a relief to the upper galleries, we can not think of confining the delicate and well educated lady there." He urged that a building be erected "with distinct accommodations for two grades of violent patients."

Both the Asylum Committee and the Inspecting Committee also stressed the same points. The Asylum Committee reported that in their belief, "many respectable females are withheld by their friends from the institution, in consequence of the mixture of the character of its inmates," and added that they had, "by the assistance and advice of the Warden and Dr. Macdonald undertaken to digest a plan whereby they think the evils can be remedied." Thus stimulated, the governors consulted in January, 1835, with Mr. Dakin, an architect, and directed him to prepare plans for "the proposed wing for female patients." Mr. Dakin's bill was $50.

Finally the committee, in May, 1835, presented drawings and estimates "of a House, which, when completed, . . . will add greatly to the comfort and facilitate the recovery of the patients, as well as give the establishment much greater respectability and thereby induce wealthy people to send their friends to the institution whenever their situation require it." [11] The report recommended that the new building should correspond with that for the men, but should be 6 feet wider and 10 feet longer, in order to provide space for a larger day room and dining room and for more sleeping rooms. They proposed that the basement should be used solely for service purposes, the "washing department" and the furnace to be located there.[12] By using the large rooms on each floor for quiet and harmless patients, forty patients might be accommodated in the building as safely and comfortably as they were in the main building. The specifications provided for a furnace with "a copper tube" for warm air, two tubs for the bathing room, two brick cemented cisterns with a capacity of 10,000 gallons each, and a smaller one of 800 gallons. The roof was to be of metal with copper gutters. Wire netting and iron frames for 17 windows and 24 cast-iron sashes were ordered.[13] The build-

[11] *Minutes of the Governors*, May 12, 1835.
[12] How this was regarded 16 years later is related in Chapter XX.
[13] *Minutes of the Governors*, May 12, 1835.

ing was completed in August, 1837, and the governors in their annual report to the legislature stated that "the noisy and violent female patients are now separated from the quiet and convalescent, and the comfort and recovery of the latter thereby greatly promoted." In the meantime, the basement of the "Brick House" had been improved by means of a four foot area along its front, with a grated door to communicate with it. Also, a yard was provided at this building for the exclusive use of the "higher pay patients," and a special stairway from the third story to give them private access to the yard.

One of the problems connected with the asylum buildings was heating. In September, 1821, the committee held a special meeting "to agree on a mode of warming the asylum." Thomas C. Taylor was instructed to "provide and put up stoves in the basement story agreeable to the original plan of warming the House." In October, 1823, additional stoves and "drums" were installed. In April, 1830, the question of burning coal instead of wood was considered, and in July, a fixture was ordered so as to use coal for cooking. In January, 1831, it was noted that the "present furnaces, even with the use of Liverpool coal, are insufficient." In October of the same year, it was found necessary to enlarge the heating flues, and in November, it was noted that the four furnaces were completed and answered well. Two months later, however, it was only "with the aid of the small stoves," that the large house was warm and comfortable, while the new house was cold, except for the lower hall. Again in November, 1835, it was recorded that the "new" stoves in the halls for women failed to heat adequately and the warden was instructed to place a stove in the basement of the east wing, similar to that in the west wing, for "warming the straw patients." Apparently, for a number of years following the opening of the asylum, there was much experimentation and considerable discomfort. "Doric" stoves and fireplaces, and Wakefield furnaces are referred to. In October, 1836, it was ordered that the latter be removed from both wings, and that Taylor and Lovett supply new ones. The next month it was noted that the furnace in the basement hall of the Brick House was of little use, and a suitable stove was ordered. On one occasion a patient escaped through an aperture made by a mason in making the "Russia stoves."

Another difficult problem was the water supply, of especial concern in the treatment of patients. From a well in the rear of the main building, a pump distributed water to cisterns. Larger pipes were installed in 1823, and in 1838, after the two new buildings had been added, the well was made deeper and additional "apparatus for leading to the houses"

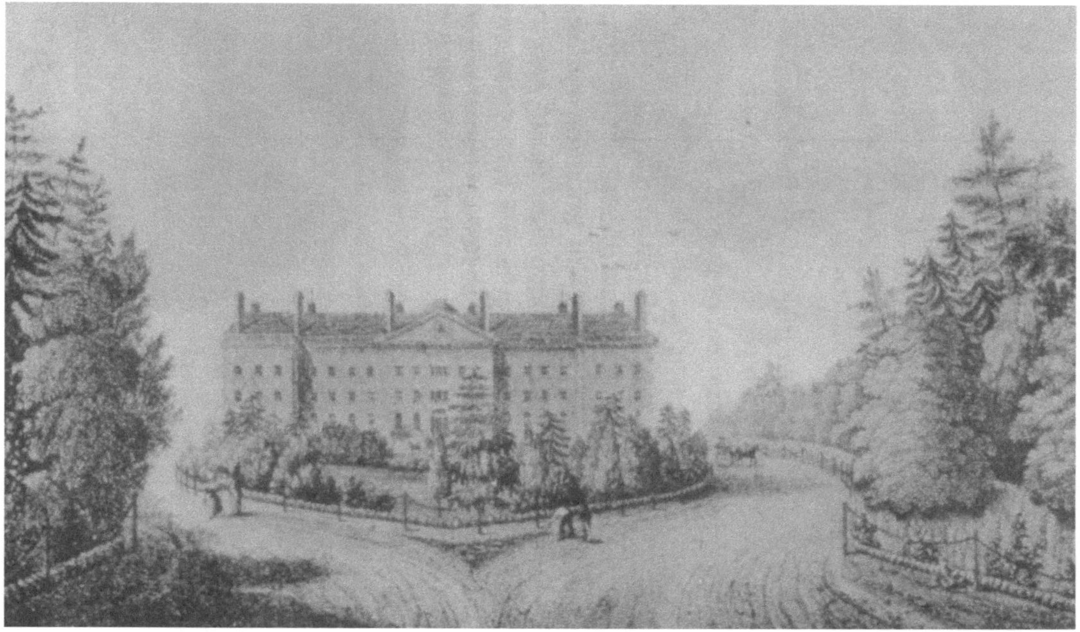

BLOOMINGDALE ASYLUM, 1821
FROM AN ENGRAVING BY JAMES SMILLIE

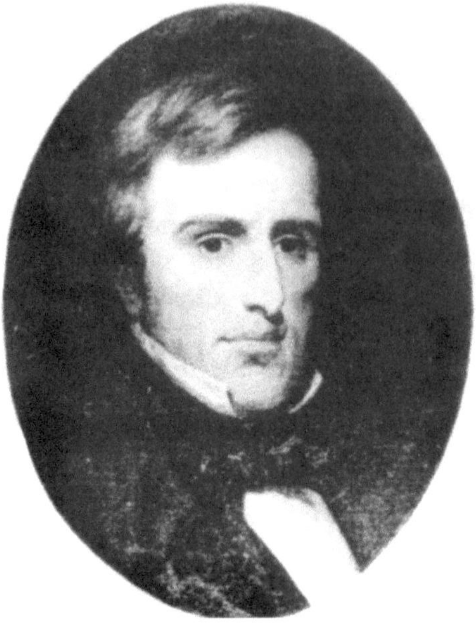

JAMES MACDONALD, M.D.
PHYSICIAN OF THE ASYLUM, 1825-1837

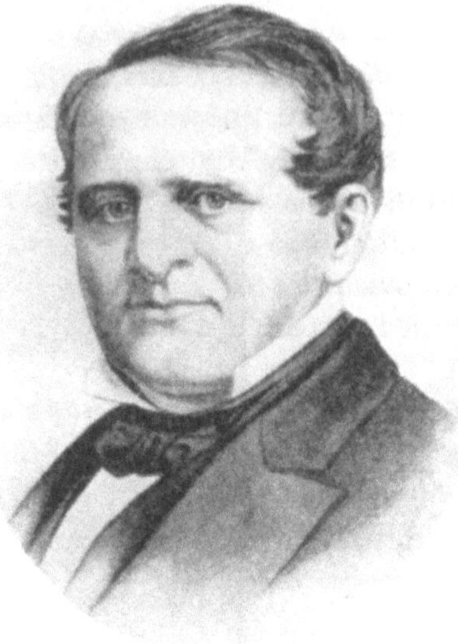

BENJAMIN OGDEN, M.D.
PHYSICIAN OF THE ASYLUM, 1837-1839

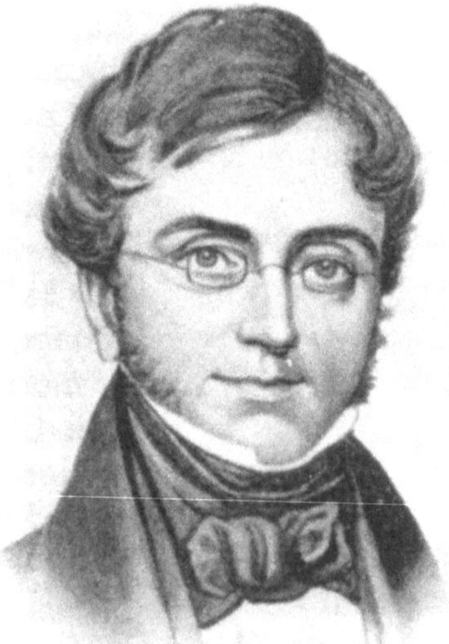

WILLIAM WILSON, M.D.
PHYSICIAN OF THE ASYLUM, 1839-1844

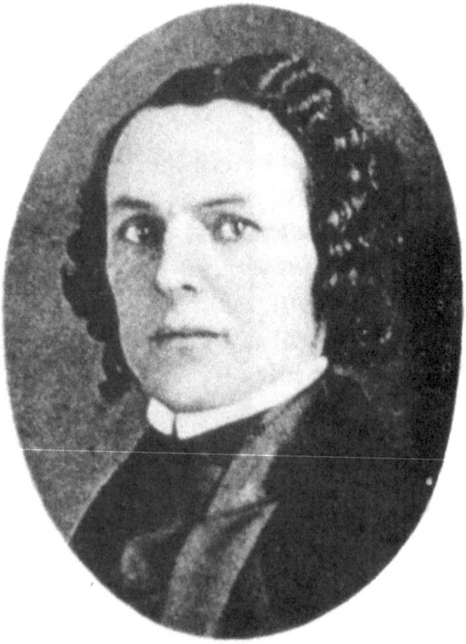

PLINY EARLE, M.D.
PHYSICIAN OF THE ASYLUM, 1844-1849

was installed. Also in 1838, a new well, 30 feet deep, was sunk near the "Female Building." There were water closets and baths in the buildings, but their number and location are not fully disclosed by the few descriptions available. As early as October, 1821, the Inspecting Committee had reported that there was "a very unpleasant and offensive smell from the water closets," especially from one "the machinery of which was out of order." An offensive smell from the opening to the sewer in the kitchen was also noted. Similar complaints appeared in later reports, and apparently the toilet facilities were inadequate and frequently offensive and unsanitary. The physicians were dissatisfied with the provision for bathing, but efforts to improve it made slow progress. Altogether, the problems of heating, water supply and toilet and bath facilities must, at least during the first two decades of the operation of Bloomingdale Asylum, have occasioned deprivations and discomforts which greatly limited and impaired the service to the patients.[14]

Attention to grading and beautifying the grounds was coincident with the start of building operations. In 1831, a plot north of the main building was set aside as a burial ground for patients without funds, and on one occasion attendance of several patients at a burial was mentioned. As opportunity arose, lawns were graded and sown, and trees and shrubs were planted. Plants from the Elgin Botanical Garden [15] were presented to the asylum in 1819, and a greenhouse was erected for their care. On a few occasions, when financing seemed difficult, various members of the board recommended that the greenhouse be dispensed with. In fact, in 1837, the Asylum Committee passed a resolution in which they recommended that the plants be sold or given away. In September of that year, however, the committee noted that

> the Governors having determined to preserve the Green House plants, the Committee concluded the following arrangement with Dr. Ogden on the subject, viz: the Fuel and repairs to be at the expense of the Institution, the Doctor to employ a Florist to take charge and care for the plants at his expense, he to be permitted to dispose of such plants and flowers as shall be raised from the cuttings, the proceeds of which, to be applied in the first place to the payment of the Florist's wages, and in the event of any balance remaining, the same to be for the benefit of the Institution.

How this arrangement operated, the records do not disclose. In any case, it preserved the greenhouse. Since then, there has sometimes been

[14] It was in fact not until after Dr. Nichols was appointed medical superintendent in 1877, that a satisfactory solution was achieved.

[15] See p. 130.

among the governors an occasional member who, failing to appreciate the value of the plants and flowers as a means of brightening the lives and promoting contentment and healing of the patients, has proposed that the greenhouse be dispensed with, but the board have, invariably, promptly refused to accede to the proposal. A grove of apple trees was cut down in 1833, but when, in 1839, some members of the Asylum Committee proposed that a number of other trees be treated in the same way, the Inspecting Committee reported to the governors that "the Committee have learned with considerable alarm that some of the Asylum Committee are desirous of prostrating the Wood in the rear Grounds. We beg their interposition of the board to prevent it." [16]

In the plan of "moral treatment" instituted by the governors when the asylum was established, the character of the grounds had an important place, and they were developed very attractively. A description was given by Dr. James Macdonald, Resident Physician from 1825 to 1837, in a paper read by him at a meeting of New York Medical and Surgical Society in 1838. To him,

> the beauty of the grounds, and the views from the main building, are almost unequalled. The approach to the Asylum from the southern entrance, by the stranger who associates the most sombre scenes with a lunatic asylum, is highly pleasing. The sudden opening of the view, the extent of the grounds, the various avenues gracefully winding through so large a lawn; the cedar hedges, the fir and other ornamental trees tastefully distributed and grouped, the variety of shrubbery and flowers; in fine, the assemblage of so many objects to please the eye, and relieve the melancholy mind from its sad musings, strike him as one of the most successful and useful instances of landscape gardening. There is, indeed, no private residence or public establishment in the vicinity of the city, which for beauty of situation, or exercise of taste in the distribution of the grounds, can compare with it.[17]

Dr. Macdonald also described the buildings as presenting "an appearance of simplicity, beauty, and strength, happily combined," but, being, he said, "constructed with reference chiefly to utility, are without those ornaments that distinguish the orders of architecture." A different impression was obtained by a committee of the State Legislature who investigated the asylum in 1830 and reported that "too large a quantity of land had been purchased, for which too great a price was paid," and that in building, "too much attention was paid to mere ornament, which increased the expense, without adding to either the comfort or the cheer-

[16] *Minutes of the Inspecting Committee*, Vol. 2, May 3, 1839.

[17] James Macdonald, "Statistics of the Bloomingdale Asylum for the Insane," *N.Y. J. Med. and Surg.* I, 310.

ful appearance of the building." [18] Dr. Macdonald's account of the interior of the building indicates that considerable attention had been given to making it attractive. One of the objects was to avoid "the semblance of a place of confinement," by using, wherever possible, cast-iron window sashes instead of bars. These sashes, it may be assumed, could not be opened wide enough to permit a person to pass through. Iron sashes, unglazed, were also used in transom openings over the doors of the patients' rooms. These openings were opposite a large window in the "gallery" to admit light and air. The rooms had "always been remarkable for their cheerfulness and the purity of their air." [19] The interior of the building, Dr. Macdonald stated, was "finished and furnished like a private dwelling. Some of the rooms are equal to any found in the best hotels." [20]

The "small cells in the basement," the windows of which, by order of the governors in 1821, were secured by iron bars, were not mentioned in Dr. Macdonald's description. They were still used, however, but when the new city asylum on Blackwell's Island was opened in July, 1839, the "pauper patients" of New York County were removed there from Bloomingdale Asylum, and the committee reported that the "basement of the main building is now unoccupied by patients." In August, however, when it was decided to admit patients who were not paupers at $3 a week, it was stipulated "that they would be treated in all respects as pauper patients, and lodged either in the basement of the main building or in the basement of the lodges." Since that day, a change has taken place in the policy of the governors relating to patients unable to pay full rates.

The provision for the mentally ill made by the Society of the New York Hospital was far from adequate for more than a very few of those in the state who were in need of hospital treatment. Throughout the state and even in New York City many were inmates of almshouses. In 1831, the City Commissioners of the Almshouse, which was desperately overcrowded, appealed to the governors to receive all the "pauper lunatics" of the city, and from time to time the transfer of considerable numbers was permitted. The governors explained, however, that, to provide for all these cases, "time must be given for preparing the necessary buildings for their accommodation." They were really averse to re-

18 New York State Assembly, Doc. 263, March 10, 1831: Report of Committee of the Legislature re New York Hospital.

19 New York City Board of Assistant Aldermen, Doc. 101, March 10, 1834. ("Communication from Dr. Macdonald, on . . . an asylum for the insane.")

20 Macdonald, *op. cit.*, p. 312.

ceiving these patients, many of whom were incurable and difficult, and often poorly clad and unclean. Public provision for the mentally ill was coming to be recognized as a clear necessity, and the establishment of state and county asylums was receiving consideration. It was evident that the state would no longer make appropriations for the work of the Society, and the governors began to shape their policy towards improving the character of the somewhat limited service which a private benevolent organization could expect to provide.

XIII

ORGANIZATION AND ADMINISTRATION

THE committee appointed in May, 1821, to draft rules for the government of the asylum, were not, like their predecessors in 1808, obliged to ask to be excused because they found themselves incompetent without at least a few months' experience. The experience gained during the thirteen years of operation of the asylum at the New York Hospital enabled the Asylum Committee, when they submitted their first report to the governors, in August, 1821, to present also a draft of "Bye-laws and regulations." They also, in September, adopted "Rules and Regulations to be observed by the keepers." [1] Together with the by-laws, which were adopted by the governors in November, these rules contain many of the principles and practices that have been followed in the administration of the service ever since. It is, however, no longer considered advisable to place a layman in charge of the management as superintendent. The place and value of medical administration in the operation of a service for the mentally ill were not at that time understood by the governors. The physician was designated simply "the Superior of the Medical Department." The superintendent, who was not a physician, was "to hire and dismiss all the nurses," as well as the other persons employed in and about the asylum. Another by-law was that

> the Patients shall be under the immediate charge and care of the Superintendent and Matron. It shall be their special duty to see that the general system of moral treatment prescribed for the patients, and the rules and regulations, as well as the special directions of the Asylum Committee and of the Physicians are carried into effect.

This will be discussed in later chapters. Although many details of administration which at that time were attended to by committees of the governors were afterwards delegated to the paid staff of the organization, the powers and duties of the Asylum Committee and the form of its organization have not been greatly changed since the by-laws first described them. The quarterly meeting specified was, however, found to be impractical, and at the request of the committee it was discontinued. On September 29, 1821, the Asylum Committee "Resolved that the monthly meeting of the Committee be held on Seventh Day [Saturday] previous to the monthly meeting of the Governors," and that has been the day

[1] For full text see Appendix p. 494.

of their meeting ever since.[2] The number of members of the committee remains as designated. The period of service has, however, not always been the same. In 1827 it was provided that only four of the six members were eligible for reëlection each year, and that the term of service of each would be three years. This is no longer the practice.

The organization of the asylum was at first very simple. In their annual report for the year 1821, the governors described it as follows:

A Superintendent, and Matron, respectable for their characters and deportment, have charge of the establishment, and the whole is superintended by a standing committee of the Governors, who visit it once a month, and by a sub-committee who visit once a week. It is also inspected monthly by another committee and monthly by the President and Vice-President; and once in every three months there is a special visitation by the Governors, and such physicians, members of the City Corporation and other respectable Citizens who are invited to attend.[3] By means of this perpetual supervision and inspection, abuses, if they should exist, cannot escape detection; and improvements are adopted whenever there seems to be room for them.

Reference was made to the "medical department . . . conducted by a resident physician who resides constantly in the house, and by an attending physician who visits it every week." In September, 1821, the superintendent reported to the committee that the monthly payroll was as follows:

Superintendent & Wife	$83.33	Baker & Dairy-maid	$9.00
2 Keepers (women) @ 8.00	16.00	Assistant	7.00
3 " (men) @ 12.00	36.00	Wash Woman	9.00
Yard Keeper	10.00	Assistant	7.00
Cook in Large Kitchen	9.00	Waiter	11.00
" " " "	8.00	"	5.00
" " Small "	9.00	Gardener	12.50
Farmer	15.00	Chamber maid	6.00
Assistant	10.00	Total	$258.83 [a]

[a] Actually, $262.83. In 1840 the corresponding amount was $531.53.

The number of patients was then about 60, for whom there were 6 "keepers," 2 of whom were women. The proportion of keepers to patients was 1 to 10. One of the keepers was designated "Yard Keeper." The wages were $8 to $12 a month, and the total amount for a month was $62. In 1829, the number of patients was 83. The term "keeper" was apparently not then used to designate those who gave personal care

[2] In 1939 this was changed to the fourth Tuesday of every month.
[3] This was discontinued in 1822.

to the patients. Fourteen "nurses"[4] were employed, of whom 10 were men and 4 were women, the proportion to patients having risen to 1 to 6. Their wages for a month were from $9 to $10, and the total was $129.50.[5]

The chief executive in the general administration of the asylum was the superintendent or warden. He purchased supplies, and had power to engage and dismiss all employees. The matron shared with the superintendent supervision of the female employees. The first persons to be employed in these positions, Laban Gardiner and his wife, were appointed in April, 1821, and remained until July, 1831. After they had left it was discovered that Gardiner was short in his accounts, and that after leaving he had continued to collect accounts due from patients. The next to occupy the positions were Ira Ford and his wife, who remained until June, 1837. They resigned because changes in the regulations deprived them of some authority.[6] They were succeeded by G. P. Pollock as superintendent and Anna Bausch as matron. In March, 1839, it was discovered that Pollock was embarrassed in his accounts, had spent several hundred dollars in furnishing his private room, and in "some other fixtures about the establishment," and was a defaulter to the amount of $1768.26. He was therefore dismissed, and soon afterwards sailed for New Orleans en route to Texas. His successor was William Boggs; Anna Bausch remained as matron.

The Asylum Committee continued to exercise vigilant and constant supervision and rendered indispensable service to the maintenance and advancement of standards. Their consideration for the sensibilities of the patients was again manifested when, in September, 1821, they decided that as visits from the whole committee agitated the patients and had a bad effect upon them, not more than two should visit at a time. The resident physician, as he grew in experience and understanding in the needs of the service, also made valuable suggestions relating to administration. Various improvements were in consequence made, from time to time, in the furnishings and facilities. Carpets were laid in many of the halls and rooms, some of the dining rooms were provided with better furniture, and knives and forks were permitted for patients who could be trusted with them. The first piano was purchased in 1835 for $170. Suitable beds and chairs were provided for destructive patients, and by order of the committee, pillows of larger size were furnished.

[4] There were no training schools for nurses at that time, nor for many years afterwards.
[5] Special Report to the Legislature, March, 1830. *Minutes of the Governors*, Vol. V.
[6] See pp. 194–195.

Many of the administrative procedures that are still followed had their origin in these early formative years.

The accounts of the asylum were kept separately from those of the New York Hospital, and a monthly report of receipts and expenditures was sent to the clerk of the hospital and entered by him in a separate account.[7] The income for ordinary current expenses was, as now, derived in large part from the rates paid for patients. Deficits were provided for by the treasurer of the Society. This accounts for the "expression of very great satisfaction" in the minutes of the Asylum Committee, in December, 1838, at the credit balance of $22.02 in the superintendent's financial report, by which, it was added, he had "succeeded in liquidating the indebtedness without calling, as has hitherto been done, on the Treasurer of the New York Hospital for aid." A very large proportion of the patients—designated paupers—were charged to the counties and towns from which they had been admitted, at a rate of $2 per week. Although this scarcely paid the cost, it was not increased until July, 1836, when it was advanced to $2.50, and in December of the same year to $3.[8] Private rates were above $3.00, though a reduction might be made after admission. The minimum rate for patients from places outside of New York State was $4.00. After the New York City "paupers" were removed to the new city asylum on Blackwell's Island in 1839, the governors reduced the minimum rate for private patients to $3. The maximum rate received during this period was $15 per week in two instances. An extra charge of $5 per week was made for a private nurse, and this was not infrequently provided. The board list for August, 1828, contained 93 patients, of whom 15, or about 17 percent, were in the $2 class. Of the remaining 78 the average weekly rate was about $4.35. The proportion of patients who were free or supported by public or charitable funds had increased from 17 percent in 1828 to 40 percent in 1838. The patients designated "free" (one of whom was a Negro) were "supported by the hospital." One of these had been admitted in 1808, and another in 1810. The average rate received from the private patients on this list was about $5.60 per week. Contrary to what has been sometimes assumed, Bloomingdale Asylum did not at any time receive maintenance support from the state. The annuity of $10,000 granted by the legislature in 1816, to be paid annually until 1857, was applied entirely to the interest and the sinking fund of the loan obtained by the governors

[7] See *Minutes of the Governors,* Feb. 5, 1833, and *Minutes of the Asylum Committee,* April 16, 1839.

[8] *Minutes of the Asylum Committee,* Dec. 31, 1836.

for the expense of the land and building and to reimbursing the corporation for amounts furnished for the same purpose from its own funds.

The problems connected with the rates charged for the treatment of the patients were the same as those met with today, and they were dealt with in similar fashion. The procedure at the meetings of the Asylum Committee resembled closely that still followed. The physician's report contained statistics and a brief account of the patients admitted since the last previous meeting, with remarks and sometimes recommendations relating to the service. The board list was presented, with a financial statement, and at nearly every meeting requests for a reduction in the rates were considered. The relation of the finances of the patient and of the rate paid, to his illness and his treatment, while not neglected, was perhaps not as clearly understood and considered as at present. Patients were assigned to rooms not only with reference to condition and needs, but also in accordance with the rate paid. Reduction to $3.00 a week might be followed by transfer to the basement or to the Lodge where disturbed patients were also accommodated. In one instance, the friends of a patient were informed that unless the rate was advanced to $7 he would be sent to "the five dollar ward." Not infrequently, however, a rate was reduced on purely philanthropic grounds, such as "it appearing that he could not afford to pay more," or as in the case of Nancy McF., "whose husband is a journeyman carpenter, and has several children to provide for."

In September, 1826, a rule was adopted requiring that payment be made for one month in advance, and payment for at least one week would be retained if the patient left within the month. In January, 1833, the period was extended to thirteen weeks, and this rule remained operative until February 1, 1916, when it was changed back to one month. The rule was, at first, directed principally to the discouragement of the too early discharge and the frequent readmission of alcoholic patients, and it was reported that it had "a salutary effect." It was also a rule that no refund would be made if the patient left without the approbation of the physician. Even if a patient escaped and went home, no refund was made, unless the patient returned. In one instance, it was agreed that the patient might return "to board out the time unexpired," which she did after two weeks at home. A patient admitted at the rate of $7 a week with an understanding that she would remain for a year, and who left in fourteen weeks, was charged at the rate of $10 a week. The rule was adhered to most closely with respect to the first payment, and was strictly enforced in alcoholic cases. Applications for a refund were sometimes "laid on the table," presumably to await further developments. Occasionally half the amount was returned. Particular circumstances sometimes led to review. Consideration was also given to the source of the funds from which payments were made, and in one instance it was directed that "in consideration of the money for Her admission having been advanced by charitable friends—that which is unexpended be returned to them." [9]

The collection of unpaid balances of amounts due the asylum for the treatment of patients was a source of much difficulty. The superintendent's financial statement at the close of the year usually showed a large part of the charge still unpaid. Notes were sometimes accepted, and from time to time the warden was directed to lay before the committee all outstanding claims due, "with his opinion of their goodness." Hopeless claims were charged off, and in rare instances, a lawsuit was instituted. The friends of patients whose bills were unpaid were, however, asked to remove the patient. When this was not promptly attended to, the warden might, as in one instance, be instructed "to send her to the residence of her husband in Long Island provided payment is not made by Wednesday of next week." [10] In March, 1833, the following form of bond was adopted by the committee:

> Upon the admission of A—— B—— of ——— into the Asylum for the Insane at Bloomingdale, I engage to pay to the Society of the New York Hospital, through the Warden of the Asylum ——— Dollars per Week for Board and Medical and Moral Treatment, I engage to make compensation for all damages done to the Windows, Bedding, or Furniture—to provide sufficient clothing for this patient,—for a removal when discharged, and in case of Death to defray the expenses of Burial.
>
> Signed: C—— D——
>
> I become responsible for the fulfilment of the above Obligation
>
> Signed: E—— F—— [11]

As the service developed, the admission of "paupers," for whom a low rate was paid by the counties and towns of the state, grew increasingly unsatisfactory. Some of the reasons for this were explained by the resident physician in his report for the year 1833. He considered that there were

> several circumstances which continue to operate unfavourably to the interests of this institution. By one of the by-laws of the New York Hospital it appears that Paupers belonging to the different towns and counties in the state are to be received for as small a compensation as they can be supported at. The rate of board established, though considered low, is higher than they

[9] *Minutes of the Asylum Committee*, May 4, 1833. [10] *Ibid.*, Dec. 16, 1837.
[11] *Ibid.*

can be kept for at home. The consequence is that the legal guardians of the poor, too often overlooking the recovery of the insane and thereby an entire future relief from their support, consult only the immediate interest of their communities and cause them to be confined in Jails or county houses till they become incurably imbecile or so violent that they destroy more than their board will amount to. Then when the disease becomes incurable, the conduct disorderly and the habits depraved, the patient as a last resort is sent to the Lunatic Asylum. The general result of the treatment of such cases must be merely an amelioration in the habits while the mental faculties of the patient are irretrievably deranged.

As it is the object of this institution to relieve where it can not cure, no stage nor form of insanity is refused admission, so that its numbers swell without increasing its character for usefulness. But it will not be denied that its intention is to cure as well as to relieve and protect the afflicted, and that incurable insanity is a great evil. The public and this institution then are equally interested in the matter.

Might not a by-law be enacted which would fix the rate of old incurable and destructive patients higher than it now is, and reduce that of recent cases, so as to induce superintendents and overseers to send them immediately to the Asylum? There is another circumstance connected with the admission of Paupers deserving of notice. From the fact that the board for town and county patients has been fixed at so low a rate, persons in easy circumstances residing in the county have in many instances gone to the overseers of the poor, advanced the necessary sum and got them to send their friends as paupers to the asylum. Several instances of this kind have happened during the past year, and those too in which the patients have been supported by their friends for a long time at other establishments. This practice is much to be regretted for the patients' sake. At home in easy circumstances; here a pauper. This consideration is sufficient to aggravate the malady of any patient who has the least self-respect left. Besides in an establishment like this, where all classes are received, a distinction must necessarily be made, in the accommodations and fare of those who pay liberally, and those supported by the public. Hence a constant source of heart-burnings, discontent and unhappiness.

A request was made to the overseers and superintendents of the poor that this practice be discontinued, and also that, in the selection of patients for admission to the asylum, preference be given those most likely to benefit from the treatment.[12]

From a very early period, the proper classification of the patients had occasioned much concern. The governors had learned that "one of the greatest and most valuable improvements of science and experience in this branch of the healing art, is the discovery of the importance and use of classification and association of patients." [13] The buildings erected

12 *Minutes of the Asylum Committee*, Sept. 3, 1836. 13 Annual Report for 1833.

in 1829 and 1837 had provided means for the separation of the noisy and violent patients from the others. Another problem was, however, occasioned by the obligation to accept patients who, irrespective of their condition and of the form and stage of their disorder, were sent to the asylum by the welfare authorities of the towns and counties. Many of these patients were suffering from advanced and incurable forms of mental illness and displayed very objectionable traits. In January, 1824, the Asylum Committee reported that the house was "crowded with pauper patients, sixty-seven of whom pay $2.00 a week and four pay nothing," and they were almost daily increasing in numbers; the annual report for the year 1833 describes as follows the principles and practice adopted in the classification of patients:

> The division of patients into classes is made according to the conduct, habits, education and station in life and state of mind. . . . In general, it is attempted to place such individuals together whose society will if possible be of mutual benefit, or at any rate will be no disservice to one another.[14]

This is sound therapeutic practice. After public asylums had relieved the Society of the New York Hospital of patients dependent upon public support, the governors were enabled, by means of private philanthropy, to adopt it to an extent that has ever since contributed greatly to the character and usefulness of the service. The advantage, and, under the circumstances, the necessity of obtaining the income to be derived from patients who could pay the full cost of their treatment, led the governors to give consideration to these patients in a way that is no longer practiced. They considered that, as there was no other institution for the treatment of the mentally ill, it was necessary to furnish "advantages suited to all classes . . . from the town pauper to the wealthy citizen who can afford to pay for extra attendance and the luxuries of life." According to the rate paid, a difference was made "in the size of the room, in the quality of furniture and of food; in associates and in the proportion of attendants to a given number of patients." Moreover, in order "to furnish

[14] In a report made to the Board of Assistant Aldermen of New York in March, 1834, Dr. James Macdonald thus classified the patients then at Bloomingdale:

	Men	*Women*	*Total*
1. Noisy, violent, etc.	18	12	30
2. Idiotic, filthy, etc.	13	8	21
3. Convalescent	13	11	24
4. Intermediate	27	14	41
Sick in the infirmary	3	3	6
Totals	74	48	122

the House so as to accomodate people of all grades and to render it attractive," [15] two "galleries" or halls were completely refurnished for convalescent and quiet patients. As early as 1822, the superintendent had been instructed to have at his own table the patients paying $8 a week or more; patients paying $5 were provided a separate table, which was appointed with some order and attention and was presided over by the principal keeper of the department. The $3 patients had a dining room in the basement, and for a sitting room had the southwest room in the basement, while the paupers had the northwest room. Separate yards were provided for "the higher rate patients." Later, when the publicly supported patients were no longer received, it was possible, without disadvantage, gradually to abandon the practice of separating the patients in accordance with the rate paid. Today it would in most instances be difficult for a visitor to the institution to determine what rate —if any—a particular patient was paying, as judged by the quarters occupied, the food, the associates, and the proportion of attendants to a given number of patients.

Few references to the dietary appear in the records of this period. In August, 1834, the Asylum Committee reported that the bread was heavy and sour, and that after a trial period a contract had been made with the baker in Manhattanville, who was furnishing "excellent bread." In April, 1837, the committee found that the meat was inferior and ordered that a better quality be purchased, even if it was necessary to reduce the quantity and to pay a higher price. Considerable quantities of vegetables were produced by the asylum farm. In 1832 apples from the trees on the property were so plentiful that some were sold. The following year, however, it was found that apples could be purchased for less than the cost of gathering them, and, as the land was more needed for hay and feed, the trees were cut down. At this period the asylum possessed a herd of cows. In October, 1835, the resident physician reported that "although improvements [in the dietary] have been made . . . [I] still consider it as neither sufficiently wholesome, nor palatable, nor as well served as the food in use by the middling classes of society at their own houses." He considered that the patients, in some instances, felt "a sense of degradation in being submitted to coarse food." He made many useful suggestions, and the committee ordered that a suitable cook be engaged to carry into effect the plan of diet recommended, and that better furniture for the dining rooms be procured. An intimation

[15] Annual Report for 1833.

of economy in the management of the dietary may be gathered from the following action of the Asylum Committee in January, 1838:

Dr. Ogden to discontinue both tables now spread in the main building for the Patients, if in his opinion no injury will arise from this measure; and that the furnishing the patients with Pies, Puddings and Cakes at each of their meals be also discontinued in part, at his discretion.

It was also directed that all patients who paid $4 a week or less were to have molasses instead of butter,

and instead of meat five days in the week, they be furnished with a sufficient quantity of mush or boiled Rice for three days, Salt Fish one day, and Soup and Boiled Meat for three days, the quantity to be regulated by the Physician, and the continuance or variance in the plan to be at his discretion.

The extent to which the rate paid by the patient determined the character of his dietary is noteworthy. The following is a sample of the dietary in 1840:

Sunday dinner. Cold beef, hot vegetables: Pies throughout the main building, Pudding in Lodges.
Monday dinner. Roast beef and vegetables. Halls 7 and 8, rice or bread puddings.
Other days. Boiled and roast meats alternately. Halls 7 and 8, pies or puddings; other hall three times a week.
Supper. Halls 7 and 8, black and green tea mixed, and cake every other night. All other halls black tea and cake twice a week.

The change that was taking place in the use of alcoholic beverages by the general population is reflected in a resolution of the governors in October, 1829, by which it was ordered that "no beer be allowed to the Patients of this House except under the direction of the Resident Physician." At the next monthly meeting of the board it was reported that the "effect of substituting water for beer as a drink for the patients . . . has been carried into full effect and thus far followed by no evil consequences—on the contrary it has been attended with every advantage anticipated by the committee." Again, in August, 1830, it was ordered that inquiry be made as to the expediency of dispensing with the "practice of issuing beer and cider to the nurses and servants." And in November, 1834, it was ordered that "wine be dispensed with at the Asylum except for the use of Patients under direction of the Physician."

The asylum was, even at this early period not immune from newspaper notoriety. On one occasion the *Evening Post* published a complaint from residents of the vicinity that patients were permitted to leave the premises unattended, and were an annoyance.[16] On investigation it was found that of the two mentally ill persons who were the subjects of the complaint, one had never been a patient at the asylum, and the other had been removed by his friends contrary to the advice of the physicians. It was also charged that a perfectly sane man had been decoyed from his house to the asylum and was detained there. Examination by physicians who were not connected with the asylum revealed that he was mentally deteriorated and had manifest delusions.[17]

The quarterly meeting of the Asylum Committee, to which the other governors, the mayor, the Common Council, the recorder, members of the State Senate, physicians, and other prominent persons were invited, was found impractical. Nevertheless, visits by these officials were occasionally made. On one occasion it was noted that they voiced "strong expressions of satisfaction with the general arrangements and good order" of the asylum. In December, 1824, Dr. Julius, who had been sent by the Kingdom of Prussia to examine United States institutions, visited the asylum.[18] In his annual message to the New York legislature in 1830, Governor Throop after describing the deplorable neglect and mistreatment of the mentally ill throughout the state, added:

> The contrast of their condition with those in the Lunatic Asylum in New York [Bloomingdale] is very striking. In the latter place everything is spacious, cleanly and pleasant to the eye; the inmates are suffered to be at liberty and range in the open air in an enclosed yard, they are treated with kindness, and their innocent whims indulged; the consequence is, that many who are placed there, are restored to reason and discharged after a short period, to enjoy the society of their friends. It speaks much in favor of the ability of the Keepers, attendants and superintendents of that interesting institution that during my visit this last summer, but one out of sixty or seventy then under their care were in close confinement.[19]

In March, 1830, a communication was received from the Clerk of the State Assembly requesting information relating to the manner in which the funds appropriated by the legislature for the support of the New York Hospital and Asylum were being used. Inquiry was made as to

> the price per week for keeping Insane Patients, with a classification of said patients, and what if any incidental charges attend said patients. The species of Insanity with which each Patient of the last Year was afflicted with the means of treating them. The rules and regulations of the Institution and

16 *Minutes of the Inspecting Committee,* June 30, 1834.
17 *Minutes of the Asylum Committee,* July 22, 1827.
18 See p. 298 re visit of General Lafayette in 1824.
19 Annual Report, New York State Lunatic Asylum, 1846.

generally such other information as may be in their power touching the important objects intended to be promoted by said Institution.[20]

The governors made as full a reply as was possible to such a comprehensive inquiry. In April the assembly passed a resolution to appoint a committee to visit the hospital and the asylum.

Resolved, That A. C. Paige, Eli Savage, Peter Gansevoort be and they are hereby appointed a committee for the purpose of investigating the manner in which the Hospital in the city of New York, and the Asylum connected therewith, have disbursed the funds which they have received from the State: and that said committee inquire particularly into the management, affairs and prospects of said establishment: the receipts and disbursements: and the propriety of making a different distribution of the funds now applied to the use, or of increasing such funds: and . . . . that they digest a system of the general and more economical distribution of such public charity; also the necessity of erecting new establishments the more extensively to distribute such charities: the proper site of such new erection, if any should be found necessary, with a plan of the same, and an estimate of the probable expense: also of requiring the physicians of said asylum to be appointed by the Governor and Senate, and that they report the result of their doings to the next Legislature.[21]

The committee report of March, 1831, was devoted almost entirely to the asylum and to the questions contained in the resolution. Although "economy was not consulted in the erection of this establishment," [22] the governors had administered with honesty and efficiency the funds appropriated by the state. The organization and the methods of treatment were described in considerable detail. Moreover,

the establishment possesses all the advantages of a cheerful prospect, and salubrious air. The grounds around it are laid out in parks and gardens. The patients have abundant opportunities for exercise, amusement and occupation, and the establishment itself is susceptible of great improvement, in carrying into more successful operation the system of moral treatment which has been found so efficacious.

After a brief review of the extent to which the state had contributed to the establishment and support of the hospital and the first asylum, the committee reported, with reference to the annuity of $12,500 to the hospital, that "without this appropriation the Hospital could not sustain itself, its means of dispensing its charities to the afflicted and diseased

20 *Minutes of the Governors,* March 16, 1830.
21 New York State Assembly, April 1, 1830.
22 New York State Assembly, Doc. 263, March 10, 1831: Report of Committee of the Legislature re New York Hospital and Asylum.

would be essentially curtailed to the lasting regret of every philanthropic citizen." In regard to the annuity granted to the asylum, the committee stated that

> upon the faith of the State in the granting of this annuity, and in its continuance to 1857, the Bloomingdale Asylum was erected. And however the Committee with others may regret the want of economy in the erection of this establishment they believe it would be a violation of the faith of the State and injurious to the interests of humanity, to withold from the Hospital the payment of this annuity.

The reply of the committee to the questions relating to the appointment of the physicians of the asylum by the governor and the senate was that

> however desirable such a mode of appointment might be thought by many, yet the Committee entertains serious doubts as to the power of the Legislature to transfer the right of appointment from the Governors of the New York Hospital to the Governor and Senate, as it might be contended that such an interference would be a violation of chartered privileges and vested rights, and therefore an infringment of the constitution of the United States.

An interest in psychiatric education was evidenced by a suggestion that

> the Governors . . . hereafter encourage the periodical publication of the cases treated at the Asylum, for the benefit of the medical profession generally, and in order to aid the researches of scientific men in the treatment of insanity, and to enable them to advance this art to a higher point of perfection than that to which it has hitherto arrived. The importance of such a publication in the interests of medical and mental science must be apparent to every individual who gives the subject a moment's reflection. In making this publication, a disclosure of the names of the patients can be avoided, and thus the great interests of humanity and science may be promoted, without wounding the feelings of individuals.

Following a rather full discussion of mental illness and its treatment in some parts of Europe and America, the committee reported that

> relying upon the favorable feelings entertained by their fellow-citizens towards all objects of charity [they] have, for the reasons stated in this report, come to the conclusion, that public establishments for the reception and cure of the insane poor, are both necessary and proper. And they therefore submit to the Legislature the expediency of providing for the erection of at least one spacious and commodious hospital, sufficient to accomodate at least 350 of the insane poor. . . . If commodious well regulated hospitals were established, the number of insane poor would rapidly diminish, by means of the recoveries that would be effected. The Part recovering would

generally cease to be a burden upon the public, and their discharge from the establishment would create vacancies for others, who in their turn would enjoy the benefits of curative treatment. . . . The building should have the appearance of a cheerful country residence, and all resemblance to a place of confinement should be avoided.

The use here of the term "hospital" instead of "asylum," and the emphasis on curability are noteworthy. These enlightened views and recommendations can hardly have been held only by the members of this committee. The problem was indeed engaging the attention of society with growing momentum.

As far as the present writer is aware, this report contains the first plan for state hospitals for the insane poor ever presented for consideration by the New York State Legislature. Twelve years elapsed, however, after the report was presented in 1831 before the first state hospital was opened in 1843, though its construction was authorized in 1836; and not until 1896—under the state care act of 1890—were all "the insane poor" provided for in state hospitals. It is unfortunate that in the development of the system the principles and recommendations of the committee of 1831 have not been more closely adhered to—so tardy is society in adopting measures of defense and remedy against the ravages of disease and misery, as of war.

It is not without interest that, in inaugurating this advance in the treatment of the mentally ill of the state, the Society of the New York Hospital had some small part. In the annual report for the year 1831, the governors expressed

pleasure that the subject of relieving the Insane has attracted the particular attention of the Executive and Legislature. They have attended to the suggestions of a Committee of the Assembly, by whom they have been visited, and they will be happy to aid in effecting the philanthropic views of the government whose almoners they are in administering the charity confided to their care.

The Society had also an opportunity to be of service to the city in connection with the establishment of the New York City Lunatic Asylum on Blackwell's (now Welfare) Island. The commissioners engaged in studying this project visited Bloomingdale Asylum in December, 1834. The resident physician of the Asylum, Dr. James Macdonald, had, in March of the same year, prepared for the Board of Assistant Aldermen a communication,[23] with floor plans, relating to the construction of the

23 N.Y. City Board of Assistant Aldermen, Doc. 101, March 10, 1834.

proposed institution, in which he gave valuable information and recommendations based not only upon his experience at Bloomingdale Asylum, but also upon a study of the asylums in Europe which he had made for the Society in 1831–1832.[24]

[24] *Minutes of the Asylum Committee*, Nov. 3, 1832. See Appendix, p. 496, for full text of Dr. Macdonald's communication.

XIV

THE BLOOMINGDALE MEDICAL SERVICE

AFTER the asylum was removed to Bloomingdale the established plan of medical service by a nonresident attending physician was continued for seven years. Dr. John Neilson was retained and visited the patients as required by the by-laws. The asylum was so far out of town, however, that a resident physician was considered to be necessary also. The first to hold this position was Dr. James Eddy, who was appointed in June, 1821. He was succeeded in September, 1822, by Dr. Albert Smith, who remained until February, 1824. No permanent successor was appointed until May, and in the interim Dr. Smith, who had taken up private practice, was called upon when necessary, and Dr. James Rogers occasionally substituted. In May, 1824, Dr. Abraham V. Williams was appointed and served for a year, with Dr. John Neilson, Jr., who had been a house surgeon at the New York Hospital, substituting on occasion. Dr. Williams became a prominent general practitioner in the Bloomingdale section of the city, and frequently when help was needed at the asylum he gave his services generously and refused to accept compensation. In June, 1825, he was succeeded by Dr. James Macdonald, who continued in the position until August, 1837, and made such a notable contribution to its advancement that a fuller account of him will be given later. Dr. Benjamin Ogden, successor to Dr. Macdonald, was a graduate of Columbia Medical School, and had been a house surgeon at the New York Hospital. He had also been physician of Bellevue Hospital, and had shown such capability that in 1837 when the hospital was infested with "typhus from top to bottom" and "eight nurses and servants had left overnight," [1] he was asked to return and cope with the situation. There were many mentally ill patients at Bellevue, and it was considered when Dr. Ogden was appointed at Bloomingdale in August, 1837, that his experience had especially qualified him for the position. When he resigned in September, 1839, he had won the strong commendation of the governors.

Dr. Neilson was faithful to his duties, but, especially after Dr. Macdonald's service was prolonged, it became evident that the resident physician, by virtue of his constant attention, surpassed the attending physician in his knowledge and usefulness in the treatment of the patients. The governors, therefore, in 1828 changed the duties of the attending physician to those of a consultant, and in 1830 that position

[1] R. J. Carlisle, *An Account of Bellevue Hospital* (New York, 1893).

was abolished. In January, 1831, they adopted a resolution that "the duties of Visiting Physician of the Asylum be performed by the resident physician." For many years thereafter, however, the authority of the physician continued to be limited by that of the superintendent. This will be considered more fully in the next chapter.

Nothing has been found in the records to indicate whether or not the provision in the by-laws that "any patient may, at the expense of his friends, be attended by his own physician," was ever resorted to. Experience has long revealed that the conditions and responsibilities of a service for the mentally ill are such that an arrangement of this kind cannot be made to work satisfactorily. The physician who is responsible for the care and treatment of the patients must be specially qualified by training and experience and must be employed by the institution.

The total number of cases admitted to Bloomingdale Asylum from its opening in 1821 to December 31, 1840, was 2,496 (including the 52 patients transferred from the asylum at the New York Hospital), an average of 124.8 cases each year. The number discharged as "recovered" during the same period was 1,145, or 45.8 percent of the number admitted. Four hundred and sixty-six were discharged "improved." Two hundred and twenty-two died, which was 8.8 percent of the admissions. It was the opinion of the resident physician that

> to the practice before admission of keeping maniacs closely confined and chained for months or perhaps years until all hope of recovery is gone and the health destroyed, and then suddenly transporting them from some of the most remote counties of the state to New York, is to be attributed many of the deaths that occur in our institution.

It is noteworthy that 446 cases (about 17.8 percent of the cases admitted) were discharged by request of relatives, and that 43 "eloped." The number still in the asylum at the close of 1840 was 131, and the largest number at the close of any year was 145 in1837.[2]

The preponderance of chronic cases was considered by the governors and by the physician to be a great disadvantage to the development of a service directed to cure. On one occasion the resident physician reported that, of 120 patients in the asylum, 102 were chronic cases. By means of statistical tables and reports, the advantages of early treatment were kept before the legislature and the public. Table 2, taken from the report for the year 1823, illustrates the form in which the ex-

[2] Figures taken from physicians' Annual Reports and Summaries in the *Minutes of the Asylum Committee*.

TABLE 2: REPORT OF THE RESIDENT PHYSICIAN [a]

	Mania		Melancholia		Hypochondriasis		Dementia		Dementia Epileptica		Imbecility Congenital	
	M	F	M	F	M	F	M	F	M	F	M	F
Remaining Dec. 31, 1822												
Old cases [c]	16	22	..	4	..	1	7	3	1	..	4	4
Recent cases [d]	1	2	2	..	1	..	1	..	..	..	..	..
Admitted in 1823												
Old cases [c]	12	13	4	4	..	..	8	3	..	..	..	..
Recent cases [d]	14	15	9	4	..	..	4	3	1	..	..	..
Total patients, 1823												
Discharged in 1823												
Old cases [c]												
Recovered	1	6	..	1	..	..	..	..	..	..	..	..
Much improved	..	4	..	1	1	..	1	..	..	..	..	..
Improved	6	2	1	..	..	..	..	1	..	..	1	..
Unimproved	2	1	1	..	..	..	2	1	..	..	..	..
Recent cases [d]												
Recovered	8	5	..	2	..	..	2	..	..	..	..	..
Much improved	1	1	2	..	..	..	..	1	..	..	..	..
Improved	2	1	1	2	..	..	..	1	..	..	..	..
Unimproved	1	..	2	..	..	..	..	..	..	..	..	..
Died	1	2	1	1	..	..	..	..	..	..	..	..
Eloped	2	2	..	..	..	..	..	..	..	..	..	..
Remaining Dec. 31, 1823												
Old cases [c]	13	28	5	5	..	1	6	4	2	..	..	..
Recent cases [d]	4	3	2	..	..	..	3	1	..	..	..	..

[a] Dr. Albert Smith.

[b] *Minutes of the Asylum Committee.* First annual report by a resident physician in these minutes.

perience with "old" and "recent" cases was presented. It also gives the diagnostic terminology.

The large number of cases of "mania," amounting to 41 percent of the admissions, is noteworthy. The terms "adventitious idiocy" and "adventitious imbecility" were in many instances used to indicate not only mental deficiency, but also the extreme grades of deterioration due to mental illness. Other terms which appear in the Register of Admissions during the period of 1821 to 1840 are: Imbecility, acquired; Idiocy,

OF THE BLOOMINGDALE ASYLUM, JANUARY 3, 1824[b]

Imbecility adventitious		Idiocy congenital		Idiocy adventitious		Hemiplegia		Mania a potu		Inebriety habitual		Total each sex		Total both sexes
M	F	M	F	M	F	M	F	M	F	M	F	M	F	
												48	43	91
6	3	..	1	5	2	1	..	..	..	..	..	40	40	80
..	..	..	..	..	..	..	..	2	1	1	..	8	3	11
												83	48	131
2	..	..	..	..	..	1	..	4	..	6	1	37	21	58
..	..	..	..	..	..	1	..	11	4	6	1	46	27	73
												131	91	222
												72	41	113
..	..	..	..	..	..	..	..	3	..	6	1	10	8	18
..	..	..	..	..	..	..	..	..	..	..	..	2	5	7
2	..	..	..	..	..	..	..	..	..	..	..	10	3	13
2	..	..	..	..	..	1	..	..	..	..	..	8	2	10
..	..	..	..	..	..	..	..	11	4	4	1	25	12	37
..	..	..	..	..	..	..	..	1	..	..	..	4	2	6
..	..	..	..	..	..	..	..	..	..	..	..	3	4	7
..	..	..	..	..	..	1	..	..	..	..	..	4	..	4
..	..	..	..	..	..	..	..	..	..	..	..	2	3	5
..	..	..	..	..	..	..	..	..	..	2	..	4	2	6
												57	52	109
10	7	..	1	5	2	1	..	2	..	..	..	45	48	93
..	..	..	..	..	..	..	..	..	..	3	..	12	4	16

[c] Of more than a year's duration on admission.
[d] Of less than a year's duration on admission.

---

acquired; Imbecility, natural; Imbecility, habitual; Imbecility acquired of infirmity; Imbecility from old age; Hemiplegia with partial delirium; Hypochondriasis with intemperance; Hypochondriasis or perverted disposition; Delirium Tremens (first noted in 1823); Drunkenness; Intemperance; Melancholia and Mania; Mania and hysteria; Typhomania; Mania typhus; Puerperal mania (first noted in 1824); Puerperal insanity. Of a case (A. S.) admitted September 8, 1832, it was recorded that articulation was "thick and awkward" with occasional stammering, the "mind quite elevated," and that it was probably "a case of Paralysie Generale of Calmeil." This was an early observation of the disease in America, made before any description of it was published here.[8]

"Recent" cases were those in which the duration of illness before admission was considered to be not more than one year, and, in one report at least, the limit was not more than three months. In their annual report for 1838 the governors stated that

> the comparative results of the treatment during the last year, of recent cases of Insanity, and of those of longer standing confirm the board in the opinion formerly expressed, of the much greater chance of success in the former than in the latter, and lead them again to urge the solemn duty of securing at an early period the advantages that the Asylum affords for the interesting subjects of this calamitous visitation. Of the whole number of seventy-three cases of recent insanity from various causes, discharged during the year, 62 recovered, 3 were discharged improved, 2 by request, and 6 died, and of 56 old cases, 11 only recovered, 19 were discharged improved, 10 by request, 1 eloped, and 15 died.

A statement of recoveries during the whole period from 1821 to 1840 showed that of 1,006 "old" cases admitted, only 111, or 11 percent, had recovered, while of 1,265 "recent" cases, 974, or 76 percent, had recovered.

After the removal to Bloomingdale the case records received a little more attention than had previously been accorded. The governors had always encouraged the physicians to keep good records, both in the hospital and the asylum. The by-laws adopted in 1821 directed that:

> The Physician of the Asylum shall endeavour to procure from the friends of every Patient who may be sent to the Asylum, a statement of his case, showing the commencement, probable cause, and character of his disease. The substance of which he shall direct the Resident Physician to enter in a Register to be kept for that purpose, in which he shall also see that the Resident Physician enters the name, age, place of residence, and occupation of each patient, what may appear to the Physician of the Asylum, the probable cause of Patient's disorder, and its History subsequently to the Patients being received in the Institution; the remedies or general course of treatment pursued in the particular case, the termination of the disease, and such other circumstances, as in the opinion of the Physician of the Asylum, may tend to elucidate the case and the nature of the disease. This register shall be kept in the Asylum, under the care of the Asylum Committee, who shall provide a proper book for the purpose; and it shall be the duty of the Asylum Committee to see that this regulation be complied with by the Physician of the Asylum, and Resident Physician, and the Committee shall report any omission in

[8] See p. 219.

this respect to the Board of Governors with their quarterly report. [Revised in 1825 to monthly report.] The Committee shall cause all remarkable cases to be reported in a proper Volume, by the Resident Physician, and as often as a volume is filled, it shall be deposited in the Library of the Asylum.

The recording of "remarkable" cases was considered by the governors to be a method of research and education. The "Register" was a large book, about a yard long when open, and was divided by vertical lines, the spaces of varying width having the following captions: Name, Age, Nativity, Residence, Married or Single, Occupation, Hair, Eyes, Nature, Conformation, History, Supposed Cause, Present Symptoms, Treatment, Diet, Result, Remarks. All the cases admitted were entered in the Register, and numbered consecutively, a method which has been continued up to the present. In a large proportion of instances, these entries constituted the only record of the patients admitted. The wider spaces were utilized for notes that became more and more extensive. Many cases were, however, reported more fully in a volume for "remarkable cases," which was kept in the library. One of these volumes contains 140 histories of patients admitted from July, 1821, to August, 1829. Another contains 79 histories of patients admitted from December, 1829, to November, 1848. These case records differed little from those kept by Dr. Handy in the old asylum.

Difficulty was experienced in obtaining histories. In November, 1828, the resident physician reported that "it is not in one case out of twenty that anything like a satisfactory account can be procured when patients are sent from a distance or when the former medical attendant of the Lunatic is not seen by the Physician of the institution." Physical examinations were no more systematic nor complete. Instruments of precision such as the thermometer and stethoscope were apparently not used. Nor were chemical examinations made. The stomach tube had not yet come into use. Patients who abstained from food were fed by means of a funnel, "a stomach pump," or a cup with a spout.

General medical treatment at Bloomingdale was not greatly different from that employed in the asylum at the New York Hospital, though the measures were perhaps less drastic. Venesection had never been practiced at the asylum to the extent prevalent in general medical practice, and in some other institutions. In August, 1826, the resident physician reported to the committee the admission of a patient who had been bled by a general practitioner every other day for a fortnight and when admitted was "a walking skeleton, with scarcely sufficient power to move a muscle, and almost deprived of the power of articulation." The treatment was characterized as "this depletory system, this professional method of murder under titled sanction, this outrage on reason and common sense." Moderate bleeding, however, was practiced at the asylum by means of cupping, and as much as a pint of blood was sometimes withdrawn. Leeches were also used, the first record noted being in 1834. Their use was continued into the first decade of the twentieth century. Blisters were still employed, and setons, in the efficacy of which Dr. Macdonald seemed to have much confidence. Blisters to the sacrum were considered to be of service in the treatment of amenorrhoea. Purges and emetics were still administered quite routinely in practically all cases; less drastically, however, than in the past. Calomel was still preferred as a purgative, but was less frequently combined with jalap or other drastic purges. Croton oil was, however, occasionally prescribed. Aloes, senna, rhubarb, and saline laxatives were more frequently used. Tartar emetic was not prescribed so routinely and was considered especially useful only when digestion was disturbed. Sedatives were used, perhaps a little more freely; caution was exercised in the use of opium. Other sedatives were hyoscyamus, belladonna, and conium. Ether and chloroform, although not yet introduced as a means of producing general anaesthesia, were sometimes inhaled to allay excitement and produce sleep. Tincture of digitalis was at this time used quite extensively. Salivation by mercury was seldom resorted to. In one instance, in 1836, the resident physician felt that only "after consultation with Dr. N—" could this treatment be employed. Evidently the more severe measures of treatment which had not yet been entirely discarded were viewed with distrust by the asylum physicians. Frequently the bad effects of those measures to which patients had been exposed before admission to the asylum were mentioned in the histories and in the reports. In one instance a patient who had, before admission, been treated by cupping, blistering, setons, frequent purging, and vomiting, was reported to have "been so drained by cathartics that he is in constant want of drinks and particularly saline fluids."

Theoretical considerations were not so implicitly relied upon as a guide to practice. It was still considered, however, that disturbance of the circulation of the blood in the brain was the principal cause of mental illness. Purges were given "to reduce the frequency of his circulation and determination to the brain." A patient in whom an intermittent fever had been allowed to take its course, was "for many weeks afterwards almost sane, but as soon as his physical health was fully established and his *vessels got to be full,*[4] mental aberration began to return." In the case of a patient whose mental condition improved following a fall from a third-story window (while he was attempting to escape, in November, 1829), it was recorded that the fall "operated similarly, though more powerfully than the Bath of surprise, it opened his eyes to a full conviction of his recent follies, and gave an impulse to his physical energies favorable to the operation of remedies." It was believed that cases originating in hot weather were more curable, "as it is then that the physical obstructions are more common"—a reminiscence of the solidists.[5]

Warm baths, sometimes for an hour, were employed, as well as foot baths containing mustard. Frequent references to the use of restraint and seclusion are found in the histories. Shower baths were used, but it was no longer considered proper to use them as a means of punishment. Nevertheless, in 1827, in the case of a patient who, in a state of apathy with extreme perverseness of disposition, "would for days observe the most perfect taciturnity and stubbornly reject medicine of every kind," it was recorded that "the shower bath, however, has in great measure overcome the habit and changed his disposition." In 1833, also, it was noted in a case history, "having destroyed clothing and done other mischief—ordered a shower bath."

Although one of the principal objects in establishing the asylum at Bloomingdale was to discard entirely the severe measures then generally considered to be appropriate and necessary in the treatment of the mentally ill, the records reveal that, though less frequently than at the old asylum, patients were placed in confinement, often in the basement—as "straw patients" (see p. 181) or otherwise—and were strapped hand and foot and fastened to the floor, or were placed in the "tranquillizing chair." It was assumed that chains would never be used; two instances, only, are recorded, one in 1823 and another in 1825.

It is interesting to find that, even in this early period, the curative effect of an attack of malarial fever in the treatment of mental illness was observed and utilized.[6] Although the location of the asylum at Bloomingdale was considered especially salubrious, it was nevertheless infested with malaria. Many cases occurred every year, in some years more than in others, depending, no doubt, upon the rainfall. It was not until 1836,

4 No italics in original.

5 See p. 7.

6 See p. 18 for an earlier observation by William Pargeter, *Observations on Maniacal Disorders* (Reading, England, 1792). Still earlier ones are mentioned in Gregory Zilboorg, *History of Medical Psychology* (New York, 1941), pp. 550–551.

however, after Dr. Macdonald had advised the governors that "moisture was a prolific source" of malaria, that the woods were cleared of underbrush and the wet places on the property drained. It was reported that during 1835 there were seventy or eighty cases in a population of less than two hundred, and that during the six months preceding the report every male attendant except one had been ill with intermittent fever. The employees were affected more than the patients in the proportion of two and a half to one. No doubt mosquitoes were abundant, but their role in malaria was not then known, and they were not mentioned in the reports. Several cases were reported in which improvement or recovery from the mental illness accompanied or followed an attack of malarial fever. In December, 1827, the physician reported that Abraham B——, who had suffered from mania for two years, had recovered and that

> his restoration was as singular as it was unexpected. . . . He was attacked in the month of July last with intermittent fever. His mind at this time having been discovered to be improved, the Intermittent was *purposely allowed to take its course*[7] and was not checked until the month of October when Quinine was employed. The consequence was, that the morbid chain of associations has been entirely broken up by another disease of a more active character on the principle that two disordered actions cannot exist in the system at the same time.[8]

In October, 1830, the physician reported "the successful result of Conklin's case . . . caused by intermittent fever or rather by a partially checked intermittent," and that, in another patient who had been ill with intermittent fever, "under its influence her mental disorder is gradually going away." Again, in October, 1836, he reported that two patients "had become almost sane" since intermittent fever was "allowed to take its course."

Other transmissible diseases also invaded the service on a few occasions. In March, 1826, a patient who was found upon admission to have typhus fever died in two weeks. There were apparently no other cases, though the means of transmission were not lacking in the asylum. In July, 1832, upon the report that "malignant cholera" cases had been discovered in Haarlem and Manhattanville, the resident physician was directed to write a public letter reassuring their friends as to the continued health of the patients in the asylum. He was also directed to prepare rooms for cholera patients, one in the northeast basement, and

[7] No italics in original.
[8] This view was held by Dr. Rush and many others.

one in the southwest basement or on the upper floor of the new building (the men's Lodge). The asylum did not long escape, and on August 11 two patients died of cholera and one was convalescing. The total number of cases was not stated in the reports to the committee. The upper story of the Lodge was, however, given over entirely to cholera patients, extra nurses were engaged, and a supply of flannel shirts ordered.

The dysentery and diarrhoea that prevailed in the summer months were attributed to the large quantity of fruit accessible to the patients on the property. In 1834 smallpox was prevalent in the neighborhood. Dr. Macdonald examined all the patients, and finding "a dozen without scars," vaccinated them. He was directed by the Asylum Committee to consult with the physicians and surgeons of the New York Hospital in regard to vaccination. It was, however, not until April and May of 1838 that varioloid and smallpox attacked the patients, seven of whom were affected. No deaths were reported and on June 2 the physician advised the governors that the house was free of the disease.

Among the forms of disorder presented by the patients admitted to the asylum, none occasioned as much concern as those produced by the use of alcoholic beverages. Many cases of "mania a potu" were also treated in the general hospital, the number in 1840 being 47, and in some other years there were many more. The cases were classified as "mania a potu," or delirium tremens, and habitual inebriety. The problem had already been the subject of much consideration at the old asylum, and the first report made by the resident physician at Bloomingdale, in June, 1822, conveyed the rather disturbing information that

> full one-third (and for the last six months nearly one half) of the cases admitted, in this institution, were the effects of Intemperance from the use of spiritous liquors—were every Institution to designate this species of Insanity in their annual reports, the results most probably would be similar. One patient has been admitted *three* times and another *twice* (since the opening of the Asylum) from this cause—perhaps the best check in such cases would be not to admit patients a second time for a less period than six months; increasing the time of residence for every admission.

The monthly statistical table of admissions kept the subject before the committee by a record of the number of cases attributed to alcohol which had been admitted during the previous month. In his annual report to the governors for the year 1833 Dr. Macdonald discussed the subject as follows:

> From the circumstances of there being no other place for the reception and reformation of the intemperate this institution has been necessarily perverted to the purpose.
>
> The mental disorder arising from intemperance is temporary and does not properly belong to the class of diseases included under the head of insanity. The proportion of this class of patients however to the whole number admitted during the past year, owing to some new and salutary regulations adopted by the committee, has been smaller than in former years. Still it is felt to be an evil that requires a remedy.
>
> The great cause of temperance has numerous and powerful advocates. The effect of their exertions is chiefly to prevent intemperance, while those far advanced in the vice are allowed to complete the work of self-destruction or continue their habits until a temporary or perhaps fatal attack of delirium takes them to the Asylum. We see around us men who if not for this disease or infatuation, if it may be so called, might adorn any station in life. Surely such men are worth saving. Might not some effectual plan be devised for their reformation? Might not the temperance society establish an Asylum where such persons could find useful employment adapted to their tastes and at the same time be under a regular course of moral discipline? It appears to me that such an institution is practicable and highly desirable.[9]

Of 1,680 admissions from 1824 to 1836, the number of alcoholic cases of all types was 391.[10] Although the psychiatric department of the New York Hospital has now solved its problem of the alcoholic by strictly limiting the number admitted and prescribing the conditions of admission and treatment, the general situation has changed little since Dr. Macdonald's report was presented.

A few cases of opium addiction were also recorded among the patients admitted. One of these, admitted in April, 1832, was described as "a very decent married female from the city. Having been habituated to the use of Laudanum by the advice of her physician during her pregnancy about two years since, she found herself utterly unable to relinquish its use, and voluntarily placed herself here to be assisted in her efforts to its entire abandonment." [11] Two other cases of addiction to "laudanum and other stimulants" were recorded, one in 1835, the other in 1840.

The governors had always realized the usefulness of a medical library, and that at the New York Hospital was liberally supported. Access to this library was, however, no longer easy for the asylum physician, and the governors encouraged the establishment of a separate library at

[9] *Minutes of the Asylum Committee,* Feb. 1, 1834. See also Dr. Bruce's report in Appendix, p. 489

[10] James Macdonald, "Statistics of Bloomingdale Asylum for the Insane," *N.Y. J. Med. and Surg.,* I, Oct. 1839, p. 307.

[11] *Minutes of the Asylum Committee,* April 28, 1832.

Bloomingdale. In August, 1823, they appropriated $16 for the purchase of books published in America, and $25 or $30 for foreign books. In November of the same year they appropriated $100 for "philosophical instruments and books," and at the same time John Clark, Jr., one of the governors, presented "several valuable medical books towards the formation of a library at the Asylum," and the governors ordered "duplicate books on insanity or diseases of the mind in the hospital library and wanted at the Asylum to be removed there." From time to time, usually at long intervals and evidently when requests were received from the physician, appropriations were made for the purchase of books. A considerable number of foreign books were imported in 1829, Mr. Hone being appointed to obtain the English books and Mr. Taylor the French (both men were members of the Board of Governors). The titles of these books were entered in the minutes,[12] and nearly all are still in the library of the Westchester Division of the Hospital. Publications from a physician of the asylum which appeared in the medical literature of the period will be referred to in the next chapter. Very few publications relating to mental illness were contributed from other sources in America, though reports of cases sometimes appeared in the *American Journal of Medical Science*.[13] Dr. Rush's treatise was still the only one by an American author. Dr. Isaac Ray's *Treatise on Medical Jurisprudence of Insanity* was published in Boston, in 1838. A treatise by Dr. J. C. Prichard of London was published in Philadelphia in 1837, and a work entitled *Observations on Insanity* by J. G. Spurzheim of phrenology fame, which had been published in London in 1817, was republished in Boston in 1833. Many publications by English, French, and other foreign authors were also, no doubt, imported.

With the exception of the New York City Lunatic Asylum (opened in 1839), Dr. Macdonald's private asylum, and a private institution at Hudson, there was still in 1840 no other organized medical service for the treatment of the mentally ill in New York State than Bloomingdale Asylum. In other parts of the country there were the Pennsylvania Hospital,[14] the Friends Asylum, the McLean Asylum, the Hartford Retreat and the Brattleboro Retreat, which were privately supported; and nine public asylums, all except one of which had been established after 1821. The awakening to the needs of the mentally ill thus manifested was due in some measure to a spreading belief that, contrary to

[12] *Ibid.*, February and April, 1829.

[13] XX (1837), 61.

[14] A separate department for the mentally ill was opened in 1841 and patients of this character had been provided for at the general hospital since 1752.

what had long been thought, many of the cases could be cured. This belief was fostered by the inordinate claims of some institutions and physicians. It was, also, however, supported by

> the really solid achievements of the early corporate hospitals (Frankford, McLean, and Bloomingdale asylums, and the Hartford Retreat itself). These institutions afforded impressive demonstrations of the truth that a fair proportion of the mentally sick *could* be cured. Their existence did much to dispel the hopeless atmosphere then surrounding the care and treatment of the insane, and contributed to the optimism necessary to the advancement of the hospital idea.[15]

Dr. Macdonald considered "that whatever improvements have since been introduced in the construction of asylums in neighboring states, the impulse was given by the Governors of the New-York Hospital, and that the plans adopted are all more or less copies of the institution founded by their humanity." [16]

The reports and records examined disclose little relating to the character and work of the nursing personnel. There is perhaps negative evidence in the fact that there was little criticism. In their annual report for the year 1840, the governors stated that there were

> nine male and eight female nurses or attendants, who are to enforce the regulations of the house, and the directions of the Physician, to see to the personal cleanliness and comfort of the patients, *to draw their attention* [17] to the amusements provided for them, and to walk with them over the enclosed ground, or in the neighbourhood; prevent their escape, and protect them from accident or injury.

There were 131 patients in the asylum when the report was made, 81 men and 50 women, making a proportion of nurses to patients of 1 to 7.7, which, while far below the standard of the present Bloomingdale service, is about the proportion now recommended for state hospitals by the American Psychiatric Association. The nurses were evidently held strictly to account for the safety of their patients, and were required to pay for the return of any who escaped, if it could be shown that the escape was due to the negligence of the nurses. It seems incredible that the patients on the halls could ever have been left entirely without supervision. Nevertheless, in October, 1835, the resident physician reported that

[15] Albert Deutsch, *The Mentally Ill in America* (New York, 1937), pp. 136–137. Reprinted by permission of the American Foundation for Mental Hygiene.

[16] Macdonald, *op. cit.*, p. 311.

[17] No italics in original. A very inadequate conception of psychiatric nursing is shown.

the nurses have hitherto been in the habit of giving the Patients their meals, and after these have been finished of going down into the kitchen for their own. These necessarily occupy some time during which the patients are left to themselves. I would suggest that the nurses be obliged to eat with all the different classes of Patients except those on Halls Nos. 7 and 8 in the Basement of the Main building and in the Brick House, and that the Committee make it a rule that in those Halls where there are two nurses, but one of them to be absent at a time.

Notwithstanding this evidence of lax supervision, the few suicides in the service seem to indicate the contrary. The resident physician in reporting a suicide on October 3, 1835, stated that it was the first in six years. The records reveal that three patients committed suicide in 1826, one in 1829, one in 1835, one in 1837, and one in 1838. Three of these patients were women, all of whom resorted to hanging as a means of death. One of the men succeeded in killing himself when "on an excursion with the resident physician." Another cut his throat with a secreted razor, which "nobody acknowledged they ever saw before." The minutes stated that "since the fatal catastrophe no patient in the Institution is allowed to shave himself or have any sharp instrument of any kind." [18]

Many patients were allowed much liberty. Of one man whose disorder "seemed likely to terminate in mental imbecility," it was reported that [19]

a love affair with a young lady in the neighbourhood, whose house he used frequently to pass in his walks, gave the first impulse to his feelings, and did more probably towards arousing his mind from the state of apathy into which it had fallen than anything else. If his mind be now disciplined by some suitable employment there is little doubt of his entire recovery.

He recovered after ten years in the asylum. An interesting account of his case ("Romance of Real Life," published in the *American Journal of Insanity)* related that the patient "returned to a life of active usefulness and never again had a recurrence of his distressing malady." The lady of his interest married and after childbirth became mentally ill. The former patient was one of those who aided in bringing her to Bloomingdale, and during her illness he "bestowed on her the kindest assiduities of a generous and delicate friendship, and eventually had the gratification of witnessing her restoration to reason and to her family." [20]

Considering the extent to which legal formalities and restrictions

[18] *Minutes of the Asylum Committee,* Feb. 3, 1838.

[19] *Ibid.,* Jan. 31, 1829. (Physician's Monthly Report.)

[20] *Am. J. Insanity,* April, 1850. A poem inspired by the story was written by Sir E. Lytton Bulwer and was published in the *Supplement to Brother Jonathan,* New York, June 11, 1842.

are now considered necessary, it seems remarkable that for many years it was found possible to treat hundreds of patients in the hospitals and asylums of New York State without resort to direct court orders or any other form of court commitment; even physicians' certificates were not required until 1842. The earliest legal document governing the admission of a patient to Bloomingdale Asylum which has been found in the records was dated July 18, 1831. The order was signed by two justices of the peace and was not directed to the asylum but to the "constables and overseers," instructing them to provide for the patient according to law. No similar orders from places other than New York City have been found in the files. Apparently, therefore, a large proportion of patients were admitted and detained without warrant of law, unless this was implicit in the authority vested in the poor authorities and the justices of the peace. Patients were, however, admitted from other states and from Canada. Some made their own application. One patient from North Carolina had selected the asylum from among others he had considered. He submitted without complaint to restrictive measures, even to "showering and strapping," after he had struck another patient.[21] The governors also felt free to send after patients who had left the asylum without permission, and, by refusing to refund advance payments, to penalize relatives who refused to deliver an escaped patient to the asylum attendant. Justices of the peace who signed orders on which patients were brought to the asylum were held responsible for providing security for the patients' support. In July, 1832, in one such case, a patient was sent to the asylum by two justices of the peace of Brooklyn; when he left without permission, the governors ordered that "these Magistrates be immediately informed that unless the necessary security be furnished forthwith or an order from the overseers of the poor of the county, that the said K— will be returned on their Hands."

Questions relating to admission and detention began to receive more particular consideration in 1840. Two patients were brought into court on writs of habeas corpus in that year, and one was declared by the judge to be sane and was discharged. In April a committee was appointed by the governors to "inquire into the practice of admitting Patients into the Bloomingdale Asylum, and should the present one be found unauthorized to apply to the Legislature for the necessary power." At the meeting of the board in May, this committee reported that they had written on the subject to G. C. Verplanck, one of the governors who was

21 *Minutes of the Asylum Committee*, Oct. 30, 1826.

a member of the legislature; no further reference has been found in the records.

When, at a later period, legislation governing the admission and detention of the mentally ill became a subject of particular attention, various circumstances led to the enactment of measures that were more arbitrary than is necessary and somewhat prejudicial to the patients' welfare and treatment. In considering revisions, it may well be advantageous to review the long period during which hospital treatment was safely and satisfactorily administered to thousands of mentally ill persons, without judicial procedures which, as now practiced, are in many instances unnecessary and are frequently prejudicial.

XV

"MORAL TREATMENT" WITHOUT MEDICAL DIRECTION

THE humane, rational principles and methods which, toward the close of the eighteenth century, began to be generally adopted in the treatment of the mentally ill, were termed "Moral Treatment." An Oxford Dictionary definition of the word "moral" as "pertaining to or operating on the character or conduct of human beings," may furnish a clue to the significance of the term in relation to measures operating on the character or conduct of the mentally ill. During the first half of the nineteenth century the term was frequently met with in psychiatric literature. The primary purpose of the governors of the New York Hospital in establishing the asylum at Bloomingdale, was to provide for their mentally ill patients the benefits of this new "moral treatment." They had evidently succeeded in convincing the legislature of its efficacy, as in their annual report for the year 1821 they announced that they had "commenced the system of moral treatment, *which the Legislature had in view* [1] when they provided for this institution." They described their object in their annual report for 1820 as follows:

> To remedy a disorder having its seat in the mind, inhuman severity and unnecessary restraint have been usually employed . . .
>
> A new method has at length been devised, and an experiment first tried at the Retreat, near York, in England, has demonstrated its superior efficacy.
>
> This consists in substituting mildness for severity, in affording to the patients salutary employment, and innocent recreation, and in using appropriate means to banish gloomy or perverted Ideas from the mind; to break morbid Associations, and to restore to the patient that command over his own thoughts and imaginations the want of which is often the immediate cause of Insanity.
>
> In the Establishment now to be opened, while no relief will be wanting which the Science of Medicine can bestow, the new mode of moral treatment will be sedulously attended to.

Although the governors did not intend to adhere to the proposal made by Thomas Eddy that the practice at the Rural Retreat should be confined "almost exclusively to a course of moral treatment," they evidently considered that this form of treatment was not exactly medical, and that medical direction was not necessary to its successful applica-

[1] Not italicized in original.

tion. The form of organization adopted is described in the Asylum Committee Minutes of December 17, 1824:

The medical department [2] receives every scientific and practical attention that is requisite, from the gentlemen who have immediate charge of it. The success that appears to attend their labors justifies this observation. The *moral department* [3] is such as warrants the belief that the patients are treated in the most benevolent and humane manner; no further personal restraint is known to be imposed other than what is adapted, the exigency of the case requiring it, nor continued longer than essentially necessary for the self-government or protection of the patient.

Although the physician, by reason of his superior knowledge and his constant professional attention to the patients, soon assumed an increasingly important position in the management of the service, the system remained unchanged officially for many years. In 1830, Dr. Guy C. Bayley, a candidate for the position of resident physician as a temporary appointment while Dr. Macdonald was visiting institutions in Europe, stated that he wrote "with the impression that the Governors of the Bloomingdale Lunatic Asylum contemplate a change in the Medical Department," and that if appointed he would have "the general superintendency of the medical department as regards the prescription of remedies and direction of moral treatment:" He was informed that "by the By-Laws the moral treatment appears to be lodged with the superintendent—*under the special direction of the Asylum Comee*. In practice it has been shared by the Resident Physician and Superintendent with the tacit approval at least of the Comee and appears not to have produced collision." [4]

Eventually, however, the governors became convinced that "moral treatment" was medical and required medical direction. Even Thomas Eddy changed his views. In a letter to Mr. Eddy's biographer, Dr. John W. Francis writes that

Mr. Eddy, in common with many other benevolent individuals, was at first disposed to place a more entire reliance on the moral management of insanity to the exclusion of all medical treatment, than, I think, the facts of the case warrant. . . . The constantly accumulating proofs in behalf of medical treatment . . . doubtless had their influence in causing Mr. Eddy . . . to adopt the opinion that the proper administration of medicinal agents, was favorable to the treatment of insanity; nay oftentimes indispensable.[5]

[2] Not italicized in original. [3] Not italicized in original.

[4] Letters on file at Westchester Division. Italics as shown.

[5] S. L. Knapp, *Life of Thomas Eddy* (New York, 1834), pp. 26–29.

In developing the service at the new asylum, the governors earnestly endeavored to fulfill their promise to the legislature that the "new mode of moral treatment will be sedulously attended to." For a long time they proceeded on the assumption that it was not medical and they gave much personal attention to operating it. The by-laws required the Weekly Committee to make a thorough examination of the house at each visitation, "to see every Patient, and . . . make a report of their having done so." This they seem to have done, and they gave particular attention to the main features of "moral treatment." Regular visits were also made by the president and vice-president and by the Asylum and Inspecting Committees. All endeavored to inculcate a kindly, friendly spirit in the service by example as well as by precept. Members of the committees sometimes dined at the superintendent's table, at which some of the patients had their meals. On December 5, 1822, Thomas C. Taylor recorded that he had dined with Captain Gardiner, in company with three of the patients, whose behavior was satisfactory. Another of the governors reported that he had "entered into conversation with several of the patients, offering such advice as, I thought, they were able to understand and to adopt." Occasionally the committee issued explicit directions for treatment:

> Dr. Bayley being in the City on business relative to the Asylum, the committee directed the superintendent to cause Mrs. Van H. to be confined in her Room in the Basement until such time as her friends may remove her from the institution, which the Committee has instructed the superintendent to advise her friends must be done as soon as possible.[6]

On another occasion comment was made on the "injurious effect of permitting Philip S. to have the liberty of leaving the grounds." Some of the governors were inclined to attribute to changes in the weather the prevalence of disturbance among the patients,[7] and in August, 1826, "change in the moon" was considered accountable.

The conception of "bad behavior," and of treatment by punishment still lingered, even among those who had accepted the principles of "moral treatment." At each visit the number of patients in "close confinement" or undergoing "personal restraint" was noted: Comments, such as the following, occasionally appeared: "Some few necessarily confined to their cells from a high state of mental excitement, but the committee feel an entire confidence that no unnecessary restraint is imposed on any,"[8] or "Polly S. had on a strait waistcoat for her bad

[6] *Minutes of the Asylum Committee*, Sept. 8, 1832.

[7] *Ibid.*, March 6, 1822.

[8] *Ibid.*, July 2, 1825.

behavior, which I approved of. I am fully convinced it is necessary at times to use the jacket as a punishment." [9] The governors seldom failed to find one or more patients in confinement or under restraint. Nevertheless, the resident physician's reports sometimes contained statements such as that "for more than two weeks not a male patient was confined in his room," or "it is now many days since either a male or female has been in close confinement." In August, 1835, it was recorded that "Mrs. S. who has been almost under constant restraint for years has not been confined for a week."

The forms of restraining apparatus are rarely mentioned, but the records reveal that straps were used to confine patients in their chairs (in one instance it was "necessary to confine him in a room with his hands strapped"), that the strait jacket was used and, occasionally, the "tranquillizing chair." On the use of chains, it was recorded (in 1823) that a patient was restrained by a chain to his leg to keep him in the center of the room to prevent him from injuring himself, and (July 28, 1825) that a woman was "in chains, in consequence of her extreme situation, which generally continues about two hours." This was apparently the end of the use of chains at Bloomingdale. Frequently, however, the notes on admission stated that a patient had, previously, been chained for varying periods, in some instances for several years, and "the salutary effect of the change from severe to mild treatment" was sometimes noted. Occasional references to "straw patients" are found in the records. This term was apparently applied to those who were so destructive, and perhaps filthy, that they were confined in empty rooms without clothing or bedding except loose straw. Efforts were made to release patients from restraining apparatus: "B. although repeatedly taken from his Room and offered everything that would soothe and gratify him still remains incapable of receiving kindness or of reciprocating the sympathy of his fellowmen. He is the only one in the House in Constant Close Confinement." The constant check kept by the governors on the use of restraint and seclusion during these early formative years of the service had, no doubt, a wholesome effect in accomplishing the limitation and eventually the discarding of routine dependence upon these forms of control.

Next to humane, rational personal relations in the treatment of the patients, "salutary employment and recreation" was the principal means of "moral treatment." The governors explained their aims and plans in their annual report for the year 1821, as follows:

[9] *Ibid.*, Dec. 5, 1822.

With a view to remove the melancholy train of Ideas, which in many cases of Insanity, takes strong possession of the mind, salutary employment is provided for the patients, and when the weather and their health permit, they walk abroad in the Garden and Grounds, accompanied by the Superintendent, Matron, Resident Physician, or keepers. Tame animals have also been procured for them, as well as the means of other innocent amusements, such as ninepins, etc.

They are permitted to dine together in classes, and their deportment at meals is much more orderly than might be expected.

The utmost cleanliness is preserved, and nothing is neglected which it is supposed will contribute to their health and comfort.

The Bible is occasionally read to them, and on the first day of the week, those whose situation will permit, are assembled to hear a Sermon, or some portion of Scripture.

Some friends of the Institution have made it a donation of books, and thus laid the foundation of a Library for the benefit of such patients as are capable of using it.

All those means which experience has shown to be efficacious in removing or alleviating mental diseases, are sedulously employed.

The problem of employment of the patients, especially the men, was, year after year, a constant source of concern for the governors and the physicians. In their first report to the Board of Governors in December, 1821, the Asylum Committee stated that

amusements of various kinds have been introduced, and a number of the women have been employed in spinning wool and Flax, sewing, knitting, etc. No employment has yet been found for the men, except that some of them have worked on the Farm and in the Garden. It is difficult to contrive suitable work for male Lunatics, but considering how important it is that they should be as much employed as their situation will permit, and considering that some of the mechanic arts have been successfully introduced in several of the Lunatic Establishments in Europe, the committee are very desirous as far as practicable to introduce a similar course of employment in our Asylum.

In August, 1822, the Asylum Committee directed the superintendent to employ a "discreet, judicious man to take out the patients." In October, 1823, the Inspecting Committee reported that many of the women were employed and they begged

leave to suggest the propriety of an enquiry whether many, if not the greater part of the men, cannot also engage in some useful and amusing employments in a greater degree and with more variety than they have heretofore been.— Cord or rope making, seine or net making with many other simple and pleasing employments could be easily introduced at a trifling expense.[10]

[10] *Minutes of the Inspecting Committee,* Oct. 31, 1823.

Following this report the governors, in December, 1823, requested the president to confer with the Asylum Committee in regard to the employment of the patients, and to authorize them to employ a person whose "special duty it shall be to attend particularly to such arrangements as may be made to carry into effect such plans as they shall devise in furtherance of this object." The committee went beyond their instructions by instructing the superintendent to employ *two* discreet persons "to take charge of such of the patients, as may from time to time, be in a situation to be amused or employed on the farm, or in walking and exercises in the open air, in classes, to be designated by the Resident Physician, *with the approbation of the superintendent.*" [11] Although, in March, 1824, two men were employed at a salary of $11 a month to attend to this duty, the positions were not constantly maintained, and no constructive development of the plan of treatment was established. At intervals, the recommendation that someone be employed for the purpose was renewed. As late as April, 1836, the resident physician repeated the request that "a person to occupy and employ the male patients in gardening, farming, etc. be employed," and also "a suitable person to superintend and have direction of the male patients in walking etc. out of doors." The plan followed in the year 1833 is described in the annual report of the governors:

As much liberty as is consistent with safety is allowed. Some are permitted to leave the house and to visit in the neighborhood, or to *amuse themselves* [12] on the farm; many others make excursions on foot in company with a keeper, or in a carriage kept for that purpose. The means for moral and mental treatment are adapted, as far as may be, to the education and taste of the patient. For the working-man, labor on the farm, or garden, or in and about the house; for the artizan, an opportunity is afforded of working at his trade, whenever it is practicable; for the pedestrian, the range of one of the most pleasing and varied spots in the country; for the lover of active or of sedentary games of amusements or exercise, there are nine-pins, gymnastics, battledoor, chess, music, etc. for those of literary habits,—books, and the papers and pamphlets of the day. The female patients are employed, so far as they are disposed, at knitting and needle and house work.

It should be borne in mind that in this period, a large proportion of the patients of Bloomingdale Asylum were farmers, laborers, artisans, and others, whose occupations involved manual labor. It was considered that, even as a form of treatment, the employment at manual labor of patients who had not previously been accustomed to it, could seldom

[11] *Minutes of the Asylum Committee,* Jan., 1824. No italics in original.
[12] No italics in original.

be undertaken. Even the women, it may be noted, engaged in handwork only "so far as they are disposed." The present system of occupational therapy in which patients are encouraged, instructed, and induced to engage in manual labor and handicrafts would not at that time have been accepted by private patients or their relatives. In the case history of Polly P. however, age 31, admitted in April, 1823, it was recorded that the physician "demanded employment of her or deprivation of food and forcible exhibition of medicines and Blisters." She had ideas of imaginary wealth, a spirit of pride and independence, despising employment. "She at first chose scanty food—but medicine and blisters caused her to choose knitting, sewing, spinning, and quilting—ordinary diet whenever she would work. But bread and water when she would not." She was discharged recovered in November, 1823, "with habits of industry."

There were some who questioned the advisability of discarding disciplinary measures to the extent that was practiced in the system of "moral treatment." The governors, in their annual report for 1825, found it wise to explain that

> the kind and benevolent treatment required to be practiced by all, towards the patients, is found not to interfere with the important and necessary policy of supporting a proper and well regulated authority over them; nor does this lessen the gratitude they frequently evince for this attention—on the contrary it induces a more ready submission to restraints at times unavoidable, which at home with their family and friends they would resist as capricious and tyrannical.

The governors had undertaken the introduction of the system of "moral treatment" for their mentally ill patients with great interest and hope. Soon after the new asylum at Bloomingdale was opened, they reported to the legislature that

> it would not perhaps, be fair to decide too positively upon the merrits of the mode of treatment that has been pursued, from the result of only six months experience; but thus far it has not disappointed the expectations that had been formed of it. It has proved eminently successful, and particularly so, with regard to the Patients, who were at first most violent and noisey, a large proportion of these are greatly improved, and sanguine hopes are entertained, that many of them will shortly be restored to their families and friends, blessed with mental as well as bodily health. Among those removed from the Old to the New Asylum, were several whom it had been necessary to subject to constant personal restraint. This is now ceased to be requisite in every instance, except that of a single Individual, who is the only patient that at present requires it.

A year later, in their report for 1822, the governors reported that "they have now the satisfaction to add, that the expectations then entertained of the efficacy and success of those means, have thus far been fully realized." In this spirit of optimism and benevolence the work of Bloomingdale Asylum was inaugurated, and it has continued to animate the service from that day to this.

The "system of moral treatment" adopted by the governors in the management of Bloomingdale Asylum would today be considered as little more than the form of administration and practice to be found in every good psychiatric hospital. Experience has shown that for successful operation the system requires the services of a well-qualified psychiatrist as director. Few, however, anywhere, were at that time aware of this. The governors of the New York Hospital were not accustomed to look to their doctors for direction in administrative matters, and probably none of these doctors would have regarded "moral treatment" as particularly a medical task. The by-laws required the asylum physician to assist in carrying out the system, and, though he had no authority over the nurses or keepers, he could hardly avoid directing them in their attention to the patients. Therefore it was not long before he was actively participating in "moral treatment." Conflicts of authority between physician and superintendent were inevitable. The first report by a resident physician covered the period from January to June, 1822, and was submitted to the Asylum Committee by Dr. James Eddy. It was principally statistical. Dr. Albert Smith, who succeeded Dr. Eddy, was requested in November, 1823, to lay before the committee "a scheme of discipline and management which may tend in some degree to secure to the patients the benefits to be derived from the application of moral remedies." A report of the service during the previous year, which Dr. Smith had submitted in January, 1824, was referred for consideration to a special meeting of the Asylum Committee in conjunction with a committee appointed to devise a plan for the better employment and amusement of the patients. On January 31, this "Joint Committee of the Governors and the Asylum Committee" reported as follows:

> They have had under consideration the plan of classification proposed by the Resident Physician of the Asylum, and however desirable it might be to adopt the classification, proposed by the resident Physician, the joint committee are unanimously of opinion, that the construction of the House, and other circumstances, render it, at present at least, impracticable.
>
> The joint committee have also duly considered the proposition of the resident Physician, to make an entire Separation of the police[18] of the House,

[18] Oxford Dictionary definition of police, "to keep in order, administer, control."

and the moral and medical treatment of the Patients, and to put these under the control of different persons.

The joint committee are of the opinion that this cannot be done advantageously. Nevertheless, the joint committee are fully impressed with the necessity of adopting measures to improve the moral treatment of the Patients.

And the Asylum Committee in pursuance of the conclusions of the joint committee, have determined to adopt means of affording to the Patients further amusements, Employments and exercises, by engaging assistants at the Institution, whose attention shall be particularly directed to these objects. . . . The Resident Physician is desired to devote a greater portion of his time and attention to the moral part of the establishment, and to communicate to the committee such improvements as his experience shall suggest to be useful and necessary in carrying into more complete effect the system of moral treatment, and to report from time to time to the committee the effect of the measures adopted.[14]

As this plan of the resident physician is not available, its contents can only be surmised. Evidently a plea was made for more authority for the physician in the "moral treatment" of the patients and in the administration; its only recorded effect was the employment in March, 1824, "with the approbation of the superintendent," of "two discreet persons" to give particular attention to the employment and amusement of the patients. Other monthly reports from resident physicians were recorded in October, 1824, and in January, February, and June, 1825. These were entirely statistical, except that in June Dr. A. V. Williams reported, in regard to the employment of patients, that "the superior utility of this system is fully illustrated by the Rapid recovery of many and the improved Condition of others, by which the importance of constant and oftentimes of severe exercise is forced upon our minds by the experience of every day." [15]

[14] *Minutes of the Asylum Committee,* Jan. 31, 1824.
[15] *Ibid.,* June 6, 1825.

XVI

TOWARDS MEDICAL DIRECTION

The appointment of Dr. James Macdonald as resident physician of Bloomingdale Asylum in May, 1825, was an event of considerable importance to the advancement of the medical character of the service. He remained longer in the position than any of his predecessors, and by his intelligence, energy, fertility of ideas, and force of character, was enabled to make a lasting contribution in shaping the policy, improving the facilities, and advancing standards of organization and administration. His father was a Scotch physician who had been in the medical service of the British army in the Revolutionary War and after the war had settled in White Plains, where in 1797 he was one of the founders and the first president of the Medical Society of the County of Westchester. James Macdonald graduated from the College of Physicians and Surgeons in 1825, at the age of 22, and received his appointment at Bloomingdale immediately after graduating. As a private pupil of Dr. Hosack he had probably learned much about mental illness, but he was without practical experience. He had, however, decided to devote his professional career to the study and treatment of the mentally ill and he applied himself earnestly to the subject.

After his appointment, the monthly and annual reports of the resident physician appeared regularly in the minutes. In each monthly report a brief account was given of the patients admitted since the previous meeting. His first report in July, 1825, was brief, but the governors were apparently impressed with his interest in the patients and their activities as they recorded that "he is encouraged to continue his undivided attention to the patients and as far as practicable to find them amusement and exercise in the open air." As he became familiar with the service and the condition and needs of the patients his reports and proposals to the governors related more and more to what had been considered "moral treatment," which was, by the by-laws, under the direction of the superintendent. In April, 1826, he reported that "the patients have used much exercise in riding, walking, and gymnastic amusements, all of which have been attended with material benefit . . . to the first from its novelty and agreeableness they are very partial. . . . The new keeper employed to walk out with the patients is found to be quite an acquisition."

In December of the same year, he proposed that a reading room for the patients, which had been considered and deferred because no suitable room was available, should be further considered and that, at least, the "papers and periodical Publications may be made very useful by forming them into something like a circulating library, and distributing them through the house." He agreed to "take the charge of circulating them upon myself." A library for the use of the patients had been started in 1822. Many books were donated by members of the Board of Governors, publishers, and other interested persons. Henry I. Wyckoff, one of the governors, presented "an elegant mahogany bookcase," and an old bookcase which answers the description is still in use at the Westchester Division. That the library was not without therapeutic value was evidently appreciated by the governors. In April, 1824, the Inspecting Committee commented that "a well selected library is an important appendage to this great institution," and in May, 1827, one of the committee reported that he was "impressed with the importance of a suitable and ample library for the various patients of the house. . . . To me it appears to be one of the essentials of moral treatment."

Dr. Macdonald kept constantly before the committee the importance of providing means of employment and recreation for the patients. In March, 1827, he advised them that "every Day's Experience has pointed out the necessity of Occupation, both mental and manual. Many Patients might be mentioned who are only unhappy and troublesome when obliged to depend upon the Resources of their own minds for Employment." In April he reported the forms of manual and mental pursuits engaged in by the patients, and added: "But daily experience confirms the want of more diversified employment, there being some patients who derive no amusement from either of these sources, one in particular I have supplied with books from the city in order to keep his mind engaged." He then brought forward again the establishment of a reading room, suggesting that a large south room on Hall 5 could be made available by transferring some patients to another hall. He proposed rules for the library and reading room, and asked for a case for books and a natural history cabinet, with opportunities for study. The committee now approved of his plan and the superintendent was authorized to make the necessary arrangements.

This dependence upon the nonmedical superintendent for carrying into effect measures for the improvement of the service and for the treatment of individual patients was no doubt considered by the physician to be a serious disadvantage; the governors were commencing to understand this. In May, 1831, the Asylum Committee expressed their views in no uncertain terms:

The physician is alone responsible for the cure of the patients, and the grand means for effecting this object is moral treatment, it therefore of right belongs to him. It is admitted that the practice has been otherwise—the Superintendent has claimed it, and except when yielded by courtesy on his part has controlled the moral treatment of the whole house—so that unless by his consent the physician has no voice in the location of the patients, their classification, exercise or amusements. He may prescribe for the physical man, but he cannot administer to the mind diseased. On this head the Resident Physican and Dr. Macdonald are equally decided—and it is probable that no physician of any eminence or due sense of self-respect will ever waive it.[1]

It was still, however, considered necessary to sustain the authority of the superintendent by providing that "all orders to nurses and keepers which the Physician may think necessary to carry these objects into effect, shall be communicated through the superintendent." Even so, however, the superintendent and matron felt that they could no longer remain in the service "under the present regulation of the house."

Dr. Macdonald had in the meantime resigned his position with the intention of entering private practice, but the governors were unable to find anyone of equal qualifications to replace him, and they invited him to return with the understanding that he would be given an opportunity to spend a year in Europe. The purpose of the trip was "to increase the usefulness of the Institution," by visiting the European institutions, "to study within their walls the different methods of medical and moral treatment, form acquaintance with the most distinguished Physicians of this branch, . . . and return qualified to advance the reputation of our own." It was agreed that after his return Dr. Macdonald would remain as physician of the asylum for five years, and that he would be given charge of the moral as well as the medical treatment. He was granted a salary of $1,500 and $500 towards his expenses. He sailed in July, 1831, and was absent about fifteen months. He visited institutions in England, Scotland, Ireland, France, and Italy. He wrote several informing letters to the governors while abroad, and upon his return made an interesting report.[2] He gave a full account of his observations of "moral treatment," which he found included "the various forms of employment and recreation, the personal influence of physicians, attendants etc., in a word every agent brought to bear directly on the 'moral' of the patient." He considered that "after classification the most important of all considerations in the management of the insane is

[1] *Minutes of the Governors,* May 3, 1831.
[2] For full text, see Appendix, p. 496.

employment." During Dr. Macdonald's absence the position of physician of the asylum was filled temporarily by the appointment of Dr. Guy C. Bayley, who retired when Dr. Macdonald returned in the autumn of 1832.

The committee had agreed that on Dr. Macdonald's return "the Asylum shall be placed under his entire control, that is so far as the curative treatment, both medical and moral, is concerned . . . and lastly that the selection of nurses and keepers shall be entrusted to him."[3] In his first monthly report following resumption of his duties in November, 1832, Dr. Macdonald recommended that the "By Laws be altered; defining the respective duties and functions of Physician and Superintendent"; and, "touching the appointment and duties of attendants." He advised that "a greater variety of occupation and amusement be afforded the patients." Patients who were mechanics and laborers, he thought might be usefully employed, but "as for amusements and mental occupation much remains to be done." His recommendations were referred to a committee with instructions that they "report such alterations in the By Laws as they may deem expedient and as early as possible." The revised by-laws, adopted in January, 1833, designated the physician "the superior officer of the institution" rather than "of the medical department" as in previous by-laws, and empowered him to "hire and discharge all the attendants on the patients, that is, all persons directly employed in the management of them." The designation "superintendent" was changed to "Warden," and instead of its being his "special duty" to see that the system of "moral treatment" was carried into effect, it was stipulated that "he shall use his best endeavors to carry into effect the general system of moral treatment, *as laid down by the Resident Physician.*"[4]

The increase in authority provided by these by-laws and their interpretation by the committee gave the physician more scope in the management of the service. He gave much attention to improving the accommodations of the patients and devising means of interesting and occupying them in wholesome pursuits. He improved the dining-room service and the furnishings in the living quarters, and obtained suitable furniture and equipment for the library and reading room. The committee warmly approved of his projects, granted an appropriation of $75 a year for periodicals, and authorized him to appoint a librarian

[3] *Minutes of the Asylum Committee,* May 25, 1831.
[4] No italics in original. *Minutes of the Governors.*

without compensation.[5] In May Dr. Macdonald reported an increase in the occupational activity of the patients, and that he had exercised his newly granted authority by discharging an attendant for unkind treatment of a patient.[6] He had appointed a patient to act as librarian and reported that the library and reading room had "answered our expectations." He established a "Singing School . . . for those who have a taste for music and are disposed to improve in sacred melody."

His annual report was presented to the committee in February, 1834. In this he referred again to the importance of employment. He proposed that the garden and farm be worked by the patients, and that hired labor be mostly dispensed with. He considered that, as

> the money now paid for labour amounts to more than would supply the establishment with vegetables, the only reason, then, for raising vegetables on the place must be to employ the patients. If such employment even cost the institution something, its beneficial influence on the insane will warrant the expenditure. But if properly managed it will not only cost nothing, but be a positive saving. . . . At any rate it may be safely said that too much is to be gained and too little to be hazarded to omit making the experiment.

The introduction of handicrafts was also urged. When one considers how many years elapsed before adequate provision for this means of occupational therapy was made at the institution, it is interesting to note Dr. Macdonald's discussion of the subject.

> Among so great a diversity of characters, tastes, and professions, a variety of employment is desirable. . . . When the mind has become diseased and the imagination fixed upon some depressing subject to the exclusion of all healthful reflection, what is better calculated to divert it from preying upon itself, and to substitute new images, than some pleasing kind of handicraft. Manual labour has these advantages; that it may be followed when outdoor employments fail and may be practiced at all times by such patients as are not capable of much locomotion, but whose idle hands are notoriously mischievous.

He cited, from a report from a Scotch asylum, 22 forms of manual occupation engaged in by the patients. He gave the occupations of 76 of the male patients prior to admission, and recommended that, besides farming and gardening, provision should be made for those who could use "joiner's tools," and that a workshop be erected with a turning lathe,

[5] *Minutes of the Asylum Committee,* March 2, 1833.
[6] *Ibid.,* May 4, 1833.

and "various sedentary and light employments in which the hands only are exercised might be introduced with advantage." [7]

He also discussed the question of religious services as a means of "moral treatment":

It has been doubted if religious exercises could be introduced with advantage into Asylums for the insane. From numerous experiments made in England and Scotland and I may add more recently at our own Institution the question is now at rest. It is a year since religious service was introduced into the Bloomingdale Asylum and it may be said to have answered the most sanguine expectations of its projectors, and it is not surprising that it has, when we consider that one of the grand principles in the management of the insane is to treat them as nearly as possible like rational beings.[8]

In his monthly report for November, 1834, he suggested that a loom be added to the occupational equipment as one of the patients and an attendant were weavers. This is probably the first introduction into the asylum of a form of occupation which is now one of the principal of the many crafts engaged in by the patients. In May, 1835, Dr. Macdonald again felt it necessary to advise the governors that the "want of proper means of diversion is still felt." His visit to asylums in Europe had increased his knowledge of the seriousness of the deprivation. He found that "those who have been at other institutions speak of it as a defect." Again in April, 1836, he repeated that the "most striking defect is the deficiency of means of diversion and useful occupation," and he again recommended that a workshop be provided. He also requested that additional attendants be employed to walk with the patients through the surrounding country, as the male attendants were too busy with housework to go out with the patients in the morning. He drew attention to the failure to use the horses and carriage to take the patients on the drives from which they had previously derived benefit and pleasure. In October, he reported that the excavation for the new building had been entirely the work of patients. He related that one patient, who was a mason, was idle, depressed, and apathetic, until he was asked to work on the new building, and "from the moment the trowel was put in his hand he became a different man." This patient became one of the best workers, and was offered wages. Dr. Macdonald recommended employing a carpenter and supplying a shop where patients could work with him. This was referred to a committee but apparently nothing came of it at that time. In the annual report for 1836, he again

[7] *Ibid.*, Jan. 31, 1835.

[8] *Ibid.*, Feb. 1, 1834.

made a plea that a trial be made, "as employment of the insane is not an experiment in institutions," and that it was desirable that, "with a due regard to the character of Bloomingdale Asylum and the well being of its inmates another year will not pass without the Erection of a suitable workshop." In March, the governors found it possible to authorize the employment of a carpenter, and the warden was instructed to procure tools for the use of the patients "at the suggestion of the carpenter who will have charge of them." Notwithstanding Dr. Macdonald's urgent recommendations and those of some of his successors, many years were still to elapse before a suitable workshop and instructors for the patients were permanently established.[9]

In July, 1837, Dr. Macdonald presented to the Asylum Committee a plan for the reorganization of the service. The chief defects in the present administration were due, he considered, to want of "unity of action," want of system, and want of employment for the patients. He proposed that the head of the institution should be responsible not only for the ordinary management of the patients, but for carrying into effect all schemes of manual labor whether on the farm or in workshops, in the house or on the pleasure grounds. He should direct and supervise all treatment whether medical or moral, and have authority to hire and discharge all subordinate persons in the employ of the institution, except perhaps those under the immediate direction of the farmer.

Indicating his appreciation of the opportunity for scientific investigations, he also proposed that, as the physician to a Lunatic Asylum was "placed in an extended field of observation," he could collect facts which would be of "immense service to his medical brethren," and that "this he cannot do satisfactorily without a professional assistant"—"in this department as well as in every other" he must have someone to attend to minutiae, and do the drudgery. (This provision was not made until twenty years later.) He warned against the danger of overspecialization: "a physician exclusively devoted to mental diseases cannot treat them medically so well as he might do with his mind enlarged by the observation of other diseases." He considered that patients should not be expected to work day after day for the mere pleasure of working, and recommended some reward, such as a delicacy of diet, an article of clothing, or money. The gardener, farmer, and carpenter should be employed with the understanding that they would furnish employment for the patients.

[9] The first workshop exclusively for men patients was erected in 1915. See p. 424.

Some of the difficulties encountered in procuring the introduction and support of occupational therapy in the asylum are intimated in Dr. Macdonald's plea that

all these schemes for the more systematic employment of the Insane may by some be deemed visionary, but when we recollect that useful Occupation has been successfully introduced into many European institutions for the insane and that it is there no longer considered as an experiment, the plan must be deemed practical.

The communication also contained an interesting account of the possible operations of one day under the proposed plan of reorganization.[10]

The proposal was attended with some dissatisfaction. On June 19, 1837, the Asylum Committee reported to the Board of Governors that they had made inquiries and were led to believe that "the evils complained of, mainly owe their origin to the appointing power delegated by the Laws to the Physician and Warden respectively." Friction was occasioned by conflicts in authority over the various persons employed. The committee considered, however, that the occurrences of which they had learned could perhaps not be eradicated except by a change of one or both of the principal officers of the institution, and they did not think that any change in the organization was necessary. They did, however, recommend that the by-laws be amended in such a way as to give the Asylum Committee control over appointments and dismissals of those employed about the establishment. They proposed that the physician should recommend to the Asylum Committee for appointment all attendants on the patients "that is, all persons directly employed in the management of them, and the persons so recommended and appointed may be discharged at his request or otherwise by the Asylum Committee." The warden should in a similar way recommend for appointment all servants employed in and about the asylum, except the attendants on the patients, and the Asylum Committee should discharge them at his request or otherwise. Evidently the warden agreed with the committee as to one means of eradicating the immediate difficulties. On May 18, 1837, he presented the following communication:

To Thomas R. Smith, Esq.
Chairman of the
Asylum Committee

SIR: from various difficulties having been presented in regard to the affairs of this institution within the year past, the duties of Warden have become

[10] For full text see Appendix, p. 507.

rather unpleasant, and of course less useful than they might be under other circumstances. I therefore beg leave thro' you to tender my Resignation to the Committee and hope a person may be procured to succeed me as early as possible.

I am dear Sir with the
highest respect your
very Hbl Serv[t]

IRA FORD

The only one of Dr. Macdonald's recommendations on reorganization to be adopted by the governors was the creation of the position of steward, or, as it was later designated, "assistant steward," as the by-laws already provided that the warden should be the steward of the asylum. The following resolution was presented:

Whereas difficulties have arisen in regard to the appointment of nurses and servants by the Physician and Warden and disadvantages resulted to the business of the establishment by the said nurses and servants claiming to be under the exclusive direction of the one or the other—Resolved that it be recommended to the Board of Governors so to alter the Asylum By-laws as to vest all appointments and renewals heretofore made by the Physician or Warden in the Asylum Committee on the recommendation of the Physician or Warden as the case may be.[11]

This was laid on the table, however, and no change was made in the methods of appointment in the by-laws revised in November, 1838. Rules adopted by the Asylum Committee in October, did extend the authority of the physician to the direction of the dietary.

Dr. Macdonald had, in April, 1837, notified the governors that he intended to retire from the service at the expiration of the term of his appointment on June 1. This was accepted by the committee, with regret that "the doctor's views seem to require this course." He remained, however, until August 15, in order to enable Dr. Benjamin Ogden, who had been appointed to succeed him, to complete his engagement in the service for the mentally ill at Bellevue. In accepting his resignation the governors expressed by resolution their thanks "for his able and faithful professional services," and "the gratification they felt with the great success that has for many years attended his treatment of the Insane Patients under his care." [12] They also manifested their confidence in his medical qualifications by appointing him in 1838 on the attending staff of the New York Hospital in which position he served with distinction until 1843. He was also honored by his medical

[11] *Minutes of the Asylum Committee*, May 24, 1837.
[12] *Minutes of the Governors*, June 20, 1837.

colleagues by election as president of the New York Medical and Surgical Society in 1843. His practical activities left little opportunity for engaging in scientific investigations or literary contributions. That he had a mind for them, however, was revealed by such contributions as his papers on statistical studies made at Bloomingdale,[13] and an excellent article on puerperal insanity based on studies and treatment of Bloomingdale cases.[14] These articles were read before the New York Medical and Surgical Society, and an account of cases presented by him also appears in the proceedings of this Society. He also gave a course of lectures at the College of Physicians and Surgeons. He was by the medical profession regarded "as the first authority on mental diseases within the reach of his medical brethren in this City," though he had "no time even for consultative practice." [15]

In 1839 Dr. Macdonald again made a visit to Europe, and in 1841 he opened a private institution for the mentally ill "in two houses, agreeably situated in Murray Hill, in the suburbs of New York." In 1845 he removed it to Flushing, Long Island, where as "Sanford Hall" it was conducted for many years. He continued, however, to aid in the advancement of the public provision for the mentally ill. As has been related, he had, in 1834, aided in the planning of the New York City Lunatic Asylum.[16] In 1847, he was appointed one of the visiting physicians of that asylum. He submitted several reports relating to it, and, with Dr. Benjamin Ogden and Dr. A. V. Williams, both of whom had previously been physicians of Bloomingdale, accomplished "the most extensive ameliorations." [17] Characteristic of his sense of values, he obtained for the institution the establishment of a library of 1,200 volumes. In 1841, he was requested by the trustees engaged in the planning of the new state asylum at Utica, New York, to suggest a plan of organization. This he did, and in 1842 he was offered the position of superintendent which, however, "after mature consideration he declined." [18] He died in 1849 of pneumonia when 46 years old. Great sorrow and regret were manifested. It was said by one of his colleagues that he "always remembered the poor" and that "his success was regarded as a public benefit, and adding new honor to the profession he adorned." [19]

13 "Statistics of Bloomingdale Asylum for the Insane," *N.Y. J. of Med. and Surg.* I, Oct., 1839, p. 307.
14 "Puerperal Insanity," *Am. J. Insanity*, IV (Oct., 1847), 113.
15 J. A. Swett, *Eulogy on James Macdonald M.D.* (New York, 1849).
16 See pp. 160–161.
17 "Life of James Macdonald," *Am. J. Insanity*, VI, July, 1849.
18 *Ibid.* See also N.Y. State Senate, Doc. 20, Jan. 11, 1841, p. 177.
19 Swett, *op. cit.*

Dr. Ogden, who succeeded Dr. Macdonald in August, 1837, was the first of the physicians appointed to the service for the mentally ill at the New York Hospital to be qualified by any previous experience. He was much respected by the governors, but the records do not disclose many suggestions for improvements that were made by him. His discussions of employment of patients and other means of "moral treatment" seem to be theoretical rather than practical. Evidently some of Dr. Macdonald's suggestions were given consideration, as Dr. Ogden was asked to report on how the new gardener and farmer was performing his duties, presumably in employing the patients, and a carpenter was engaged "to be subject to the direction of the Physician" as well as of the warden. Dr. Ogden reported the difficulty experienced in employing the male patients of the "higher classes of society," and mentioned walking, bowls, gardening, athletic exercises, reading, billiards, chess, and cards as activities in which they engaged. Under the new rules, his relations with the new warden were satisfactory: in June, 1838, the committee invited the Board of Governors to visit the asylum, and note improvements "since its management under the care of the present officers." His service was, however, comparatively uneventful and he remained for less than two years. His successor was Dr. William Wilson, whose service will be described in a later chapter.

Bloomingdale Asylum and the Friends Asylum were the first to be established in America expressly for the purpose of adopting in the treatment of the mentally ill, the humane, sensible system of "moral treatment" which, in various institutions, notably the Quakers' Retreat for the Insane at York, England, was supplanting the fearsome methods that had long been employed. The project in New York originated with the governors of the hospital, particularly the Quaker Thomas Eddy, and medical considerations or medical advice had at first little to do with the planning and introduction of the system. The governors themselves gave much personal attention to its operation, and charged the nonmedical superintendent and the matron with the responsibility of seeing that it was carried into effect. In time, however, experience in the operation of the service enabled the governors to recognize that "moral treatment" was medical and required medical direction, and the authority of the physician was gradually extended accordingly. The deliberate purpose which animated the governors in establishing this benevolent form of service, the interest and zeal with which they endeavored, by personal attention, to develop it, and the manner in which "moral" and medical treatment were eventually merged under the direction of the physician, constitute a striking example of the evolution of psychiatric hospital administration and service, and went a long way in determining the character of the Bloomingdale service and the lines followed as its development proceeded.

PART FOUR
A Transition Period
1840-1852

XVII: A PRIVATELY SUPPORTED BENEVOLENT SERVICE

When Bloomingdale Asylum was established, the widespread movement for better provision for the treatment of the mentally ill was steadily gaining momentum. The number of medical institutions for this purpose in the United States increased from five in 1821 to seventeen in 1840, and to nearly double that number in 1852. In New York State, where at first Bloomingdale was the only such institution, a private asylum was established at Hudson in 1830, the New York City Asylum in 1839, Dr. Macdonald's private institution in 1841, and the State Asylum at Utica in 1843. In promoting these developments, the psychiatric service conducted by the governors of the New York Hospital had a part. Reference has already been made to its influence in the movement for public provision for the mentally ill, and to the contributions of Dr. Macdonald in the planning of the first city and state asylums.[1] Services rendered by Dr. William Wilson and Dr. Pliny Earle will be mentioned in a later chapter.

The establishment of public asylums, and the consequent withdrawal from Bloomingdale of publicly supported patients, necessitated full dependence upon private interest and support for the maintenance of the service. The New York City "paupers" had been removed when the City Asylum on Blackwell's Island was opened in 1839. A further depletion occurred with the opening of the New York State Lunatic Asylum at Utica in 1843 and of the New Jersey State Asylum at Trenton in 1848. Special provision, of a sort, was also made at some of the almshouses in the more populous counties, and references to the Kings County Asylum and to the Westchester Asylum are occasionally met with in the Bloomingdale records. In August, 1849, the "last county patient" at Bloomingdale Asylum died,[2] and the inaugural phase of public medical treatment of the mentally ill in New York came to an end. Good standards were adopted in the establishment of the state asylums, and

[1] See pp. 95, 160, 174, 196.
[2] *Minutes of the Asylum Committee*, Sept. 1, 1849.

privately as well as publicly supported patients resorted to them. In 1843 the governors of the New York Hospital considered that the establishment of the State Asylum at Utica and of Dr. Macdonald's private institution in New York City had "deprived Bloomingdale Asylum of the most profitable class of patients." [3] Following the successive openings of the institutions mentioned, there was, on each occasion, a marked fall in the number of patients at the asylum. At times this occasioned some concern, and in order to encourage admissions the minimum rate for private patients was reduced to that formerly charged the public authorities. The reception of patients at low rates had always been regarded by the governors as "one of the most valuable features of this establishment." [4] They explained this in their annual report for 1852:

> This Asylum is not now to any great extent used for the entirely gratuitous reception of the insane poor. . . . But the charge for support and care is fixed at a rate much below that which any private enterprise could afford, and not more than sufficient to defray the expense of personal support. Thus it has brought the means of probable cure or relief, and certainly of comfortable retreat, within the reach of families of limited means, who can here support a child or parent, afflicted with mental disease, under the best medical care and with all the external aids to its efficacy that wealth could command, at a charge, not exceeding that of the support and care of such patients at home, without hope of recovery. The value of such an establishment near a great city, and within the reach and supervision of the friends of the insane, is evident.

The number of low-rate private patients steadily increased, and in 1847, when the census reached 146, the physician advised the governors that the asylum was "as full as it ought to be, consistently with the comfort, health and judicious treatment of the patients." [5] The number of "low paying" men became so great that they could not be accommodated in the Lodge, and it was necessary to remove eight of them to the basement of the main building and to employ an extra attendant. Following the opening of the New Jersey State Asylum, there was again a great reduction in the number of admissions to Bloomingdale. In 1849 only 95 patients were admitted, and the number in the asylum on some days was 100 or a few over. The number of incurables continued to be large, and on one occasion the physician reported that of 142 patients in the asylum, 120 were of this type.[6] In October, 1847, he reported that "the House is filled with a mass of chronic and incurable cases," and that aside from alcoholics, not a dozen were susceptible of cure.

[3] *Ibid.*, April 1, 1843.
[4] Annual Report for 1848.
[5] *Minutes of the Asylum Committee*, May 29, 1847.
[6] *Ibid.*, Sept. 4, 1847.

In April, 1846, the physician reported to the committee that "it is a fact worthy of notice that in thirteen days of the month of March there was an equal number of male and female patients, and one day there were more females than males." What made this observation noteworthy was that since the establishment of the service the number of male patients had invariably greatly exceeded the female. In his annual report the physician noted that there were more females under treatment than in any previous year. In December, 1848, he reported that "for the first time since the institution was opened, the monthly average of the female patients is greater than that of the males." After that the proportion of women continued to increase, and in October, 1852, of 118 patients in the asylum 72 were women. This change in the proportion of men and women patients was evidently related to the change in the source of support, and it has persisted to the present day.

The admission and commingling of patients from every walk of life, and of every form and grade of mental illness, had always been considered prejudicial to satisfactory treatment, and the withdrawal of publicly supported patients quickened interest in the problem. The question of classification, which had always been present, assumed a new aspect, and became more pressing. In accordance with a policy previously referred to,[7] the rate received for the treatment of a patient determined his accommodations, food, and nursing attention. This led the physician of the asylum, Dr. William Wilson, when suggesting in April, 1842, additional accommodations for noisy and violent patients, to remind the governors that, as low-priced patients were admitted with the understanding that "they are, in general, to be placed in one of the Lodges," they were compelled to associate with noisy and boisterous patients "of their own class as well as those of other classes," even during their convalescence. This, he considered, tended to retard recovery, and might be of permanent injury to some. It was not because many of the patients were poor, but that some of them were "from the lowest ranks of society." [8] There seemed to be no prospect of being relieved of these patients. The State Asylum, then in course of construction, would not receive them, as it was designed for curable patients and the law forbade the reception of cases of long standing, and limited the stay at the asylum. Dr. Wilson suggested that a one-story building, 40 feet square, be erected for each sex, each building to accommodate twelve patients, and the basements to be constructed so as to provide workshops, "should some systematic plan of occupation be

[7] Pages 145, 151.

[8] Convicts from the state prison were admitted.

introduced among our patients, to which subject I would most respectfully ask your consideration." His report was "laid over for future consideration." In the following June, he again drew attention to the importance of the subject, and to the impossibility, under the existing conditions, of separating the noisy, dangerous, and filthy patients from the others. He directed attention to the establishment of other asylums, "with the latest improvements," and suggested that Bloomingdale "should not be undone by rival institutions for public favor." He was thereupon requested to furnish a sketch of a plan with an estimate of probable cost. This he did, and after it was revised on a smaller scale, the committee referred it to the Board of Governors. After consideration by the board in October, "the whole subject was laid on the table," and seven years elapsed before it was again revived.

During the interval, with the increasing admission of patients of different economic and social levels, the question became more involved. In his annual report for 1849, Dr. Charles H. Nichols, who had recently been appointed physician of the asylum, advised the governors that

> a thorough classification, in view of the most effective moral treatment cannot, I think, be made, except in the absence of the necessity of considering, or temptation to consider, the social position and wealth of those under care. If it is impossible for sane people of widely different tastes and means to associate agreeably together, no one need be surprised at the wounded pride and bitter envy which patients from the two extremes respectively experience when brought together in close proximity in an asylum for the insane. . . . The most effectual application of the most extensive facilities that could be made available in the moral treatment of insanity, requires a scale of expenditure of which poorhouse rates for the poor, and hotel rates for the rich, afford no criterion.

He also advised the governors that there was an "abatement of prejudice" against asylums for the mentally ill among the "higher classes," that the average board rate had increased, and that there was "an increasing social uniformity among the patients which renders the direction of their treatment more successful and more satisfactory to all concerned."

Three years later Dr. D. Tilden Brown, who had succeeded Dr. Nichols, suggested to the governors, in his annual report for 1852, that the character of the institution as "a great public charity" was not generally known or appreciated by the community. He advised that it be

> exhibited by stating that one half of all its inmates are maintained at prices varying from twenty to forty per cent. less than the average cost of their

support. Were it not for the larger remuneration afforded by the more wealthy class of patients, this large number would be deprived of many of their present enjoyments and the good effected be materially diminished.

Thus the policy which today governs the operation of the service began to be definitely formulated. Financial considerations had a part in shaping it, but the fundamental aim was then, and has continued to be, to provide the best treatment for the mentally ill that could be devised, and especially to accomplish for persons of limited means the benevolent purpose for which the institution was established.

No addition to the accommodations for patients was made during this period. New construction for other purposes, however, included a building for a bowling alley and a shuffleboard, which the physician regarded as a "valuable acquisition." The need for a residence for the physician arose, when in 1849, a vacancy in the position having occurred, it was found that all the candidates were married. After steps had been taken to provide the residence, however, a candidate applied who was not married, and, as he proved to be the best qualified, he was appointed. The governors, in confirming the appointment in June, 1850, expressed the hope "that Dr. Nichols will be enabled within the present year to comply with the wishes and expectations of the Governors as expressed and understood at the time of his appointment in regard to his soon becoming a married man." The hope was unfulfilled: Dr. Nichols remained unmarried during his short term of service, and it was not until 1852, when he was succeeded by a married physician, that the house was painted and furnished for occupancy.

The better classification of the patients continued to be a source of constant concern, and in 1850 the project of extending the accommodations, which had been abandoned in 1842, was revived. In August of that year the Inspecting Committee, after making rounds with Dr. Nichols, reported that "increased accommodations for the more violent class of patients in this department is recommended to the favorable consideration of the Asylum Committee; it can probably be effected at a moderate outlay, and obviate the present disadvantages." In June, 1851, Dr. Nichols again brought the subject to the attention of the committee, and recommended an additional building connected with the women's Lodge, for "the use of highly excited and noisy patients." In July the vice president of the board, after visiting the asylum, reported that "he entirely united in opinion with the Physician and Committee that an additional building for violent female patients is necessary."

In January, 1852, the Weekly Committee presented a plan for two brick buildings of two stories as additions to both the men's and women's Lodges, and the Asylum Committee recommended to the board that the plan be carried into effect. The estimated cost was $20,800, and the Asylum Committee referred to the Board of Governors the question whether "it would be wise to enter upon improvements at the present time involving so large an outlay." [9] The only other recorded reference to the subject during that year appeared in the Weekly Committee Minutes of December 9, when "the absolute necessity of apartments for the reception of the violent was again forcibly impressed upon the notice of the committee." In their annual report to the legislature for 1852, the governors also directed attention to the need of additions or alterations to the buildings and other expenditures for the more complete classification and comfort of the patients. The difficulty in procuring funds for a project so long and urgently needed may in some measure account for a reference in the *American Journal of Insanity*, in 1850, to "the reproach sometimes thrown upon the Bloomingdale Institution as being 'behind the age' in improvements." [10] Judged by the standard specifications adopted by the Association of Medical Superintendents in 1851, Bloomingdale Asylum at that time was deficient in: 1) Accommodations (all apartments used for patients should be entirely above ground); 2) Gas lighting; 3) Steam or hot water heating; 4) Forced ventilation; 5) Boilers in detached building.[11]

Notwithstanding the delay in providing these improvements, substantial contributions were made to the comfort and convenience of the patients, and to the facilities for their treatment. The introduction of Croton water into the buildings in 1848, after negotiations begun in 1846, was declared by the asylum physician to be "one of the most important improvements ever made in the institution." [12] The cost of the installation was $1,350, and it was agreed that the charge per year would be $75. Hitherto, the water supply came from wells and from the rainfall on the roofs. A few water closets had been installed on the first floor of the main building when it was erected. In December, 1842, Dr. Wilson, in recommending that a water closet be placed in each hall, stated that at that time the patients were obliged to use chambers in their bedrooms or resort to a privy in the yard, generally at a great distance. After sundown all were in the habit of using chambers, "which

[9] *Minutes of the Asylum Committee*, May 1, 1852.
[10] *Am. J. Insanity* VII (1850), 173.
[11] *Ibid.*, VIII (1851), 79–81, 87.
[12] Physician's Annual Report for 1848.

was a cause of frequent and just complaint." The only bath tub was in the basement. In 1843, at the request of the physician, a bathtub, a shower bath, a wash basin, and a water closet were installed on the second floor. In 1847 there was a water closet on each floor of the main building, and a bathroom on the second floor only. There were also bathrooms in the basements of the main building and of the Lodges, one in each wing of the former, making six in all. There were apparently no water closets or other water facilities in the Lodges. In 1849 the physician was authorized to install baths and water closets throughout the wings of the main building, and in January, 1850, the Inspecting Committee reported that "they were particularly struck with the great improvement in the Baths and water closets, which are now completely finished, and form a gratifying contrast with the former imperfect and annoying condition of these accommodations." They considered that "credit is due to Dr. Nichols who planned it, and under whose constant supervision it was carried out by common mechanics." Again in August this committee reported that they were "much gratified with the thorough and effectual manner in which the water for bathing and other purposes had been arranged in the main building," and they recommended "an early introduction of more water facilities."

The heating arrangements were also, at this period, still quite unsatisfactory. From year to year different varieties of stoves, "drums," and furnaces were tried. Complaints were usually followed by an increase in the number of heating units. In 1843 the physician visited the new State Asylum at Utica, and was informed by its superintendent that the heating system was remarkably satisfactory. The governors thereupon installed the same system in the "middle house" of the main building and in the women's Lodge. The annual report for 1843 announced that the year was the first in which hot-air furnaces were operated in heating the asylum, and that "advantages are evidenced in the increased and regular temperature afforded — improved ventilation — greater safety, and in the economy of fuel." Nevertheless, it was soon necessary to increase the number of furnaces, and at one visit the committee reported that, while heat and ventilation were satisfactory in the main building, the Lodges were "deficient in both." As late as December, 1851, it was found necessary to provide fireplaces in the dining rooms in the basement of the main building, and, with an outdoor temperature of one degree below zero, the Weekly Committee reported "all apartments warm." In the earlier periods it was considered that a furnace producing a uniform temperature of 52° to 62° in the halls and "a few degrees lower" in the bedrooms "rendered them comfortable."[13] In 1850 a committee of the governors visited hospitals and asylums in Boston, Trenton, and Philadelphia for the purpose of examining their heating and ventilating systems. Large sums were spent in improving these and also the water supply, and toilet facilities at both the general hospital and the asylum, and for this purpose it was found necessary to borrow $40,000.

Another improvement was the removal of the heavy iron guards from the windows. In May, 1844, Dr. Pliny Earle, who had recently been appointed physician, reported that the rooms of the second floor of the men's Lodge were "barricaded with iron as if they were the cells of a penitentiary."[14] He recommended the substitution of iron sashes, and was authorized to have this done. In November he reported that eight windows had been changed, with great improvement without and within. The new casings were made by a patient, the iron guards had been sold, and the net cost of the change in the windows was $4.97½. Thereupon, the governors readily consented to have other windows treated in the same way, especially those of the women's Lodge. In order that the quiet patients on the second floor of the men's Lodge might avoid commingling with the turbulent on the lower floor, an outside stairway leading down to the yard was erected. To add to the safety of the patients, lightning rods were, at the suggestion of Dr. Earle, attached to the buildings. At the suggestion of his predecessor, Dr. Wilson, a portable fire engine had been purchased for $45, and eighty feet of leathern hose at forty cents a foot. The pipes leading from the tanks were prepared for the hose, and the attendants and servants were instructed in the use of the equipment.

To make the asylum more inviting to private patients, the entrance hall of the main building was refurnished, blinds were placed on many of the windows, floors that appeared "naked and uncomfortable" were covered with carpet, at a price limited to eighty cents a yard. Twenty dollars were appropriated for prints for the patients' rooms, and $200 for a pianoforte. A number of bedsteads were replaced, mattresses were renovated, the hair picking being done by the patients, and straw mattresses were substituted for loose straw "under beds." A new carriage for the patients' drives was made to order, from a "draft furnished by the committee," by Levi Adams of Harlem, for $450. In 1851, through Mr. James Beekman, a member of the Asylum Committee, a "set of valuable Engravings published by the American Art Union," and the

[13] *Minutes of the Asylum Committee,* Dec. 3, 1842. [14] See p. 139.

next year a large number of books and periodicals, were received from Dewit and Davenport for the use of the patients. Through "General Fleming" (Augustus Fleming, one of the governors) two hundred volumes "suitable for the patients" were received from D. Appleton & Co. Mr. Fleming had, in 1841, presented to the library forty volumes and three periodicals.

Various purchases and sales of asylum land were made during this period, for the purpose of straightening the borders of the property, and from considerations relating to the possible opening of streets and to taxation. The largest transaction was in 1849, when fourteen acres were sold for $10,000. Portions of the property were sometimes placed on the tax list by the city assessor. On one occasion (in 1844) a plot was sold for nonpayment of taxes, without notice to the governors. When the governors protested they were told by the City Comptroller that "the Hospital had a great many pay patients," that the asylum "never received any one without pay," and that they had been "exempt from taxes heretofore from courtesy, and not by law," as neither hospital nor asylum was mentioned in the law, only almshouse.[15] After consulting dictionaries, the governors informed the Corporation Counsel of the city that "the Institution of the New York Hospital which includes the Asylum for the Insane at Bloomingdale is a charitable Institution in the true sense of the word, and is defined by the most authentic Lexicographers as synonymous with Alms House." This was apparently convincing; the lots which had been sold were redeemed by the city and restored to the asylum. To avoid further embarrassment, the warden of the asylum was instructed to examine the tax list once a year and report to the committee. In 1848, when it was proposed that all the asylum land except that on which the buildings stood should be taxed, an appeal to the legislature was contemplated. The supervisors thereupon exempted the property. When, in 1849, it was announced that Eleventh Avenue was to be opened, the governors joined with other property owners in a protest. The avenue was 400 feet nearer the asylum than was Bloomingdale Road. Opening it would entail a loss of privacy and quiet for the patients, as well as some of the open space used for exercises. The erection of a twelve-foot stone wall around the portion of the property between 114th and 120th Streets and Tenth and Eleventh Avenues had already been considered. It was, however, decided that it would be inexpedient to build this, as nearly half the farm, part of the garden and orchard, the field between Eleventh Avenue and Bloomingdale Road,

15 *Minutes of the Asylum Committee*, Dec. 31, 1844.

and three quarters of the barn and coach house would be outside, separated from the rest of the property and an "invitation to the vexatious question of taxation." [16]

In the annual report for 1847, the property was described as consisting of 55 acres, 30 of which were under high cultivation, "laid out and planted in one of the most approved styles of English gardening," and bearing "a strong resemblance to the beautiful homesteads of the wealthy, in the rural, cultivated districts of England." The central portion of the main building contained offices and apartments for the officers. The wings, east for the women and west for the men, were identical. A central corridor 10½ feet wide extended the whole length of the wing with apartments on each side. At the end of each hall there was a dining and sitting room. There were seven sitting rooms 25 feet long and 18 feet wide. The sleeping rooms, of which there were 68, contained from one to four beds. There was a water closet on each floor, and a bathroom on the second floor. One hundred and fifty feet in the rear of the main building and parallel with the western extremity was the men's Lodge, a brick building of three stories, 57 by 38 feet, with a central corridor 10 feet wide in each floor, and rooms of uniform size, 9 feet 2 inches by 7 feet 2 inches. It contained 59 rooms for patients. The sitting-rooms were 21 feet long, 15 feet wide and 10 feet high. A similar building, parallel to the eastern extremity, was a Lodge for women. The laundry was in the basement of this building, with two floors above for patients. The building measured 66½ by 38 feet, with a central corridor 9½ feet wide and rooms 9½ by 6½ feet. Every department occupied by patients was heated by "air furnaces" with the exception of sitting and dining rooms in the main building, in each of which there was a grate or stove with a coal fire. The greenhouse was said to contain "about seven hundred plants, many of them rare and beautiful exotics." [17]

Although the annuity appropriated by the State Legislature in 1816 was, by law, to be continued until 1857, a revision of the state constitution required that all appropriations should be for no more than two years, and the question of discontinuing the annuity was, from time to time, proposed by new members of the legislature. In their annual report for 1849 the governors explained that "in pursuance of permanent acts" the annuity had formerly been paid regularly, but since the revision of the constitution it was

[16] *Ibid.*, Nov. 4, 1848.

[17] Description of the property from Annual Report for 1847.

regarded by some members of late Legislatures as a subject open to be examined anew on grounds of expediency or economy. . . . The conditions of the grant have been faithfully complied with on the part of this Corporation, by the application of means and services to the public object in view, much beyond anything that the monies granted by the State could have effected, these annunities, so long as the duties resulting from the grant are faithfully performed, are vested rights in this Corporation, to which the faith of the State is as much pledged as for the payment of its public debt.

In an earlier report they had pointed out to the legislature that

on the faith of these grants, not only were spacious buildings erected, large debts contracted for their construction, but private contributions were and still are given, earnings obtained from other sources and arduous professional and other services gratuitously rendered; all which, if reduced to the form of a money calculation, would far exceed in amount the payments received from the State Treasury.[18]

The annuity for the asylum was, as already related, applied to the interest and sinking fund of the debt incurred for purchasing the land and erecting the main building. The last payment on this debt was made in 1845, and in September, 1847, the treasurer of the Society reported to the governors that there was now "no bond or mortgage debt against the Society." As, however, it had been necessary for the Society to employ some of its own funds in establishing the asylum, the annual payments made by the state until the expiration of the annuity in 1858 were applied to reimbursing these funds.[19] Apparently, none of the annuity was used directly for the maintenance of Bloomingdale Asylum. Nor has the asylum ever, up to the present, been blessed with more than a nominal income from endowment. The first bequest for this purpose was received from Elizabeth Demilt in 1850. On January 7, 1851, the bequest was accepted by the governors and the following action was taken:

Resolved and it is hereby ordained that the bequest to the Society of the New York Hospital, of the late Elizabeth Demilt of the sum of $10,000, receipt of which has been acknowledged by the Treasurer thereof, be and the same is hereby wholly set apart and constituted a permanent Fund and Endowment; to be kept forever undiminished and inviolate, for the purposes and uses of said Society; and that the income or earnings thereof shall be paid over, from time to time, to the Treasurer for the time being of said Society; one half for the use of the Hospital in the city and one half for the use of the Bloomingdale Asylum according to the intention of the Testatrix.

[18] Annual Report for 1848.
[19] Annual Report for 1850.

The bequest was said to be the largest that had been received by the Society since it was established. The president, vice president, and treasurer were appointed a committee to "invest and manage the said Fund, and any other sums, or property, which may be given, or bequeathed, to the said society and added by a vote of the Governors to the said Fund."

In November, 1840, the asylum was inspected by a commission appointed by act of the legislature, which, after the visit, advised the governors that "the Commissioners beg permission to bear the fullest testimony to the perfect order, cleanliness, and propriety of the Asylum, and to the good management of the committee, and the several persons under their government." [20] In July, 1843, the governor of the state, Hon. William C. Bouck, in company with five members of the Board of Governors, "carefully examined" the asylum and made a "rigid inspection," at the close of which and a "light collation" the governor said that he was "highly gratified with what he had seen." Another noteworthy visit to the asylum during this period was that of one of the commissioners who were planning the New Jersey State Asylum, in 1845.

Owing to the diversion to recently established public and private asylums of many patients who would previously have been admitted to Bloomingdale, the number of patients and the income of the asylum were fluctuating. The income from rates paid by patients fell from $34,992.82 in 1848—the year in which the New Jersey State Asylum was opened—to $27,511.37 in the following year. At the close of the period, in 1852, it had increased to $30,949.67, and the following year it was $37,507.85. The number of patients, which also diminished as other asylums were opened, soon increased, and in his report for the year 1851 the physician was able to report that "the House was constantly well filled." Although the annuity from the state was applied to the interest and sinking fund of the debt, it was entered in the accounts as part of the asylum income. In July, 1843, the Asylum Committee reported that they had on hand $3,000 more than they needed and they were instructed to pay it to the treasurer. This policy of transferring to the general funds credit balances appearing on the Bloomingdale accounts was continued until 1911. In May, 1846, Dr. Earle the resident physician asked that the full amount of the asylum earnings be devoted to the institution and to improvements, and he quoted from Dr. Bell of the McLean Asylum:

[20] *Minutes of the Asylum Committee.*

> It is manifest that if we would hope to keep our institutions up to the recent level of those of England, France, and Germany, it must be done by unremitting activity; by never resting satisfied with present attainments, and by keeping the community well advised of the absolute necessity of liberal means to meet this great end.[21]

The importance of keeping this necessity constantly in mind can scarcely be overestimated.

The necessity of continuing to provide for public patients at a low rate prevented the rise in expenditures required for the intensive treatment of a selected group under private support. The prosperity and advancement of the service were thereby retarded. The necessity of economy was so pressing that the governors, through their committee, gave much attention to it by personally engaging in the purchase of supplies and in the management. In 1843 the position of farmer was abolished and a foreman who would sleep in the basement with the other "hands" was substituted. In the same year, which was that in which the State Asylum at Utica was opened, the cost of the dietary was lowered by substituting meal and rice for meat in the Lodges, reducing the amount of food at breakfast, and omitting pastry entirely. In the main building meat was served twice a week in the upper halls, and once a week in the others. The private kitchens were closed. Dr. Wilson, in 1843, advised the governors that the proportion of attendants to patients was less than in other asylums of equal standing. Dr. Earle, his successor, in June of the following year compared the proportion with that of the Friends Asylum at Frankford, Pennsylvania, where for 58 patients there were 9 attendants, while at Bloomingdale there were 9 for 108 patients. The governors, however, felt unable to authorize more than one additional attendant for each sex. Reporting that wages were below those paid in other asylums, Dr. Earle proposed an increase, with a gratuity on occasion for particularly satisfactory service. The payroll for 1845, when the average daily number of patients was 120, was: Physician $1,800, Warden $1,000, Matron $250, Chaplain $150, Apothecary $100, Attendants $2,503.20, Domestics, carpenter, etc., $2,103.10, Farmers $870.06; total $8,776.36.

The policy adopted in regard to the rates paid for the care of patients was adhered to pretty closely. A rate of three dollars a week necessitated residence in one of the Lodges, whatever the condition of the patient. There were exceptions, however, and the rate for a physician's daughter

21 *Ibid.*, May 2, 1846.

was reduced without change of quarters.[22] It was noted that the requirement of payment for three months in advance seemed, in some instances, to convey the impression that three months was the total period for which hospital treatment would be required, and in consequence patients were removed prematurely.

Some minor occurrences during the period seem to be worthy of note. The practice of designating the months by number (Quaker style) instead of by name, or as well as by name, was continued by different secretaries of the board until 1845.[23] In December, 1844, instruments for meteorological observations were installed and the apothecary was instructed to report regularly to the State Board of Regents. The observations were recorded in the Minutes of the Board of Governors until December, 1849.

22 *Ibid.*, June 3, 1843.

23 *Minutes of the Governors.*

XVIII

TREATMENT METHODS AND THE GENERAL STATE OF THE SERVICE

IT may, perhaps, be appropriate to repeat here that, in introducing a system of "moral treatment" in their service for the mentally ill, the governors of the New York Hospital regarded it as an administrative rather than a medical undertaking. The York Retreat in England, which had been held out to them as a model by Thomas Eddy, had been founded and conducted by a benevolent layman. The Bloomingdale committee considered the system of "moral treatment" to be under their own particular direction, and they undertook its operation through the warden and matron. The physician was, by the rules adopted, expected only to coöperate. This was a different form of organization from that followed in the new asylums that were steadily increasing in number throughout the country. With few exceptions, of which one was the Friends Asylum at Frankford (also patterned after the York Retreat), the plan adopted provided for a medical superintendent to control and direct the whole organization. The adherence of the governors to a form considered defective by those best able to judge, was probably prejudicial to the reputation of Bloomingdale, impaired its influence, and retarded its advancement as a medical and scientific service.

Notwithstanding the agreement with Dr. Macdonald that he would have charge of "moral treatment," [1] and the gradual extension of the authority of the physician, the governors continued to maintain a particular degree of supervision. Rules adopted in 1846 stipulated that "as the supervision of the moral treatment of the patients, is placed by the by-laws with the Asylum Committee, it would seem to be proper that the physician should report his plans and operations in this respect, with the result of such plans, to the said committee." [2] The governors continued the practice of seeing all the patients at each of their visits, and of noting in their minutes the number in mechanical restraint or isolated in rooms. They also noted the activities of the patients in useful and recreational pursuits, and defects and needs of the service that were brought to their attention by the physician or observed by themselves. The Inspecting Committee were especially independent and frank in their observations. In February, 1852, they reported that

1 See pp. 189–190.

2 *Minutes of the Asylum Committee,* Feb. 28, 1846.

the sympathies and feelings of the Committee were a good deal outraged by the condition in which they found a male patient in one of the Lodges —being in an appartment which for want of facility for heating and ventilating during the inclement season they would hardly have appropriated to a favorite dog—they were informed by the Dr. it was the best appartment he had for a patient of that class.

Such supervision, however, no doubt contributed to the introduction of better facilities and to the establishment at Bloomingdale of the humane "system of moral and medical treatment of which it gave one of the earliest examples on this side of the Atlantic." [3]

The physician's particular task was, therefore, still considered to be individual medical treatment, consisting principally in the prescribing of medicine and diet, in various medical and nursing procedures, and in the direction of the nurses and attendants. In this task, he had little skilled assistance. It was not until 1833 that an apothecary was employed, the first being Jarvis Titus. The position of consulting physician had been abolished in 1830, and, despite Dr. Macdonald's recommendation in 1837, that an assistant physician be appointed, the post had not been established.

Little advance in the methods of medical treatment occurred during this period. There was further mitigation, and in some instances abandonment, of the extreme depletion that had for years been routine practice. From the time of Pinel most physicians engaged in asylum practice had condemned excessive bloodletting and had attributed to its effects some of the failures in the treatment of the mentally ill. In his annual report for 1844 the asylum physician, Dr. Earle, stated that "the abstraction of blood from the veins or arteries of those who are suffering under mental derangement is but little practiced in lunatic asylums, either in Great Britain or the United States. The lancet has probably confirmed and perpetuated more cases of insanity than it has cured." He considered, however, that there were "undoubtedly cases which require the use of the lancet, but they are rare," and it was the "indiscriminate employment of this method of depletion" that was "highly injurious and reprehensible." In regard to a patient from whom two quarts of blood had been taken before his admission to the asylum, he noted that the "violence of the symptoms probably warranted this treatment." [4] The employment of general bloodletting was nevertheless

[3] Govenors' Annual Report for 1853.

[4] *Minutes of the Asylum Committee*, May 31, 1845. (Physician's Monthly Report.) See also Dr. Pliny Earle's "Bloodletting in Mental Disorders," *Am. J. Insanity*, X (1854), 287.

practically abandoned at Bloomingdale by Dr. Earle. The local abstraction of blood by "cut-cupping" was, however, still practiced. Considerable confidence in the use of blisters and setons was also retained. Purgatives were still adhered to as routine practice, though the more drastic doses and forms were no longer administered. Croton oil was, however, considered a useful remedy by Dr. Wilson. Vomiting was no longer produced as a general depletory measure, though wine of antimony, tartar emetic, and ipecac were still used in moderate doses. Mercury to the extent of producing salivation was no longer considered good practice. In 1845, however, Dr. Earle reported that, in a case of "repeated paroxysmal mania," salivation prevented a pending attack, and there was no further recurrence, though the patient remained voluntarily at the asylum for a year, in fear of an attack.[5]

In an article on "Baths and Bathing" published by the medical superintendent of the Friends Asylum, it was stated that

> the days in which it was considered necessary to treat every case of disordered cerebral circulation by a resort to depletory measures have happily passed by, and the end which was sought to be attained thereby, may be answered, in many cases of insanity, by other means, including the use of the warm bath.[6]

This form of treatment was, indeed, approved at Bloomingdale, but the inadequate bathing facilities in the Lodges where the more disturbed patients were treated rendered the effective use of the bath scarcely practicable. The cold bath in any form was not employed in the treatment of the patients. The shower was used by Dr. Earle only with the patient's consent, and it was entirely abandoned as a means of punishment. Some writers, however, still approved of it, on the ground that "as a means of positive punishment, nothing is equal to the cold bath, as used in the douche, bath of surprise, etc." [7]

Sedatives were used perhaps a little more freely. Conium was employed by Dr. Earle, after he had tried it himself. Iodine in the form of Lugol's Solution was introduced in the treatment of cases in which it was thought that the brain was organically affected. A rather novel remedy used experimentally in some asylums was sulphuric ether by inhalation,[8] which had recently been introduced as an anaesthetic. In a few cases admitted to Bloomingdale, the cause of the mental disorder was at-

[5] *Minutes of the Asylum Committee*, May 31, 1845.

[6] J. H. Worthington, M.D., "Baths and Bathing," *Am. J. Insanity*, VII (1851), 207.

[7] John R. Allan, M.D., "On the Treatment of Insanity," *Am. J. Insanity*, VI (1850), 277.

[8] See "Inhalation of the Vapor of Sulphuric Ether in Cases of Insanity," *Am. J. Insanity*, IV (1847), 73.

tributed to habitual ether inhalation. In the administration of medicine, Dr. Earle in 1844 introduced "the single dose system." Instead of having bottles and boxes of medicines in the halls, single doses were distributed in small glasses on a tray.[9] This method was followed until 1911, when the introduction of nurse training and skilled supervision made it possible to keep medicines in the halls without danger. The problem of nourishing patients who refused food was seldom mentioned in the Bloomingdale records of this period. The stomach tube was apparently not yet introduced nor hypodermic medication.

Many of the patients were suicidal; some had before admission made serious attempts at taking their own lives, but the number who succeeded in the asylum was small. This seems especially remarkable because the supervision, especially at night, was very imperfect. As has been related, patients were left unattended when the attendants were at meals. At night they were locked in their rooms, the only sanitary convenience being a metallic chamber which could be used as a weapon. It was customary to place a suicidal patient in a room with another patient, sometimes of the same type. A night watchman was not always employed, and when he was, he passed through the halls not oftener than once an hour. On the women's service, the only night supervision was that of a nurse who slept in an adjoining room. Seven patients committed suicide during the period of 1840–1852. Three of these were men and four were women. All of the women and two of the men resorted to strangulation, usually by suspension, though in one instance a sheet and in another a cravat attached to the bedstead were utilized. One man obtained a razor by breaking into a drawer and cut his throat. There was some publicity in this case,[10] which Dr. Nichols deprecated because, he reported to the governors, "suicide is contagious by imitation." Some writers, he said, "have supposed that the affection of the brain causing the suicidal form of insanity, is subject to epidemic agencies like most other kinds of bodily disease," and added that the fact that the record of suicidal cases "gives a startling interest to almost every daily print, certainly corroborates the supposition to which allusion has just been made." [11] Dr. Earle believed that entire prevention of suicide in the asylum was impossible. He considered that "should every patient suicidally disposed be placed constantly under corporal restraint, asylums would become hideously deformed with straps, wristbands and

[9] *Minutes of the Asylum Committee,* May 4, 1844.
[10] *New York Tribune,* March 29, 1850.
[11] *Minutes of the Asylum Committee,* March 30, 1850.

muffs." He referred to a woman in another asylum who was deprived even of her clothing but succeeded in strangling herself with her hair, and to observations at Bethlehem Asylum in London, where it was reported that from 1750 to 1770, when every patient was under restraint, the suicide ratio was 1 to 202 patients, while in the twenty years just preceding the report, when restraint was seldom used, the ratio fell to 1 to 963 patients.[12]

The routine recording of patients' histories was still confined principally to the registers. Dr. Earle's "Register of Discharges," was introduced in 1845. Entries in this book were pretty full during Dr. Earle's service. After he left, however, there were omissions under some of the headings, notably under "Corporal restraints," "Worked," "Attended religious worship," "Attended School," "Attended lectures," "Attended weekly parties." In 1846 Dr. Earle also introduced a book for "Case Records." The pages were spaced by means of vertical lines, and entries were made under the following captions: "Name and Date," "Previous history," "State when admitted," "Symptoms and treatment in Asylum." Cases were recorded in this volume from July 2, 1846, to April 20, 1853. Until December, 1849, the monthly reports of the physician to the Asylum Committee contained brief accounts of the patients admitted and discharged during the month. The governors, however, directed that the full report of the physician should thereafter be omitted from the Minutes of the committee but should be recorded at the asylum. After that the Minutes contained only a statistical statement from the physician. The full reports were recorded in a separate book, designated "Physician's Reports," which contains, however, only those from December 29, 1849, to May 1, 1852, which were made by Dr. Nichols. The annual reports of the physicians have been printed separately from those of the governors since 1843. In authorizing this for the first time, the governors recorded that it was "for extending generally a knowledge of the benefits of the institution." [13] They contain no information relating to individual patients and their treatment.

The case histories during this and preceding periods were not kept systematically. The registers, however, contain the names and a few other facts relating to all the patients admitted to the service since it was organized in 1808, and available space in them was, in some instances, utilized for recording clinical observations. Expensive, specially printed and ruled books were purchased on recommendation of a physician,

[12] *Ibid.*, Nov. 30, 1844.

[13] *Ibid.*, April 1, 1843.

only to be discarded by some successor, with a large part of the volume without an entry. The practice of recording the histories of "remarkable" cases in a special volume [14] was continued until 1849, though none has been found for the years 1826 to 1836. Many of these histories are quite full but contain little to indicate progress. The patient's appearance is described in general terms, including whether he was tall or short, thin or stout, the color of hair, skin, and eyes, and the temperament. The state of the pupils began during this period to receive notice pretty regularly. Instruments of precision were not mentioned. The previous history and behavior of the patient were recorded in colloquial language without much regard for systematic presentation. The treatment and the course of the illness were often recorded quite fully, though in many instances the intervals between entries were long. The symptoms described were not essentially different from those of present-day patients and it is quite possible to obtain a fair understanding of the character of many of the cases.

Religious ideas continued to have a larger place than at present in the troubled thinking of the patients. Depressed patients had "no hope of salvation," "must go to that bad place," "grow more sinful every day," "seven evil spirits are crawling over her body," "the devil has torn her to pieces," it is "sinful to eat," her child "was not made by God, he will not smile on it," she is "commanded by Heaven to kill it," and so on. In a separate book in which Dr. Earle recorded his statistical studies, delusions are classified as: *Titles, Riches, Poverty, Religious, Spirits (Devils, Witches, the Stars etc.) Suspicions, Illusions of the Senses, Destructiveness* (*Homicide, Arson etc.*), *Love, Bodily Organs, Pennance* (*Mutilation*).

The number of alcoholic cases was greatly reduced. In 1848, eleven cases were admitted. Many cases of delirium tremens were, however, treated at the general hospital, as well as occasional cases of other forms of mental disorder. In January, 1850, the Committee on Ventilation (General Hospital) reported that "Lockup room (so-called) No. 2 in the basement of the North House, being a room altogether appropriated to Delirium Tremens cases . . . is entirely without ventilation," and they recommended a window. In May, 1851, Dr. Swett recommended "that the windows of the third story of the North House be better secured in order to prevent the patients laboring under insanity from jumping out, as has recently happened." Seven cases of opium addiction

[14] See p. 167.

were admitted to Bloomingdale during this period. One woman's illness was attributed to excessive smoking.

In August, 1844, a case recorded in the register as general paralysis was admitted.[15] Dr. Earle made a special study of this disease, and in April, 1847, he reported eleven cases, nine with autopsies, in the *American Journal of Medical Sciences.*[16] This was the first article on the subject to appear in a general medical publication in America. Dr. Luther V. Bell, medical superintendent of McLean Hospital, had, however, in his annual report for 1843, given an account of the disease, and stated that a number of cases had been admitted to the McLean service. He noted as

> a somewhat curious fact, that it is only in the last three years that this disease has been admitted to this institution. As late as my visit to Europe in 1840 it was unknown within our walls. Nor having seen it so often manifested there, can I recall a case in our register which would at all meet its characteristics, rendering it certain it was not overlooked.

As early as 1819, however, a case described in the records of the service for the mentally ill of the New York Hospital can be identified as general paralysis with reasonable certainty, and, in 1823, a case designated "paralysie generale of Calmeil" was recorded.[17] A case of another form of disease, which was at that time not generally recognized, was admitted to the asylum in February, 1848: the diagnosis was *Mania accompanied by St. Vitus' Dance.* The patient was a woman of fifty whose father, brother, and sister had been affected with the same disease. The father had committed suicide, and the brother and sister had "both become imbecile." [18] The form of disease in these cases was apparently that now well known as "Huntington's or Hereditary Chorea." Although cases had been described in medical literature as early as 1816, it was not until 1870, after an account of a group of affected families on Long Island had been published by Dr. George Huntington, that the distinctive character of the disease was generally recognized. Cases affected by it are not infrequently admitted to the institutions for the mentally ill, though, until many years after he published his article, Dr. Huntington was not aware of this.[19]

15 *Minutes of the Asylum Committee,* Aug. 3, 1844.

16 Pliny Earle, M.D., "Cases of Paralysis Peculiar to the Insane: the Paralysie Générale of the French," *Am. J. Med. Sci.,* New Series, XIII (1847), 333.

17 See pp. 110, 166.

18 *Minutes of the Asylum Committee,* March 4, 1848.

19 Personal conversation of the writer with Dr. Huntington.

It was still customary, whenever anything considered significant was learned, to attribute mental illness to some particular "participating cause." Apparently, the statements of the patients or their relatives were accepted as sufficient evidence. The causes might be physical or "mental and moral," and the variety of each was considerable. In his statistical tables Dr. Earle listed 46 kinds of physical causes and 29 "mental and moral." One of the principal physical causes was intoxicating liquors, which, Dr. Earle reported, "are so cheap that the labour of a few hours will procure enough to addle the brain for a week, and prevent the healthy exercise of reason perhaps a much longer period." It was also his belief that

> the comparative ease with which the products of both nature and art in every quarter of the globe are here obtained, have a direct tendency to foster a luxurious life. . . . The almost unavoidable effect of the artificial mode of living thus produced, is either a debility of the system, or an augmentation of nervous excitability, either of which facilitates the invasion of mental disease. . . . Children, before the body has acquired sufficient tone, or the brain sufficient firmness to endure much mental exertion with impunity, are placed in schools where the intellectual faculties are unduly urged, while the physical exercise necessary to the due development of the frame is too often neglected. Under these circumstances, the head will expand, but the body cannot grow in size or vigor sufficiently to maintain "a balance of power." [20]

In June, 1849, he reported an "instructive case" to illustrate his thesis. Suppressed secretions, repelled eruptions, and the healing of long discharging sores were still assumed to be "causes." Masturbation was included among the physical causes and attributed only to the male sex. Mesmerism was mentioned as a physical cause in a case admitted in August, 1844; the patient had fallen into a state of "maniacal delirium and excitement" while "under the manoeuvres of a practitioner of 'Mesmerism.' " In reporting the death of a patient whose mental illness followed childbirth, Dr. Earle said that such cases were generally curable and that he had never before lost a case.[21] Among the mental causes, religious excitement and worries had a large place. The illnesses of three women were attributed to "novel reading." Fear of cholera was considered to be the cause in two other cases. There was considerable difference of opinion among physicians in regard to the relative importance of physical and mental causes. Dr. Earle was of the opinion

[20] *Minutes of the Asylum Committee*, Feb., 1846. (Physician's Annual Report for 1845.) Compare with references to education on page 11.

[21] *Ibid.*, Jan. 31, 1846.

that the latter operated most frequently. He believed that physical conditions such as "cerebral disease, epilepsy, typhus fever may be induced, and frequently are, by mental influences." [22] Dr. Nichols, however, believed that "it is not the mind itself, but its immediate instrument, the brain whose functions are first disturbed in cases of insanity." [23]

Dr. Earle's statistical studies included many subjects, such as heredity, and suicidal and homicidal propensities. These studies, especially those relating to the curability of insanity, received much attention, and probably contributed substantially to the establishment of the broad statistical studies of mental disease and defect which have since been made in this country.

With one exception, the general health of the asylum population was, during this period, free from any great prevalence of infectious disease. In November, 1847, a female patient was reported ill with typhus fever. No further cases were reported until about the first of February, 1848, when a recent immigrant, who had been admitted to the men's Lodge, was found to be ill with the same disease. This probably was the patient of whom it was noted at the time of his admission in January that "his disease was apparently delirium accompanying ship fever." He and six others who soon contracted the illness were isolated in the upper floor of the Lodge. The disease spread, and in the first week of February, 1848, all the cases, which then numbered eleven, were transferred to the general hospital. Three died there, and five who were returned on the 19th had to be sent back to the hospital because their recovery was not complete. The Lodge was then cleaned and ventilated and there were no new cases.[24] At the New York Hospital the number of cases treated during this epidemic was 1,034 with 136 deaths.[25]

Apparently malaria was no longer so prevalent at Bloomingdale as it had been in previous years. In September and October, 1842, the Inspecting Committee reported that several patients were ill with "intermittent bilious fever," and in September, 1843, the physician reported that two nurses were ill with the same disorder. The patients were, however, on that occasion said to be entirely exempt, and no other cases were reported during the period. Smallpox was, apparently, quite prevalent in New York in 1845. The patients and employees of the asylum were vaccinated, however, and no case occurred. One case of typhoid fever was reported in November, 1844, and in March, 1848,

[22] *Ibid.*, Feb., 1846. (Physician's Annual Report for 1845.)
[23] *Ibid.*, Sept. 1, 1849.
[24] *Ibid.*, Nov., 1847 to March, 1848.
[25] Governors' Annual Report for 1847.

influenza prevailed extensively among the patients. On one occasion cholera was also reported in the neighborhood, but no case occurred in the asylum.

Previous to 1842 mentally ill persons were admitted and detained in the asylum without being subjected to any well-defined legal procedure. In that year the act creating the New York State Lunatic Asylum was passed; this was "the first definite step towards seeing the proper commitment of patients to asylums." [26] The act provided that neither justices of the peace nor superintendents or overseers of the poor, who had previously been empowered to confine a "lunatic," would any longer exercise this right "without having the evidence of two reputable physicians, under oath, as to the alleged fact of insanity." [27] But even after the act was passed, "it was still customary to send pauper patients to institutions without certificates of insanity or any formality beyond the simple order of the superintendent of the poor, which in fact only guaranteed the payment of necessary expenses." [28] At Bloomingdale the law was strictly complied with and the legal papers of all patients admitted since the act was passed are preserved at the Westchester Division. The limit of state jurisdiction was not observed as it is today: in January, 1843, the Asylum Committee, in ruling that "pauper" patients from New Jersey would be admitted at the same rate as those from New York, stipulated that the "warrant for commitment required by the Laws of the State of New Jersey will be indispensable." Many patients were accepted by authority of these warrants.

The legality of the restraint required for the proper treatment of a mentally ill person was not often questioned. During the period 1841 to 1852 only five patients were produced in court on writs of habeas corpus. In March, 1844, a patient from Sing Sing prison was, on a writ, returned to the prison because of a technical error in the manner of his transfer to the asylum. In October, 1845, a patient in whose case a writ had been issued, was released "by consent of the parties." In October, 1846, it was recorded that two men had been "removed from the Asylum by writs of habeas corpus," and in June, 1848, another case was removed by the same process. The records seem to indicate that these proceedings were not opposed and they occasioned little concern at the asylum.

Although previous to the act of 1842 there was little or no legal

[26] Henry M. Hurd, *The Institutional Care of the Insane in the United States and Canada* (Baltimore, 1916), I, 323.

[27] *Laws of the State of New York Relative to Lunacy* (New York, 1842), Section 22.

[28] Hurd, *op. cit., I*, 323. As late as 1897 orders of this kind were the only official documents relating to some of the patients in the New York state hospitals.

authority for the detention of a patient at Bloomingdale against his will, personal applications for admission were occasionally received. The only formalities related to support. The first formal application in writing was made on December 14, 1844. The application, which was witnessed by Dr. Earle and two other persons, stated that the patient had come to the asylum from New York of his own free will, and wished "to be under the Medical care of the physician to the Asylum aforesaid, until such time as it shall be thought best for me to leave" In a separate statement, also witnessed, he promised to conform to all the rules and regulations. The person who accompanied him to the asylum certified that "David B. informed me that he wished to go to the Bloomingdale Asylum as a boarder, and furthermore that I accompanied him there." There is indication here that, notwithstanding the freedom from legal restrictions which had for so many years attended the treatment of the mentally ill, a period had now been reached in which precautionary measures had become necessary. Patients who had gone home for a period were, however, readmitted without renewal of "the permit." In October, 1846, the patients from Sing Sing prison were transferred to the State Asylum, no doubt much to the relief of the governors and officials at Bloomingdale.

Although the standard of expenditures for board and treatment of the patients was at this period extremely low, the main obstacle to advancement of the service was the inadequacy of available funds. The reduction in the number of patients occasioned by the establishment of public asylums was, indeed, temporary, but the rates received for private patients were in many instances as low as those paid by the counties. As late as 1851 only 6 patients were paying as much as $10 a week, and 38 were paying only $3 a week. [29] The total income from patients in that year was $29,174.21, and the total number treated was 198.[30] The governors, however, were indefatigable in their attentions to the service, and the committees constantly endeavored to maintain existing standards and to direct attention to needed improvements.

They fully realized the importance of an adequate nursing service. They talked with the patients from time to time, noting their classification, and the number of nurses. In July, 1844, they reported 62 patients in the main building: 28 were in the women's wing, of whom 11 were on the first floor, 10 on the second, and 7 on the third, with one nurse for each floor; and 34 patients in the men's wing, 11 on the first floor, 13

[29] *Minutes of the Asylum Committee*, Jan. 4, 1851.
[30] Governors' Annual Report.

on the second, and 10 on the third, with one nurse to each floor. In the women's Lodge there were 21 patients, 11 on the first floor and 10 on the second; and in the men's Lodge 27, 18 on the first and second floors and 9 in the basement. Two nurses were reported in each Lodge. This gave a total of 110 patients, and 10 nurses. There were also two private nurses. When in April, 1852, three nurses at the general hospital, one of whom had been in the service for 14 years, one for 15, and one for 25 years, all widows without means, were notified by the superintendent that their services would no longer be required, the Inspecting Committee reported that they were

> under the impression that the Governors of the Hospital . . . had adopted the policy of holding out inducements, by extra wages and a system of bounties, for nurses to continue a long time in the Hospital, as well as to faithfully discharge their duties, while there, with an implied assurance, that such extra wages and bounties, would be the reward of long and meritorious service . . . one twenty-five years, the latter being now entitled to the highest bounty, that the former Governors have thought proper to give, for the very purpose of securing long and faithful service . . . they are precisely in the situation, that must have been anticipated by former Governors, who fixed their highest wages and largest bounty on nurses after twenty years, of Hospital services in their employ. If these views of your Committee are correct they cannot but think, there is at least an implied contract, with these Nurses and that they cannot now be sent away without doing an act of great injustice.[81]

The satisfaction felt by the governors in the asylum service was frequently manifested. On June 29, 1848, the Inspecting Committee reported that their visit was attended with "more than usual interest from its being the first ever made by one of the committee, H. Chauncey. The good order that prevailed throughout the buildings, the comfort of the patients, the beauty and order of the grounds deeply impressed him and was a source of great gratification to the committee." Possibly the custom of attending an office hour at the New York Hospital—now a daily practice—may have originated at this time, as the Inspecting Committee, on their visit of September 3, 1849, made note of the absence of the physician and added "it being the day in which he visits the city."

Equipment requested by the physician was invariably granted. Books were, from time to time, purchased for the medical library, sometimes in Europe, and medical journals were subscribed for, one of which was French. Dr. Earle made a catalogue of the library in 1846.

[81] See *Minutes of the Governors,* Feb. 6, 1821.

The physician was from year to year given leave of absence to attend the annual meeting of the Association of Superintendents and to visit other institutions. The first meeting of the Association was attended by Dr. Earle in October, 1844. Upon his return he gave an account of the meeting to the Asylum Committee, and of the sixteen committees appointed. These committees were naturally concerned almost entirely with the treatment of the mentally ill in asylums. For years afterwards the avowed object of the Association was to "alleviate the condition of the insane in every part of the country" and to devise and introduce efficient methods and forms of organization. The proceedings were devoted principally to these objects. In May, 1848, the Association met in New York, and Dr. Earle proposed to the governors that the hospitality of the asylum be offered for one evening. The Visitors Book of the asylum contains, under date of May 12, 1848, the signatures of fourteen members of the Association.[32]

Few physicians besides those engaged in asylum practice gave much attention to mental illness, and scientific study of the subject made slow progress in America. Nor was much if any provision made for teaching the subject in the medical schools. The *American Journal of Insanity,* in 1847, called for "a distinct course of Lectures on Mental Maladies, at every Medical School," and at the same time announced that Dr. Samuel M. Smith had been appointed Professor of Medical Jurisprudence and Insanity at Willoughby University, Columbus, Ohio.[33] This was, apparently, the first appointment of this character in America. In Germany, however, Heinroth had been appointed Professor of Psychiatry at Leipzig University in 1811. The example was not generally followed, and even at the few schools in which some provision was made, the instruction was quite inadequate.

In October, 1847, Dr. Earle submitted to the governors an historical and statistical account of the asylum and requested that it be printed. In January, 1848, the printing of 750 copies was authorized.[34] The governors hoped that "the experience of this Institution will furnish many facts and results of great value to the study of the phenomena, causes, and cure of mental disease," and for many years this account of the asylum was the principal source of information relating to the early history

32 This book contains also the signatures of other distinguished visitors, notably that of Miss D. L. Dix on July 10, 1849—which was two years before her inspection and report on Bloomingdale conditions (see p. 249). The book contains entries from July, 1845, to Nov. 27, 1850.

33 *Am. J. Insanity,* IV (1847).

34 Pliny Earle, *History, Description, and Statistics of the Bloomingdale Asylum for the Insane* (New York, 1848). Also in Appendix 1847 Annual Report.

of the institution. It was said to contain "the fullest account of the operations and results of an American asylum which had ever been published" and the "statistics in new forms, after much labor in tabulation, made it the first essay in the reformation of statistics of insanity in America." The review of the measures employed in the "moral treatment" of the patients and the statistical studies of the period from 1821 to 1844 are both interesting and suggestive.

Several other publications by Dr. Earle appeared during this period. He contributed to the first volume of the *American Journal of Insanity* an article on the "Poetry of Insanity" and some translations from the French of case histories; to the second and third, contributions to the pathology of insanity; and in the fourth, an article on "Causes of Insanity," together with an account of a case under the title "A Leaf from and for the Annals of Insanity."

During this period, and for many years after, general interest and effort in behalf of the mentally ill of America were confined almost entirely to providing suitable institutional treatment for those who were most urgently in need of it. In this endeavor the general medical profession in some places contributed valuable services. It was through the interest and efforts of the Connecticut State Medical Society that the Retreat at Hartford was established in 1824, and the State Medical Society of New York had a large part in the establishment of the first State Asylum in 1843. The annual address of the president at the meetings of the New York State Medical Society in 1844, 1847, and 1848 was on a psychiatric topic. Dr. Samuel White, president in 1844, presented an address on "Insanity." In 1847, the president, Dr. John McCall, discussed "Mental Manifestations," and included consideration of the baffling questions of "responsibility" and the "irresistibility of the insane impulse" in criminal cases. Dr. Thomas W. Blatchford, president in 1848, discussed "Temperaments." In that year also, Dr. Joseph Bates made an address to the Columbia County Medical Society on "The Influence of Mind on Disease." In this he discussed the influence on the production and relief of illness of faith, imagination, fear, grief and other emotions, and of belief in astrology and superstitions. He considered that "the physician has it in his power to a very great degree, to convert mental emotions into agents of life or death." In 1843, Dr. C. B. Coventry, professor of obstetrics and medical jurisprudence in the Medical Institution of Geneva, New York, and one of the managers of the State Asylum at Utica, addressed the State Medical Society on "Insanity, Its Causes, Pathology, and Treatment." [85] The address was general in character. A noteworthy feature, however, was the manifest influence of phrenology in the views expressed. Dr. Coventry held that the mind was made up of "several separate and distinct faculties. These faculties are manifested or exerted through separate portions of the brain—that these portions being the instruments of the several faculties, may properly be called organs." Insanity, therefore, could not be regarded as a disease, as it was only a symptom or evidence of disease in one or more of these organs. This was the doctrine of phrenology which went so far as to profess ability to evaluate the various "faculties" by means of the "bumps" on the skull which were supposed to demarcate the underlying "organs." Many people were disposed to think that there might be some degree of truth in this teaching, among them some physicians engaged in the study and treatment of the mentally ill. In the view of Dr. H. A. Buttolph, medical superintendent of the New Jersey State Lunatic Asylum,

> phrenology bears the same relation to insanity, that physiology does to pathology . . . to the prevalence of this system are the insane mainly indebted for the well defined and philosophical views of mental and moral treatment now in vogue. That some have adopted the maxims of phrenology without admitting, or perchance even knowing their obligation to the science, may occasionally be as true of physicians, in treating insanity, as of professors and divines in teaching science and theology. . . . "By revealing the nature, number and origin of the human faculties, the conditions of their operations, their mutual influence, their modes of acting, and the natural laws by which their manifestations are regulated," phrenology has assisted to elucidate and more fully to establish the correct system of moral treatment of the insane, than any and all former systems of mental science.[86]

No indication that these views had any influence in the service at Bloomingdale has been found in the records.

The psychiatric literature of the period, in America, related principally to institutional problems and to the study and treatment of patients of the types received at the institutions. Most of the contributions were published in the *American Journal of Insanity*. Some, however, appeared in other journals, and the annual reports of some of the medical superintendents of this period contained interesting accounts

[85] All the addresses presented at the state or county medical societies were published in *Transactions of the State Medical Society*.

[86] H. A. Buttolph, "Relation between Phrenology and Insanity," *Am. J. Insanity*, VI (1849), 128, 134.

of current views and of the methods employed in the study and treatment of patients. The only book on mental disease, by an American author, to be published during this period was *The Treatment of Insanity* by Dr. John M. Galt, superintendent and physician of the Eastern Lunatic Asylum, Williamsburg, Virginia.[37] This consisted of a review of the treatment employed in mental illness in various places and by various physicians from 1689 to the date of publication. The section on American asylums describes pretty fully the treatment employed during the period under consideration in this chapter. It contains an interesting account of treatment at Bloomingdale written by Dr. Earle. Dr. William Sweetser, in 1843, published a book entitled *Mental Hygiene or, An Examination of the Intellect and Passions designed to Show How They Affect and Are Affected by the Bodily Functions and Their Influence on Health and Longevity*. A noteworthy publication in 1845 was the translation of Esquirol's treatise on mental disease by Dr. E. K. Hunt.[38] An American edition of Dr. Alfred S. Taylor's work on medical jurisprudence, edited by Dr. R. E. Griffiths of Philadelphia, is also noteworthy.[39]

[37] John M. Galt, *The Treatment of Insanity* (New York, 1846).
[38] E. Esquirol, *A Treatise on Insanity*, trans. E. K. Hunt (Philadelphia, 1845).
[39] Alfred S. Taylor, *Medical Jurisprudence*, ed. R. E. Griffiths (Philadelphia, 1845).

XIX

THE PHYSICIANS OF THE ASYLUM

DR. WILLIAM WILSON, who succeeded Dr. Ogden as physician of the asylum in September, 1839, was of "old Colonial stock" of New York and a graduate of Columbia College. He was thirty-four years old, and there is nothing in the information obtained concerning him to indicate that he had previously had training or experience in the treatment of the mentally ill. He was evidently, however, an earnest student and practitioner and his services seemed to be entirely satisfactory to the governors. He made many recommendations relating to the safety, comfort, and good treatment of the patients.

In 1842 he, like his predecessors, recommended that the accommodations for noisy and violent patients which were in the original plans be supplied. After he had presented the subject several times, he was requested to prepare plans and estimates.[1] The project was, nevertheless, not undertaken until several years after he had left the service. He endeavored to improve the "moral treatment" of the patients, and soon after his appointment the governors appointed a committee to confer with him on the subject. He allowed many of the patients to walk out unattended, and reported that the privilege was rarely abused. In the employment of the patients, the women did much housework and sewing, making all the articles of bedding and clothing. Any of the men who were "disposed to engage in some useful employment," were "cheerfully accommodated" with garden or farm work, or in the carpenter shop. In his annual report for 1843 he urged "the erection of suitable workshops for different avocations, and particularly the enlargement of our carpenter's shop." He approved of physical exercises, games, and amusements, but considered that they were "not to be compared, as regards the beneficial effects on the mind, with the occupations in which a man labors to some useful end." [2] Dancing parties or balls were, he believed, a source of interest and pleasure and had "a decided remedial influence, inducing in all an uncommon degree of self control." [3] He recommended an increase in the number of attendants.

He was the first to publish statistical studies of the patients in his annual report,[4] though he was aware that the information on which the statistics were based was "not fully to be relied upon, still as approximat-

1 See p. 201.

2 Physician's Annual Report for 1841. 3 *Ibid.*

4 Physician's Annual Report for 1839. Dr. Macdonald's article containing statistics of the service was published in 1839. See p. 196, above.

ing the truth." In his annual report for 1840 he presented, by request of the Bloomingdale committee, fourteen tables relating to patients admitted and discharged during the year and to all in the asylum. Ages, civil state, occupations, causes of illness and of death, time in the asylum, and other facts were tabulated. The forms of disorder were classified as mania, monomania, dementia, and idiocy. The principal causes to which the illnesses of the 239 patients treated during the year were attributed were: "hereditary" in 35 cases; intemperance, 30; pecuniary embarrassment, 18; domestic troubles, 16; religious excitement, 15; disappointed affection, 12; puerperal, 12; succeeding fever and other diseases, 10; with smaller numbers attributed to seventeen other causes, and 37 without known cause. In computing percentages of recoveries, the cases in which the duration was not more than one year were designated "recent" and were considered separately from the "old" or chronic cases. Dr. Wilson advised in his report for 1841 that "the public should be made acquainted with the almost certain curability of recent cases of insanity, when early subjected to treatment in an asylum judiciously managed." In the following year he showed that 46 percent of all the patients treated were not over thirty-five years of age. He also noted that 23.7 percent were farmers or the wives and daughters of farmers. In this report he referred to mechanical restraint and his "constant endeavour to obviate its use as far as possible." He added that "the use of the ordinary leather straps for the wrists and ankles comprise the means for the purpose. Frequently we have not a patient under restraint, and the [daily] average for the year would certainly not exceed one of each sex." He considered religious worship to be a "source of pleasure" to the patients, and "to some, at least, not without a profitable tendency in maintaining in their minds the kindly influences of religion on the heart, as well as the habits and associations of their former lives." He served until April, 1844. He evidently gained some reputation as a hospital administrator as the report of the trustees engaged in planning the first state asylum contains a communication from him relating to organization.[6] Following his retirement from the asylum in 1844 Dr. Wilson was a much respected citizen and practitioner in New York City. He died in 1872 and it was stated in his obituary that he was "honored for his skill in treating cases of lunacy, of which he made a special study."

The establishment of other institutions for the mentally ill had now enabled the governors of the New York Hospital, when filling vacancies

[6] New York State, Senate Doc. 20, p. 169. Letter of Nov. 15, 1841.

in the position of physician of the asylum, to consider candidates qualified in asylum practice. Dr. Wilson was the last to undertake the service without the advantage of previous experience, and a step toward complete medical direction was made. Many years elapsed, however, before this was fully accomplished. Dr. Pliny Earle, who succeeded Dr. Wilson in April, 1844, brought to the service an established reputation based on considerable study and experience in mental disease. His age was 35. His graduation thesis at the medical school of the University of Pennsylvania, in 1837, was on insanity and was published in the *American Journal of Medical Sciences* in 1838 under the title "Researches in Reference to the Causes, Duration, Termination and Moral Treatment of Insanity." Following his graduation he spent about two years in Europe, where he engaged in medical studies, and in visiting a number of the principal institutions for the mentally ill. An account of his observations was published in the *American Journal of Medical Sciences* for November, 1839, with the title "A Visit to Thirteen Asylums for the Insane in Europe with Statistics." Soon after his return to America in the spring of 1839, after a few months of general practice in Philadelphia, he entered the service of the Friends Asylum at Frankford, Pennsylvania, where he remained until his appointment at Bloomingdale. His experience in asylum practice, and his liberal opportunities for study and observation enabled him to assume his duties with understanding and ability, and he contributed substantially to the advancement of the medical character of the service. In August, 1844, the president of the Board of Governors, after an inspection of the asylum, reported that it was "much improved since placed under the charge of the present Physician."

Dr. Earle at once directed particular attention to the personal treatment of the patients by the attendants, and to the advancement of order and system in the administration of the service. One of his first official acts was to address a letter [6] to the male attendants, five in number, all of whom he had engaged since his appointment. Apparently it was still customary to use the term "keeper," because he wrote that he considered that the term "savours too strongly of the jail"; nor did he consider it appropriate that they should be called "nurses," as that term "is more applicable to women whose occupation is exclusively in the room of the sick." It was apparently considered that the attention required by the mentally ill was not exactly "nursing." He regarded the term "attendant" as most appropriate and wrote that it was his wish that "it may be intro-

[6] *Minutes of the Asylum Committee*, May 4, 1844.

duced." He enjoined them that to strike a patient would be a sufficient cause for dismissal and that neither shower bath, douche, nor water from the pipes which supplied the bath was to be used as punishment, "unless ordered by myself." He directed that "if a case occurs that seems to require it, I should like to be immediately informed before other measures are taken than such as are necessary for the security of those concerned." He advised them that if they never allowed themselves to be "looked out of countenance," there would be no danger of the patients thinking that they were afraid of them. He suggested that the patients appear "decent in their dress and condition," and that "to contribute to the good looks of the halls," they remove their hats when within doors, and so "keep their heads cool in hot weather."

He also proposed to the governors that rules and regulations for the attendants be adopted, similar to those at the Pennsylvania Hospital, the McLean Asylum, and the Massachusetts State Asylum. In June, 1844, he presented a comparison between the service of Bloomingdale and that of the asylum at Frankford. He drew particular attention to the employment at the latter of two special attendants who gave individual attention to excited patients, and to four whose time was exclusively devoted to "moral treatment." A month later, he was authorized to employ an additional attendant of each sex. In August, a *Guide for the Attendants* which he had prepared was adopted by the governors and 250 copies were ordered.[7] In the Preface he advised the attendants that "it is expected that no one will occupy the place of Attendant who does not make it his aim to secure to himself the highest possible respectability of character, and, by prudence and judicious economy, to attain a sufficient pecuniary provision for the advanced period of life." The rules were preceded by the following *Maxims for the Halls of the Bloomingdale Asylum:*

1. A place for everything, and everything in its place.
2. A time for the performance of each duty, and each duty to be performed at its appropriate time.
3. No place is clean if it can be made cleaner, and no place is in good order if it can be put in better order.

The *Guide* remained unchanged for fifty years. In 1894, however, when the asylum was moved to White Plains, it was revised by Dr. Lyon, medical superintendent, and reënacted by the governors. In his Preface to the revision Dr. Lyon commented that, "it is interesting to note how

[7] *Guide for the Attendants at the Bloomingdale Asylum for the Insane* (New York, 1844). Copy at the Westchester Division of the New York Hospital.

little the general principles of the ordinary and routine care and management of patients by their nurses has changed with the passage of years."

Dr. Earle proposed[8] that the wages of the attendants be increased from $13 a month to a sum at least equal to that paid by other institutions. He mentioned particularly the difficulty of securing the services of competent women, and suggested a gratuity of two dollars at the end of each month for satisfactory service. He explained to the governors that no institution should be without a night watch, but that if the attendants' wages were increased, they might, without detriment to their other duties, remain on duty at night, one for each night during the week. In November he reported that the plan was working satisfactorily. The watchman made a tour of every hall in the male department, in both the main building and the Lodge, through the attics and basements and around the outside of the main building and the women's Lodge, "at least four times between the hours of 10½ p.m. and 4½ a.m., at which latter time the apothecary is generally up." This arrangement was continued until July, 1848, when the position of night watchman was established. Dr. Earle reported, however, that the man appointed would also teach in the school for patients in the afternoons. The small number of attendants had always been an obstacle to getting the patients out of doors. In August, 1844, Dr. Earle assigned a man and a woman whose whole duty was to walk out with the patients, assist in their "moral treatment," and "relieve tedium." In May, 1846, he reported the appointment of a "walking attendant," at $16 a month, who accompanied the physician on his morning visit to the patients, kept a record of the prescriptions, did cupping, and carried the medicine to the men's department. In the winter he also taught in the school for patients. At that time the attendants' wages were about the average paid in all the principal asylums of the country.

Dr. Earle reported[9] that, while they endeavored to procure persons of intelligence, education, and "disciplined passions," he hoped that the time would come when attendants would be specially trained for their work, "as teachers are educated in the normal schools, or as nurses are taught in France." He made no concrete recommendation, however. He referred to a society which had been formed in London, in 1842, for "the advancement of the moral, intellectual and professional education of the immediate attendants on insane patients," and suggested that "the

[8] *Minutes of the Asylum Committee,* August 31, 1844.
[9] *Ibid.,* Feb. 23, 1846. (Physician's Annual Report for 1845.)

same subject presents an uncultured field to the philanthropists of the United States." He nevertheless reported that "the attendants now employed in the Asylum are industrious and faithful, discharging their important duties with much credit to themselves, and to the comfort and welfare of the persons entrusted to their care." In 1847, he reported that "nearly all the young men who have been so employed during the last few years, were from the country, and so well educated that they have been accustomed to teaching school in the winter." He drew attention to "the numerous advantages of attendants of this kind over those who are ignorant, and whose only ideas of exerting control over others, are measured by the strength of their arms," and added that "he who has once tried the former, would greatly deplore the exigency which should render it necessary to return to the latter." [10] How much more would we of the present day, when the training of nurses and attendants in the treatment of the mentally ill has become an established practice, deplore an exigency which might render it necessary to revert to the conditions which prevailed at the time in which Dr. Earle was writing!

In endeavoring to follow the principles and practices of "moral treatment" in the operation of Bloomingdale Asylum, much attention was given by the governors and the physician to limiting or dispensing with coercive measures, especially mechanical restraint. That this spirit prevailed throughout the service is indicated by Dr. Earle's statement in his first annual report, that he found the attendants "fully disposed to second our views in regard not only to the use of mechanical restraints, but in the general management of the patients." [11] The forms of restraining apparatus which he found in use when he assumed his duties at the asylum were leather straps, anklets, muffs, mittens, wrist bands, and an apparatus for confining patients in bed which was called "Dr. Wyman's bed strap" or a "saddle." This apparatus was the invention of Dr. Wyman, superintendent of McLean Asylum. It consisted of a sheet of leather, 30 by 18 inches, which was secured by straps to the rails at the head and foot of the bed. The patient was laid upon it, and straps attached to it were passed over his shoulders and across his chest. His feet were fastened to the straps at the foot of the bed by means of anklets and his hands were placed in a muff. The patient was then confined in a horizontal position but he could turn partly over from one side to the other. Another form of restraining apparatus was the "tranquillizing chair," "tranquiliser," or "composing chair," of which there were apparently two. It had "a high back with a method of securing the

[10] Physician's Annual Report for 1847. [11] Physician's Annual Report for 1844.

patient to the back. On the side each hand and forearm went into a box where it could be locked, and made a very secure arm rest. The feet also went into a box and they could be locked and fastened." [12] There were slight differences in the designs of these chairs. Very soon after entering upon his duties, Dr. Earle reported to the committee that he had removed from the floors of three of the buildings the spikes to which patients were sometimes attached by means of straps.[13] In his annual report for 1845, he stated that the tranquilizing chairs had been discarded for a year and eight months,[14] and that thirteen months had elapsed since the muffs, mittens, wrist bands, straps and all other forms of leather apparatus had been removed from the halls to the office of the physician and that not once during that period had any of them been carried into the men's department. Restraining apparatus made of canvas was, however, still used, especially in the women's department, in which it was resorted to more frequently than in the men's. During the thirteen months referred to, the only instances of restraint in the latter were the use of a camisole to protect a delirious patient from exposure to cold air, and to control another while a blister was "drawing."

In the annual report for 1846 the governors summed up the situation by stating that "chains are never used, and even the mildest forms of restraint are seldom resorted to." The use of mechanical restraint in the treatment of the mentally ill, was, at that time and for many years afterwards, a controversial subject among physicians of the institutions.[15] Even the most extreme forms, such as chains and manacles, the crib bed with a cover, and all leather straps, had defenders and even advocates. At the meeting of the Association of Medical Superintendents in 1852 it was recorded that Dr. Nichols was among those who defended the use of the crib and that "the opinion of those present seemed to be in its favor." Although Dr. Earle abolished the use of all forms of leather apparatus from the service at Bloomingdale, in his annual report for 1847 he refers to "the invaluable apparatus invented by Dr. Rufus Wyman . . . a means of insuring sleep, and of saving the life of the

12 This description and that of the "saddle" are from a letter from Dr. John B. Chapin which appeared in *Mental Hygiene*, X (1926), 143.

13 *Minutes of the Asylum Committee*, May 4, 1844.

14 In a discussion of mechanical restraints at a meeting of superintendents in June, 1870, Dr. Earle said in regard to tranquilizing chairs that "I threw these chairs out of Bloomingdale Hospital in 1844." He used the term "French restraining chair." *Am. J. Insanity*, XXVII (1870), 206.

15 Albert Deutsch, *The Mentally Ill in America* (New York, 1937), p. 213. See also issues of the *Am. J. of Insanity* and *Transactions* of the Am. Assn. of Supts. of Institutions for the Insane (now the Am. Psychiatric Assn.).

patient. It is a method of restraint with which every institution should be supplied." The physicians of this period were apparently either unable to anticipate what was later accomplished by means of intelligent trained nurses and attendants and of adequate treatment facilities, or they felt hopeless of obtaining them at that time. This excuse is, however, not valid for those states, municipalities, communities, and private organizations which, even today, are, by failure to provide adequate financial and social support, perpetuating coercive and repressive forms of treatment of the mentally ill which have long been discarded by more progressive institutions and communities.[16]

Dr. Earle's views on the practice of "moral treatment" of the mentally ill were briefly expressed in his annual report for 1844, and in later reports. He considered that "kindness is more powerful than 'stripes and a dungeon' in the management of the insane," and he endeavored to maintain this principle in the service at Bloomingdale. The particular methods of "moral treatment" were "religious worship, instruction, manual labor, recreation and amusements." Worship, he stated, "disposes to calmness, quietude and reflection, wins the mind from the visionary fancies of disease and renders the individual happier and more contented." Cases in which there was overabsorption in painful religious thoughts were, he found, exceptional. As a means of instruction, he considered the patients' library, with its many volumes of scientific, historical, and miscellaneous works, to be most useful. A number of newspapers, quarterlies, and other periodicals were subscribed for, and were freely used by the patients in the reading room. A supply of newspapers and books were also kept on tables in some of the patients' halls. "The benefit derived therefrom," he described as "astonishing to ourselves . . . there are but very few of the patients who have not made use of them." There had been little damage to the books; probably much less than would have been caused by as many children. He also instituted a series of instructive lectures which he considered to be

> a simple method of exerting disciplinary restraint, simultaneously, over a large number of patients; [as] a means of fixing the attention and withdrawing the minds of comparatively a multitude from the delusions incident to their disease, we believe there is no other plan, hitherto adopted in the system of moral treatment, which will prove more generally and extensively useful than that of judicious and well managed lectures.[17]

[16] Reports of surveys made by the National Committee for Mental Hygiene and the U.S. Public Health Service.

[17] Physician's Annual Report for 1847.

The lectures were given in the evening and were attended by about seventy patients. Ten or fifteen boys from the adjacent Leake and Watts Orphan Asylum also attended. The subjects were: Sketches of Greece and Malta (which he had visited); the Elements and the Analogies of Physical, Intellectual and Moral Beauty; National and Local Peculiarities; Physiology of the Eye and the Phenomena of Vision; Physiology of the Muscular System; Physiology of the Brain and Nerves; of the Heart and Bloodvessels; of the Organs of Breathing; of the Ear and of the Organs of Speech; Electricity; Descriptive Astronomy; Chemistry, Oxygen, Hydrogen, Nitrogen; Descriptions of Several European Cities; Characteristics of Americans and Europeans; Recitations of Poetry. Thirty-eight or more lectures were given during the winter, and they were illustrated by means of diagrams, pictures, and experimental demonstrations. Apparatus and equipment were purchased at various times, and, when Dr. Earle resigned, the governors purchased from him sixty muslin charts presenting three hundred illustrations. Equipment, listed in the annual report for 1847, consisted of an air pump, a set of "Mechanical Powers," a magic lantern, an orrery, an electrical machine with its implements, a pneumatic trough, receivers, retorts, and other articles used in chemistry, 146 diagrams on bleached muslin illustrative of the human and lower animal frames, 20 diagrams explanatory of the laws and phenomena of light, 25 astronomical diagrams, and 100 diagrams illustrating various subjects.

Dr. Earle also established a school for the instruction of patients. This early essay in adult education as a therapeutic measure was first undertaken in October, 1845, and was continued each winter while he remained at the asylum. It was located in the basement and was attended by twenty or thirty patients. The subjects taught were the ordinary English branches, with some chemistry and natural philosophy. The Weekly Committee, after a visit to the school in January, 1846, reported that the patients in attendance were "apparently happy and contented." The school was considered by Dr. Earle to be, like the lectures, a means of exercising moral control over a considerable number at the same time, and of subduing excitement, rousing the inactive, and giving a new content to the thoughts. A similar school was established at the State Asylum at Utica, and at some other institutions in the United States. One at least was still in operation at the close of the nineteenth century, and in the annual report for 1896 a school at Bloomingdale was again described.[18] On a visit to an asylum at Stephansfeld in Alsace in

[18] See p. 372.

1849, Dr. Earle found a similar school. It had been established in 1842, and was attended by almost 100 patients, one fourth of the total number in the asylum.[19] There were several others in European asylums.

Dr. Earle held that "of the means included under the head of Moral Treatment, manual labor—useful employment with the hands—justly claims pre-eminence over all the others." [20] Like his predecessors at Bloomingdale, however, he met with great difficulties in finding satisfactory employment for the men. The women did domestic work and sewing, and it was generally possible to keep most of them occupied. A few of the men also assisted with the housework, and a few others engaged in farm work, well described, perhaps, by a Weekly Committee report in April, 1847: "some of the patients were amusing themselves in giving their assistance in the work of the farm." Occasionally one or more worked in the mattress shop, the carpenter shop, or in other departments of the asylum. It was found, however, that "a large proportion of the inmates are from the classes unaccustomed to manual labor. These, with very rare exceptions, will never commence any employment of the kind, while at the Asylum." The plan pursued was "that patients are advised, and, if possible, induced to apply themselves to some useful occupation, but no compulsory measures are resorted to for the purpose of enforcing it." [21] Dr. Earle was of the opinion, however, that "there are some patients—a class of patients—who can be cured by labor, and apparently by nothing else," [22] and that it should be enforced if necessary. He confides in his *Memoirs* that "he did not allow a supposed public opinion (probably non-existent) to prevent him from administering labor as a remedy and a means of discipline." The editor of the *Memoirs* added that "whether this had aught to do with his short term of office at New York I have never heard, but it is conceivable." [23] In the Bloomingdale reports the only inducement to employment mentioned is a " 'lunch' or some other trivial privilege out of the ordinary course," which "often opened the way, in this manner, to a complete restoration of the person diseased." Dr. Earle felt that "could some light occupation, requiring but little mechanical ingenuity or skill, be carried on in all the wards of the men's department, the number of laborers on that side might be materially augmented." [24] The asylum

[19] *Memoirs of Pliny Earle, M.D.*, ed. F. B. Sanborn (Boston, 1898), pp. 179–180.

[20] Physician's Annual Report for 1844.

[21] Physician's Annual Report for 1847.

[22] *Memoirs*, p. 160.

[23] *Ibid.* (There is no evidence in the Bloomingdale records to support the editor's statement.)

[24] Physician's Annual Report for 1844 and for 1847.

records fail to show that he had any better success than his predecessors in introducing occupation as a means of treatment.

Nor did he add materially to the means of treatment by recreational measures, unless the lectures and the school are so considered. He used all available resources, however, with great energy, and quickened interest in measures which influenced favorably the adjustment of the patient to wholesome personal and social interests and activities. Walks about the surrounding country were engaged in daily, some of the patients unaccompanied and others accompanied by attendants. One attendant was employed especially for this and other recreational tasks. High Bridge, Harlem, and the receiving reservoirs are mentioned as places visited. The number of drives was increased and reference is made to the beauty of the surrounding country and the numerous roads along "the Harlaem river passing through cultivated vallies and between abrupt and precipitous hills," [25] to Hell Gate with its rocks and whirlpools, and the broad reaches of the Sound studded with islands and projecting points. Bowling, quoits, bagatelle, chess, chequers, cards, "Doctor Busby," and other games were engaged in. A "rocking boat," with rockers and a seat at each end, and an "elastic board having its ends laid on two benches" served as "gentle exercise and amusement for the females." Dogs, a peacock, and a goat were provided as pets. A building, or "enclosed shed," was erected in the principal airing court of the men's department to house the bowling alley and a shuffleboard. On one evening in every week a social party was held in the "family parlor"; it was attended by the officers of the asylum and fifteen or twenty patients, and refreshments were served. At the balls given once a month and attended by about sixty patients; "There was cheerfulness without extreme hilarity; gaiety without boisterousness, and a pervading disposition to participate in the enjoyment—to please and to be pleased." [26] Dr. Earle was, in fact, of the opinion that "a large majority" of persons affected with mental disorders "enjoy life as much as the average of people in the community." Some of Dr. Earle's personal visitors attended the dancing parties; in a letter to his biographer, one of his nieces wrote, "I remember one of the dancing evenings at Bloomingdale, at which Margaret Fuller, William Henry Channing, Marcus Spring and I were present." [27] Two of these names, at least, are surely noteworthy.

The dietary of the asylum was apparently subjected to few changes during Dr. Earle's term of service and seemed to be considered satisfac-

[25] Physician's Annual Report for 1844.
[26] Physician's Annual Report for 1844.
[27] *Memoirs*, p. 314.

tory. In May, 1846, he reported that it was good and that complaints were rare. It was, he stated, of the usual variety of meat, vegetables, pastry, fruit, generally found upon family tables. The Weekly Committee also reported in October, 1852, that they had visited the dining rooms at meal time and that the patients seemed to be "quite satisfied with the fare." Special dietaries were apparently seldom provided. The principle and practice pursued were that

no patient is placed upon "diet" excepting those laboring under acute mania. The insane, as a class, require more food than other people. The organs of nutrition appear to be in a morbid state, somewhat analagous to that of the nervous system which renders necessary a greater quantity of medicine to produce a given result than in other persons, and which also enables them to sustain unaffected, remarkable degrees of heat and cold.[28]

This apparent adherence to a belief in the insusceptibility of the mentally ill to extremes of temperature, which in practice had resulted in much neglect and suffering, seems rather remarkable.

Dr. Earle is characterized by his biographer as of an "arithmetical turn of mind." He not only continued the statistical studies instituted by Dr. Wilson; he extended and analyzed them. The tables presented with his annual reports were accompanied with explanatory notes and comments. He followed the custom of separating the statistics of "recent" cases from those of the "old" or chronic cases. He questioned, however, the value of the classification, because of the difficulty of determining accurately when the illness began. He noted that, while the recovery rate of "recent" cases might be 70 percent or higher, there was, nevertheless, a recovery rate of 20 percent of the "old" cases. He observed also that many of the cases discharged "recovered" were soon readmitted, in some instances several times, and he began to doubt the validity of all current statistics on curability. In fact, this was the period of the "cult of curability," to which Deutsch in *The Mentally Ill in America* devotes a whole chapter.[29] The wide acceptance of the principles and practice of "moral treatment," and the rapid development of medical institutions for the mentally ill, were attended with astonishing optimism regarding the curability of the patients. Many of the physicians, some of whom had, previous to their appointments, had little experience with mental illness, seemed to compete with one another in reporting recovery rates, until, in one instance, a rate of 100 percent was reported. Dr. Earle shared in the prevailing optimism, but his inquiring turn of mind led him to examine carefully the records of readmission, and

[28] Physician's Annual Report for 1844.

[29] *Op. cit.*, Chapter VIII.

eventually the whole question of curability. In a separate book he recorded those who had been admitted and discharged more than once, with their diagnosis and condition when discharged. He noted that one woman had been discharged 22 times, and a man 14 times. A man who, from December 5, 1829, to March 2, 1833, had been admitted 12 times, had been discharged "cured" 7 times and "relieved" 5 times. He found that 2,150 persons admitted to the asylum during the first twenty-three years of its operation were registered as 2,937 cases. Of these, 322 were inebriates who had been admitted 594 times and had contributed over 500 "recoveries" to the statistics. These he did not consider to be cases of insanity and he eliminated them from the statistics. Of the remaining 1,841 persons, registered as 2,308 cases, he noted that 726 had been discharged "recovered" and 18 others were reported to have recovered after their discharge. Relapse had occurred, however, in more than 105 of the cases, some of whom died while mentally ill. The permanent recoveries, therefore, amounted to less than 34 percent.[30] Dr. Earle's interest in the subject continued for many years. He wrote many articles relating to it, and much discussion resulted. Years after he retired from Bloomingdale he assembled his articles in a volume entitled *The Curability of Insanity,* which was published in 1887.[31] The "cult of curability" lasted for only a few years and, according to Deutsch, to Dr. Earle "must be given the credit for dealing the fallacy its death-blow."

It was during the period of Dr. Earle's service at Bloomingdale Asylum that two events occurred of particular significance and importance to the progress of psychiatry in America. In both of these he had an active part. In 1844 the Association of Medical Superintendents of American Institutions for the Insane was founded by thirteen medical superintendents of whom Dr. Earle was one. This Association has grown in numbers and usefulness, so that now (1944) it is an organization of over 3,000 members; its name has been changed to The American Psychiatric Association. In the same year, Dr. Amariah Brigham, the first superintendent of the State Lunatic Asylum at Utica, New York, established the *American Journal of Insanity,* the first of its kind in America and one of the earliest in the world. This periodical is now the *American Journal of Psychiatry* and is the organ of the Association. Dr. Earle was the first colleague to whom Dr. Brigham confided his intention. He wrote: "I shall look to you and hope to interest you in the work . . . and shall want your opinion, advice and assistance." Dr. Earle was an

30 *Memoirs of Pliny Earle,* pp. 157–158.
31 Pliny Earle, *The Curability of Insanity: a Series of Studies* (Philadelphia, 1887).

early and frequent contributor to the pages of the *Journal*. In 1847, Dr. Brigham, whose health was failing, wrote to him that the subscriptions to the *Journal* covered the cost of publication, and he asked him to take it over as owner and editor. Dr. Earle was, however, unable to consent.[82]

He was professionally active in the community as well as in the asylum and was frequently called to give testimony in court. He was highly regarded by his medical colleagues and when the New York Academy of Medicine was founded in 1847, he presented the first paper that was read before it, "History of Insane Hospitals in the United States."[83] In this paper he gave to Dr. Eli Todd, first superintendent of the Hartford Retreat, the credit of having "practically introduced into this country and made extensively known here, the moral and medical treatment recommended by Pinel, Tuke, and Willis." Dr. Todd's annual reports, and an extremely laudatory account of the Retreat published by Captain Basil Hall, an Englishman who visited the institution in 1827,[84] were doubtless means by which the treatment mentioned was "made extensively known here." Consideration should also be given, however, to Thomas Eddy's communication on "moral treatment" to the Board of Governors of the New York Hospital in 1815, and to the establishment, before the Hartford Retreat, of the Friends Asylum at Frankford, and of the Bloomingdale Asylum, for the avowed purpose of introducing a system of "moral treatment," especially that followed at the Retreat in York, England, which was founded by William Tuke.[85] In 1847 Earle was appointed on the visiting staff of the New York City Lunatic Asylum. After one visit, however, it was felt that it was inexpedient to spare the time from his regular duties.

Dr. Earle's career throughout was one of distinction and permanent value. Although the service at Bloomingdale was not extended under his direction, he made improvements in the facilities and contributed substantially to the character of the service. He was one of the most eminent psychiatrists of his time. He resigned in April, 1849, in order to pursue further his studies and observations of the treatment of the mentally ill in Europe. A reference to him as "Superintendent and Physician" in the Governors' Minutes, instead of "Physician of the Asylum" or "Head of the Medical Department," which were the usual designa-

[82] *Memoirs*, p. 295.
[83] New York Academy of Medicine, *Proceedings*, I (1847).
[84] Deutsch, *op. cit.*, p. 135.
[85] See Chapter X. See also Annual Reports of the Governors to the Legislature, 1821 and after; Deutsch, *op. cit.*, pp. 99–102.

tions, may perhaps indicate his influence on the general administration of the asylum. The position of Medical Superintendent was not officially established until 1877.

After leaving Bloomingdale Dr. Earle in 1852 opened an office for consulting practice in New York. He was again appointed on the visiting staff of the city asylum, and lectured at the College of Physicians and Surgeons. He published several articles and a treatise on "Blood-letting in Mental Disorders." He left New York in 1854 and spent some time in Washington, preparing an introductory chapter for the "Census Statistics of the Insane" for 1860. He traveled much. During the Civil War he assisted in the service of the Government Asylum for the Insane. In 1863 he was appointed Professor of Psychologic Medicine in the Berkshire Medical Institute. He continued to be frequently employed as a medical expert in court. In 1864 he was appointed medical superintendent of the Northampton, Massachusetts, State Asylum, where he gained further distinction in the treatment of patients and as a student and author. He died in 1892.

In selecting a successor to Dr. Earle, the governors turned to the physicians of the New York Hospital for counsel and assistance. A large majority of them met with the committee, great interest was manifested and a special meeting was held to enable them to deliberate and make inquiries. All were agreed that, other qualifications being equal, a married man should be selected. Inquiries were addressed to the state asylums at Worcester and Utica and to Dr. Kirkbride of the Pennsylvania Hospital. The applicants considered were Dr. S. P. White, Dr. T. W. Powers, Dr. W. T. Buel, and Dr. C. H. Nichols. Dr. Buel and Dr. Nichols received the same number of votes, and it was thought that it would be necessary to submit both names to the governors. Additional testimonials relating to Dr. Nichols were, however, received and he was nominated to the board and elected. He was at that time twenty-nine years of age, and had for the previous two years been an assistant of Dr. Brigham, superintendent of the State Asylum at Utica, by whom he was highly recommended.[26]

Just as Dr. Earle was said to be of an "arithmetical turn of mind," it may perhaps be equally correct to say that Dr. Nichols was of a me-

[26] *Minutes of the Asylum Committee,* March 8–13, 1849. Apparently Dr. Nichols was under consideration as Dr. Earle's successor in 1847 as in December of that year Dr. Brigham wrote to Dr. Earle that he considered that Dr. Nichols had not sufficient experience. Dr. Brigham had in April written to Dr. Earle a letter of inquiry relating to Dr. Charles H. Nichols of Lynn, Mass., who had given Dr. Earle as a reference. Letters at the Westchester Division.

chanical or architectural turn of mind. Soon after entering upon his duties, he proposed improvements in the sanitary conditions and with approval of the governors he planned, supervised, and, with the aid of "common mechanics," greatly increased the number of baths, basins, and toilet fixtures in the main building.[37] By proceeding in this way the work was done in a "better and more durable manner than . . . under the usual contract system," and a saving of $200 was accomplished.

Dr. Nichols's reports to the governors of the defects and needs in the provision made for the classification and care of the patients, and the plans, explanations, and demonstrations of improvements he furnished were, probably, his greatest contributions to the service during the short period in which, at that time, he was physician of the asylum. His recommendation for new accommodations for "noisy" patients will be discussed in Chapter XX. He defined a policy by which the service could be adjusted to the social and therapeutic needs of selected patients along lines that were afterwards followed. His main effort was directed to improving facilities without which adequate personal treatment could scarcely be accomplished. He tried to impress upon the governors, and, by his published reports, upon the public, an understanding that "the elaborate and expensive arrangements called for in the curative treatment of the insane, are not needless luxuries, but needful means to one of the most desirable ends." His work was remembered, and 25 years later he was reëmployed, as medical superintendent.[38]

Dr. Nichols apparently accomplished little towards advancing the personal treatment of individual patients. In some particulars there may have been some regression. During the summer he discontinued the meagre night service instituted by his predecessor. He also considered it necessary to resort to the use of straps and other forms of leather restraint discarded by Dr. Earle. No reference has, however, been found to any further use of the tranquilizing chair or the Wyman bed strap. Apparently he discontinued the school and the lectures which Dr. Earle had considered especially valuable as a means of group treatment. He suggested that, instead of providing employment for the patients in merely industrial pursuits, better results would be obtained "if they could be subjected to continuous and systematic bodily and mental training, by persons fully competent for such a duty," [39] thus anticipating the present system of occupational and recreational therapy. Apparently,

[37] *Minutes of the Inspecting Committee*, Jan. 2, 1850.

[38] See p. 302.

[39] Physician's Annual Report for 1850.

however, no progress was made in the use of these measures during his administration.

He was well aware of the importance of an adequate nursing service, believing that, "if the number of attendants is deficient, among other and not less serious evils it becomes necessary to resort to straps and mittens." In February, 1851, at the request of the governors, he presented a report relating to the attendants. He pointed out what is painfully apparent to any student of the records of that period, namely, that there is "no means of ascertaining the precise number of attendants in former years." He concluded from what he could learn that two had been added to the male department during the previous seven years. These were a watchman and a dining-room attendant added by Dr. Earle. The present number in the male department was nine, including the watchman and the coachman. One, who also acted as librarian and choir master, was paid $18 a month. Two were paid $16, one $15, three $14, one $13, and one, the dining-room attendant, $10. In the female department there were eleven attendants. Six were hall attendants, and five were seamstresses who also assisted in the care of the patients. Five of these attendants were paid $10 a month, four $8, and two $6. Some of the patients paid for dresses made for them by the seamstresses. "Our most genteel ladies are now having their dresses made here, and several of our gentlemen their shirts etc. which saves annoyance and mischief, and is most satisfactory to themselves and their friends."

Like his predecessors, Dr. Nichols advised the governors that the proportion of attendants was less than in the McLean Asylum and Pennsylvania Hospital. He added that twenty more patients could be given equally good care without adding to the number of attendants, because "a certain system requires to be kept up, and it does not make much difference in the labor required to maintain it, whether it be applicable to a few more or less patients." He advised them that "the Institution is recommending itself to the higher classes upon whom it is obvious that it must hereafter materially depend for support," and he pointed out that it would be "of incalculable advantage to have an extra attendant of each sex to be devoted to particular cases." He had, he said, "when the exigency of a male patient seemed to require it," detailed the watchman for the purpose, and kept "such night watch as I have deemed necessary, myself." He added, "I have done in this respect what very few individuals would do, not because I could boast of more devotion to my afflicted friends, than others possess, but because I am blessed with a physical constitution that has hitherto almost unfalteringly born[e] every effort to which it has been subjected."[40]

Dr. Nichols presented his resignation to the governors on January 31, 1852, and left the service on May 29 to take the position of superintendent of the new asylum for the mentally ill which the United States Government was establishing in Washington, D.C. On that day the Asylum Committee recorded in their minutes that they "have much pleasure in bearing their testimony to his invariably exemplary deportment, and to the faithful and intelligent manner in which he has discharged the duties devolving upon him." In their annual report the governors referred to his resignation of "the situation, which he had filled since May 1849, with great skill and fidelity." The vacancy was filled temporarily by Dr. James R. Merritt, who had "had the advantage of some months service at the Institution for the Insane at Flushing and the Committee considered themselves fortunate in securing his services."[41] It was arranged that Dr. A. V. Williams, a private practitioner in the neighborhood and formerly physician of the asylum, should make a visit every day in consultation.

[40] *Minutes of the Asylum Committee,* Feb. 1, 1851.
[41] *Ibid.,* May 29, 1852.

XX

DOROTHEA L. DIX SURVEYS BLOOMINGDALE IN 1851

Dr. Nichols's communication of June, 1851,[1] with that of Miss Dix which was presented a few weeks later, is a remarkably realistic portrayal of conditions in what was one of the best of the asylums of the period, and enables one to appreciate, in contrast with the Bloomingdale of today and, in essential respects, with all of the modern hospitals for the mentally ill, the great progress that has been made. Dr. Nichols referred particularly to the building known as the "women's Lodge," in which noisy and violent patients were housed on one floor, and on another, irrespective of their mental condition, patients who paid three dollars a week or less. He reported that "perhaps the most crying defect in the architecture of the present building is the entire absence of any arrangements whereby the noise of excited and vociferous patients can be shut off from those who are quiet." The noise of the disturbed patients could, he said, be heard throughout the whole institution, and during the warm season, no one could sleep for an average of as many as five nights out of seven.

Patients and their friends generally have an unconquerable prejudice against the "lodge." . . . As I now write a patient leaves us, who has prevailed upon her husband to remove her, chiefly on account of the suffering she has experienced from loss of sleep and from hearing almost constantly by day and by night blasphemous, vulgar and invective declamation.

Of the basement bathroom, the only one in the Lodge, he wrote:

It is wholly improper to take such patients into a cold room and strip and wash them there—that room being often at the temperature of freezing, and sometimes lower. I have often been under the absolute necessity of administering stimulants to patients either before or after a bath on account of the coldness of the bathroom and the distance to reach it.

The lack of water circulation and toilet facilities throughout the Lodge was such that "nearly half of our female patients enjoy only its most ordinary comforts and benefits—such as are enjoyed in all the shanties which line the ungraded avenues and dot over the commons in our neighborhood." In the absence of circulating water,

every ounce of the great quantity of water that is or should be used on the Halls in keeping them clean and in the ordinary washing of the patients'

[1] Physicians Reports, Bloomingdale Asylum, 1849–1852. (Special Report, June 28, 1851.)

faces and hands, and in cleansing them from their hourly accidents of nature, is carried by hand up one or two flights of stairs and used in little half effectual slops at any point about the Halls where a stove with a basin upon it can be set down in temporary safety. During at least three days of every week all the hot water used is brought by hand in pails all the way from the main centre building.

There was no water closet in the building: "The privy, which is placed at a little distance in the rear, is reached by a covered walk or passage with lattice sides." It was "objectionable in affording patients frequent opportunities to get out of the view of their attendants." It was necessary for an attendant to accompany a much demented patient on each occasion. In winter the feeble were obliged to use chambers in their rooms, tending "to render the air foul and unpleasant." He also described the effects of the defective heating and ventilating provision in the Lodge, in consequence of which,

during our coldest months many of our patients suffer exceedingly, particularly at night, and, in order to make them as comfortable as possible, we are obliged to tie the worst in their habits and feeblest into bed at night, and tie their clothes upon them—a species of restraint which is calculated to induce filthy bodily habits and to confirm those already existing.

The draft of the furnace was so poor that every morning and evening "when the fire is replenished" it was necessary "to throw open the windows . . . and let the patients shiver through a couple of hours" until the air was free of coal gas.

He deplored the lack of night supervision by the attendants of the patients in the "associated dormitory."

Such a thing as an associated dormitory in the Hall occupied by the worst class of patients is, under the best arrangements, wholly wrong. . . . Into it from four to six of the worst class of patients are locked at night and the attendant is out of sight and hearing (accustomed as she is to sleep, unless the noise be very near or very extraordinary) and whatever accidents occur among them, no one is wiser for it till morning.

The chief, and ordinarily the only, night service provided was what could be given by an attendant who slept in a room adjoining the rooms occupied by patients. The remedy proposed was that "the attendant's room should be adjacent to the associated dormitory and separated from it only by a lattice door, through which all disturbances could be readily heard and seen."

With this report Dr. Nichols presented a plan and explanation of a proposed addition to the women's Lodge. Two months later, in August,

1851, he substituted, at the request of some of the governors, a more complete plan for additions to the main building, in which provision was made for eight distinct classes of patients of each sex. He recommended that the lodges should be demolished. In his monthly report for November he gave an account of some effects of the inadequate heating provision on individual patients; two had been confined to bed at night by bed straps on account of their feeble condition and the low temperature of their rooms. He added, "We could have used bed-straps in other cases to great advantage, and should probably have done so, had we happened to have more of these instruments on hand." It should be borne in mind that at that time no provision was made for heating the bedrooms, and Dr. Nichols stated that though he considered it an "axiomatic truth that feeble and excited insane patients cannot be made even safely comfortable unless their sleeping as well as day rooms can if necessary be maintained at a temperature of from 60° to 70°," he fully concurred in "the generally received opinion that all well persons and perhaps the majority of the inmates of an asylum for the insane, should sleep by night in *un*heated apartments."

Among the immediate results of this report were the supplying of circulating hot and cold water to the bathroom in the women's Lodge and the installation of a small stove. A water closet was not "deemed essential by the Doctor, till the determination of the Board as to future improvements shall be made known." A convenient water closet was, however, installed in the men's Lodge. It was also recorded that "a new smoke flue has been made to the Furnace, which has so improved the draft, that the House is relieved from gas, and much more heat obtained than heretofore." Grates were supplied in the "Gentlemen's Dining Rooms" in the basement of the main building.[2] The governors found "no very serious ground of complaint, except for the want of additional accommodations for the excited patients, and there can be no doubt that such are imperatively called for at the earliest day practicable."[3] Later an appeal for funds was made to the public, and various improvements were made.

In the fall of 1851 the asylum was visited and inspected by Dorothea L. Dix, that remarkable woman who devoted a great part of her life to learning by personal observation the manner in which the mentally ill were provided for and treated, and to obtaining the interest and support of public officials, legislators, and private citizens in establishing

[2] See p. 205.
[3] *Minutes of the Asylum Committee*, Dec. 5 and 20, 1851.

suitable institutions for them. Her success was phenomenal. She was instrumental in the establishment of more than thirty institutions in the United States, Canada, and Great Britain. Accounts of her interesting and useful life have appeared in many publications,[4] and it seems unnecessary to do more than invite attention to it as an informing and inspiring revelation of the nobility and power of human endeavor at its best. At the time of her visit to Bloomingdale she had been occupied in her undertaking for ten years. The records offer no evidence as to whether her visit to Bloomingdale was at her own initiative or by invitation, the length of her stay, and whether or not she resided at the asylum at the time. She had already visited it in 1849, and now made a thorough investigation. At a meeting of the governors on November 4, 1851, a communication from her was referred to the Asylum Committee "with a request that they would thoroughly examine the statement of the wants and defects of the Asylum and the suggestions of improvements made in said communication, and report fully to this Board." A few years ago a "General and Concise Summary" [5] in Miss Dix's handwriting, and signed by her, was found tied with blue ribbon among some old papers at the Westchester Division. It was framed and now hangs in the office of the medical director. Whether a fuller report of her inspection was presented to the governors, or only the summary, is not stated. The report relating to it which was presented to the governors by the asylum committee on December 2, refers only to the latter, though subjects that do not appear in the summary are mentioned.

Miss Dix evidently directed her attention particularly to the discovery of defects, and it is not surprising that the committee felt "constrained to say that in their judgment the defects of the Institution are materially magnified and its many merits overlooked." She noted the architectural defects, the crowding in some of the "lodging rooms," the lack of suitable accommodations for "the highest class of patients," and the contiguity of "strong rooms" to the common dormitories. The insufficient toilet and bath facilities, and the inadequate heating and ventilation which have been described, were soundly condemned. The food service was attended with "confusion and discomfort" and with exposure to severe and inclement weather in reaching the Lodges. The lack of a dumb waiter, and the consequent carrying of heavy trays up several flights of stairs from the basement kitchens, occasioned unsuitable congregation

4 Francis Tiffany, *Life of Dorothea Lynde Dix* (Boston, 1891). Albert Deutsch, *The Mentally Ill in America* (New York, 1937), pp. 158-185.

5 For text of this and Dr. Nichols' report see Appendix, pp. 512, 516.

of nurses and attendants, and often of patients, in the passages, and left excited patients unguarded and the more quiet unprotected in the absence of the nurses and attendants. Attention was directed to the fire hazard of some of the heating and lighting arrangements. As for the Lodges, besides insufficient warmth and ventilation, they had "no bathing rooms, wash sinks, and other requisite accommodations for invalids and excited patients." In the basement of the women's Lodge, the laundry was an offensive nuisance and unhealthful; the noise of the steam engine disturbed the quiet patients, and stimulated to violence the excited. The patients were also in danger of the boiler exploding.

Miss Dix was particularly concerned with the inadequate supervision. There was no supervisor and no night watch in either Lodge, and the inspection and supervision by the officers of the asylum were entirely insufficient and infrequent. Among "absolute wants" she mentioned competent supervisors in every department, and the appointment of an assistant physician. She considered also that enlargement of the asylum was needed for the comfort and advantage of the patients and for the admission of a larger number. She saw little hope of remedying the defects under the form of organization which she compared to three commanders[6] leading an army, three captains commanding a ship, and three magistrates ruling a city. She commented on the number of physicians employed since the asylum was established, with an average duration of professional connection of about three years, and asserted that none had entered upon his duties at Bloomingdale Asylum approving its organization, none had retired from his charge without great dissatisfaction, without having made efforts for improving its condition, and without a conviction of the impossibility of carrying out the greatest good under the existing organization. "No physician, respecting his own reputation, strictly conscientious; respecting the rights and claims of his patients, and his obligation to their friends, and to the community at large, will ever long hold the office under the present system,"[7] which, she said, had the "disapprobation of medical men—well informed and experienced in the treatment of the Insane." Her closing comments were as follows:

6 The asylum committee, the warden, the physician.

7 Soon after Miss Dix's visit, Dr. Nichols resigned and was appointed medical superintendent of the U.S. Government Asylum for the Insane in Washington, D.C., the establishment of which was brought about largely by Miss Dix's efforts. At the meeting of the Association of Medical Superintendents in 1888 he stated that it was on Miss Dix's recommendation that he received the appointment, and added, "I consider myself greatly indebted to her for the opportunity of a wider career and perhaps greater usefulness than was otherwise likely to come to me." *Am. J. Insanity*, XLVI (1888), 147.

. . . Finally the Institution should accomplish good it does not accomplish; should take a rank it does not now hold; should reflect honor, not ask reproach on its Officers and Governors, tho all have done too much that is well, not to advance to that which is greatly better. The Institution they direct should do honor to their City, to their State, to their Country:—it now does neither.

Excuse me Gentlemen, if I seem severe; I am only truthful.

A passing glimpse of some of the personality traits of this gentle, valiant, and high-minded woman is afforded by this communication. She belonged to the period of "The Flowering of New England," and had spent several years in the home of William Ellery Channing, as tutor of his children.

The Asylum Committee to which Miss Dix's communication was referred held at her request a special meeting "to examine and discuss the various topics of her memorial." The whole committee attended. The vice president of the board introduced Miss Dix and was requested to remain for the meeting. A full and deliberate examination of the first part of the memorial was made. At a second meeting and interview, two days later, the reading and commenting upon the memorial were concluded, and two members of the committee were appointed to prepare a report to the board. This report was presented on December 2, 1851. Architectural defects that would not be present if the buildings had just been erected were admitted, though the committee considered that in its general arrangements the main building was convenient and comfortable. They believed that the occasions were very few, if any, in which a sufficiency of heat was not obtained both for health and comfort in this building; that "the dormitories can not well be otherwise than comfortable, provided a sufficiency of bed-clothing is furnished, and a proper care observed in closing windows"; and "the water arrangements are certainly both as regards bathing tubs and water closets very complete." Dumb waiters might be convenient, but were not essential, "nor does the want of them effect the convenience or comfort of the patients.' Undesirable commingling of male and female attendants in procuring food, and of patients on stairways, was preventable by proper supervision. In regard to the Lodges the committee found that "candor will lead them to name many defects." Relating to the criticisms of the men's Lodge and its inmates, "should enquiry be made of the Physician and other officers and attendants, facts would be revealed showing censurable circumstances too numerous to detail and too unpleasant or offensive to record"; furthermore, "the Board will judge as to the propriety of such strong language in relation to it." As to the lack of night attention, the committee commented that

Dr. Earle soon after he took charge of the Asylum employed a watch in the male department whose duty it was to pass through the men's hall and Lodge once in each hour of the night. Dr. Nichols has dispensed with a watch during the summer, but employed one in the winter; a man is now in the house engaged for that duty.

In regard to improvement in the classification of the patients, attention was directed to the consideration that had long been given to the question by the governors, especially during the previous few months. The several members of the board who in former years had served on the asylum committee and were familiar with its management were believed as capable of forming a sound judgment on this head as those now on duty, but "the committee, however, will say, *they are not in favor of enlarged power in the hands of the Physician.*" [8] They believed Miss Dix's statement that no physician had ever entered upon his duties at the asylum approving its organization, to be a mistake, and added that

the rules of government now existing were drawn up by the late Dr. Macdonald after his visit to European Asylums and it is believed was in entire accordance with his judgment as to what was wise.[9] Dr. Earle when commencing his duties at Bloomingdale expressed his satisfaction in being relieved from responsibility of duties to be performed by the Warden.

The secretary of the board was directed to send a copy of the committee's report to Miss Dix and to inform her of the action of the board thereon, and that the subject was under their consideration. The vice president also presented the following for consideration at the next meeting:

It being acknowledged by all, that the arrangements for bathing heating and ventilation in the Lodges, is defective:—and that no proper classification of the patients can be made, without an enlargement of the establishment:

[8] No italics in original.

[9] It seems appropriate to quote from a letter of Dr. James Macdonald written to the trustees of the New York State Asylum in January, 1841, in which, at their request, he proposed a plan of organization. In this he stated: "As the supreme object of the institution, to which every thing in its construction and government directly or indirectly tends, is the improvement and recovery of the insane; I propose that the *physician in chief*, who may also have the title of Director, shall be its first officer, the *head*, in name and in fact of the whole establishment, so that all other officers, under the board of trustees, shall be subordinate. The physician and director should be the main spring of the whole machine, the master spirit of the entire institution . . . He should have power to hire or dismiss all subordinate persons in the employ of the institution: and all superior officers should be so far under his control as to receive instruction from him."

and it being also the opinion of persons best informed on the subject of the Insane; that very great additional accommodations are absolutely necessary, because all the Asylums are now full to overflowing—therefore

Resolved that it is expedient and necessary, to enlarge the Bloomingdale Asylum by the addition of wings to the Main building, *or* to the Lodges; as soon as means for the purpose can be obtained.

Resolved that to accomplish this purpose, a Committee of Governors be appointed to make an appeal to our liberal minded fellow citizens to contribute of their abundance the sum of $100,000, which it is estimated the largest and most desirable improvement will cost; and failing in *this* appeal, the smaller sum of $20,000 required to enlarge and improve the Lodges—will undoubtedly be furnished.

Resolved that the Asylum Committee be requested to make such temporary improvements in the Lodges, in respect to heating, Ventilation and Bathing, as may be done at a moderate expense, until the proposed enlargement and improvements can be completed—said committee is also further requested to devise and prepare the best plans for said enlargement and improvements and submit them to the Board at some future meeting.

And on motion Resolved that the Asylum Committee be requested to make such temporary improvements to the Lodges in respect to heating, ventilation, bathing and water closets as they may deem expedient.[10]

The resolution relating to an appeal for $100,000 was withdrawn in January, 1852, but at the same meeting the Asylum Committee was instructed to carry out the views of the governors expressed in these resolutions. Dr. Nichols's plans and estimates for additional buildings were submitted by the committee, but, as already related, no further action was taken at that time. In November, however, an appeal to the public for $150,000 for the general hospital and $100,000 for the asylum was issued. In this appeal attention was invited to "the necessity for enlarged accommodations etc." [11]

10 *Minutes of the Governors,* Dec. 2, 1851. See Appendix, p. 519, for full text of committee's report.

11 *Address of the Governors of the New York Hospital to their Fellow Citizens, Nov. 2, 1852* (New York, 1852).

PART FIVE

Planning for Classification and Removal State Supervision and Laws 1852-1877

XXI: BUILDING FOR CLASSIFICATION

THE governors of the New York Hospital had long been impressed with the place and importance of classification of the patients. Classification was one of the objects in establishing their first "medical asylum" in 1808,[1] and it seems to have been rather successfully accomplished. In 1818 when the new asylum at Bloomingdale was planned, provision was made for "noisy patients" in a separate building remote from the others. Unfortunately, lack of funds prevented the construction of this building. At first, disturbing patients were lodged in the basement. This was unsatisfactory, however, and it was partially remedied by the erection of the "Lodges" described in a previous chapter.[2] In 1851 Dr. Nichols proposed that additions be made to the Lodges and presented plans to the governors, which were approved. An appeal for funds was made to the public; $150,000 for the hospital in the city, and $100,000 for the asylum. The amount subscribed was $136,852, and the soliciting committee reported that the "high price of money discourages any further efforts at the present time." Part of this amount was used in the erection of the new South Building at the general hospital, which was opened in 1855.

In April, 1853, Dr. D. Tilden Brown, who had succeeded Dr. Nichols as physician of the asylum in June, 1852, presented revised plans which were adopted and the additions to the Lodges were completed in 1854. In his annual report for the year Dr. Brown reported that these additions were occupied and all anticipations of usefulness realized. The new buildings were described as spacious, of two stories, about 100 feet long, and specially constructed with reference to classification. The governors

had for some time felt, that whilst the increase of patients demanded more room, such addition should not be restricted to a mere extension of the buildings, with more chambers and apartments; but should also be so constructed as to give the means of more perfect classification, and of shutting out en-

[1] See p. 49. See also *Minutes of the Governors* and the Annual Report for 1805.
[2] See pp. 138–142.

tirely from convalescents and patients of calm and orderly habits, the annoyances of other classes. . . . It was also desired to provide for more liberty and room for exercise and occupation for the noisy and excitable. . . . The halls or galleries of the additions are remarkably cheerful, having, on one side only, a range of rooms for patients, which are, in many respects, the most desirable in the house.[3]

The new additions accommodated 150 patients, and cost about $52,000. In his report for the next year Dr. Brown described "accommodations for the present number of patients as ample as could be desired . . . and will probably postpone indefinitely the removal of the asylum from these premises." This is the first intimation found in the records that removal of the asylum from Bloomingdale had been contemplated. Rather plaintively, it was added that the consideration hitherto accorded the institution could no longer be expected, as "ours is no longer a monument of local and laudable pride, for our community has outgrown its distinctive elemental character."[4]

A further improvement in the women's Lodge was brought about by the removal of the noisy engine and laundry of which Miss Dix had complained, and the basement was then assigned to the farm laborers as a dormitory. The new laundry was a separate three-story building, 75 feet long and 40 wide, the third story being occupied by domestics as a dormitory.[5] Notwithstanding the evident satisfaction occasioned by the improvements, further causes of complaint soon occurred. The heating arrangements proved inadequate, and additional furnaces were required in both buildings. A fire in the state asylum at Utica directed attention to fire protection, and Thomas B. Stillman, one of the governors, personally superintended the installation of new pipes and of a hand pump in the garret.

The distance between the Lodges and the main building prevented the early transfer of patients and exposed them and their food to inclement weather. To overcome this Dr. Brown, in January, 1857, proposed the erection of still another building to connect the women's Lodge with the main building and to accommodate the physically sick, the suicidal, and patients who could afford to pay for extensive apartments. An architect was engaged, and in August the plans were ready. Evidently, however, no action was taken by the board, and in February, 1858, Dr. Brown again brought the project to their attention: "The separation of the buildings and the consequent distribution of the patients

[3] *Minutes of the Governors,* Feb. 6, 1855.
[4] Physician's Annual Report for 1855, *Asylum Committee Minutes,* Feb. 2, 1856.
[5] *An Account of the New-York Hospital* (reprinted with by-laws, 1856), p. 12.

into two principal classes, without those intermediate grades which the superior architectural arrangements of other institutions permit, is regarded by every Asylum Physician as a serious defect in our institution." Even if the expediency of the project appeared doubtful, "on account of the apprehended necessity of abandoning the location within a comparatively few years," it was nevertheless advisable to retain the present site as long as possible and to make improvements that would aid in maintaining the reputation of the institution. Dr. Brown believed that the expense would be compensated for by an increased income. He estimated that as the populated city was approaching the asylum at the rate of only three streets per annum, it would be twenty years before the institution would be seriously affected. Central Park was within easy walking distance for the exercising of patients, and was "as safe and attractive a resort as any country road." He felt that consideration of the asylum as only a tenant at its present location,

> liable any year to be expelled by the caprice of political power, has rested like an incubus upon the best interests of this asylum, retarding its progress in improvements, and thereby impairing its usefulness and in effect tarnishing its early fame. . . . It is no longer named with those of modern construction as a model establishment ingeniously adapted in all its parts to the most efficient fulfillment of its designs, and comprising all the adjuncts which the benevolent zeal and ingenuity of recent times has introduced into its sister institutions.

The Asylum Committee were "unanimously of opinion that the improvements recommended are of great importance." They asked the board for an appropriation of $15,000, but, as a studied estimate increased the cost to $27,110, the request was withdrawn.[6]

The project continued to occupy the interest and occasional attention of the Asylum Committee, but it was not until March, 1860, that they again addressed the board with a more urgent form of request:

> On motion it was unanimously resolved—that the present crowded condition of this Institution and other similar Institutions in the United States and the increasing demand for Asylum treatment for the insane, justify and demand additional accommodation for the insane at the Bloomingdale Asylum; and that impressed with the constantly increasing necessity of enlargement, the Asylum Committee will present to the Board of Governors at their monthly meeting in May next, plans and estimates for the construction and cost of an additional building on the Asylum grounds.

These were presented at the June meeting; the plans were adopted and $30,000 was appropriated. The committee suggested that the funds be

[6] *Minutes of the Asylum Committee,* May 29, 1858.

obtained by means of a mortgage on the "Bloomingdale fields" between 11th Avenue and Bloomingdale Road, and 116th to 120th Streets. The governors voted, however, that the cost would be paid by the treasurer, and a few months later a mortgage was placed on the property of the Society in the fifth ward of the city.[7] The building with its "superior class of apartments" was completed by the end of 1862. It was described in the annual report as a three-story structure, 110 feet long and 42 feet wide. A central corridor 10 feet wide extended from end to end of each of the principal floors. This was broken in the center by an alcove 12 feet wide, and was lighted at each end by a window extending from floor to ceiling. On one side of the corridor there were a dining room, a bathroom and rooms for sick patients, with communicating rooms for attendants. On the opposite side there were eight single rooms of "unusual size," 12 by 14 feet. Accommodations were provided for forty patients. The third floor, finished in 1867, with an appropriation of $3,000, contained a large lecture room, and a "diversion room" for entertainments. In 1864 Dr. Brown reported that the building was "in every respect well adapted to its purpose." The governors reported that the completely connected wing permitted the division of the female patients into thirteen classes in independent suites of apartments, "thus providing unusual facilities for a primary necessity in the treatment of insanity." It was evidently considered that the long-standing problem of classification had been solved for the women's department. The provision of corresponding accommodations for the men was discussed, but was deferred while the asylum remained at its present site, as "the time for this disappearance can be already foreseen." Dr. Brown suggested, however, that consideration be given to providing for women only in the present accommodations and making provision for men in another location on the grounds or elsewhere.

Besides the major improvements described, others of less magnitude were made. In 1854 the attic of the main building was finished so as to provide a chapel and sleeping rooms for employees "who now sleep, to the great injury of health, in the basements." The windows at the front and ends of the main building were lowered and bays were constructed. Much of the cost of this improvement was borne by John David Wolfe, one of the governors. In 1856 the first urinals were installed. Lighting by gas was provided in 1858. This was declared by Dr. Brown to be the principal improvement of the year, "promotive of cheerfulness and of evening occupation, and therefore of mental health." In 1858 also "a

[7] *Minutes of the Governors,* Jan. 2, 1861.

little building [was] constructed on the grounds as a smoking room." This, said Dr. Brown, "suggests to Asylum Orthodoxy a most heretical usage." He explained, however, that smoking was restricted to those already addicted, that the indulgence was well regulated, and was the "only unalloyed pleasure" of the habitual smoker in the asylum.[8] In 1865 a "handsome organ" was presented by Otis D. Swan, one of the governors, to "assist the religious services." It was replaced with a new organ in 1876. In 1872 the billiard room was extended at a cost of $3,725, and the men's dining rooms in the basement were abandoned. Yale cylinder locks were installed in the main building and in the Lodges in 1873. In the same year a fence was erected on the north and east boundaries of the property, and many minor improvements were made within the buildings. In 1875 a conservatory of brick, wood, and glass, containing a plant house, aviary, and aquarium, was erected at a cost of about $7,350. The notes of the committee contain references to the pleasing effects of flowers in the patients' halls and rooms, and the physician reported that the conservatory was a resort for the patients, who enjoyed the flowers, the aviary, and the aquarium. In the same year, noting that the older portion of the women's Lodge was in bad condition, the vice president and the Inspecting Committee recommended that it be rebuilt. No action was taken, however, at that time. The Croton water supply was improved, also in 1875, by a connection with the high service reservoir, and pumping was dispensed with.

It seems probable that the prospect of early removal of Bloomingdale Asylum to a different location was, as Dr. Brown believed, prejudicial to progress and even to adequate maintenance. However, the steady approach of the populated streets, the frequent assessments, as well as the encroachment on the property when streets were opened or improved, the withdrawal of state support, and the constant menace of repeal of tax exemption warned the governors that removal would, sooner or later, be inevitable. The first intimation that it was becoming a consideration in the development of the institution appeared, as has been noted, in the annual report for 1855. The removal did not take place until nearly forty years later. It seems probable that the prospect would have had little immediate effect, had it not been that the removal of the hospital on Broadway from its original location was also receiving serious consideration. The majority of the physicians and surgeons of the hospital were in favor of moving uptown; Dr. John Watson in 1858 wrote to the governors that he recommended the re-

[8] Physician's Annual Report, *Minutes of the Asylum Committee*, Jan. 29, 1859.

moval of Bloomingdale Asylum to a new location "not far remote from the city," as the sale of its present site "would be sufficient for the support of more than one city hospital, equal in capacity to the present institution." The governors were, however, averse to moving the general hospital, or to obtaining funds in the manner proposed. For several years they made strong appeals to the legislature to enable them to retain it in the business part of the city, near the docks and railways. Their appeals were in vain. Nor were they more successful in obtaining private subscriptions; they were told that ample funds could be raised for the hospital by leasing or selling the present property and moving to a less expensive location. In April, 1866, therefore, it was

> Resolved, that financial relief from existing indebtedness and future pecuniary need, as well as greatly extended usefulness in the charitable operations of this Corporation can be permanently secured by the sale or lease of the present site of the Hospital buildings and by the erection of suitable buildings for the accommodation of the sick and injured on a portion of the grounds belonging to this corporation at Bloomingdale.

It was considered that the adoption of this plan would necessitate a change in the medical organization of the hospital and the employment of paid resident medical and surgical directors or superintendents, assisted by a staff who would receive no pecuniary compensation. It was also proposed that a "receiving house" be provided in the city, and an ambulance service established. Although this plan was not acceptable to the physicians and surgeons of the hospital, the governors proceeded with preparations to carry it into effect. In December, 1866, it was

> Resolved, that it be referred to the Asylum Committee to take into consideration the expediency of selecting a suitable location for the Asylum beyond the city limits and to report to the Board.

In July, 1867, a special committee reported that "the best course open to the governors would be to appropriate the present buildings of the Bloomingdale Asylum to the purposes of a hospital proper, after preparing a new building for the insane on such site 'beyond the city limits' as may be selected." This committee recommended, in the organization of the proposed new hospital, "the appointment of a permanent Resident Physician and Surgeon in a single person," with "a salary proportionate to the responsibility devolving upon him." The successful operation of Bloomingdale with full-time, salaried resident physicians was cited. The medical and surgical staff of the hospital were requested "to inspect the Bloomingdale Asylum buildings and grounds with a view to report whether the same can be economically adapted to Hospital uses." In November the staff made a unanimous report that "the present buildings at Bloomingdale could be made suitable, without very great expense, for the treatment of medical and surgical patients to the number of 150." They added, however, that "Bloomingdale would be too remote from the centre of the commercial and manufacturing activity of the city, and from the dwellings of the poor." Some of the governors suggested that a hospital be built on the "pavilion plan" proposed by Dr. John Jones for the first hospital in 1773, and that six such pavilions "be erected without delay on the southerly portion of the Bloomingdale Asylum Grounds." [9]

In the meantime the committee which was searching for a new site for the asylum was not inactive. In his annual report for 1866 Dr. Brown reviewed the situation at Bloomingdale and called the appointment of the committee "most timely and judicious." He recommended that they seek a location 1) where the institution might remain undisturbed for at least another fifty years; 2) where not less than fifty acres could be appropriated for exercising grounds for each sex, with a liberal allowance for gardening, farming, long walks, and a drive; 3) within a short distance of a village or other settlement having a railroad station, the nearer the better provided the grounds were sufficiently spacious to insure the requisite privacy; 4) with an unfailing supply of good water. He added that "no place can be considered too beautiful or too valuable for the temporary refuge or permanent home of insane persons."

As early as February, 1858, Dr. Brown had emphasized the importance of accessibility, "within carriage reach," for patients, visiting relatives, and governors. In regard to the last mentioned, he said that "the history of many such benevolent institutions proves that whenever the cordial and active personal interest of its managers begins to waver, progress is arrested . . . retrogression commences simultaneously with the arrest of progress." He recalled that the governors who established Bloomingdale Asylum, although they knew few precedents, felt that they should not "limit their plans simply to an effort for the mitigation of the old-time discomforts." They recognized the importance of making the institution attractive. They went so far as to consider that the building should "resemble a palace rather than a gaol," and they proposed using marble for its exterior. Although this was found to be too expen-

[9] *Minutes of the Governors,* Nov. 27, 1868.

sive, the building erected was of "noble design and admirable workmanship," resembling in many of its features the City Hall which had been built a few years previously. He recommended that the new asylum should be planned with reference to the needs of two classes of mentally ill persons who were "inadequately provided for in existing establishments." Patients who were wealthy were "either kept at home, or placed in small private Asylums." He considered that the system of private asylums was founded on a "wrong basis," and had "led to great evils in other countries, and must almost inevitably do so here." He recommended, therefore, that adequate provision be made for patients of this class. A greater need was presented by the "respectable indigent insane," those "of cultivated minds and refined habits of life." He mentioned especially the families of clergymen and other professional persons, teachers, businessmen who had experienced reverses, and dependent unmarried women. These cases, he said, were "too often compelled to forego all the benefits of hospital treatment, rather than accept that offered by the City." He reminded them that some of the governors had themselves supplied the means to support persons of this character in the asylum. He contrasted the liberal provision made for the sick poor in "the generous and admirable" hospital accommodations in New York with the inadequate assistance extended to the indigent mentally ill. He felt that "if this Institution possessed a fund for the assistance of such persons, it would find many a worthy object for relief, and would accomplish a measure of good not excelled by any general hospital for the sick." Evidently the policy and plan of service which had its inception when the admission of publicly supported patients was discontinued was now becoming established.

The committee reported in December, 1867, in regard to three sites. Saxton's Woods, not far from White Plains, had been offered on liberal terms, one of the owners being willing to donate his half interest in the property. The committee considered, however, that the site (now a Westchester County park) was "too secluded" and that the cost of clearing the land would be too great. The Hunter's Island site contained 167 acres, and was connected with the mainland by a causeway 475 feet long, but it was remote from a railroad station, the buildings were very expensive, and the price asked was $250,000. The best prospect, the committee reported, was the farm of Samuel Faile at White Plains. It presented the following advantages: 1) a healthy location; 2) proximity to a railroad station at which all expresses stopped, the time to 26th

Street being an hour and five minutes; 3) the village of White Plains was in a central position in the county; 4) the site was near the village but well elevated; 5) it was centrally located in a system of walks and drives; 6) it contained 300 acres, which would permit the construction of ample walks and roads on the premises "for the use of patients who cannot properly be allowed to appear upon the public roads"; 7) the supply of water from springs and brooks was in excess of all needs; 8) the grounds could be made attractive. The price of $450 per acre could be wholly met by the sale of three and a half acres of the Bloomingdale property between 11th Avenue and Bloomingdale Road.

At the January, 1868, meeting of the board, the committee reported further that the actual acreage of the property was 292.57, which at $450 per acre would cost $131,656.50. A mortgage of $100,000 at 7 percent for from two to five years would be acceptable, and Thomas H. Faile, a member of the committee, had offered to advance the cash needed, on a second mortgage. They had learned that the proceeds from the sale of half of the Bloomingdale land west of 11th Avenue would exceed the price of the farm, and the value of this land would be greatly increased by the projected public drive. The vote on the purchase of the property was twenty in favor, and three against. A year later a special committee was appointed "to devise and prosecute the ways and means for constructing suitable buildings at White Plains for the reception and treatment of insane patients." It was designated "Executive Committee on White Plains Asylum Buildings." In October, 1869, the governors again passed a resolution acknowledging that the present site of Bloomingdale Asylum was the most eligible for a new general hospital and directing the committee on the White Plains property to proceed with the erection of buildings. Five of the governors voted against the resolution.

It was not, however, until April, 1871, that ground plans for a building, which had been prepared from the original plan of Dr. Brown, were submitted and approved by the board. The proposed building was of irregular form with diagonal wings to secure the best exposure to sun and air and to diminish opportunities for annoyances among the patients. Separate buildings were recommended for men and women, but this was considered impractical for the number of patients to be at first accommodated, which was 150.[10] Unfortunately, no plans have

10 Communication from Dr. Brown to the Executive Committee on White Plains Asylum Building, Dec. 8, 1870.

been preserved. In the course of a discussion at the meeting of the Association of Superintendents in June of that year, however, Dr. Brown stated that

in anticipation of the erection of new buildings for Bloomingdale Asylum on a new site, it became my duty to consider whether it seemed best to modify the usual system and to separate the buildings into groups, or to erect smaller buildings apart from the main building. After abundant and disagreeable experience of nearly twenty years I had no intention of repeating that system unless there should seem to be reason adequate to overcome my own impressions. Therefore I had several conversations with Dr. Kirkbride about the matter and concluded not to have separate buildings. . . . At Bloomingdale Asylum there are separate buildings and there is a prejudice against them in the minds of the patients as well as among the friends of the patients. They all feel that there is a disparagement somewhere.[11] They desire to be near or within the main building, for they think the nearer the centre the better the accommodations and the better the service. I proposed to have small buildings . . . but . . . we determined to have those buildings connected with the main structure rather than separate. . . . On general principles I would be unwilling to place any near friend of mine in any cottage or other building beyond the immediate supervision of the principal officers of the institution. I could not feel easy or justified in entrusting such friends to the care of such attendants as I should find even in the buildings least removed from the main structure.[12]

Competitive plans were obtained from three architects, and that of Richard M. Hunt was accepted. The cost of the building was limited by the governors to $600,000.[13] Another year passed without the beginning of construction. In March, 1872, George Cabot Ward, one of the governors, without preliminary explanation introduced the following resolution:

Resolved, That it is the sense of the Board that the property situated on Broadway and its revenues, should be applied, primarily, to Hospital purposes, and the property at Bloomingdale and its revenues, to the purposes of the Asylum.

This, however, was laid on the table. Its adoption might have expedited the development of the psychiatric work of the New York Hospital in later years. At the April meeting of the governors, the White Plains committee was again directed to proceed with building operations, the appropriation was increased to $1,200,000 and the committee was

[11] There *was* an actual disparagement owing to classification in accordance with rates as well as with the condition and behavior of the patient.

[12] *Am. J. Insanity*, XXVIII (1871), 329–330.

[13] *Minutes of the Governors*, June 6, 1871.

authorized to contract a mortgage of $1,000,000. By October considerable progress had apparently been made in the preparation of plans, as Thomas H. Faile resigned from the committee in protest against the expensive and ornate building that was proposed and the employment of three architects to prepare plans at a cost of $6,000.

Not all the governors were satisfied with the site, and in February, 1870, a special committee was appointed "to inquire and report whether a more eligible site for the proposed Lunatic Asylum cannot be found." It was evidently felt that the more picturesque Hudson River region with its beautiful views would be a more desirable location. This committee reported in April that the residents objected to selling land for the establishment of a lunatic asylum. They recommended, however, that consideration be given to the property of Cyrus Field, on Broadway, between Dobbs Ferry and Irvington. It contained 140 acres of a beauty superior to that of the White Plains property, and had a fine view of the river. There was a plateau which was suitable for building sites, an extensive quarry, and a landing on the river. Good springs on the property and the rights to another spring, elevated above the building sites, would furnish an ample water supply. There were five houses on the property and the price asked was $250,000. At the next monthly meeting the committee asked that consideration be given to the Church property at Scarborough. This seems to have been the only serious attempt, at that time, to abandon the White Plains property as a site for the new asylum, and the governors, after receiving the report, discharged the committee from further consideration of the subject.

The property at White Plains was of some expense to the Society. It was a farm, but could hardly be operated advantageously as such by the governors. For some reason not given in the minutes, some additional land was purchased, four acres on "the new Mamaroneck Avenue to be opened," [14] and eight acres from Mr. Platt for $5,000.[15] For the opening of Mamaroneck Avenue the property was assessed $2,485.[16] A topographical survey and map were authorized. Buildings were renovated and a shed for stock and tools was erected. A man and his wife were appointed to live on the property. In August, 1871, right of way through the property was requested by the New York, Housatonic and Northern Railroad.

The physicians and surgeons of the New York Hospital were irreconcilably opposed to the plans of the governors for removal of the

[14] *Ibid.*, June 7, 1870. [15] *Ibid.*, Nov. 1, 1870.
[16] *Minutes of the Asylum Committee*, Dec. 4, 1869; *Minutes of the Governors*, Dec. 7, 1869.

hospital to Bloomingdale. In January, 1869, a "remonstrance" prepared by them was published in the *New York Times,* much to the annoyance of the governors, who ordered the Visiting Committee to ascertain who was responsible for the protest. The physicians were also opposed to the proposal for a pavilion or cottage hospital, or for a number of small hospitals in different parts of the city instead of one large hospital. In regard to the latter a special committee, in February, 1874, reported to the governors that they had held several conferences with a committee representing the board of physicians and surgeons and had found that

in their opinion a General Hospital should be established with a capacity of at least two hundred and fifty beds with sufficient land for the enlargement of its accommodations as necessity should require; and the principal reason assigned for this policy was that by this means the Society would perpetuate the well earned reputation of the New York Hospital as a School of Medical and Surgical Science.

The committee considered, however, that as there were seven other general hospitals in the city,

the importance of affording Medical and Surgical instruction through the agency of this Society, as a primary consideration, does not seem to be apparent. . . . The first consideration of the Board should be, by what application of the funds under their control, this Society can be most helpful to the sick and disabled poor of this city. If in the discharge of this primary obligation medical and surgical instruction can thereby be imparted under favorable conditions and the cause of science advanced, the past history of this Society affords abundant evidence that the active co-operation of the Board of Governors will not be wanting to provide every proper facility for professional culture.

They added that they were "compelled in reaching a decision to look at this subject from a different point of view" than that of the physicians, "and our dissent from their conclusions is not due to any lack of respect for their arguments. Our obligations as Trustees require us to regard as of primary importance the necessities of those for whom the Institution was organized and to subordinate all other considerations to this." The governors had previously found it necessary to recall the primary purpose of the hospital to the physicians particularly interested in utilizing it for teaching and scientific study. In the annual report for 1851 they had expressed their views as follows:

The Governors of the New York Hospital have repeatedly expressed their desire, which they still entertain of rendering the Institutions under their charge auxiliary to the improvement of medical science, and the courses of public and private medical instruction given in this city. But they have always felt, that the care and comfort of the numerous patients under their charge formed their primary duty, as these were the main objects of the original establishment of this hospital, and they have been led, by the experience of some of the great foreign hospitals, to the conviction that these primary objects of duty and humanity may be hazarded, and sometimes sacrificed, by any system which makes the curative treatment and care of the patient merely subservient or secondary to the purposes of medical instruction or science.

In March, 1870, a second "remonstrance" against closing the hospital and transferring it to Bloomingdale was presented by the physicians. The original charter of the hospital was therein stated as granted for

"relieving the diseases of the indigent and preserving the lives of many useful members of the community." It is true that the care of insane patients was subsequently added to its work, but it was in order that the work of the General Hospital might be carried on more effectually that the Legislature was petitioned for means to erect an asylum at Bloomingdale. . . . If it were necessary to close either of the Institutions under your charge, which we cannot believe, it must be admitted that the Asylum for the Insane could be suspended with less injury to the public welfare. All its inmates could be at once well provided for in other institutions, and no serious inconveniences could result either to the patients or their friends, while to close the doors of the General Hospital would involve the transfer of the majority of the patients to pauper establishments, break up an administrative force that has been disciplined by years of service, and worse than all, deprive the victims of disease and accident of the care and treatment to which by the terms of your charter they are justly entitled.

Apparently these physicians did not consider, as the governors always had, that "relieving the diseases" for which the charter of the hospital was granted included treatment of the mentally ill. One wonders also, whether at that time the city asylum on Blackwell's Island, to which, if Bloomingdale were closed, it would be necessary to transfer most of its indigent patients, was considered to be better than the "pauper establishments" mentioned. A perusal of Chapter X of this volume, or of the governors' annual reports of the period, will reveal more accurately than this statement of the physicians the considerations and motives which led to the establishment of Bloomingdale Asylum, which do not seem to have been primarily that "the work of the General Hospital might be carried on more effectually."

A week after the "remonstrance" was presented, at a meeting of the governors and physicians one of the governors suggested that provision be made in the new general hospital for a certain number of incurables.

One of the physicians disapproved however, on the grounds that "the Charter of the Hospital made no allusion to an Asylum for the Insane or a Home for Incurables." No further discussions of these controversial issues appear in the records. The proposal to establish the general hospital in the asylum buildings at Bloomingdale or in pavilions on the asylum grounds, and the proposal to replace it with several smaller hospitals in different parts of New York City were both discarded. A new hospital of 163 beds was built on the Thorne property on West 16th Street, and was opened in 1877. The asylum remained at its Bloomingdale site until 1894, when it was transferred to its present location on the Faile farm, which had been held by the Society for the purpose since 1868.

XXII

CHARGES AND INVESTIGATIONS

FOR many years the laws of New York contained little or no provisions governing the confinement and treatment of the mentally ill.[1] Not even physicians' certificates were required until 1842.[2] It is noteworthy that, during the long period in which patients were received and treated without formal court commitment, no injustice to the patients and no embarrassment in the operation of the institutions seem to have been experienced. It was not until March, 1844, that the first appeal to the courts for the release of a patient from Bloomingdale Asylum occurred. The patient had been discharged from the state prison and admitted to the asylum by order of the Recorder of the City of New York. He was brought on a writ of habeas corpus before the mayor, who ruled that the Recorder did not have jurisdiction and ordered that the patient be returned to the prison.[3] Thereafter, writs of habeas corpus were occasionally issued for patients in the asylum. No publicity had resulted, however, and the question was easily disposed of.

This happy state of affairs did not last, however. On September 13, 1869, the New York *Tribune* published an article entitled "Alleged False Imprisonment in Bloomingdale Asylum," which was followed a few days later by an account of a patient for whom a writ of habeas corpus had been issued. In an editorial entitled "Suspected of Sickness," it was asserted that a man "charged with insanity may be committed by a magistrate on very slight testimony, and without warning or opportunity to present his own story, may be hurried to an asylum before he can communicate with his friends, and once there may be imprisoned for ever," unless he could reach a lawyer. It was added that "it makes no difference who the physicians are, how little they know about insanity, or how much they have seen of their patient," and that the directors of the asylum probably "assume him to be crazy merely because he has been brought there, and wait for time to justify or refute their assumption." [4] This was apparently the start of an undertaking by the *Tribune* to bring about changes in the provision governing the treatment of the mentally ill, some of which were unquestionably needed. Unfortunately, very reprehensible means were resorted to and, as so frequently occurs, in endeavoring to correct one evil new ones were created in the form of

1 Laws of 1788, 1809. See p. 73 of this volume.

2 See p. 222.

3 *Minutes of the Asylum Committee*, March 2, 1844.

4 New York *Tribune*, Sept. 18, 1869. Note "charged with insanity," a form which still prevails in some parts of this enlightened land.

extreme legal measures which proved unnecessarily prejudicial to medical management, as well as to the peace of mind of the mentally ill and their relatives.

Three years later, in August, 1872, the *Tribune* renewed its undertaking by a violent attack on the management of the asylum. Under the heading "Strange Developments Promised—Sane Persons Released by Habeas Corpus from Bloomingdale Asylum—Painful System of Cruelty to Inmates," an account was given of a "once prominent banker" who was alleged to have been confined for sixteen months "though to all appearances, and according to the admission of the keepers, he is unquestionably sane." The lawyer in the case was the one mentioned in the *Tribune* story in 1869. He informed the newspaper that it was the practice at the asylum for the superintendent, in order to avoid public inquiry, to discharge a patient as soon as it was known that proceedings were to be taken in court, and to make a return of "not in custody." In the present instance word was sent that the "prisoner" was sufficiently recovered and had been released. This was not denied by Dr. Brown, who explained that, knowing the condition and needs of his patients, his object was to screen them from general curiosity and remarks.

A second article in the *Tribune* was entitled "A Tale of Horror." The character of the article may be gathered from some of the captions: "An Infernal Institution," "Was This Man Murdered?" "Dirt and Filth Abundant," "Devilish Treatment of the Insane," "Another Person Alleged To Have Been Killed." [5] It was related that at the instigation of the "once prominent banker," who declared that they were sane, the lawyer had obtained writs for two ladies. One was a nun "forcibly taken from a convent in this city and confined as a lunatic." The "female who attended her . . . swears of her own knowledge that the patient is perfectly sane . . . that she was committed for complaining that a priest in attendance at the convent had made insulting proposals to her." It may be said here that this patient, who had been at the asylum for over a year, was considered incurable and was transferred to the New York City Asylum.

The *Tribune* article contained an affidavit by a former attendant at the asylum, charging the physicians with neglect of their duties and the attendants with ignorance and brutality—the women with "lewdness of the worst description." The affidavit also condemned the lack of facilities for classification and for adequate heating, he described the kitchen as "in the dirtiest condition" and the food as not only of the cheapest and

[5] New York *Tribune*, Aug. 6, 1872.

commonest but also improperly cooked, and charged that the death of a patient caused by mistaken medication was not reported to the coroner. It characterized the treatment of some of the patients by the attendants as "devilish," consisting of kicking, choking until blood came from the patient's nose, leaving patients unchanged in filthy beds for twenty-four hours, and forcing the dirtiest part of the attendants' duties upon the patients. An accompanying affidavit by the former attendant's wife supported these statements. She complained particularly of the ill treatment of patients by the attendant in charge of the hall on which she had been employed, resulting, in one instance, in death.

The *Tribune* carried its crusade still further. In order "first to test the medical and scientific knowledge of insanity by regular physicians in ordinary practice and of experts at the asylum; second to test the nature of the law of commitment and the manner of its administration; third to make personal examination of the condition of the institution and the method of treating patients," [6] a reporter was delegated to feign insanity. He registered at a hotel and, after giving orders "of more or less absurdity," maintaining a sullen silence when addressed or shaking his head in helpless fashion, and walking up and down with his hands clasped about his temples, he was seen by a physician who was called in by a friend. The reporter pretended to recognize the physician and when questioned answered in "unsatisfactory whispers or dubious shakings of the head." The physician suspected the influence of a drug and suggested that the man's relatives be summoned. Then, considering it unsafe to leave him at the hotel he took him to his own house, where he was under constant attention. Meanwhile the friend and "an uncle" consulted Dr. Arthur Lockrow, and then brought the reporter to his office. Dr. Lockrow admitted that he did not understand the case, although he suspected "a species of brainal disorder." He recommended Bloomingdale Asylum, "the best retreat in this city for curable patients notwithstanding the reckless charges to the contrary made in the newspapers." The reporter was lodged at a hotel for the night, in charge of a "professional [male] nurse," who claimed to have been for ten years employed at the New York Hospital and to have had experience with insane patients. The reporter made assaults on the nurse, engaged in rambling conversation, aroused other guests of the hotel, and so frightened the nurse that he asked for help. The physician then engaged a medical student to watch the reporter closely through the night. He also "made every effort to do justice to the case," by visiting the patient

[6] *Ibid.*, Aug. 29, 1872.

frequently and by learning from the nurse the character of his symptoms and conduct. In the morning Dr. C. E. Billington was engaged to assist in the formal examination for certification. The two physicians then proceeded to the Jefferson Market Police Court, signed the certificate after the "uncle" had applied for the commitment of his "nephew," and the judge issued the order. The procedure thus far hardly seemed to confirm the assertions of the *Tribune*. There was delay in obtaining a "permit" from a member of the Asylum Committee, and finally the reporter was taken to the asylum at five o'clock without one. He was accepted conditionally for the night, and the permit and the advance payment required were delivered next day. No examination was, it was asserted, made by the admitting physician, except of the pulse. "No information was solicited in regard to the features of the case and no inquiries were made concerning the temperament, constitution, or personal habits of the man or the probable cause of his derangement." The expense, including payment for thirteen weeks in advance, was about $350.

The reporter was admitted on August 14 and discharged on the 26th. The account of his experience was published in the *Tribune* of August 31 and September 3. The character of his story is indicated by the headlines of the first instalment:

> Among the Maniacs. Four Days in the Excited Wards of Bloomingdale. A Night of Horror Among Raving Patients. Sleep Disturbed by Agonized Cries of the Dangerous Idiots. Close Cells, Uncomfortable Beds and Chairs. Scanty and Foul Food. Filthy Baths and Rude and Vulgar Attendants. No Amusements, Games or Reading Matter. Imbecile Boys exposed Naked to the Sun and Venerable Blind Man Beaten by Enraged Keepers. Instances of Brutal Treatment Witnessed by the Tribune Reporter.

The story revealed that the reporter saw what he came to see; he ignored the earnest efforts to manage difficult and delicate conditions and situations with kindly consideration and skill. After four days he was transferred to the main building, in which his room was "in great contrast" to the Lodge room. His attendant "always treated the patient civilly." The meals were "vastly more enjoyable," the library contained many valuable books, and an "extensive collection of foreign and a few American Reviews." A newspaper was furnished daily except Sunday on each hall, and several patients received papers of their own. He had access to a comfortable sitting room, with pictures and a beautiful view. The billiard room was a "source of real enjoyment." Patients were, he said, allowed to write when they pleased, but he was evidently critical of the physician's caution in regard to sending letters out and admitting visitors other than relatives. The reporter charged that some of the patients he met were not insane. As he was no longer feigning mental illness, he considered that when he was evidently sane, the rigid questions to which the physician subjected his friend should have been asked in a previous interview. He considered the medical examination "farcical," and mentioned, significantly, the cautious remarks of the physician in regard to the possibility of relapse, the reluctance to permit him to walk out in the grounds, and other natural and wise precautions in the treatment of a patient whose case after ten days' observation was still puzzling. As it was planned to test the procedure of habeas corpus, especially whether it was the custom at the asylum to evade return to the writ by discharging the patient as soon as it was learned that one had been applied for, a writ was obtained on August 24 and served on the same day. Dr. Brown advised the reporter's friend that a return to the writ would be made and the patient produced in court, but the man appeared to be perfectly sane and could be discharged without the publicity of appearing in court if the writ were withdrawn. This advice, with some show of reluctance on the part of the reporter, was followed and he was discharged, many innuendoes as to the physician's motive being contained in the narrative.[7]

Some of the other newspapers were not disposed to accept too seriously the *Tribune's* charges. The New York *Times,* commenting editorially on the *Tribune's* story of August 6,[8] remarked that "from this highly sensational story it seems that the chief amusement of the attendants . . . consists in pounding the male lunatics and choking the female lunatics. It is also averred that the physicians in charge either neglect the patients for months at a time or else serve out medicines indiscriminately and so kill off the weaker ones." The editor warned his readers that, though the charges should be investigated, it must not be forgotten that "in every lunatic asylum in existence the unfortunate patients say that they are unlawfully detained and in many instances that they are brutally treated. Very frequently the patient who is discharged as nearly cured retains the hallucination that he has been subjected to hideous cruelties." A *Times* reporter also visited the asylum,

[7] This reporter afterwards published an account of his alleged observations and experiences in book form—Julius Chambers, *A Mad World and Its Inhabitants* (London and New York, 1877). Much in the book fails to correspond with his *Tribune* story of 1872. The transfer to satisfactory service soon after admission was omitted. The book contains a congratulatory note from Charles Reade, the novelist.

[8] P. 270.

where he obtained particulars of the "once prominent banker" who had been discharged after a writ of habeas corpus had been issued. He was also shown over the institution. He reported that he found it to be "in admirable condition," everything clean and comfortable. The provisions he saw were first class, but he considered "the refectories and the lower range of rooms altogether too low and dark," the "*tout ensemble* . . . gloomy and dispiriting." Some of the other papers, however, praised the *Tribune* for its "journalistic enterprise" and references appeared relating to attempts to establish legislation for trial by jury before confinement in an asylum for the insane.

On the day that the first *Tribune* article appeared, the governors of the New York Hospital appointed a special committee of nine members to investigate the charges. The committee report of September 3, 1872, denied the charges, stating that they had known the physicians for many years and during that time had been in almost daily intercourse with them, finding them never absent except for health or in the interests of the asylum. The committee believed that there were "no three men of their profession more conscientious or faithful in the performance of their duties or more entitled to the confidence of the friends of the patients." The patient who had made the original charges, they reported, had once before been in the asylum, and when temporarily improved had been discharged. In the present instance he had again improved and his friends had been notified that a trial at home would be advisable, and he had been given freedom of the grounds. After careful inquiry, the committee reported themselves satisfied that the charges of violence to patients were without foundation beyond hallucinations of certain patients. They were unable, after the fullest investigation, to discover any occurrence to substantiate the charges of social irregularities. The former attendant, whose affidavit appeared in the *Tribune* story, had been discharged for intemperance. As to cleanliness, the committee believed that no one acquainted with the asylum need be told that the charge relating to it was without foundation. They described in some detail the close supervision by the governors, which, by weekly and other visits, gave them constant opportunities for observing the patients and conversing with them. It was impossible that evidences of injury or violence or of alienation between the patients and attendants would pass unnoticed. A number of the employees had been in the service many years; and the committee thought that no institution had a more faithful and deserving staff.[9]

[9] *Minutes of the Governors*, Sept. 3, 1872.

The character of the charges, however, the publicity given them, and the general attitude of the public in regard to confinement in the asylums for the mentally ill and the treatment received there, led the Governor of the state to appoint a commission to investigate the charges, and any others that might be laid before them, and to visit and inspect all the asylums for the mentally ill in the state. In his letter of appointment on August 20, 1872, the Governor advised the commission that

> charges of abuse in the Bloomingdale Lunatic Asylum have lately been made in the public prints, by parties who give their names, and avow their ability to prove their allegations. . . . Our laws permit the confinement of alleged lunatics as well in these private institutions as in the public asylums of the State. . . . This condition of the law giving opportunity for abuses, I have, more than once, asked the Legislature to correct. At the last session, two bills passed the Assembly, furnishing better safeguards in connection with the commitment and care of lunatics; one of these provided (very properly) that no person or institution should undertake the care of lunatics, except when licensed by the State Commissioners of Charities and thus subject to their inspection; this bill failed to pass the Senate. It was publicly asserted (and not denied) that the failure of the bill in the Senate was due, chiefly to the personal efforts at Albany, of the chief physician of Bloomingdale Asylum. An aversion, thus manifested, to proper supervision of the public authorities, makes it the more important, as well to the repute of the institution itself, as to the public interests, that the charges now made should be investigated.

The commissioners were Attorney-General Francis C. Barlow, M. B. Anderson, LL.D., President of Rochester University, and Thomas Hun, M. D., of Albany. They made their report in February, 1873.[10] It was on broad lines and directed 1) at the fear created by the complaints and charges in the public prints that the insane asylums were made instruments of oppression by the incarceration of persons who were not of unsound mind; and 2) at the apprehension excited by the stories of abuses in the treatment of the patients. In regard to the first they were "of opinion that there is no just foundation for the apprehension that persons not insane are improperly confined in these institutions. . . . We do not hesitate to say that, in our opinion, the public anxiety on that point is wholly unfounded." In regard to the second question they mentioned the difficulty in finding persons of kindness, patience, and consideration who were willing to spend their time in the care of the insane. They believed that instances of abuse occurred in all asylums and that "all that can be required of managers of such in-

[10] See *Am. J. Insanity*, XXIX (April, 1873), 591, for full report.

stitutions is an active and vigilant scrutiny into all cases of complaint." A very small part of the report was directed specifically to Bloomingdale. It was as follows:

In regard to the charge made against Bloomingdale Asylum in the public prints, we think that in order to do justice, both to the institution and the public, we may fairly say this: That the gross cases of mismanagement and misconduct charged against it have not been substantiated, and that great injustice has been done to the institution in representing it as the scene of outrages and habitual maltreatment of patients. At the same time we are compelled to say that some instances of the improper treatment of patients by attendants have been fairly proven before us, and that we do not think that the utmost vigilance in detecting and guarding against this kind of abuse has prevailed in this asylum during the past summer. Nothing but the sternest discipline, and the most careful watching over attendants, and the most searching and prompt investigations into, and suggestions or suspicions of harsh treatment by them, should be tolerated in an institution of this kind, and we think there has been some laxity in this respect. It is proper to say that one of the attendants charged with improper treatment of patients, had been discharged before our visit to the asylum, and that any relaxation of discipline during the past summer may have been the result of the absence of the superintendent for a considerable period by reason of the illness of himself and family, and of the illness and death of one of the assistant physicians. We are bound to state the facts as we found them.

To remedy the conditions revealed by their investigation, the commission recommended a system of licensing of privately conducted asylums for the insane by the State Board of Public Charities, and the appointment of a state commissioner in lunacy to visit and inspect them. They presented a bill containing these provisions. It was passed by the legislature and became a law which provided for the appointment of a commissioner by the Governor with the consent of the Senate. He was constituted an ex-officio member of the State Board of Charities, to which he made his reports. The first commissioner was Dr. John Ordronaux. These measures had been long advocated, and in 1862 a bill providing for a commissioner in lunacy had been introduced in the legislature.[11] It was, however, the undeserved tribulations of Bloomingdale that precipitated the passage of this needed legislation.

The New York *Tribune* of February 18, 1873, in commenting on the report, considered that the commission dealt with the subject in "a very gingerly manner, yet they substantially admit the accuracy of the Tribune's reports. . . . The measure which they propose is a proof that additional safeguards are necessary both to protect sane persons from

[11] *Am. J. Insanity,* XIX (1863), 479.

being shut up by conspiracy and to shield the insane from brutal treatment." An editorial on the following day added that the report was "lame and impotent as we anticipated from the first," also that it was "a whitewashing report rather than an exposure of abuses," and that the editors were still convinced that commitment to asylums took place without proper care in examinations and by "negligent and unscrupulous judges," that classification of patients was poorly carried out, that the nurses were coarse and the nursing rude, the cells [12] repulsive, cold, and not infrequently damp and injurious to health, that the food was supplied with greater consideration to economy than to the health of the patients, and that releases and transfers of patients were as loosely conducted as the commitments themselves.

The governors instructed the secretary to cause the report of the investigation by the committee of the board to be published. The *Tribune* printed it in inconspicuous type and place at a charge of $420.[13] The governors recorded their gratification at the appointment of the commission by Governor Hoffman, and instructed the Investigating Committee of the board to extend to them every facility within their power for the immediate and thorough prosecution of the investigation.[14] A visit of the commissioners to the asylum was noted in the Asylum Committee's minutes of October 21, 1872. In their annual report the governors stated that the charges were unfounded and that "This Board feels confident that the report of the Commission cannot seriously disparage an Institution which has ever been conducted upon principles of enlightened humanity."

The asylum physician, in his annual report, denied the accusation of Governor Hoffman that he had opposed the enactment of legislation to provide state supervision of the asylums for the insane. He explained that his opposition was directed against a different provision "tending to obstruct measures for the early treatment of mental diseases," which had originated in the impression that the present requirements were inadequate to prevent the confinement of sane persons, when, in fact, they were more rigid than in any other state. In regard to the *Tribune* story he declared:

That an ingenious and enterprising young newspaper reporter, by connivance with other parties, should succeed in simulating mental derangement so far as to convince two respectable physicians, that a man who behaved like

12 Patients at Bloomingdale had not for years been placed in "cells."

13 *Am. J. Insanity*, XXX (1873), 241. New York *Tribune*, Aug. 9, 1872.

14 *Minutes of the Governors*, Sept. 3, 1872.

a lunatic for two days and nights continuously, may appropriately be lodged in a lunatic asylum, does not prove the insufficiency of the present law regulating the isolation of the insane.

The judicial investigation in 1869, occasioned by the habeas corpus cases which had lasted several weeks, and the numerous newspaper editorials unfavorable to the management of the institution, had induced more or less uneasiness in the public mind respecting the possible confinement of sane persons under the charge of insanity, and also the care of the insane themselves. The asylum physician had found that in the habeas corpus proceedings

> the legal aspects of the question were the only ones considered; the medical conditions being wholly ignored or subordinated . . . the laws are already so stringent as frequently to discourage resort to the best method of caring for persons attacked by insanity, until the period of curability has passed away . . . the best efforts of philanthropy and of medical science are also liable to be occasionally thwarted by the authority of law, which esteems the maintenance of its own principles, as of more importance than the health or life of an isolated individual.[15]

At the annual meeting of superintendents of asylums which was held in May, 1873, however, the physician reported that the only apparent influence of the charges and publicity on the relations with patients and their relatives was confined to one instance in which a patient was removed by her brother. He brought her back the next day, saying that she had refused to go to bed until she was returned to the asylum, thereby satisfying him that she could not have been ill treated. Dr. Brown also reported that the habeas corpus cases on which the *Tribune* had based some of its charges were all decided by the courts in accordance with the views of the asylum physicians. In fact, one of these patients told the court that she wished to remain at the asylum until her relatives considered it proper for her to leave.[16] It is remarkable that, a few months after publication of the charges, Dr. Brown was consulted in regard to the illness of the editor of the *Tribune,* and advised his admission to a private institution for the mentally ill, at which he soon afterwards died. Dr. Brown noted that this was not the only editor of the *Tribune* who had been under his professional care.[17]

This was, unfortunately, not the last experience in investigation and newspaper publicity to which the asylum was subjected during this period. On September 30, 1876, Dr. John Ordronaux, State Commis-

15 Physician's Annual Report for 1869. 16 New York *Tribune,* Aug. 14, 1872.
17 *Am. J. Insanity,* XXX (1873), pp. 241–243.

sioner in Lunacy, notified the governors that he had received a complaint of ill treatment of a patient at the asylum and wished to investigate. The governors immediately offered their full coöperation and provided every facility required for the investigation. The patient, who had been discharged more than a year before making the charge, asserted that she had been roughly treated by an attendant, placed in a camisole, and that her throat had been lacerated and permanently deformed in attempts to feed her forcibly with a spoon. Examination of her throat revealed that it was deformed by scars and adhesions, and it was conceded by the asylum physicians that these might have been produced in the manner described in the complaint. At that time physicians had not learned a satisfactory way of performing forcible feeding, and the flexible tube and facility in using it had not come into universal use. The patient, who was probably not fully recovered, was exploiting her experiences at the asylum in appealing, with some other persons, for funds with which to establish a private institution for the mentally ill. She later brought a lawsuit against the asylum.

At the close of his investigation, the commissioner made his report in December, 1876. He requested the members of the Board of Governors to assemble to hear it, and to invite reporters of the New York *Tribune* and the New York *Times*. He reported that the patient's mental state while at the asylum rendered the statements of her experience there not entirely reliable. There seemed, however, to be no question that her throat was injured in the manner claimed. He exonerated the attendant of any wrong intent. She was endeavoring to the best of her ability to perform a proper and necessary procedure. He blamed her, however, for failing to report the signs of injury, bleeding, and inflammation. He also found that the organization, discipline, and administration of the asylum were at fault. He recommended, or ordered, that a supervisor should be appointed whose sole duty should be to supervise and instruct the attendants. He said that, "the experiment above suggested has already been tried and with good success for the past year, in the male wards of the Willard Asylum." How strange this "experiment" appears in these days of nurse training and better nursing standards! [18] He also considered that "more particular reports should be required from attendants daily," and that "it would seem, therefore, that for better protection both of the good fame of asylums as well as of the safety of the insane committed to them, more details of the daily life and occur-

[18] Miss Dix in her report on the asylum in 1851, drew attention to the lack of supervisors and recommended their appointment. See p. 251.

rences to the patients should be entered upon the case books of these institutions." He drew attention to the law of 1874, by which every superintendent of an asylum was required "to make entries from time to time of the mental state, bodily condition and medical treatment of such patient, together with the forms of restraint employed during the time such patient remains under his care," and concluded:

> The respondents having also through the Chairman of their Committee, Mr. Beekman, anticipated my action in the premises by themselves, soliciting suggestions, tending to the more efficient administration of their trust, I deem it sufficient to announce my conclusions to them, believing that they will carry the same weight in their estimation as attaches to a legal promulgation. I shall issue no order, therefore, under the statute, provided the respondents shall, within the next sixty days, furnish me with satisfactory evidence that they have carried the above suggestions into operation.

In May, 1877, the Asylum Committee reported to the commissioner that they had appointed, "a man for the male department and a woman for the female department, neither of them having any other duties to perform than to supervise their several departments and to bear communications from the Insane Patients to the medical officers of the Institution." They also reported that "a Register has been kept of all the cases in the Institution which is written up to date. Directions have been given to have entries made from time to time . . . which were formerly kept in accordance with the By-Laws for governing the Asylum, in a separate book, which has been inadvertently neglected for some time past."

The *Tribune,* in commenting on the case, was much more moderate than on previous occasions. An editorial of December 19, 1876, which opened with the statement, "The Bloomingdale Lunatic Asylum is in trouble again, another patient having made charges of cruelty against her attendants," was devoted principally to a general discussion of the character of those employed in the position of attendant. It was conceded that the "Visiting Committee" of Bloomingdale Asylum was made up of "gentlemen of the best character for benevolence, integrity and shrewdness," that Dr. Brown had "a high reputation in his profession," and that "nobody who knows Dr. Brown will for a moment suppose that he could possibly be guilty of cruelty." Reference was made to the failure to instruct the attendants in their duties, and the extent to which the patients were in their power, by which much neglect and harsh treatment might be engaged in without its coming to the attention of the physician, who could not be everywhere and see everything. In accordance with Dr. Ordronaux's recommendation, it was suggested that "upon each floor there should be one man or woman well fitted to act in case of emergency, well informed, and of an established reputation for humanity and good sense." In regard to newspaper publicity it was stated that "there is a chronic public suspicion of neglect, violence and cruelty," and that "newspapers, often from an honorable sense of duty, are prompt in giving publicity to all *prima facie* cases of abuse." It was called "next to useless to ask for anything like a generous consideration on the part of the public on the perplexing position of the officers of these asylums . . . the traditional reputation of madhouses and bedlams is against them." [19]

The law providing for the licensing of private institutions for the mentally ill became effective in 1873, and in August of that year the governors were requested by the State Board of Charities to apply for a license. The application was referred to the law firm of Evarts and O'Conor, with a request for an opinion on the position of the asylum under the terms of the act. Their opinion was "that the corporation of the Governors of the New York Hospital in the maintenance and conduct of its Asylum for the insane, as a part of its public and chartered charity, is not subject to the provisions respecting licenses contained in the Act of 1873, but is expressly exempted therefrom." This opinion was based on the exemption from license provided in the Act of any corporation for charitable purposes which was already, when the Act was passed, operating on a charter granted directly by the state government; "a charter from the Legislature, expressly giving authority for the maintenance of an Institution or Asylum for the insane, was intended to exempt such an institution or asylum from a necessity of a license, to be and to be managed, from the State Board of Charities, itself a creature of the Legislature." [20] The Attorney General of the state, the Honorable Francis C. Barlow, in a counteropinion, considered that the intent of the law was to exempt only institutions which were conducted at public expense.[21] He advised that the objections of Evarts and O'Conor were not so clear as to justify omitting to apply the licensing law, and he proposed to bring suit not for the purpose of inflicting punishment but in order to obtain a judicial determination of the question. Apparently this course was not followed, and the institution has continued ever

19 New York *Tribune*, Dec. 19, 1876.

20 *Minutes of the Governors*, Sept. 2, 1873.

21 *Ibid.*, Jan. 6, 1874.

since to operate under its charter. It is, however, regularly visited and inspected by the State Department of Mental Hygiene and their rules, regulations, and recommendations are strictly followed.

An account of the sensational misleading newspaper stories and of the investigations to which Bloomingdale Asylum was subjected during a period of seven years, from 1869 to 1876, is of more than local historic interest. It presents a sample of what many of the other asylums for the mentally ill throughout the country were experiencing. These asylums were regarded by the newspaper reporters and story-writers of the period as a fertile source of material for sensational news items. An eminent psychiatrist of the period, in discussing the alleged confinement of sane persons in asylums, wrote in an article published in the *American Law Review* in January, 1869:

> The prevalent notion on this subject has been derived in some measure from novels and periodicals . . . It only indicates the change in modern civilization whereby much of the old machinery of the poet and story-teller has become effete, and thus it happens that the castle and convent and poor-debtors prison, as places for confining luckless heroes and heroines, have given way to lunatic asylums. . . . Their walls are strong, their windows barred, their doors locked, and though utterly devoid of cells and dungeons, it required no great stretch of the imagination to conjure them up.[22]

It must be added, however, that the institutions have since then been greatly improved and humanized in their structural character and in their organization and administration. Also that the governmental and social provisions for managing the problems occasioned by mental illness are now more appropriate and effective, and the public is more enlightened on the whole subject. There can be little doubt that the widely published charges against the management of Bloomingdale Asylum and the treatment of the patients were of immediate disadvantage to the reputation and successful operation of the institution. They probably contributed in some measure to making the word "Bloomingdale," in the minds of the uninformed and credulous public, synonymous with "Bedlam"; a disorderly "mad-house" and a place of horrors instead of the haven of relief and cure for many sick and troubled persons that it always has been.

Some advantages were, however, gained. The appointment of supervisors in the nursing service, which was apparently at that time an "experiment," was a step towards the form and character of nursing organization which was eventually developed. The keeping of systematic

[22] Quoted in Physician's Annual Report for 1872.

case histories, which, though always required by the by-laws, had not been adequately attended to, became a more consistent and progressive practice. The misfortunes of Bloomingdale were also a means of advancing the treatment of the mentally ill throughout the state, through the introduction of the licensing system of private institutions, and the regular visitation and inspection of all the institutions, private and public, by a medical state commissioner. To Dr. Brown the anxiety occasioned by the charges, the newspaper attacks, and the investigations, was a devastating experience, which will be described in the next chapter.

XXIII

TWENTY-FIVE YEARS OF MEDICAL SERVICE AND A TRAGIC SEQUEL

FROM 1852 to 1877 the medical direction of Bloomingdale Asylum was exclusively the work of Dr. D. Tilden Brown. His term of service was much longer than that of any of his predecessors, and embraced virtually the full course of his professional career. At its close, full medical direction, although not officially adopted, had been extended to nearly every detail of the administration, and many decisions and responsibilities which had previously been assumed by the Asylum Committee or left to the warden were referred to the physician. Dr. Brown's annual reports covered "the general operations" of the asylum, and he was occasionally referred to as "superintendent."

Prior to his appointment at Bloomingdale, Dr. Brown had been an assistant physician at the State Asylum at Utica, at the Vermont Asylum, and at the New York City Asylum. He had also, during a period of impaired health, been in Central America, where he was interested in opening a route across Nicaragua for emigrants to California. He negotiated the first treaty which secured the right of transit across that isthmus.[1] For a short time he was associated in private practice with Dr. Willard Parker of New York. Dr. Brown was a graduate of the College of Physicians and Surgeons, New York, and at the time of his appointment was thirty years of age. Others who were considered for the post were Dr. Benjamin W. McCready, Dr. Gray, and Dr. Van Arsdale.[2]

When the new physician entered upon his duties, plans for additions to the asylum buildings had already been made by Dr. Nichols. The extent to which Dr. Brown's efforts were directed to this, to improving the facilities for comfort and good treatment and the operation of the service, and to the selection of a new location for the asylum and the preparation of plans, has been described in an earlier chapter. In the last few years of his administration he was subjected to the crude and unjust charges, the sensational newspaper publicity, and the investigations which have been recounted. He was a sensitive, tender-minded man, and his health was not robust. There was also sickness in his family which, on several occasions, necessitated his absence from the asylum.

1 Howard A. Kelly and Walter L. Burrage, *Dictionary of American Medical Biography* (New York and London, 1928).

2 The first names of Dr. Gray and Dr. Van Arsdale were not given. Dr. Gray was probably John P. Gray who afterwards became very prominent as the able superintendent of the New York State Asylum at Utica, N.Y.

One of his sons died in 1870, and another was severely ill in 1872. The warden of the asylum was aged and infirm and was given unlimited leave of absence early in 1877.

Dr. Brown was also unfortunate, during the most difficult period of his service, in some of his assistant physicians. Until 1857 he, like his predecessors, was without medical assistance. Dr. James Macdonald had, in 1837, recommended that the position of assistant physician be established.[3] In 1854 the Inspecting Committee made a similar recommendation which was approved by the Asylum Committee. It was, however, not adopted by the Board of Governors until 1856 and it was 1857 before the position was established and an appointment made.[4] The number of patients accommodated had, in the meantime, been considerably increased. The first assistant physician was Dr. Charles Corey. He served until June, 1866, when he resigned and was succeeded by Dr. Horace K. Wheeler. He, unfortunately, proved to be affected with tuberculosis and, after a period of frequent inability to attend to his duties, he died at the asylum in May, 1868. In June, 1867, Dr. Edward E. Porter, who had previously been on the staff of the Hartford Retreat, had been employed temporarily to assist Dr. Wheeler, and in August, 1868, he was given a permanent appointment. He was, however, also tuberculous, and died in October, 1872. In the meantime after the institution had been further enlarged, the position of second assistant physician was established in 1869, and filled in July of that year by the appointment of Dr. Dwight R. Burrell, who had previously been on the staff of the New York City Asylum. He was, following Dr. Porter's death, advanced to the position of principal assistant, and in April, 1873, the position of second assistant was again filled by the appointment of Dr. William H. McDonald, who had also been on the staff of the New York City Asylum. Dr. Burrell resigned in November, 1876, to become superintendent of Brigham Hall, a private asylum at Canandaigua, New York, where he remained for many years. Dr. McDonald was promoted to the place of first assistant and was still in the service when Dr. Brown resigned.

The painful and wearing experiences to which Dr. Brown had been exposed for several years had evidently seriously affected his physical and mental health. In February, 1877, he advised the governors that for some time past he had felt "an infirmity of health which has made the performance of my duties extremely difficult, and has at last led me

[3] See p. 193.
[4] *Minutes of the Governors*, Feb. 3, 1857.

to seek rest at the house of my friend Dr. Choate." [5] This was a private institution for the mentally ill. He was immediately granted three months leave of absence. Dr. McDonald was placed in temporary charge of the service, and Dr. James C. Hallock, Jr.,[6] was engaged as a temporary assistant. In May, Dr. Brown's resignation, which had been presented in February, was accepted. In their annual report for 1877 the governors recorded that he "had administered the office of Resident Physician . . . to the entire satisfaction of the Governors, maintaining by his ability and devotion the already high reputation of the Asylum, and earning for himself an eminent position among the professional men in his specialty."

It seems appropriate to present a brief account of his further history containing an example of the newspaper standards of the period relative to mental illness and the institutions for the mentally ill. Dr. Brown went to Europe and in May, 1878, was received for treatment in the Royal Edinburgh Asylum. He remained there for nine days only and was discharged to return to the United States in the care of his wife.[7] He afterwards was a patient in a private institution in Batavia, Illinois, and later purchased some property in Batavia, where for many years he lived in retirement. He did not engage in medical practice, and apparently made no contributions to medical literature. He would probably not have been heard of again except by his intimate friends, had not a reporter of the New York *World,* for some inscrutable reason, in August, 1889, "with instructions to find Dr. David Tilton Brown," after some difficulty obtained access to him and endeavored with no success to induce him to review his New York experiences. The reporter's communication to his paper was published, on August 25, under the heading "The Dead Alive." In the same issue a small picture of Dr. Brown appeared and an article, the character of which may be gathered from the opening paragraph:

To rise to the highest pinnacle of one's ambition; to become an authority in a great profession; to lose one's mind and position in the hour of greatness; to be buried alive in a madhouse; to die and be forgotten; to return to life as if by a miracle; to exist only as a sacred confidence to one's most trusted relatives; to melt out of the social sunlight of fashionable New York and after years in the purgatory of an Edinburgh maniac ward, to reappear amid the mellow atmosphere of a lonely farm near a straggling country village in Illinois—such is the romantic, tragic story of David Tilton Brown,

[5] *Minutes of the Asylum Committee,* Feb. 3, 1877.

[6] He was afterwards physician of the State Emigrant Hospital on Ward's Island, N.Y.

[7] Letter from Prof. D. K. Henderson, Physician in Chief, Morningside Hospital, Edinburgh, December, 1942.

Doctor of Medicine, formerly chief of the Bloomingdale Asylum for the Insane.

There followed what purported to be an account of his personal characteristics and his position at Bloomingdale. It was also stated that he had long been given up as dead by his New York friends, and a letter which, it was asserted, had been written by a Scotch physician who was a "friend and counsellor to the unfortunate man," was quoted, in which he was said to have "breathed his last in a corner of his cell, under his cot, with his hands madly clutching crumbs of bread, while his poor parched lips piteously pleaded for food." This and much of the rest of the article was, of course, grossly untrue. One of the governors of the New York Hospital, who was interviewed by a reporter of the New York *Times,* said that Dr. Brown was

> as competent a Superintendent as Bloomingdale ever had. At the time of the exposure of the alleged outrages there in 1874 or 1875 the confidence of the Governors in his integrity was never shaken. . . . He was a particularly sensitive man, however, and it was undoubtedly those attacks which made it necessary for him to go abroad to be treated for insanity. Since his return to America he has been in constant communication with his friends here.[8]

The end of the story soon followed, as on September 4, 1889, Dr. Brown ended his life by hanging. A full account of his death in the *World* was headed "He Was Insane to the Last," and referred to his history as the "Story of a once brilliant mind shattered by contact with the insane." The interview with the reporter was referred to; not, however, with any intimation of impropriety, responsibility, or regret. In an account of his death published in the *American Journal of Insanity* in October, 1889, his suicide was attributed to the revival of the painful experiences in his past life, and the publicity with its sensational headlines. The reporter was described as

> a prying emissary of a New York newspaper in the performance of one of those feats of journalism upon which "the largest daily circulation in the world" is directly dependent. This prurient and wanton purloiner bore away in triumph the forgotten story of our departed brother's breakdown, regardless of his natural desire to be alone with the sad secret of his life in a secluded home of his own seeking and finding; sensationalism held high carnival with attractive headlines; scandal-mongers smacked their lips over the tidbit purveyed by the "smart" reporter,—and alas! poor Dr. Brown died. Was this suicide merely?

[8] New York *Times,* Sept. 7, 1889.

It was added that "to the credit of several fearless organs of public opinion in New York and elsewhere be it said, their editors have not hesitated to call this 'journalistic feat' by its right name."

During this period from 1852 to 1877, little if any advance seems to have been made in the clinical service of Bloomingdale Asylum. In fact, there may have been some retrogression. The brief accounts of cases admitted and discharged previously given in the monthly reports of the physician to the Asylum Committee no longer appeared in the minutes after 1849. The governors also gradually discontinued the practice of noting in the minutes of their visits the patients in restraint and seclusion, and their observations of the occupation of patients. In 1866, the patients were seen "as far as was expedient to do so," whereas theretofore *all* the patients had been seen. From time to time, however, the continued concern of the governors in "moral treatment" was revealed by such observations as that of the Inspecting Committee in February, 1858, when very many of the patients were "listless and indifferent, and wholly unoccupied." This was followed in June, 1859, by a report that "if the Asylum Committee could contrive any additional sources of amusement or occupation it would be a matter of congratulation." In March, 1873, the subject was again considered and a committee was appointed to provide means of amusement and instruction for the patients. They merely recommended that more illustrated papers, monthly magazines, novels and travel books be furnished, that an inexpensive piano be purchased for the women, and that carriage hire be paid by the institution for friends who might be willing to provide lectures and exhibitions. Following this, it was noted in the physician's annual report for 1873 that friends had contributed musicales, readings and recitations, exhibitions of "natural magic," and scientific experiments. In 1860, a magic lantern had been purchased for $300 and the committee recommended that additional slides be provided. In February, 1877, a committee was appointed to examine the organization of the outdoor services.

In their annual reports the governors frequently repeated that

> the Asylum continues to be administered upon that system of classification and separation, and of moral and medical treatment, of which it gave one of the earliest examples on this side of the Atlantic. This system, now general in all similar institutions of the higher order, has here received, and continues to receive, all the improvements which the many skillful and humane persons at the head of similar establishments in this country and in Europe are constantly presenting or suggesting for the relief of mental disease.

Several of the forms of occupation, instruction, and amusement introduced by former physicians of the asylum, were, however, apparently discontinued; both the governors' and the physician's reports contained less than in previous years in regard to the character and treatment of the patients. There was, however, no diminution in the regularity and fidelity with which the governors discharged their duties in visiting and inspecting the asylum, and in contributing to the good treatment of the patients. On some occasions members of committees arrived at the asylum early enough to inspect the breakfast. To facilitate the transaction of business, it was ruled in July, 1874, that any number of the members of the Asylum Committee present at a meeting would constitute a quorum for the regular routine of business prescribed by the committee. In November, 1868, the Weekly Committee was authorized to reduce rates instead of waiting for the action of the Asylum Committee at their monthly meeting. Needs and defects noted by the committees were brought to the attention of the board with recommendations.

The Inspecting Committee reported also that there were too few nurses employed in the asylum, there being at that time (March, 1854) 11 for 59 male patients and 9 for 66 female patients. The payroll in June, 1875, showed some improvement. It listed the names of 14 male and 23 female attendants. The number of patients was then about 190, 84 men and 106 women. The proportion of attendants to patients was, therefore, 1 to 6 for the men, and 1 to 4.6 for the women. Monthly wages ranged from $20 to $30 for men, and from $14 to $18 for women. References to the nursing service in the reports of the governors and the physician indicate that it was considered satisfactory. The state commissioners had found occasion to point out defects in the service, but it was probably not inferior to that of other institutions for the mentally ill at that time.

Apparently, even before the disclosures of the investigations by state authorities, the governors were concerned in regard to the medical service. On two occasions the president and vice president reported that "an undue number of officers were frequently absent from the premises at the same time." [9] The medical histories during the period were at first rather meager. In 1871, however, "Case Books" were introduced and, especially after the investigation made by State Commissioner Ordronaux in 1876, contained more frequent entries. An innovation in these case books was a five-line form printed at the top of each page and followed by a blank space for notes. Previous to this, the only provision for

[9] *Minutes of the Governors,* Jan. 2, 1872; March 7, 1871.

history notes was on printed forms, some of which contained many items. The "Warden's Register" contains the names and dates of admission of all the patients from the establishment of the department in 1808. The "Register of Discharges," [10] introduced by Dr. Earle in 1845, contained headings of great number and variety, and, with the exception of six of the sections, was kept up by Dr. Nichols and Dr. Brown. There was no provision, however, for a full account of the patient and his illness. In 1866, when a new volume became necessary, the items which had not been utilized were omitted, and a column headed "Special Observations" was added. In 1866 also, a "Medical Register" of admissions was introduced by Dr. Brown. This, like the "Register of Discharges" was, when open, a book about a yard in length. The pages were spaced vertically, with the following headings:

(1) No.; (2) Name, Nativity, Residence; (3) By Whom Supported; (4) Sex; (5) Age; (6) Stature; (7) Color of Hair; (8) Color of Eyes; (9) Temperament; (10) Original Disposition and Intellect: (11) Single or Married (12) No. of Children; (13) Occupation; (14) Degree of Education; (15) Profession of Religion; (16) Habits of Life; (17) No. of Admission; (18) Date of Admission; (19) Date of Discharge; (20) Time in the Asylum; (21) Age at First Attack; (22) No. of Previous Attacks and Their Duration; (23) Duration of Present Attack; (24) Class in Regard to Duration; (25) Apparent or Alleged Cause of Disorder (Predisposing,—Hereditary, Others; Exciting); (26) Form of Mental Disorder; (27) Particular Propensities and Hallucinations; (28) Accompanying Bodily Disorders; (29) Changes in Form of Disorder before Discharge; (30) Result; (31) Supposed Cause of Death (P.M. signifies that a Post Mortem examination was made); (32) Observations.

The form, it will be noted, made little provision for any history of the case after admission. In 1873, still another book entitled "Histories" was introduced, in which all admissions were entered. On one page was a printed list of questions which added somewhat to the medical character of the information called for in the other books. Some of the questions were:

(1) When were the symptoms first manifested and in what way? (2) Is the disease variable? (3) Has the patient had any acute disease or received a bodily injury? (4) State of health at accession of mental disease? (5) Conduct at home or abroad? (6) Conduct as regards business? (7) Habits of eating, drinking and sleeping? (8) Character of delusions? (9) Nature of treatment received?

The page opposite the form was left vacant for the entry of notes, but was seldom utilized except, on occasion, for recording the observations

[10] See p. 217.

in the certificate of the physicians who examined the patient for commitment. It has been considered advisable to present these details, because, in the absence of better information, they reveal what, at that time, was considered by the physicians to be particularly important, and also the expedients which were resorted to in this period of medical recording without clerical assistance.

Altogether, the entries came far short of presenting a full account of the patient and his illness and treatment. There are signs, however, of better differentiation in the formal classification of mental illnesses. Several varieties of mania are mentioned, such as periodical, circular, partial. Dementia is designated acute or chronic. General paresis is a frequent diagnosis. A brief account of the development of the illness is usually given, but there is still an attempt to assign a definite exciting "cause" in each case.

The physical examination was apparently quite superficial. The general appearance, nutrition, and the condition of the skin were noted, also the character of the pulse, and usually the pupils. In the case books introduced in 1871, an occasional note of the treatment was entered. From these and from entries under various headings in the forms used, it may be gathered that the drastic medication and other measures formerly practiced had been abandoned. Sedatives prescribed were chloral in doses as high as thirty grains, with beer; morphine, and potassium bromide, with brandy; cannabis indica and asafoetida. Croton oil was still resorted to as a purge. Castor oil was given in farina. Quinine and iron were given as tonics. Notes of the course of the illness were in many instances very meager or lacking. When they began to appear in the 1871 case book, it was, after the first few notes, usually at long intervals, and seldom or never produced a complete history. Occasionally a note was made of the condition of patients who were heard from or seen at varying periods after discharge.

Observations on the use of mechanical restraint and seclusion and the occupational and recreational activities of the patients appear less frequently in the records of this period than in those of the preceding periods. Probably little change occurred, and both the governors and the physician may have seen little occasion for noting what had become routine. Occasional notes reveal the character of mechanical restraint employed, such as "she was put in a camisole," or "she wore a camisole at night." One patient was noted to have "slept in restraint," one was referred to as "tied to a seat," another as "no longer restrained in bed with a sheet," and still another was "often in restraint." The "oesophageal tube" was used for feeding patients who refused to eat; through it, meat broths, farina, and wine were administered. There is nothing in the records to reveal the extent to which occupations and recreational and social activities were engaged in by the patients. A suggestion of their pursuits may be obtained from a note by the committee in April, 1876, that the ladies were engaged in dancing, "after their weekly sewing society." Probably little or no change from previous customs was made. Patients were apparently allowed considerable liberty. One was noted as having a key, and coming freely into the center building. He also made a practice of attending funerals. Patients went into the city, and it is noted that, on one occasion, one of the physicians accompanied a patient on a trip to Niagara.

The statistical tables which had been published with the annual report since 1839 were discontinued in 1848. They were considered by Dr. Brown to be "devoid of special interest for unprofessional readers." He explained, however, that, as the register introduced by Dr. Earle was continued, the "materials furnished by these records will, doubtless, be again arranged and preserved in some appropriate form when they shall become sufficiently copious to afford a basis for safe generalization." [11] Most of Dr. Brown's annual reports were exceedingly brief, so much so that in January, 1863, the editor of the *American Journal of the Medical Sciences* commented that "it must have required labour to make the report of the Bloomingdale Asylum, what with one-third of a page of margin at its beginning, and one-quarter of a page at the end, it occupies two pages." Dr. Brown explained that he regarded the annual report solely as a means of informing the local community, and that, in a city as large as New York, other means of spreading information were available and were more effective.[12] By most asylum physicians of this period the annual reports were considered a means of publishing, for the benefit of the medical profession and the public, information concerning the nature and treatment of mental illness; in many instances the reports were not confined merely to the operation of the asylum to which they particularly related.

In his annual report for 1853 Dr. Brown emphasized the necessity of preserving individuality in the treatment of the patients, as follows:

> In the Lunatic Hospital as in society and in the state, the individual must be prominent. The very disease for which he is admitted tends ultimately to destroy individuality. For this reason his identity must be preserved, his

11 Physician's report for 1855, *Minutes of the Asylum Committee*, Feb. 2, 1856.
12 Physician's report for 1862.

just claims recognized, his self-respect encouraged, and his mind incited to useful or refining occupation.

In his annual report for 1854 he expressed his views of the prevalence of physical disease in the mentally ill. He considered that the insane

as a class are unsound alike in mind and body. They inherit the multiform varieties of scrofula, and among them abound the Protean forms of nervous diseases, hysteria, chorea, neuralgia and epilepsy. Some are victims to depraved appetites unrestrained by an enlightened and vigorous will, and suffer the torments of alcoholic poison which has paralyzed alike their physical energies and their moral sense. Cardiac, hepatic, renal and uterine affections are common among them, excite and shape their delusions and generally shorten their lives. Their sensations being enfeebled or perverted they disregard extremes of heat and cold, and become indifferent to danger; but while the mind may betray no indication of pain, their bodies suffer like those of sane men. . . . Obstinate derangements of the digestive and assimilative organs are induced by prolonged abstinence or excessive and unmasticated food; the circulation is languid from muscular inactivity; the extremities are cold and livid; slight abrasions of the skin become alarming ulcers and serious visceral disease insidiously establishes itself, too often successfully resisting medical aid. These patients become prematurely old, their intellectual perceptions and moral emotions disappear with healthy sensation; they sicken and die, often without an intimation of suffering or an expression of concern.

They were, however, he believed, remarkably exempt from prevailing epidemics, in proof of which he mentioned the freedom of the asylum household from cholera when it prevailed in the neighborhood.[13] With the exception of his annual reports, few publications by Dr. Brown have been found. He participated in a revision of the *Elements of Medical Jurisprudence* by Dr. T. Romeyn Beck,[14] and wrote part of the section on "Mental Alienation." In the proceedings of the Association of Superintendents of Asylums for 1856, it is recorded that Dr. Brown read a paper on "Acute Dementia," in which "important facts" were elicited. No discussion was recorded, however, and the paper was not published. An address before the alumni of the College of Physicians and Surgeons in 1862 was published but was not medical. Dr. Brown was appointed Lecturer on Psychological Medicine and Medical Jurisprudence at the college in 1868, but, so far as has been learned, his lectures have not been preserved. In May, 1863, he made a report to the Association of Medical

13 Physician's reports for 1854 and 1866.

14 Published in 1823. Dr. Curwen, in an address before the American Medico-Psychological Association in 1894, referred to Dr. Brown as being in the first ranks of medico-legal experts. See the *Transactions* of the Association, I (1894), 66.

Superintendents of American Asylums of a meeting of the corresponding British Association which he had attended in London during the previous year.[15]

He attended nearly all the meetings of the American Association of Medical Superintendents during his service at Bloomingdale, and occasionally took part in the proceedings. His remarks were sometimes related to conditions and experiences at Bloomingdale. At the meeting in 1853, during a discussion of night service concerning which there was evidently some difference of opinion, he mentioned that the asylum had managed without a night watch for thirty years, except during a short period, and that there was none at the time he spoke. At the 1854 meeting, he mentioned having used ether and chloroform in the treatment of patients with good effect. This is the only positive evidence that has been found that these anaesthetics were used at Bloomingdale.

In a discussion on mechanical restraint at the 1855 meeting, Dr. Brown said that he was responsible for the construction of the first covered crib bed in the United States, under the direction of Dr. Brigham at Utica, New York. During this discussion Dr. Nichols said that he did not use the covered crib at Bloomingdale, because he found several sets of Wyman's straps there, which were "enough to effect coercive recumbency in all cases that ever at any one time required it." Dr. Brown approved of the crib in the treatment of emaciated, restless, aged persons. At this meeting, in discussing a paper on "The Treatment of Periodical Insanity," he stated that he lived in a malarious region "where all diseases exhibited more or less an intermittent type," and though he never employed emetics as recommended by the reader of the paper, "he had used quinine in large doses with apparent benefit in cases of insanity. The popular belief that mental disease yields to an invasion of fever and ague he had, however, not found verified." [16] Dr. Brown also spoke of his experience with the use of the prolonged bath for two to three hours "with the most evident good result." [17] In a discussion in 1860 on the commingling of the sexes in asylum social activities, he said that this had been allowed three or four years previously, but had been discontinued. Two patients who had met in this way had married. At the meeting of 1866 he said that nearly all the patients at Bloomingdale were under commitment, but that some came voluntarily, and were not detained if they subsequently desired to leave. At another meeting in 1873, Dr. Nichols said that there were a few colored patients at Bloom-

[15] *Am. J. Insanity*, XX (1864), 270.
[16] See pp. 169–170.
[17] Meeting of Association of Superintendents, 1854.

ingdale when he left there in 1852, he thought less than half a dozen.

Dr. Brown was evidently much respected by his colleagues in the medical profession and had an attractive personality. When he died, the *New York Medical Journal* of September, 1889, described him as an "alienist of high attainments and a man of extraordinary nobility and gentleness of character." That he had a tender solicitude for the patients is indicated by a note of the Weekly Committee that "Dr. Brown and the matron had been up all night with a dying patient." He was frequently called in consultation by private practitioners, and to give testimony as an expert in court. He was also considered to be especially qualified in institutional planning, so much so that in 1862 when the trustees were contemplating the establishment of the Sheppard Asylum near Baltimore, he was asked to visit and inspect institutions in Europe in order that he might aid the trustees with their plans. He was given leave of absence from May to September, and, on his return, he made a report which was published in the *American Journal of Insanity* in October, 1863.[18]

Dr. Brown visited institutions in England, Scotland, France, Holland, and one in Germany, and considered them no better than those in America. The only one which seemed to be "identical in its design and other peculiarities" with what was proposed for the Sheppard Asylum was the "Prefargier Asylum" at Neuchâtel, Switzerland. He learned that in the organization of European asylums, "after undergoing every conceivable modification" and "innumerable experiments of divided authority and responsibility," the plan generally adopted consisted of a board of managers and a medical superintendent in entire charge. His plan for the Sheppard Asylum, designed in collaboration with an architect, was awarded only third prize, though much of the design "formed the nucleus of the plans which . . . were finally adopted." [19] He was also consulted in regard to the plans for a new state asylum at Morristown, New Jersey.[20] It is interesting that, among the places visited by Dr. Brown in Europe was an institution at Bloomingdale, near Haarlem, in Holland, in regard to which he reported that "the exact coincidence in name and neighborhood with the location of our own institution, added another to the agreeable impressions derived from the beautiful situation of one of the very best establishments it was my pleasure to see." [21]

[18] *Am. J. Insanity*, XX (1863), 200.

[19] H. M. Hurd, *Institutional Care of the Insane in U.S. and Canada* (Baltimore, 1916), II, 561. See also *Am. J. Insanity*, XXXII (1876), 291.

[20] *Am. J. Insanity*, XXXII (1876), 295.

[21] Physician's report for 1862.

During Dr. Brown's administration the asylum was free from epidemic disease. Cholera prevailed in the vicinity in 1854 and 1866, but both the patients and the personnel of the asylum escaped. In 1866, malaria, which was for many years an annual visitor, was unusually prevalent during the summer. Tuberculosis was a frequent cause of death among the patients, and, as has been mentioned, among its victims were two of the asylum physicians. A considerable number of patients, many of them affected with extremely acute forms of mental illness, died very soon after admission. In one year, 1867, it was reported that five had died within five days, and four others within two weeks, and in 1853 it was reported that seven patients had died within eight days after their admission. The advances in medicine and in nursing and hospital standards since that period, would probably permit the saving of many such patients, and their restoration to mental and physical health. Feeding of resistant and indifferent patients is also better managed now, and patients whose deaths were attributed to "specific cachexia," "exhaustion from acute mania," "gradual exhaustion and marasmus," and other equally vague "causes," would probably be more frequently restored. Fifteen patients died by suicide during the period, three of them in 1873; one man and two women, all by strangulation by suspension. Four others died by the same means, one "by wounds," and one by drowning after escape from the asylum. In six instances the mode of suicide was not mentioned. The number of deaths from suicide at the New York Hospital during the same period was much greater, though, no doubt, nearly all of them were admitted after the self-injury had been inflicted. A considerable number of cases which were designated "insanity" were, however, admitted (18 in 1866), and some were retained for considerable periods. Many cases of delirium tremens were also treated there, (99 in 1853). Among the patients who died at Bloomingdale was the last survivor of those who had been transferred from the asylum at the New York Hospital in 1821. He died in 1872. Two sisters, Sally and Betsy B., one of whom had been admitted to the old asylum in 1808, the year it was established, and the other in 1812, also died during the period, one in 1863 and the other in 1865. Betsy's age at death was said to be about 95, and she had been 57 years in the asylum.[22] The records indicate that both had been free patients for many years. Of a patient who died in 1853, attention was directed to "her relationship and marked resemblance to the 'Father of his Country.' "[23]

[22] *Minutes of the Asylum Committee*, July 31, 1865.
[23] *Ibid.*, Feb. 4, 1854. (Physician's report for 1853.)

Among the visitors to the asylum during the period were the Governor of the state and several members of the legislature and of state commissions. The Association of Medical Superintendents were entertained at the asylum in 1857, and were "pleased with the condition of the institution." Some of the most distinguished members also visited at other times, including Dr. Kirkbride, Dr. Ray, Dr. Bell, Dr. Earle, and Dr. Nichols. Miss Dorothea O. Dix, who had inspected and rather severely criticized the condition of the asylum in 1851, accompanied the governors on a tour of inspection in 1866, and "expressed her satisfaction with its condition." [24] In 1860 Dr. Emily Blackwell, who was one of the first women physicians to practice in New York, was a visitor with the Weekly Committee. She was one of those who in 1877 proposed to the governors that "a separate ward to be attended by female surgeons" be established.[25] Another visitor of considerable importance was Dr. John C. Bucknill, "Lord Chancellor's Visitor of Lunatics," of England. He spent the day of May 29, 1875, at the asylum and made several suggestions as to treatment, amusements, and so on. In his *Notes on Asylums for the Insane in America* published in 1876, Dr. Bucknill wrote that Bloomingdale "is under the careful and skillful superintendence of Dr. Brown. . . . I saw no restraint here . . . and only one patient in seclusion—a case in which to my mind it was obviously needful. . . . There is no place but the Bloomingdale Hill from which you can look down upon the harbors and the great river of New York." He considered the asylum "very well managed," and added "there is no intention of selling it and removing the institution further into the country." He disapproved, however, of

> the plan of placing noisy and excitable patients in what are called "lodge-wards," apart from the main building. . . . The number of patients whose noise is incessant and annoying is very small, even in a large asylum containing many hundreds of inmates. There might, perhaps, be some reason for providing a small ward out of ear-shot of other patients . . . but it seems to me that excitable lunatics, being those who most need frequent medical observation, ought, in the arrangement of a hospital for the insane, to be brought as near to the medical staff as convenient architectural arrangements will permit.

He also noted that

> at Bloomingdale, on a glorious genial day, I did see some male patients in one of the airing courts, but as a rule the asylum population was persistently within doors, and there were unmistakable signs that this was the habit and

[24] *Ibid.*, March 13, 1866.

[25] *Minutes of the Governors*, April 3, 1877.

custom of the land. The airing courts were untrodden, and the pathways in the fine grounds but little used, like those of some absentee nobleman in our own country. Of course I mean all this as comparative only, for I did see a solitary patient now and then out of doors, but such a sight as one sees on any fine day from the Great Western Railway passing by Hanwell was totally and conspicuously absent in the States.[26]

A notable visit to the asylum, which was not recorded in the Minutes of the Governors, was referred to by Dr. Nichols at a meeting of the Association of Medical Superintendents in 1872. He mentioned that "an estimable gentleman who was a patient in the Bloomingdale Asylum . . . made an address of welcome to Lafayette when he visited that institution in 1824." Lafayette visited the hospital on September 10, 1824, and was elected an honorary member of the Society.[27]

The fiftieth anniversary of the establishment of Bloomingdale Asylum was celebrated in 1871. It was recorded that 6,325 patients had been admitted during the period, of whom 2,767 had been discharged "recovered" and 1,460 "improved." In March, 1871, the governors, for the first time,

Ordered that all patients hereafter admitted, be furnished with commitments, either before or after admission, as the case may be and that all commitments of patients now in the Asylum or who may be hereafter received, be filed in a book prepared for the purpose and in the order of their dates.

It is noteworthy that it was ordered that *all* patients admitted be furnished with commitments. It was, however, not until September, 1872, that the Minutes of the Asylum Committee noted that "the commitments of the new patients were examined and found in order." Thereafter it was noted at each monthly meeting that the commitments were "exhibited," "inspected," or "approved." The practice of examining commitment papers by the committee or one of its members was continued until 1932.

A rather singular incident in November, 1860, was the reception by the Asylum Committee of a letter from the attorneys of Dr. William T. G. Morton requesting compensation for infringement of Dr. Morton's patent on the use of sulphuric ether as an anaesthetic. It was stated that the patent had not been extended and Dr. Morton's "health has been destroyed by his exertions in relation to this discovery and he is destitute of the means of support." In July, 1858, the governors had do-

26 J. C. Bucknill, *Notes on Asylums for the Insane in America* (London, 1876). Also *Am. J. Insanity*, XXXIII (1876).

27 *Am. J. Insanity*, XXIX (1872), 177. New York *Commercial Advertiser*, Sept. 11, 1824.

nated $500 to a fund for Dr. Morton's benefit. Another occurrence of some interest was the participation of some of the governors and of some of the physicians of the New York Hospital in the management of the Inebriate Asylum which was established at Binghamton, New York, in 1859, as members of the board of trustees.[28]

The operation of Bloomingdale Asylum was apparently little affected by the Civil War. In 1861 a reduction in income was attributed to "wide-spread pecuniary reverses compelling the removal of many patients to State and municipal asylums," [29] and, in 1864, a general advance was made in the rates charged. In consequence the monthly income rose from $4,568 in January, 1864, to $8,629 in January, 1865. Although the New York Hospital engaged extensively in the treatment of wounded soldiers, the Bloomingdale records are singularly free from reference to members of the military forces among the patients.

The period of 1852 to 1877 was one of great activity in institutional construction and organization throughout the country, and much of the effort of the physicians of asylums was directed to problems not directly concerned with clinical and scientific work. So impressed was Dr. Bucknill with some of the conditions and practices which he observed at the asylums that, in his published account of his visits, he stated that the "superintendents of American Asylums are far better men than their present work would indicate." He found the New York and Philadelphia asylums "lamentably deficient in resources." [30]

The programs of the Association of Medical Superintendents of American Asylums furnish a guide to the subjects of particular interest in this period. Although institutional architecture, internal arrangements and economy received considerable attention at the meetings, the programs contained in increasing numbers communications and discussions relating to the study and treatment of patients. By 1860, treatment by venesection, tartar emetic, and shock-producing cold baths seemed to be almost entirely discarded. Salivation by mercury was still a subject of discussion in 1865. The treatment of excited and violent patients was given much attention, and the question of mechanical restraint, strong rooms, padded rooms, covered crib bedsteads and other restraining apparatus, occasioned much discussion. Dr. John Conolly's book on *The*

[28] In 1866 Dr. Willard Parker, one of the physicians of the New York Hospital was elected president of the Board of Trustees of the institution, succeeding Dr. Valentine Mott. S. W. Francis, *Biographical Sketches of Distinguished Living New York Surgeons* (New York, 1866), p. 150.

[29] Physician's report for 1861.

[30] Bucknill, *Notes on Asylums for the Insane in America* (London, 1876), pp. xii and xi.

Treatment of the Insane without Mechanical Restraint, which was published in 1856, and Dr. R. Gardiner Hill's work on the same subject, which was published in 1857, excited much interest and difference of opinion. At the 1854 meeting of the association, Dr. Brown spoke of his experience with prolonged warm baths in the treatment of excited patients, but his request for information in regard to the experience of others met with no response. Drugs mentioned in the course of discussions at the meetings were opium, conium, belladonna, hyoscyamus, gelseminum, bromides, chloral, digitalis, phosphorus, nitrite of amyl, and ergot (in chorea). Two types of feeding tubes were in use; the English tube contained a spiral wire and was rather stiff and hard, the French was soft and flexible.[31] One speaker considered brandy punch to be a satisfactory substitute for the tube, as, when placed to the lips, it "has a very fascinating influence."

Much interest was manifested in the medical jurisprudence of insanity. Numerous papers were presented; cases cited in the discussion indicated that the speakers had experience in testifying as experts. From time to time attempts were made to draft a law relating to criminal responsibility and insanity with a view to its adoption by the different states. The members were, however, unable to agree on the terms of the law, and in 1873 when a proposal to renew the project was made, it was considered by many to be futile and was abandoned. Epilepsy, together with its relation to crime, was another subject of particular interest. "Emotional disorders," hysteria, hypochondriasis, goitre, kleptomania, amnesia, hallucinations, "emotional insanity," and aphasia, were also discussed. In 1868 Dr. Edwin H. Van Deusen, superintendent of the state asylum at Kalamazoo, Michigan, used the term neurasthenia, which was new at the time, in a paper on "Forms of Nervous Prostration Culminating in Insanity." [32] An article by Dr. A. O. Kellogg on "Reciprocal Influence of the Physical Organization and Mental Manifestations," [33] in 1855, seemed to foreshadow later views relating to physical types and mental reactions. Considerable attention was directed to inebriety and its treatment. There was a difference of opinion as to whether it should be regarded as a disease or a vice. The association was interested in the establishment and management of special asylums for inebriates. Several were established; the one located at Binghamton, New York, in 1859 was afterwards transformed into a state asylum for the insane. An "Association for the Cure of Inebriates" was organized in 1870. In 1863

31 *Am. J. Insanity,* XVI (1859), 73.
32 *Ibid.,* XXV (1868), 445.
33 *Ibid.,* XII (1855), 30, 111, 305.

communications relating to anatomical studies began to appear on the program and in the *Journal of Insanity*. Dr. E. R. Hun was appointed pathologist at the New York State Asylum at Utica in 1868, and was succeeded by Theodore Deeke, his technician, in 1873. Dr. Gray, the superintendent of the asylum, considered that physical disease was invariably the cause of mental disorder, and he expected to prove this by anatomical investigations.[34] Much attention was given to general paresis and brain syphilis. A review of a work on the prevention of mental illness [35] appeared in the *Journal* in 1859, and in the same year an article with the title "Mental Hygiene" was contributed by Dr. George Cook. When Dr. Ray's book of the same title was published in 1863, a reviewer in the *Journal of Insanity* considered that it was based on theories of a purely materialistic philosophy and the doctrine of phrenology. Spiritualistic phenomena were discussed at some of the association meetings. In 1855, Dr. Brown proposed that the members should attend "a circle." Phrenology also still lingered as an influence in conceptions of the functions of the brain. Other subjects discussed at the meetings were suicide, heredity, surgery in the insane, pellagra, and senile, traumatic, and juvenile insanity. In 1855, a communication relating to decayed teeth as a cause of insanity was presented. Some attention was given to the question of uniform statistics, on a national and even international scale.

Very little periodical literature relating to mental disease was produced in America during this period. In 1867 *The Journal of Psychological Medicine* was established with Dr. W. A. Hammond as editor. It survived only until 1872, and was resumed in 1874 with the title *The Psychological and Medico-Legal Journal. The Journal of Nervous and Mental Diseases* was established in 1874 and still flourishes under the able editorship of Dr. Smith Ely Jelliffe, who in 1898 was for a short time in the service of Bloomingdale Asylum. No general treatise on mental disease by an American author was published. Dr. Hammond's *Treatise on Diseases of the Nervous System,* which was published in 1871, contained, however, a chapter on "Insanity." A popular book entitled *Plain Talk about Insanity,* by Dr. T. W. Fisher of Boston, was published in 1872. Griesinger's *Treatise,* translated into English in 1867, exercised considerable influence on psychiatric thought and practice in America.

[34] John P. Gray, "The Dependence of Insanity on Physical Disease," *Am. J. Insanity,* XXVII (1871), 377.

[35] George Robinson, *On the Prevention and Treatment of Mental Disorders* (London, 1859).

PART SIX

A Medically Directed Private Charity
1877-1894

XXIV: RELATION TO STATE AND CITY

THE number of patients in residence at Bloomingdale Asylum increased from 162 at the close of 1877 to 302 at the close of 1893. The total number treated was also increased from 255 in 1877 to 470 in 1893, and the number admitted from 81 to 164. The appointment of Dr. Charles H. Nichols as medical superintendent in May, 1877, inaugurated this period of expansion and of renewed activity and progress in the life of the asylum. It will be recalled that he had been resident physician from 1849 to 1852, and during that brief period had proposed extensive improvements, some of which were accomplished after he left. He resigned to accept the position of medical superintendent of an asylum which the United States Government was preparing to establish in the District of Columbia.[1] In this position, which he held for twenty-five years, he displayed unusual ability in planning and supervising construction, and in organizing and administering a great institution. He was held in high esteem by his medical colleagues, and at the time of his reappointment at Bloomingdale he had, for four successive years, been elected president of the Association of Medical Superintendents of American Institutions for the Insane (now the American Psychiatric Association), and he continued to occupy that position for two more years. While at Washington he visited Bloomingdale occasionally, and the governors were no doubt well informed concerning his qualifications and achievements. When Dr. Brown retired, Dr. Nichols was apparently the only candidate considered for the position, and he was appointed at the meeting at which Dr. Brown's resignation was accepted. He was no doubt remarkably well qualified by experience for undertaking the further expansion of the service and its eventual removal to another location, which was known to be inevitable.

Although, in practice, medical direction of administration had, for many years, been gradually extended into all the departments, the form of organization had not been officially changed. The appointment of Dr. Nichols, therefore, with the title of Medical Superintendent, firmly

1 Now St. Elizabeths Hospital. See p. 251 note.

established the medical character of the asylum, and opened the way for the development of a sounder and more effective psychiatric service. On May 1, 1877, the Board of Governors adopted the following amendment to the By-laws:

> That Sec. 1 under the head of Physician be amended so as to read as follows,
>
> There shall be elected annually by the Board of Governors at the regular meeting in the month of June a Physician who shall be a married man to be called the Medical Superintendent of the Asylum.
>
> That Sec. 3 under the same head be amended so as to read as follows,
>
> He shall be the chief executive officer of the Institution and shall be responsible for the proper discipline and government thereof and for the medical and moral treatment of the patients.
>
> He shall have control over all the other officers and servants subject only to the direction of the Asylum Committee. He shall nominate to the Committee such assistant Physicians as may be required and also suitable persons for Steward and Housekeeper and shall have power to suspend any such officers at his discretion.
>
> He shall have authority under the direction of the Committee to hire and discharge all attendants upon the patients and all other servants employed in and about the Asylum.
>
> He shall make requisitions for such supplies as he may deem necessary and if required shall purchase the same under the direction of the Committee.
>
> On motion of Mr. Trimble it was unanimously Resolved that the By Law requiring a month's notice of action upon a proposed amendment be suspended and that the above ordinance be now considered. The ordinance was then adopted and ordered to be recorded in the Book of ordinances.

The title of Warden was changed to Steward, and the position was entirely subordinated to the medical superintendent. The first to occupy this position was James R. Lathrop, who was appointed in 1878 and resigned in 1884 to become superintendent of Roosevelt Hospital.

Dr. Nichols entered into the duties of the new position on July 7, 1877. Fresh from a service in which his attention had been directed principally to obtaining adequate accommodations and facilities for the treatment of patients, it was natural that his first consideration at Bloomingdale should be along the same lines, and evidently there was ample scope for his interest and capability. At the meeting of the Asylum Committee on August 4, he presented his views on heating and ventilation. These were subjects which had greatly concerned the governors since the institution was established. Dr. Nichols recommended that no further attempts be made to operate or extend the existing distributed equipment, and that all fires throughout the different buildings be dispensed with and a central heating plant provided. He had recommended this in 1851 also. An appropriation was promptly made for the erection of a suitable building for the purpose, and also for a central kitchen in a separate building, with a second story to be a suitable hall for entertainments. This building was located so that the entrance to the hall was at the ground level, and the porch from the old New York Hospital was installed at its doorway. The adjoining laundry was raised two stories, and a dormitory for maids was provided in the upper story. In September, 1878, an additional appropriation was made to equip and furnish the new buildings, for passages to connect the kitchen with the halls, for tramways for the conveyance of food to the dumb-waiters, and for air ducts leading from the fans in the heating plant. These ducts provided ventilation for the sewers and plumbing system and were connected with the ventilation section of the central smokestack. There were no traps in the toilets, the downward draft created by the fans being considered sufficient to exclude emanations and to aid in ventilating the rooms. The new assembly room was formally opened on March 20, 1879, with a special evening entertainment in honor of the governors. This was "numerously attended by the Governors, including the venerable vice-president of the Board, Mr. Willetts." Several were accompanied by members of their families. The hall was, thereafter, used regularly for entertainments for the patients.

During the first eight or nine years of Dr. Nichols's administration, the physical condition and appearance of the buildings and grounds and the administrative standards of the asylum were completely transformed. He was so well qualified in regard to building requirements that a contractor was seldom employed. A former employee [2] has a vivid recollection of the doctor, wearing a top hat and a long black coat, high up on a ladder inspecting new construction. The annual report for 1878 mentioned more than twenty-five pieces of work which had been accomplished for the improvement of the sanitation, comfort, durability, appearance, and convenience of the buildings, grounds, and facilities. Some of the principal items were the replacement of the old stone sewers and cesspools with well laid pipes and cement construction. The water supply was improved and better fire protection provided. In 1882 a telephone was installed at a charge of $186 a year. Walls, fences, and roads were renovated and extended. A tower clock and cupola were a gift from the treasurer of the Society, Mr. Macy. The bell struck the hours and half hours from 7 A. M. to 7 P. M. and was then silent until the

[2] James Welch, blacksmith and locksmith 1878–1937.

next morning. The three illuminated dials were visible from every hall at all hours. This description corresponds to a considerable extent with that of the present tower clock, and, in fact, Mr. Macy's clock was transferred to the tower of the main building at White Plains. In October, 1879, Dr. Nichols presented a "schedule of further Improvements necessary to put Bloomingdale Asylum in proper condition for the satisfactory residence and treatment of patients of culture and means." This consisted of fourteen items directed principally to renovations and renewals. In July, 1880, he was able to report that the greater part of the work had been completed. Among the more important alterations was the complete replacement of the heat distribution equipment throughout the buildings. Flues which had previously served as chimneys for furnaces, stoves, and fireplaces were found to be suitable for conveying warm air from steam radiators in the basements.

Another important accomplishment was the reconstruction and refurnishing of the Lodges which had been the object of complaint and criticism for many years. The walls of these buildings were replastered. The dining rooms were reconstructed and provided with dumb-waiters and hot and cold water. Floors were renewed and sound-proofed with ashes between the joists; partitions were removed to increase the size of bedrooms, and, to provide accommodations for private nurses, connecting doors were installed between some of the rooms. Lavatories and water closets were reconstructed and their number increased. The whole place was painted "in cheerful colors," and "appropriately and handsomely furnished." These buildings were cheaply constructed, but were reported by Dr. Nichols to have now "an air of respectability, cheerfulness, and comfort, and are fairly convenient and satisfactory," though still below the standard that would be provided in new buildings. Similar improvements were made in other parts of the asylum.

The windows in many halls were lengthened, and the area around the main building was extended so as to render the basement "dry and properly habitable." The cement floors of some of the basement rooms were replaced with wood under which an excavation paved with concrete was made for the passage of pipes. These rooms were considered to be lighter than most rooms in the compact part of the city, and suitable for lodgings for "out-ward" employees and for industrial and administrative purposes. In 1885 a substantial brick building was erected as a general mechanics shop. The second story of this building was arranged for lodging male "out-ward" employees, and the cellar was used for meats, vegetables, and other foods "requiring cool, sweet air." The transfer of employees to the lodgings thus furnished released space in the basement of the east building which, it was considered, would, after means of easy egress to the open air had been provided, be suitable for "aged, feeble, quiet patients to whom it is a great boon to be able to go out and in without ascending or descending one or more flights of stairs." This basement provision, however, proved to be a source of some embarrassment when, a few years later, an investigation was made by a committee of the legislature.[3] A third story on the old chapel, and the addition of two stories on the bay connected with it, provided a direct communication between the front and east buildings and space for billiard rooms accessible from each hall. A Mansard story on the east building provided accommodations for fifteen patients of the chronic class who were considered to "have the requisite vigor to ascend three flights of stairs," and in May, 1886, the Asylum Committee recorded that these quarters were proving "of great advantage, being very light and in every way desirable." The attic story of the wings of the main building was finished and furnished in 1883, one wing providing accommodations for about twenty attendants and releasing sleeping quarters on the halls for about fifteen more female patients.

In making provision for adding to the capacity of the asylum, consideration was constantly given to better classification. A substantial contribution to this consideration was made in 1880 by the opening of the Green Memorial Building. This was donated by the widow and other residuary legatees of John C. Green, who, at the time of his death in 1875, was president of the Society. It was for women patients, preferably recent and probably curable cases; discrimination was to be made "in favor of those of good character and of such antecedents, education, and refinement, as to render a hospital of more select character than a public institution necessary to their comfort." [4] The cost of the building was $130,000. Before it was opened an additional gift from Mrs. Green and the other residuary legatees provided an endowment of $200,000, the income to be used for "the maintenance, treatment and support, in whole, or in part," of selected patients "unable in person or by the assistance of their friends or family to adequately provide for their own support." [5] The opening of this building was regarded by Dr. Nichols as "the most important event of the year." It was connected with the west wing of the main building to which it corresponded in architectural

[3] Investigation by Committee on Taxation and Retrenchment of the State Senate, p. 312 this volume.

[4] Annual Report for 1880.

[5] *Minutes of the Governors*, March 2, 1880.

design. It was attractively furnished and provided liberal accommodations for patients at the higher rates. Dr. Nichols, in his annual report, considered it unnecessary to describe the building, as he planned to prepare a special report on this and other structural improvements, with illustrations.[6] Unfortunately no copy of this report has been found, and there is in the minutes no record of its presentation. All that can be said of the building, therefore, is that there were four stories above a high basement, all of which were occupied by patients. The opening of the Green Building was followed by an increase in the number as well as the character of the applications. The governors in their annual report for 1882 attributed this increase also "to the freedom with which the Governors have been able to respond to the many demands for increased appliances for the efficient treatment, the comfort, and the diversion of the inmates, intelligently utilized as these means have been by the skill and devotion of the Medical Superintendent and his assistants."

Dr. Nichols considered that only second in importance to the opening of the Green Building was the transposition of the sexes in their location in the buildings. As the most suitable location for the Green Building was found to be on the west side, it was decided that it would be advisable to assign all of the accommodations on that side to the women, and to transfer the men to the east side. It was considered also that the sex which spent more time indoors, and was confined to a somewhat narrower range when out-of-doors, was most entitled to the more picturesque and varied views that were to be seen from the west side accommodations.[7]

Although the additional accommodations facilitated classification of patients, this was not yet considered satisfactory, especially for the men. In March, 1884, the Asylum Committee reported that "as the Asylum now stands, the classification of patients is not as thorough as would be desirable, there being but eleven grades of women and nine of men, while as many as twenty on each side of the house would be advantageous." This condition was at least slightly relieved in 1885 by a gift of $25,000 from the president of the Society, Mr. Macy. It was designed for the erection of a building for "a few gentlemen who are able and willing to pay for such special accommodations as it will afford." [8] Mr. Macy hoped that he would live to see the building completed under the supervision of Dr. Nichols, "as I think him peculiarly

[6] Annual Reports, 1878 and 1879.

[7] Annual Report for 1880.

[8] *Ibid.*, 1885.

well qualified for the undertaking."[9] It was completed in 1886, and was described in the annual report as "a very spacious and substantially built edifice; its interior finish and furniture are handsome and convenient, . . . its sanitary arrangements the most complete that are known to sanitary science." It was located east and slightly south of the main building.[10]

In his annual report for 1887, Dr. Nichols reported that the villa had been occupied by eleven patients, and that it had been praised by "many experts in provisions for the insane." He considered that "excepting an infirmary and mortuary, and three or four cottages for the isolated treatment of a few patients, as many buildings have now been erected on these limited grounds as they will properly accommodate,"[11] and in July, 1886, the Inspecting Committee reported that "the whole Institution in its present condition is now worthy of its past history and reputation, and the Committee recommend that at an early day the whole Board be invited to visit and inspect the remodeled Institution." At this time the asylum had evidently reached the peak of its development and activity within the city. Not only the buildings but also the grounds had been greatly improved. Heavy masonry walls, or substantial iron or wooden fences, enclosed the whole property. A drive and walk a mile long encircled the grounds inside the walls and fences, providing an excellent means of systematic exercise for the patients. Many trees and shrubs had been planted, and the courts and shelter houses were kept in good repair and beautified. The north section of the property, termed "the woods," the drainage of which had baffled repeated efforts from an early period, was at last thoroughly drained, producing " a delightful and salubrious park." At this period the property consisted of about forty acres, and extended from 112th to 120th Streets between Tenth Avenue and the Boulevard. Some lots west of the Boulevard were also owned by the Society. Part of the property was still used as a farm. The 103 odoriferous swine, however, were dispensed with in 1880. In 1889 the land between 112th and 114th Streets was sold at auction for $501,400.[12]

Questions concerning the relation of the state to the asylum, to taxation and to the opening of streets through the property continued to be a source of constant concern to the governors. In January, 1878, the governors received the following communication from the president of the Department of Charities and Correction of New York City:—

[9] *Minutes of the Governors,* March 3, 1885. Mr. Macy died in May, 1887.
[10] This building still stands east of the Low Library of Columbia University.
[11] Annual Report for 1885.
[12] *Minutes of the Governors,* May 2 and 7, 1889.

To the Governors of the Society of the New York Hospital

GENTLEMEN.

The overcrowded state of the several Lunatic asylums within the Department of Charities of the County of New York, and the difficulty of obtaining appropriations of a sufficient magnitude to secure enlargements commensurate with the rapid increase of the Insane, lead us to address your Board for the purpose of ascertaining whether you can not aid us in providing additional accommodations for the pauper insane of the County of New York.

Understanding that in the early years of the New York Hospital pauper lunatics were received in its wards, we accordingly ask whether some portion of the Bloomingdale Asylum could not be set apart for that class of patients, or some suitable building for their accommodation erected within its grounds by your Board.

An early reply to this communication is solicited.

Very Respectfully
THOMAS G. BRENNAN, *President.*[18]

To this, after much consideration, the governors replied as follows:

Thomas G. Brennan Esq.
President Board of Commissioners
Department of Public Charities & Corrections

SIR.

Your communication of 21st ultimo addressed to the Board of Governors of the New York Hospital, was referred by that body to the Asylum Committee, and has today been made the subject of careful consideration by them.

In the earlier days of its history the Bloomingdale Asylum was able to treat and did treat a large number of pauper patients, assisted by an annual grant of $10,000 by the Legislature of the State.

About the middle of the present century the continually increasing demands upon the Asylum by the class of patients for whose benefit it was more particularly intended viz: those able to pay a small sum towards their support, had become so pressing, and the bounty of the State having been withdrawn it became necessary to limit as far as practicable the admission of patients to those of that class. Up to the present time its wards have been thus filled to their full capacity, a few being always retained as free patients, and many more at a rate far below the outlay incurred in their support.

While the management of the Asylum are desirous of contributing to the public good so far as their resources will allow, they feel that they will best fulfill their mission by pursuing at least for the present the feeling above indicated.

There are however improvements already in progress looking to the accommodation of an increased number of patients. In the light of experience it seems probable that the demands upon the Asylum will keep pace with

18 This and the governors' reply copied from the *Minutes of the Asylum Committee,* March 2, 1878.

the contemplated enlargement, but should the result be otherwise a still further extension of its benefits to the purely indigent will become a subject well worthy of consideration.

Upon receipt of this the president of the Department of Public Charities sent copies of the correspondence to the State Commissioner in lunacy, with the following note:—

Honorable John Ordronaux, *State Commissioner in Lunacy:*

DEAR SIR—As you are well aware the several lunatic asylums belonging to the county of New York under our care have long been over-crowded, despite every effort made by us to secure additional accommodations for the pauper insane.

Being informed that in the early part of the century the Society of the New York Hospital received annual appropriations from the State for the purpose of providing accommodations for the pauper insane of this county, we accordingly addressed them a note, asking whether they could not aid us in any way in ministering to the wants of this class for whom we now have such inadequate means of providing. Their reply gives us no encouragement for any relief in that quarter, and we accordingly feel it our duty to report these facts to you, believing that you will see in this an endeavor on our part to ameliorate the condition of the insane beyond the degree now permitted by our means.

I beg leave to inclose herewith copies of the communications addressed them and their reply thereto.

Respectfully yours,
THOMAS S. BRENNAN, *President.*

Thereupon the commissioner in lunacy, in March, 1878, made a report to the legislature [14] the purport of which was that "the several acts of the Legislature of 1806 and 1816, granting subsidies to the Society of the New York Hospital for the purpose of founding, erecting, and maintaining an Asylum for the Indigent Insane of the City and County of New York, constituted the State the original founder of the Bloomingdale Asylum," [15] and that, consequently, the state had power to appoint a board of governors for its management. After an extensive presentation of facts and arguments in support of his opinion, the commissioner recommended

that it be referred to the Attorney General to determine—First.—What duty the corporation of the New York Hospital owe to the State in respect to making provision for the pauper insane of the county of New York; Second.

[14] Report of State Commissioner in Lunacy to the legislature on the relations of the State to the Society of the New York Hospital, March 27, 1878. (Vol. I, Annual Reports of the State Commissioner in Lunacy, Senate, No. 17, State Library, Albany, N.Y.) The two preceding letters are contained in this report.

[15] *Ibid.*, Supplemental Brief.

—What legislation is necessary to enforce such duty, and, Third.—Whether the State has power to appoint, as founder of the Bloomingdale Asylum, a board of governors for its management.

The Attorney General, in expressing his opinion, pointed out that the Society of the New York Hospital had never in its history been required by its charter or otherwise to receive patients without compensation. A law was passed, in 1809,[16] which authorized the authorities of the several counties to contract with the Society for the admission and treatment of "pauper lunatics," at the lowest rates at which patients were received. This practice was continued until provision was made at Bellevue, and "when other lunatic asylums had been erected in the State." There had been, he stated, no "breach or neglect of any duty owing to the State or the County of New York." The average cost of $12.05 per week, he stated, "appears to be high, but it is claimed to be only an equivalent for the comforts and attention furnished, and it has not been shown to be an abuse, or a subject of complaint." [17] In reply to the third question, the Attorney General considered that, in appropriating funds for the establishment of Bloomingdale, "the State gave these sums, not to found or establish a society for the care of the insane, but to aid an existing corporation chartered for that purpose, in conducting its operations on a larger scale." He added, however, that

whether the State can be regarded as the founder of the Bloomingdale Asylum from the circumstance that it has made donations of money to a private charity, or whether assuming the relation of founder to exist, the right to displace its chartered management, by legislative enactment, and appoint other governors, are questions which may afford scope for much interesting discussion, but are not now material. I therefore express no opinion and make no recommendation upon those points.[18]

In 1884 the city was prohibited by law from opening the streets, 115th to 119th, which would traverse asylum property.[19] In 1886, 114th Street was opened and the half of that portion of Bloomingdale Road adjoining the asylum grounds, which had been purchased by the governors for $250 when the road was closed in 1878, was fenced in. In 1886, however, agitation over taxation, the opening of streets, and the removal of the asylum from the city, assumed more formidable dimensions. A bill providing for repeal of the special acts which exempted the property

16 See p. 73. 17 The rate for "pauper lunatics" was never more than $3 per week.

18 Opinion of the Attorney-General of the State of New York, on certain matters concerning The Society of the New York Hospital and The Bloomingdale Asylum, April 9, 1879. (Report to the Senate of N.Y. State.)

19 *Minutes of the Governors,* March 4, 1884.

from taxation was introduced into the legislature and committed to the Committee of the Whole.[20] This bill provided for taxation of the asylum property, with the exemption of $10,000 for each poor insane person committed to the asylum by the Department of Public Charities and Correction of New York City, and cared for without charge for one year previous to the preparation of the assessment rolls, and proportionate for part of the year. In their endeavor to defeat the bill, the governors issued a circular entitled "A Bad Bill," in which they explained the character of the institution and protested against what seemed to be an attempt to compel the admission of "insane thieves, vagrants, and prostitutes," and to reduce it to the status of an institution solely for paupers. They also, in March, 1886, issued a communication addressed "To the Public" entitled "Shall the Bloomingdale Asylum Be Destroyed?" This presented an historic review of the asylum and of the policy pursued in the admission and treatment of patients and the manner in which the charitable object of the institution was established and maintained. The governors explained the necessity of an open area for the seclusion, recreation, and exercise of patients, and protested that the opening of streets through the property would result in the *"destruction* of the Institution." They objected to being "singled out" for taxation while other institutions with no greater claim were exempt. The bill failed of passage, and though again introduced at the next session of the legislature, it was never passed.

In February, 1888, a memorial was presented to the State Senate by the Morningside Park Association, "a voluntary association of persons interested in real estate," in the vicinity of the asylum. The memorial requested the senate to investigate certain questions relating to the Society of the New York Hospital and its management of the Bloomingdale Asylum.

1st. Whether the governors of the hospital deny to the State Board of Charities the right of visiting the asylum. 2nd. Whether the governors have the right of perpetual succession. 3rd. Whether the asylum is conducted as a public charity, and whether or not free patients are admitted there, or have been during the past five years. 4th. What property belongs to said society. 5th. As to what streets are now closed; and what street or streets should be opened. 6th. Whether the asylum is detrimental to property in the neighborhood, or unsafe for persons residing, or who might reside there. 7th. Whether the said asylum is or is not properly conducted, and whether its finances are judiciously and providently administered. 8th. Whether any madhouse or asylum for lunatics should be maintained in the city of New York.

20 Assembly Bill No. 213.

The memorial was referred to the Committee on Taxation and Retrenchment of the Senate, which on March 10th proceeded to conduct an investigation. Both the memorialists and the governors employed counsel and much testimony was taken. The investigation was continued for about a month. The testimony presented by the memorialists was directed to proving the statements and implications contained in the memorial.[21] Those who testified were practically all real-estate owners and brokers interested in neighboring property. The aim was to show that the asylum "casts a blight upon the whole west side of the city and prevents the erection of buildings in its vicinity," and that the expenditure was so unnecessarily extravagant, the income from patients so great, and the number of free patients so small that the institution could not be considered a public charity, and should therefore be taxed. To prove extravagance and injudicious financial management, comparison was made with the New York City Asylum, at which the cost of maintenance of 1,693 patients for a year was $203,302, while at Bloomingdale the cost of maintenance of 272 patients for the same year was $219,887. It was also asserted that the State Board of Charities had been denied right of visitation of the asylum. It was requested that power should be given to the Board of Street Openings to open various streets across the property whenever they thought proper, and that the asylum be removed "within a reasonable time."

In reply to these allegations and implications, the Society presented testimony to show that the development of the area was retarded by its relative inaccessibility and inadequate transit facilities, and not the asylum. The testimony of real-estate dealers and of the City Park Commissioner was presented in proof of this. Dr. Edward Cowles of the McLean Asylum and Dr. Stearns of the Hartford Retreat compared these institutions, of which they were the medical superintendents, with Bloomingdale, showing that there were no extravagances at the latter, that their plans of financing and administration were similar, and that the asylum could not be successfully operated if the area were reduced and streets were opened through it. Dr. Alfred L. Loomis, a practicing physician of the city, testified as to the necessity of an asylum for the mentally ill in the city; he knew of "no asylum that is better conducted than the Bloomingdale, and, I think, as far as my experience goes, that it receives the poor and the rich." He considered it "one of the most

21 See Testimony Taken before the Senate Committee on Taxation and Retrenchment, New York, March 10, 1888–April 7, 1888. (Printed Reports Relative to Bloomingdale, N.Y. Hospital.)

noble charities New York has ever had," and felt that it was of public benefit when patients who were able to pay were expected to do so. It was quite important that in a large city like New York there should be an institution to which the acute insane could be readily taken. There were accident hospitals and there should similarly be "acute insane provisions." Dr. E. C. Spitzka, a specialist in nervous diseases, testified that he had sent many patients to Bloomingdale, and none had been refused admission. Some had been admitted for as low a rate as two dollars a week. He considered the average rate received from patients to be scarcely sufficient to pay the expense of adequate treatment. He regarded the asylum as a charitable institution, and added, "We should not know in this city what to do without Bloomingdale." He felt that the asylum was in the right place for the present. "In my experience, they have always preferred to take curable . . . cases, and if they took chronic or incurable cases, they have taken them upon trial, with the proviso that they were to transfer them to the proper institutions when the time came." Dr. Nichols testified that "we should not hesitate to take a patient for nothing, or whatever the patient was able to pay," particularly if the case was "recent and presumptively curable."

Merritt Trimble, a member of the Asylum Committee of the Board of Governors, explained fully the form of organization, administration and financing of the asylum and of the other branches of the New York Hospital. He referred to the classification of patients by which the professional treatment and dietary were in all cases the same; patients were located with reference to their condition and needs rather than to the rate received—those paying the highest rates might be given better accommodations and, possibly, private attendance. Access to and inspection of the asylum by the State Board of Charities had never been refused by the governors. However, the administration of the institution by the Board of Governors was stipulated by the charter, and a license under the State Board was not required.[22] With a view to showing that, although much of its income was derived from rates paid by the patients, the asylum was a public charity and therefore not subject to taxation, it was claimed that

> Charity means not simply alms . . . but it means relief to the distressed. . . . An institution which, taken as a whole, . . . devoted to public charity its entire income, including that received from charges to patients . . . is, in the strictest and best sense, a public charity. . . . Any definition of charity

[22] Opinion of William M. Evarts and Charles O'Conor, August 11, 1873. See p. 281.

which would exclude the idea of relief or assistance would exclude a large part of the wise charities of the world.

In support of this view, various cases in which it had been judicially considered were cited. One of these concerned the Massachusetts General Hospital, which operates, at McLean Asylum, a service identical with that of Bloomingdale. It was in that case stated by the judge that

its affairs are conducted for a great public service, that of administering to the comfort of the sick, without any expectation on the part of those immediately interested in the corporation of receiving any compensation which will enure to their own benefit, and without the right to receive such compensation. This establishes its character as a public charity. The fact that its funds are supplemented by such amounts as it may receive from those who are able to pay . . . for the accommodation they receive, does not render it less a public charity.

In their report to the Legislature in May, 1888,[23] the Committee on Taxation and Retrenchment found that the Society had not denied to any officer of the state, or properly authorized board or body, the right of inspection. As to the assumption by the Society "that the management of the charity . . . was confided by charter to the governors," the committee found that "there were no subsisting questions between the authorities of the hospital and any public board or officer of the State, and it seems hardly necessary . . . to assume to dispose of theoretical public questions, which had not been shown to exist and which might never arise." In regard to whether the asylum was conducted as a public charity, the committee reported that "it cannot be said . . . that there is a particular charity known as the Bloomingdale Asylum, because the asylum is but a branch of the charitable work of the Society of the New York Hospital. That institution is *the charity*." Various details from the testimony and the numerous exhibits presented at the hearings were cited, and the committee reported that

both free patients and patients who pay moderate sums have been and are taken at the asylum, and that no reason has been shown why the New York Hospital, in all its branches, should not now be considered, as it has heretofore been considered, a public charity in the true sense of the term, and entitled to the support of the State and of the public.

In regard to exemption from taxation, the committee considered that whether any part of the property was not used for the purposes of the charity was "purely a question between the local assessors and the

23 New York State Senate, Doc. 61.

corporation." In regard to the effect of the asylum on property in the surrounding area, the committee said that it seemed "to be a question whether public necessity demands the removal of the asylum at this time, or whether there is, as is claimed by the authorities of the hospital, no pressing necessity for such removal." The committee added, however, that they had

> reached the conclusion, on the whole, that under existing circumstances, the public interest would not be subserved by the cutting through of streets to the injury, if not to the destruction of the buildings upon the asylum property, or the bringing of the buildings of the asylum into close proximity to public streets, and that in the present condition of affairs there is no pressing need for the opening of the streets [115th and 116th] referred to in the memorial.

The committee also reported that no evidence was produced to warrant the charge of mismanagement of the finances of the asylum, nor to sustain the charge of extravagance. They considered "from the evidence of experts and otherwise, that there is no doubt of the good work accomplished by the asylum at the present time, and that its destruction would be a serious injury to the city of New York." They suggested, however, that as the governors had for some time past been anticipating removal, and that within a few years the opening of the closed streets would become a necessity, "such preparations be made for the removal of the asylum to some other locality, as can be made without detriment to the spirit, aim, and sound financial administration of the charity."

The newspapers of the city also recommended that the asylum be removed. The *Times* of April 8, 1888, commented that

> Bloomingdale Asylum ought to move on and locate itself where property is less valuable and where it will not be in the way of the city's development; and if it insists on staying where it is it should pay taxes on some of its vast amount of real estate, the value of which is due to the city's growth and not to anything which it has done.

Apparently the writer was not aware of what such an institution contributed to making growth of the city worth while. The *World* believed that it was "thanks to the World's work in pointing out some of the abuses in that institution" that the investigation of Bloomingdale Asylum by a Senate Committee had been undertaken.[24] Headlines in this paper on March 7, 1888, characterized Bloomingdale as "The Retreat for Rich Insane People, and the Poor who may not enter its doors help to support it—A Wealthy and Powerful Corporation Buoyed up by the

[24] New York *World*, March 10, 1888.

Public Purse for Private Gain." It was plainly intimated in the article that the governors had the right under the law governing the institution to administer the property for their own benefit. It was also asserted that "Time and again charges have been made that people have been sent to Bloomingdale by their relatives in order to get rid of them." After the Senate Committee had made its report, however, the *World*, on May 11, under the heading "A Victory for Bloomingdale," gave a fair resumé of the conclusions, without comment.

Numerous references in the minutes of the Board of Governors and of the Asylum Committee, and in the annual reports show the earnest purpose of the governors to administer the asylum as a truly charitable institution. They considered that to render financial aid to worthy mentally ill persons who were unable to bear all or perhaps any of the expense was a more effective service than merely to duplicate the work of public institutions. In March, 1884, the governors requested the Asylum Committee, by resolution, to make a report on the question of receiving free patients. At the next meeting the committee reported that the asylum was overcrowded, with 268 patients in accommodations that could only with some inconvenience provide for more than 240. More than half the applicants during the previous month had been declined because of lack of room, and the committee were "now finding forced upon them more urgently than at any former period during the history of the Institution, the necessity of discrimination in favor of those, whose cases present the strongest claims, regard being had to probable curability and personal requirements, based upon education and previous manner of life." They feared that any indiscriminate infusion of free patients would be likely to aggravate the difficulty. The amount spent not only for the support of free patients, but also of those who were paying rates below the cost of maintenance, represented the charitable aid extended to this class of patients. Many of the free patients were pay patients when admitted, and when their families or friends ceased to pay the charges the burden was assumed by the institution; some of them could be transferred to public institutions, but the change might well prove a greater hardship to these particular patients than to those who were originally admitted free. The committee felt, therefore, that the indiscriminate admission of free patients for long periods might involve the rejection of others who were as much in need of treatment and were able, at least for part of the time, to pay something towards the cost. They considered that under the present system the best use was made of the accommodations, and recommended that an appropriation applied to an increase of accommodations instead of for the indiscriminate admission of free patients "would tend towards effecting the object sought . . . in a more enlightened manner, and with more eventual beneficent results." [25]

[25] *Minutes of the Asylum Committee,* March 29, 1884; *Minutes of the Governors,* April 1, 1884.

XXV

MEDICAL SERVICE, 1877–1894

At this period the standards of medical study and treatment of the mentally ill in America did not in asylum service demand as high a degree of personal psychotherapeutic attention as at present. Consequently, no great necessity seems to have been felt for an increase in the number of physicians to keep pace with the increasing number of patients. Although the number of patients admitted increased from 81 in 1877 to 176 in 1885, and the total number treated from 255 to 420, the number of physicians remained the same as it had been in 1869. In 1885, however, the position of clinical assistant was added, the period of service being six months and the salary fifty dollars a month. A further addition was made in 1886 when Dr. Samuel B. Lyon was appointed assistant medical superintendent. He did not participate regularly in the clinical service.

Some advance apparently occurred in the qualifications of the physicians appointed. All of the assistant physicians, and many of the clinical assistants, had been in the service of other asylums. Dr. Sanger Brown (1880–1886), Dr. Henry S. Williams (1889–1892), Dr. Charles E. Woodbury (1880–1881), Dr. William E. Dold (1881–1898), Dr. Charles E. Atwood (1892–1905), and Dr. Albert Durham (1892–1914) had already had considerable experience. Some of those who resigned did so in order to accept advanced positions elsewhere. Dr. William B. Goldsmith (1877–1881) became medical superintendent of the Danvers State Hospital in Massachusetts and was afterwards appointed to a corresponding position in the Butler Hospital. In 1882 Dr. Woodbury was appointed medical superintendent of the Rhode Island Hospital and later became the state inspector of institutions in Massachusetts. Dr. G. F. M. Bond, who finished his term as clinical assistant at Bloomingdale in 1888, was appointed acting medical superintendent of the New York City Asylum on Ward's Island. Dr. William Noyes (1885–1889) was, in 1889, appointed pathologist of the McLean Asylum, "for which position his studies and practical work well fit him." [1] He was later medical superintendent of the Boston State Hospital for fourteen years. Dr. Henry Smith Williams (1889–1892) resigned to accept the position of medical superintendent of the Charitable Institutions of New York City on Randall's Island. He later retired from medical practice and gained literary distinction as the author of a *History of Science,* and other publications and as an editor of the

1 Medical Superintendent's report for 1889.

Encyclopedia Britannica. Some of the clinical assistants gained promotion by appointments as assistant physicians in state hospitals, and two in succession were appointed to the position of second assistant in the Butler Hospital.[2] Two of the assistant physicians, after resigning to spend a year of study in Europe, returned to Bloomingdale.[3] In 1890 Dr. Edwards J. Pinto of Costa Rica spent several months at Bloomingdale "as guest and assistant," before returning to assume charge of the government hospital for the insane in Costa Rica.

Dr. Nichols's view of what he considered to be "positive" medical treatment of the mentally ill was described in his annual report for 1878:

> I have purposely used the word *uncured* in referring to this class of cases, because of the remark of a distinguished medical friend, in a note addressed to me in the course of the year, that he thought it a more or less prevalent impression in professional circles that the physicians of asylums and hospitals of this character rely largely upon Nature for the recovery of their patients. I think such an impression an erroneous one, if it supposes that the patients of most American institutions for the insane do not receive a positive medical, hygienic, and moral treatment. The expenditure last year of $1,367.05 for medicines and medical supplies, and $2,608.09 mainly in the material means of diversion and exercise, renders such a supposition, in respect to this institution at least, highly improbable. Indeed, in the progress of our knowledge of the causes, nature, and phenomena of insanity, the treatment of the insane is not only more positive, special, and persistent than it was twenty-five or thirty years ago, but more meliorative, if not curative. If a less proportion of the current invasions of mental derangement are cured, it is because disorders of the mind are oftener accompanied with great nervous debility and organic affections of the brain, and with less general recuperative power than they formerly were. I apprehend that it has been the aim of intelligent practitioners, ever since medicine could fairly claim to be a liberal profession, to co-operate with the *vis medicatrix naturae* in the exercise of their art, but the heroic treatment of the past often dealt the healing power of Nature as severe a blow as it did the disease it was intended to cure, and more or less impaired the vital constitution. The truer science and wiser practice of our time, as I believe, effects better results by first clearing away the obstacles to the recuperative energy of the constitution, and then by directly aiding the restorative processes by the prudent use of all those drugs that have a specific power to antagonize certain morbid actions and conditions.[4] It can hardly be claimed that there are any specifics in the treatment of insanity, like bark in fever, but all of the numerous agencies—surgical, medicinal, hygienic, and moral—that restore and maintain physical health, are in the daily and efficient use of alienist physicians, while all the nerve tonics, stimulants, and sedatives, separately or in combination, are directly,

[2] Drs. William J. Schuyler, 1887, and David H. Sprague, 1888.

[3] Drs. William B. Goldsmith, 1880, and William E. Dold, 1887.

[4] This seems to hark back to discarded theories. Cf. p. 14.

if not specifically, effective in bringing the functions of the nervous system to their normal condition.

He also, in his report for 1881, informed the governors that,

in the direction in which I believe the improvement of American institutions for the insane now mainly lies, the endeavor has been steadily made to conduct this Institution more and more as a hospital for the efficient treatment, medical, hygienic and moral, of active disease whether recent or chronic, though not any less as an asylum or proper residence for chronic, passive cases. With the former end particularly in view, a skilled apothecary and special nurses have been employed, and it has been made a point to consult with specialist physicians of the city when there seemed to be occasion. The maintenance of the habits and amenities of refined social life and the bodily exercises that promote appetite, digestion and sleep has been sedulously continued, with great and nearly equal benefit of all classes of patients.

It is noteworthy that the psychotherapeutic value of these measures was not mentioned. The clinical records indicate that much attention was given to medicinal treatment. Hypnotics and sedatives were, however, used sparingly, seldom for more than one to three patients on any day, and frequently not at all. Hyoscine was occasionally used, beginning about 1890. In the course of a discussion at a meeting of the Association of Medical Superintendents in 1883, Dr. Nichols said, "I have of late used less hypnotics than I formerly did, and think I have got better results, both as respects sleep and the support of the patient, from tonic baths, stimulant nutrition and massage, than from the soporific drugs." [5] Tonics were administered to many of the patients, and the number receiving "stimulants" in the form of beer or wine rose, on some days, to sixty. At a meeting of the British Medico-Psychological Association, which he attended while spending a vacation in Europe in 1884, Dr. Nichols stated that in the treatment of insanity in the United States there had been

a more general recognition that it has essentially a physical pathology than was formerly the case, and that the general aim among us is to place the patient in a sound physiological state, and at the same time to give the cerebral disorder and the mental derangement such special treatment as appear to be indicated in each case. We probably resort to medical treatment as often, perhaps oftener, than we formerly did, but I am glad to believe that it is much more delicate and discriminating, and less gross and routine than it formerly was.

He considered that opium was curative in a limited number of cases of mania and of melancholia, and, in combination with the bromides,

[5] *Am. J. Insanity,* XL (1884), 264.

chloroform or hyoscyamus, advantageous in allaying excitement and promoting sleep. Long-continued use, he said, should be avoided. Warm baths, with cold applied to the head ("taking great care not to frighten or distress the patient") and followed by rubbing with alcohol, he considered "will often procure sleep more satisfactorily than any drug administered internally." Counter irritation to the shaven head had been given up, as it was considered that equally good effects were obtained from cupping and blisters over the nape of the neck, temples, and behind the ears. He was personally, he added, "an earnest believer in the value of medicines in the treatment of insanity." [6] Laxatives were given only when indicated and there appears to have been no gross purging with a view to "clearing away the obstacles to the recuperative energy of the constitution." "Medical baths" were employed, as many as fifteen on some days; also massage.

The clinical records had undergone many changes since the asylum was established. Some of these have been described in previous chapters. The recommendation of the State Commissioner in Lunacy in 1876 had no doubt a stimulating influence. In 1877, however, the case histories were still far from complete. In 1879 a "Daily History of Cases" was adopted. In a well-bound book a daily record was made of the physical and mental condition of particular patients in the various halls. An index of patients was made on the front pages of the book showing where entries relating to each could be found. Other information was entered in "Histories on Admissions," and "Male [or Female] Patients Present" in which the record was "continued from the Daily History." By compiling the notes made in these various books, an account of the character of the case and its progress could be put into connected form. At different times from 1871 on, a few attempts were made to introduce a systematic record of complete histories, but not until 1891 was it permanently established, to form the beginning of the vastly improved histories now kept. As the years passed, more and more information was recorded. The active attention received by the patients is manifest in many of the case histories. In 1891 a clinical chart appeared in some instances, recording in graphic form the temperature, pulse, respiration, stools, and urination. Beginning in 1885, a photograph of the patient was frequently attached to the history. Of particular interest in "Daily History of Cases" were the daily statistics of the number of patients receiving various measures of treatment such as hypnotics, tonics, and the use of baths, outdoor and other exercise.

[6] *J. Mental Science* (London), XXX (1884), 474.

These are the only daily records of the use of restraint and seclusion during the period. They show that in 1879 as many as twenty-three patients were under mechanical restraint and seven in seclusion on some days. The forms of apparatus used were the Wyman bed strap, the camisole, muff, wristlets, and chair straps. Sheets were also used over the shoulders and around the ankles to tie patients in bed. The reasons given for resort to restraint were masturbating, undressing, forcible feeding, violent and restless, excited and indecent, to secure sleep, and to secure quiet. Seclusion was employed on account of violence, noise, attempts to escape, "exposing himself to others' violence." Some progress was made in reducing or eliminating the use of these measures: in 1882 the Weekly Committee reported that "all implements of restraint are now removed from the wards. In this respect there is a marked improvement from what it was a very few years since"; and in his annual report for 1883 the medical superintendent informed the governors that "no mechanical restraint was used in the course of the year," and no seclusion except of one powerful man who was in confinement for three months. This record was not maintained continuously, though for months at a time the service would be entirely without resort to these measures. Dr. D. Hack Tuke, who visited Bloomingdale in 1884, stated that he examined "the journal" and that only two men were under restraint between January and October of that year, and that on the women's side no restraint had been used for the last two years and no seclusion during 1884.[7]

In his report for 1882 Dr. Nichols presented his views and practice in regard to restraint and seclusion as follows:

> I am in full accord with what may be properly called the American doctrine and practice in the use of mechanical restraint and seclusion in the treatment of the insane, which is, as I understand it, that neither mode of treatment shall ever be resorted to unless, in the opinion of a competent and responsible medical officer, protection in particular cases against violence, exhaustive activity, the removal of surgical dressings, etc., etc., can be effected more easily, completely, and beneficially to the patient than the necessary end can be attained by either the hands of attendants, medicinal agents, showers and douches which I consider inadmissible except in a very limited number of cases, or "packs," wet or dry, which are obviously a very positive form of mechanical restraint, though their therapeutical advantages may now and then be superior to any substitute for them—and that it is the duty of the practitioner to resort to mechanical restraint or seclusion whenever he clearly sees that it is needed upon the grounds stated. Of course, the actual practice

[7] D. Hack Tuke, *The Insane in the United States and Canada* (London, 1885).

in the use of restraint varies more or less in different institutions in this, as I believe it does, actually and necessarily, in every other enlightened country, and is governed, as are other measures of treatment, by the training and character of the medical officers in charge, the opinion and support of trustees, the number and character of patients with respect to the extent and quality of their accommodations, proportion of attendants to patients, scale of expenditure and other agencies of treatment. The restraint needed in the same institution will vary greatly according to the varying conditions of patients. While I still conscientiously entertain the views just expressed, in common with the great majority of my American brethren, and am entirely unwilling to be governed by a prohibitory dogma or an arbitrary proportion to patients in the use of restraint, I am of the opinion that the circumstances that justify its average use in more than 2 or 3 per cent. of the cases under treatment must be quite exceptional. Seconded by the present assistant physicians of the Institution, who have been earnest and efficient in their co-operation in this undertaking, the effort has been made this year to see how far restraint, either by mechanical instrumentalities or seclusion, could be reduced without violating the principles just laid down, and on the men's side of the house restraint by camisole or bed strap, or by seclusion, was resorted to in the course of the year in only 11 different cases, 1 time in 3 cases, 3 times in 2 cases, 4 times in 2 cases, 5 times in 2 cases, 6 times in 1 case, and 7 times in 1 case, for periods varying from 1 to 12 hours. On the women's side of the house more restraint was used in the early part of the year, but in the last 7 months it was used in only 2 cases, 3 times in 1 case and 4 times in the other, for periods varying from 1 to 10 hours. In the foregoing list of restraint used, is included the seclusion of 3 different cases of paroxysmal mania in men and 1 of general paralysis, 4 times in 2 cases, 5 times in 1 case, and 1 time in 1 case, for periods varying from 2 to 6 hours. Seclusion was not resorted to in any other case, and the habit of voluntary seclusion into which certain old cases are inclined to fall, has been entirely broken up. I desire it to be distinctly understood that the reduced use of restraint has not been attended by an increased use of nervous sedatives or hypnotics, which have in fact been very sparingly used. On the contrary, I have depended more than ever before upon the composing and indirect hypnotic effects of tonic and stimulant treatment and the use of warm medicated baths and massage at bed time.

It should be mentioned that while about the usual proportion of excited patients has been treated this year, there have not been any cases of acute delirious mania or other cases of extreme violence in which it is most necessary to husband the strength by confinement to the bed; and that the minimum use of restraint that is consistent with the welfare of active cases of mental derangement requires a large corps of superior attendants. The number employed at Bloomingdale in the year has averaged 1 attendant to 2⅔ patients, including 2 supervisors, 2 trained nurses and 8 regular night attendants.

In the course of a discussion at a meeting of the Association of Medical Superintendents in 1877, Dr. Nichols stated that "it wounds my sense of human dignity to see any patient under mechanical restraint." He added, however, that "the use of such vital sedatives, as tartar emetic and digitalis, in energetic doses, cold douches, or even very large nervous sedatives and hypnotics, is utterly inadmissible as substitutes for mechanical restraint." [8]

The statistical tables which had formerly appeared in the annual report had, long before Dr. Nichols's appointment in 1877, been omitted. In 1891, however, Dr. Lyon, who succeeded Dr. Nichols in 1889, presented tabulated statistics of the forms of mental disorders of the patients admitted. The forms listed were: acute mania, acute and chronic melancholia, primary dementia, chronic, senile and epileptic dementia, primary delusional insanity, alcoholic insanity, paresis, and moral imbecility. The table also showed the condition of those discharged under the same classification, and the condition of those who were still in the asylum. In his report for 1892 Dr. Lyon added tables of age, civil condition, hereditary tendency, exciting causes, and the physical diseases of the patients admitted during the year. The report for 1893 contained corresponding tables. Here also, because of "interest which is now felt in the remote or immediate connection between Syphilis and General Paresis," brief abstracts were presented of the histories of 22 cases admitted during the year, in which the diagnosis of paresis had been made. In twelve of these cases a positive history of syphilis had been obtained, and in three others the evidence was strongly probable. In seven no evidence of syphilis was obtained. From a third to a half of the patients who died each year were victims of paresis. In 1891 the medical superintendent's annual report stated that "no doubt we get a larger proportion of paretics than most institutions" and added that 21 percent of the men and 11 percent of the women were paretics. The paretic cases in 1893, one of which was a woman, constituted over 13 percent of the total number of patients admitted that year. (The death rate during this period was frequently 8 percent of all patients treated, and the number of paretics in the asylum was very large.) Quite a number of "acute" cases among the patients admitted also died within a month.

Although measures directed to engaging the patients in wholesome activities were not well organized, their value as "moral treatment" continued to be understood and their use encouraged by the governors. In 1882 the Asylum Committee reported that they had "observed with great satisfaction the salutary effects of the increased efforts made for the amusement of the patients and the occupation of their minds under the

[8] *Am. J. Insanity*, XXXIV (1877), 243.

present administration," and in his annual report for 1885 Dr. Nichols stated that "at no time under my executive administration have the diversified means that your Board has here provided for the treatment of mental alienation, been used with more earnestness, diligence, and skill." The Asylum Committee frequently commented on the large proportion of the patients observed out of doors; in his annual report for 1883 Dr. Nichols referred to visits of the committee when not a single patient was found within the halls. Lawn games were provided, and more liberal provision was made for carriage drives. A few patients were allowed to ride horseback. The property at White Plains was utilized for excursion parties of ten to forty patients, who twice a week drove to the farm to spend the day, accompanied by a physician and a requisite number of attendants. Similar excursions were made to the seashore, presumably Long Island Sound, and on the Hudson River boats. The only unfortunate experience on these excursions was a drowning accident, the cause of which was believed to be a sudden illness and not a suicidal intent.[9] In 1887 a dining and amusement pavilion was attached to the farmhouse at White Plains, and also a wing containing one single and nine double bedrooms. This provided accommodations for patients and attendants to remain overnight, and in the following year it was reported that forty-three patients had resided there for an average of seven weeks each. It was particularly noted that they enjoyed "the sense of freedom" there. It was, however, not only patients who were benefited, as it was reported that "the opportunity which the Farm affords of sending to it for rest, attendants who are run down with confinement and exhausting work, has been of marked advantage to the ward service." [10]

In 1882 the practice of boarding patients in private families was adopted, with the understanding that no other boarders would be accepted. In 1883 it was reported that four men and eight women had been provided for in this way, and that in five of the cases recovery had been promoted. In 1885 the annual report stated that "38 different patients have had the manifest benefits of residing in the country or at the seaside an average of 10½ weeks." This experience with a "boarding out system" for the mentally ill is of particular interest today, in view of its introduction as a means of reducing the number of patients in the state hospitals.

Among the means of entertainment provided were "hops," plays, readings, music, or prestidigitation, two or three times a week. Some of

[9] Medical Superintendent's report for 1883.

[10] *Ibid.*, 1887.

the entertainments were provided by friends of patients. A performance was given by the Madison Square Theatre Company, "one of the troupe being the wife of a patient," [11] and the New-York *Tribune* of May 4, 1894, remarked that "the presence of W. J. S. at the Bloomingdale Asylum is certainly a boon to the other inmates. Since he has been there, there has been a succession of variety entertainments," some under the auspices of Mrs. S. and one under the auspices of Mrs. Tony Pastor. One of the singers, Maggie Cline, was given a "rousing reception" that "somewhat startled her." Parties of patients with their attendants also attended plays and other entertainments, and visited exhibitions in the city. An orchestra and a baseball team were organized among the employees. In 1878 six pianos were purchased, and in 1884 eight others. The weekly committee reported in February, 1885, that "it was evident that the recent addition to the former number of these instruments had greatly increased the enjoyment of the patients."

In the medical superintendent's report for 1886 it was stated that "a useful school, the pupils of which have been female patients and attendants, has for several years been conducted at Bloomingdale by the Female Supervisor, Miss Johnson, with manifest pleasure and advantage to most of the limited number of patients selected to attend it." No other reference to this school was found.[12] Provision was also made for indoor games and athletic exercises in the gymnasium, instruction being given by the young physicians and the attendants. Religious services were well attended, "the excellent Sunday music of the choir" being especially enjoyed. One of the governors who attended the service in June, 1887, reported that he was impressed by the suitable sermon of the Reverend Mr. Peters. The governors were apparently apprehensive lest secular entertainments might encroach upon religious observances, as in April, 1894, they requested the Asylum Committee "not to permit any theatrical entertainment for the amusement of the patients in the Asylum to be given therein on Good Friday or on Sunday."

The problem of providing the patients, especially the men, with the benefits of satisfying productive occupation continued to be baffling. In December, 1885, the Inspecting Committee reported that they were impressed with the desirability of giving, if practicable, more occupation to the patients. Although it was reported that in 1890 40 percent of

11 *Minutes of the Asylum Committee*, Feb. 9, 1893.

12 It will be recalled that Dr. Pliny Earle, when physician of the asylum, 1844 to 1849, established a school, which he considered was a valuable resource in group treatment. It was discontinued, however, by his successor.

the men, and 54 percent of the women engaged in some manual employment, no forms were mentioned except sewing and housework. Reference was made to the "difficulty in providing other kinds of work and in inducing patients to take part in them." Dr. Lyon, the medical superintendent, felt that "the city habits and tasks of the class of patients at Bloomingdale precluded gardening or farming, or work on small handicrafts" such as were successfully practiced in institutions in manufacturing districts. He considered that "occupations of the mind . . . are perhaps more natural than those for the hands to patients of our class." The hope was expressed in his report for 1892 that, "at the new Institution . . . better and more convenient work will be done, and that the larger fields for diverse occupation, both as treatment and as mental resource, will be available."

It was during this period that the movement for the establishment of training schools for nurses was accomplishing great advances in the standards of personal care of patients in the general hospitals. This movement, however, which originated and derived much of its support from outside the hospitals and was bringing into the service women of education and refinement, was not directed to the needs of the mentally ill and to the hospitals and asylums in which they were treated. In his report for 1879 Dr. Nichols warned the governors that "without intelligent and faithful attendants, all other provisions for the best care of the insane will prove nearly worthless." In his 1886 report he commented on the "display of devotion, fidelity and tact in the discharge of what I regard as one of the most trying duties of life." The New York Hospital Training School, which was one of the earliest in America, was established in 1877, and furnished many superintendents for schools in other hospitals. Moved by a strong desire to procure equal benefits for the mentally ill, physicians attempted to introduce similar training schools into the institutions under their direction. The first to be established was at McLean Hospital in 1882, and in the following year another was established at the State Hospital in Buffalo, New York. By 1892 there were nineteen training schools at mental hospitals throughout the country.

Influenced, perhaps, by these developments, and especially by the difficulty met with in procuring qualified nurses for mentally ill patients in private homes, for which occasion not infrequently arose, Dr. Nichols, in his annual report for 1883, proposed that three to six months' training and practice in an institution for the insane be added to the curriculum of training schools for nurses. He offered

> with the approval of the Asylum Committee . . . to undertake to give the graduating nurses of the Hospital 3 or 6 months training and service at Bloomingdale. . . . The Asylum would gain something from the instruction and methods the nurses would bring with them from the Hospital, and [I] should hope that the nurses would derive a full equivalent for the time they might spend in the Asylum.

No record of the way in which this proposal was regarded by the training-school authorities has been found. Thirty years elapsed, however, before it was put into effect. In 1890 an indication of advancing awareness of the dignity and importance of the nursing service was manifested in the adoption of a "neat and pleasing uniform" for the attendants of both sexes. This was followed in 1891 by the establishment of a course of weekly lectures on their practical duties to be given to the male attendants by the assistant physicians; the head attendants were to be given more advanced instruction than the others. The object was "to give such instruction as would make, of the material available to the Institution for nurses, as good and efficient and kind attendants as possible," in other words "to improve the service." It was in this way that all the schools in the hospitals for the mentally ill were started. There was no support from without, and candidates of greater education and refinement than the attendants engaged in the work were not available. In his annual report for that year Dr. Lyon stated that it was expected that the course would be extended to the women. He considered that it was "too early in the experiment as yet to judge fully of its results," and that the course was "not sufficiently wide or deep to entitle it to be classed as a training school."

As the facilities of the asylum were expanded, and an increasing number of patients admitted, the number of attendants was correspondingly increased. In 1877 the average number of patients under treatment was 75 men and 92 women, and there were 15 male and 24 female attendants. In 1893, when the average number of patients was 145 men and 157 women, there were over 50 attendants of each sex. Improvements were also made in the organization. It will be recalled that on the recommendation of the State Commissioner in Lunacy, a supervisor was appointed for each service in 1877, and it was regarded as an experiment. In 1883 an assistant supervisor was added to the women's service, and in 1885 to the men's. In 1890 a "first attendant" was designated for each hall, and in 1892 the title was changed to "head attendant." A "night watch" was appointed in each service in 1877, and by 1882 the number assigned to night duty was four on each service.

The general sanitary condition of the asylum was greatly improved by the changes made by Dr. Nichols and appears to have been remarkably good during the period of 1877 to 1894. Malaria, which had once been extremely prevalent at Bloomingdale, was no longer mentioned in the records. The only infectious diseases of which there were cases were scarlet fever, from which two female employees were ill in 1879, without spread to others, and a few cases of measles in 1887.

It seems remarkable that only two suicides occurred in the asylum during these seventeen years. Frequent references to suicidal propensities appear in the records, and evidently great precautions were exercised. Dr. Nichols's views on the prevention of suicide are set forth in his annual report for 1879:

It is a common impression that the singular disposition to take their own lives that the insane frequently manifest is to be thwarted by the absence of the means of effecting their purpose. I think this view fallacious and often literally fatal. The suicidal insane should be carefully kept from all such ready opportunities to effect their purpose as open unguarded windows, precipices, bodies of water, razors and other sharp or pointed instruments, and from ropes and poisons; but the furniture of their apartments and their ordinary surroundings should be, in the main, suited to such mental conditions and manifestations as are independent of the disposition to personal violence. Suicides are very ineffectively prevented by mere lack of mechanical opportunity. Cases in large numbers could be cited in illustration of this fact. The only mechanical means of preventing suicide which I have much confidence in, are the muff or camisole and the Wyman bed strap. Suicides are most effectively prevented by the observation, night and day, of faithful attendants. Such observation should be intelligent and vigilant, but not so obtrusive as to excite the spirit of rivalry in vigilance between the patient and attendant. The necessity for a special attendant at night for each case may be avoided by placing all such cases of one sex under treatment at one time, in an associated dormitory or suite of rooms, and have them overlooked by one night attendant. His vigilance may be rendered almost absolutely certain by the occasional calls of the regular night attendant. This plan of preventing suicides is rendered practicable by the fact that the determinedly suicidal cases are rarely so turbulent as to disturb the rest of near neighbors. I may add, that I think more can be accomplished than was formerly thought practicable to alleviate the distress that looks to death for relief, by medical and dietetic measures, and by cheerful apartments, associations and exercises.

No copies of the dietaries of this period have been found among the records. Evidently, however, great improvement resulted from the new kitchen and food distribution system provided in 1878. In the annual report for 1879 this is referred to with the statement that "the food is now well cooked and served hot." This was confirmed by reports of the committees; on June 28, 1882, the Inspecting Committee particularly observed the preparation of food and commented on the contrast "with the customs many years ago."

It will be recalled that during his first term of service as physician of the asylum in 1849 to 1852, Dr. Nichols had promoted the policy by which the resources of the department would be devoted especially to the treatment of patients of a greater degree of "social uniformity," than was possible before public asylums were established.[13] He believed that this would render "the direction of their treatment more successful," and he proposed improvements by which the service would be made satisfactory to better educated and more refined patients than most of those who were supported by public funds. The new construction, the alterations and renovations, the added facilities, and improved organization by which he was "in a large measure, the recreator" [14] of Bloomingdale, were shaped with a view to this purpose. He obtained from the governors and other benevolent persons the means of providing accommodations for a limited number of patients who could afford liberal rates. His main interest, however, was to aid the "deserving indigent insane." He considered that the asylum, "like a benevolent citizen, . . . economizes in its expenditures in order to maintain or increase its charities, and is the almoner of the gifts of others for the same purpose." [15] He interested the governors in making provision for curable patients whose resources were exhausted before they were well enough to be discharged properly, and in his annual report for 1879 he said, "I trust that the day is not distant when pecuniary considerations will not compel any patient to leave our protection and care so long as the case gives promise of recovery or material further relief." The following year he was enabled to report:

> I take great pleasure in being able to inform you that no premature removal took place because of the inability of friends to support the patient—not that the friends of some such patients have not been in moderate and even straightened circumstances, but in every such case the Committee has promptly proffered from the resources of the Institution, the pecuniary assistance necessary for the treatment of the case as long as it continued hopeful; and in most instances the proffer has been very gratefully accepted.

He also reported that, due in some measure to a reduction in the rates to "worthy people in reduced circumstances," there had been an

13 See p. 244.
14 Medical superintendent's annual report for 1889.
15 *Ibid.*, 1878.

increase in the number of admissions. In 1882 the governors reported an increasing number of applications from "the more educated and refined classes." In 1884 the number of cases assisted pecuniarily was larger than ever before, 171 of 268 patients being cared for free or below cost.[16] In his report for 1885 Dr. Nichols directed attention to the care taken

> on the one hand that the wealthy do not crowd out the poor, and on the other hand that the poor have the benefit of all donations and of all that the rich pay above the cost of treatment. The remunerative and unremunerative cases are made to balance each other, as it were, and are nearly equal. An increase of accommodations, and of the number of patients who are able to pay liberal rates for the benefits of the Institution, and that munificent donation a few years ago for the benefit of indigent insane women (the John C. Green Memorial Fund) enable the Institution to treat, in the most liberal manner, even a larger number of free and low-paying patients than it treated when the average rates charged were much lower than they are now.

Dr. Nichols took advantage of every proper opportunity to remind the governors of this fundamental principle and aim in the operation of the service, and did so with evident success, for Tuke records that "the great feature of this institution is the large amount of good it effects for the indigent classes who are socially above the poor."[17] The theme was taken up by Dr. Nichols's successor, who, in his report for 1890, in anticipation of the removal to White Plains, advised the governors that "it is earnestly to be hoped that this Institution will, before many years, be able to extend its aid to a greater number of those who, by reason of their insanity, have become proper subjects," and in his report for 1892, when construction was undertaken, he expressed the hope that the new hospital would be better prepared to meet the demand of an increasing number of applicants for admission and "to do its proper charitable work, among the self-respecting insane, who are become dependent, by reason of their insanity; which may have disabled the bread winner, or which may have made the income, formerly adequate for the modest support of the family in health, insufficient under the new affliction." By means of these reminders and their ready acceptance by the governors, the policy which has been long followed in the admission of patients and in their support in the service was firmly established.

The governors and the medical superintendent found it advisable, on occasion, to give some attention to measures pending in the legislature, not all of which related directly to Bloomingdale. The licensing provisions of the insanity law of 1890, and the rules and requests for in-

16 *Minutes of the Asylum Committee*, March 29, 1884. 17 Tuke, *op. cit.*, p. 143.

formation of the newly established State Commission in Lunacy, created needs for new adjustments; some misapprehensions remained until the adjustments were made. A similar condition was experienced by the state hospitals. This situation was of short duration, and, as mentioned in the preceding chapter, harmonious relations were soon established. The exclusion of pay patients from the state hospitals—a policy which was not long followed—occasioned an increase in the applications for admission to Bloomingdale. This led Dr. Lyon, soon after the asylum had been removed to White Plains, to address to the governor of the state a plea for the transfer of the city asylums to state jurisdiction in order that "New York County's partially dependent insane, of refined instincts and good character," might have the same privilege as their fellow citizens in other parts of the state of admission to the state hospitals at "a small rate of board, sufficient to preserve their self-respect, to relieve them from the odium of pauperism." [18] These institutions were transferred soon afterwards.

In 1891 a bill providing for a jury trial before commitment to a hospital for the mentally ill, "to be conducted in all respects as a trial for a felony," [19] was opposed by the governors and the medical superintendent and was defeated. The medical superintendent served on occasion as a medical expert in court proceedings, and in 1881 Dr. Nichols was summoned to Washington to testify for the defense at the trial of Guiteau, the assassin of President Garfield. Dr. Earle, formerly physician at Bloomingdale, also testified. Resort to writs of habeas corpus for the release of patients in the asylum seems to have given little trouble to the administration during this period. Of some interest is a case reported to the governors by Dr. Nichols in 1883. The patient was declared sane by a jury, despite the evidence of five physicians, three of whom were experts in mental disease and well acquainted with the case, the opposing testimony being that of two laymen and one physician who was not an expert. After the patient was declared sane and had promised the jury he would return to his home, he refused to leave the asylum although told that he must go. Resort to force was considered inadvisable, and the patient remained for seven months. His condition then grew worse and he was arrested as a trespasser, taken to Bellevue, and admitted to another asylum at which he committed suicide.

18 Letter from Dr. Lyon to Gov. Levi P. Morton, May 28, 1895. New York Hospital, Westchester Division.

19 Minutes of the Committee on Law, Feb. 27, 1891. (State of New York in Senate, No. 238, Feb. 11, 1891.)

For many years the main problem relating to the mentally ill in the United States was the expansion of facilities for care and treatment. In the fifty years before 1894 the number of new asylums or hospitals established was 125. In New York State 11 of 12 state hospitals were established during the same period. There were also in New York, by 1893, 11 private institutions. In the last decade of the 19th century, however, scientific and clinical study was beginning to receive increasing attention. The articles and references in the *American Journal of Insanity,* which continued to be the principal channel for contributions to the literature, were becoming, both in quantity and quality, more fully clinical and scientific. It was a period of great progress in general medicine, and this was reflected in the increasing attention given to physical conditions met with in the mentally ill. Pathological laboratories were established in some of the institutions. The role of infections in mental disease received more attention. Hydrotherapy, massage, faradism, and other forms of physical therapy were given a larger place in treatment. The role of the ductless glands began to receive consideration, and thyroid extract was administered on occasion. Cannabis indica and sulphonal were introduced as hypnotics. Rest treatment by confinement to bed was practiced in the treatment of mentally ill patients both in hospitals and in private practice.

The medical profession generally, and particularly specialists in neurology, were developing a greater interest in the mentally ill. The teachings of Charcot and others had awakened a more active interest in the less incapacitating forms of mental illness or neuroses. Psychotherapy in the form of hypnosis was practiced by a few. A mass meeting was held in Cooper Union in December, 1879, for the discussion of various problems of lunacy reform, particularly the need for establishing a state commission in lunacy. Following the meeting, a "National Association for the Protection of the Insane and Prevention of Insanity" was organized, with a view to educating the public concerning the nature of mental disease, the advantage of early treatment, and the improvement of the methods of management. Other aims were the adoption of an enlightened state policy, more complete supervision of institutions, the allaying of public distrust,[20] and "the encouragement of special clinical and pathological observations of the nervous system by the medical profession generally, as well as by those connected with asylums for the insane." The association survived only four years, but accomplished much good, par-

20 State supervision and licensing of private institutions for the mentally ill and the position of State Commissioner in Lunacy had, however, been established in New York in 1873.

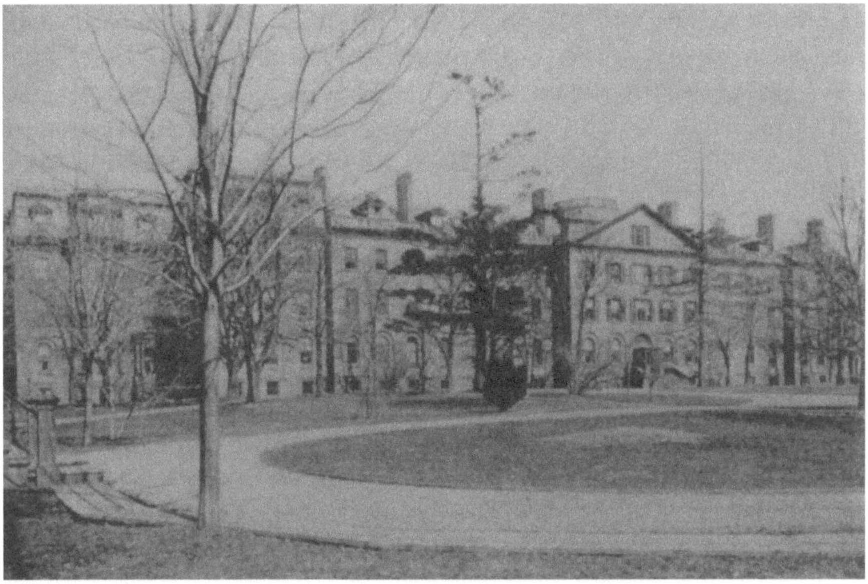

BLOOMINGDALE ASYLUM, 1881

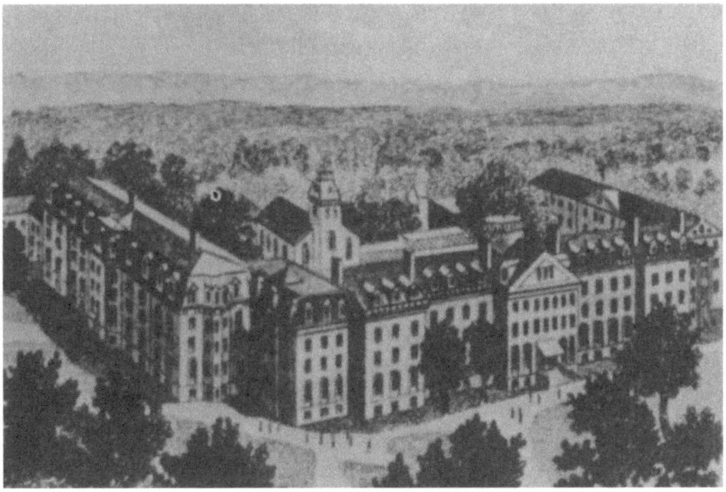

BLOOMINGDALE ASYLUM, 1885

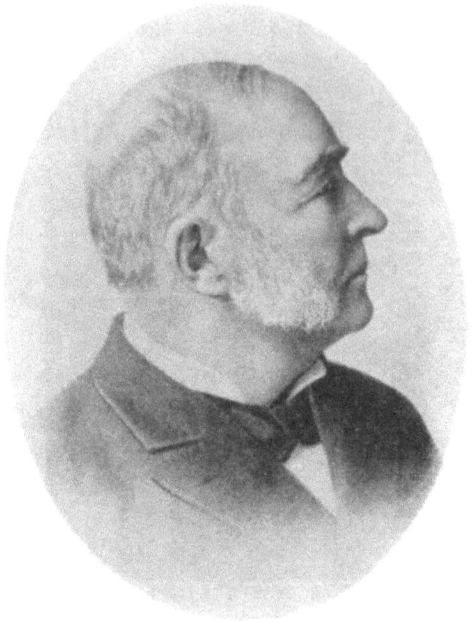

CHARLES H. NICHOLS, M.D.
PHYSICIAN OF THE ASYLUM, 1849-1852
AND MEDICAL SUPERINTENDENT, 1877-1889

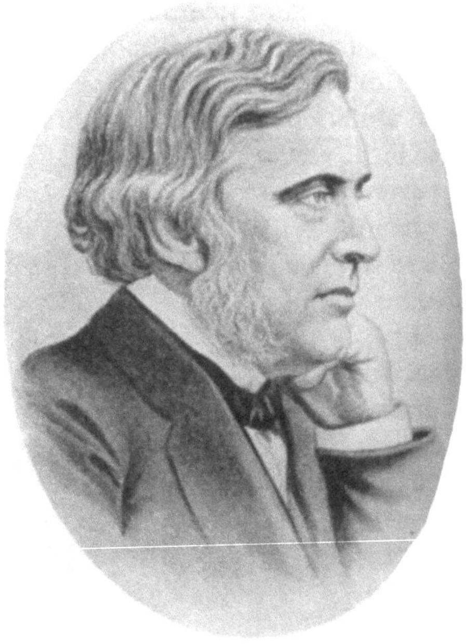

D. TILDEN BROWN, M.D.
PHYSICIAN OF THE ASYLUM, 1852-1877

ticularly in New York, by exercising a keen vigilance in matters of institutional care, and by agitating for legislative inquiries wherever the existence of abuses was known or suspected. For a year it published a quarterly entitled *The American Psychological Journal.* Its failure to survive was due, in some measure, to the antagonism of the medical superintendents of the institutions for the mentally ill, which was aroused by the campaign of exposure, legislative investigations, and proposals for central supervision and control of state institutions.[21]

Few contributions to scientific literature were made by the asylum staff during this period. Dr. Nichols participated actively in discussions at the meetings of the Association of Medical Superintendents; an address which he had delivered at the International Medical Congress at Philadelphia in 1875 was published,[22] but while he was at Bloomingdale no other article from his pen appeared in the literature. An article by his successor, Dr. Lyon, entitled "Present Hospital Care of the Insane," was presented at a meeting of the American Neurological Association and was published in the *Journal of Nervous and Mental Diseases* in 1894. An article entitled "A Few Psycho-Somatic Base-Lines," written by Dr. Henry Smith Williams, one of the assistant physicians, was published in the *American Journal of Insanity* in 1891, and a second article by him, "The Dream State and Its Psychic Correlatives," appeared in the same journal in April, 1892.

The literature of the period contained the first general treatises on insanity to be published since that of Dr. Rush in 1812. In 1883 general treatises were published by Dr. William A. Hammond and Dr. Edward C. Spitzka. In 1882 a smaller work entitled *Insanity and Its Treatment* by Dr. S. Worcester was published. Other publications were *Insanity, Its Causes and Prevention* by Dr. H. P. Stearns, superintendent of the Hartford Retreat, and *Insanity Considered in Its Medico-Legal Relations* by Dr. T. R. Buckham, in 1883. In 1885 Dr. Tuke's account of *The Insane in the United States and Canada* was published. Other books of less significance also appeared. The awakened interest in the less incapacitating mental disorders or neuroses was shown by the publication of various articles and of such books as *A Practical Treatise on Nervous Exhaustion* by Dr. G. M. Beard in 1880, and *Brain Rest* by Dr. J. L. Corning in 1883. That the need of training nurses for the mentally ill was recognized by others than the physicians of the asylums is shown by

21 Deutsch, *The Mentally Ill in America* (New York, 1937), pp. 311–314.

22 "On the Best Mode of Providing for the Subjects of Chronic Insanity," *Transactions* of the International Medical Congress, Philadelphia, 1876.

the publication in 1887 of *The Nursing and Care of the Nervous and Insane* by Dr. Charles K. Mills. Other publications of the same character were *How to Care for the Insane—A Manual for Attendants in Insane Asylums* by Dr. W. D. Granger of the Buffalo State Hospital, and a junior and senior *Text Book on Nursing in Bodily and Mental Disease* by Drs. R. M. Phelps and S. L. Phelps. Several new periodicals were established during this period. The *Medico-Legal Journal,* a continuation of the *Bulletin* of the Medico-Legal Society of New York, which had been first issued in 1879, was established in 1883. *The Alienist and Neurologist* edited by Dr. C. H. Hughes, was established in 1880 and survived until 1920; it contained several useful translations of foreign literature. *The American Journal of Neurology and Psychiatry,* edited by Dr. T. A. McBride in association with Drs. L. C. Gray and E. C. Spitzka, established in 1882, was discontinued in 1885. *The American Journal of Psychology,* edited by Dr. G. Stanley Hall, was established in 1887. The *Review of Insanity and Nervous Disease,* edited by Dr. J. H. McBride, was published from 1890 to 1894, and then discontinued.

Little or no progress in the medical teaching of mental disease was made during this period. A few of the medical schools had lecturers and even professors of nervous and mental diseases in their faculties but the time given to the subject was almost negligible. In 1890 Dr. Henry Hurd was appointed professor of psychiatry at the Johns Hopkins Medical College. In his History, Dr. Hurd states, "In June 1879, four clinical lectures on insanity were given at Ward's Island for medical practitioners and general students. These were probably the first lectures of the kind ever given in a hospital for the insane in New York." Twenty attended and two hundred patients were demonstrated.[23]

Significant of the broadening field of psychiatric interest and practice was, perhaps, the change in 1892 of the title of *Association of Medical Superintendents of American Institutions for the Insane* to *The American Medico-Psychological Association.* The title *American Psychiatric Association* was suggested, but it was feared that it would mystify the public; it was adopted several years later.[24]

23 Hurd, *Institutional Care of the Insane in the United States and Canada* (Baltimore, 1916), III, 205.

24 Proceedings of the Association, 1891, *Am. J. Insanity,* XLVIII (1891), 105, 106. For Constitution and by-laws adopted see Proceedings of 1892, *Am. J. Insanity,* XLIX (1892), 282 ff.

XXVI

REMOVAL TO WHITE PLAINS

For many years the steady growth of the city in the direction of Bloomingdale was a constant reminder that the day of removal of the asylum to another location was irresistibly approaching. As early as 1858 Dr. Brown felt that the prospect "rested like an incubus" on the progress of the service.[1] About that time the question of removal of the New York Hospital from its original site on Broadway was commencing to receive attention. Proposals to sell the asylum property or use it as a site for a new general hospital were so favorably accepted that in 1868 property was purchased at White Plains, an architect engaged, and plans made, with a view to removing the asylum there. As has been recounted, the project was abandoned, but the White Plains property was kept.[2] Eventually, as the built-up streets approached and as the number of applications for the admission of patients increased, the question again became an issue.

In his report for 1885, Dr. Nichols stated that applications had been received for twice as many suitable patients as there was room for. The number treated that year was 420, and at the close of the year 272 were still under treatment. This report was followed by a communication from Dr. Nichols in which, after reviewing the situation, he proposed that a branch of the asylum be established in the country. His proposal was made "without special reference to any proposition to altogether abandon the use of this site for your department for the insane and to establish it on another site in the country." He did not think it practical, however, to provide on the present property additional accommodations for the reception, classification, and treatment of a large number of patients. He estimated that there were many patients "of the medium class in respect to fortune, and of the indigent but not pauper class, whose care in a sufficiently accessible institution well adapted to their means and needs would be one of the greatest boons to themselves and their friends that wealth and benevolence could bestow."[3] Dr. Nichols considered the White Plains property suitable for a branch or as a site for the whole institution. He advised the governors, however, that, if it was considered necessary to investigate further, "having first resolved to

1 P. 257.

2 See Chapter XXI.

3 *Minutes of the Governors*, July 6, 1886. It is noteworthy that the needs of the patients and families who could afford to pay only moderate rates were the principal objects of consideration. This had been the main interest of the governors from the foundation of their department for the mentally ill and it has continued so to be.

establish the greatly needed branch of this department in the country," they should, "with the least practical delay and as definitively and irrevocably as possible, fix upon a site for the purpose." His proposal was favorably considered, and in July, 1886, the following resolution was adopted:

> Whereas the Medical Superintendent of the Bloomingdale Asylum in a communication to the Governors of the Society of the New York Hospital has stated that the present accommodations at Bloomingdale are not adequate to meet the claims upon the Asylum of those seeking and entitled to admission, and suggesting that a branch of the Institution be established in the country,
>
> Therefore Resolved that the Board of Governors will establish a branch of their Asylum for the Insane in the country outside the limits of the City of New York at a place to be selected which shall be of sufficient extent to receive the entire department for the Insane in case the Society is hereafter compelled to remove from its present site at Bloomingdale—and further resolved that it be referred to the Asylum Committee to enquire and examine as to a suitable place for the establishment of such a branch of the Asylum and to report thereon to this Board.

At the August meeting the governors requested the Asylum Committee "to lay out a general plan of improvement with elevations, plans, and estimates for cost of such structures as may be contemplated." In December the attorney of the Society was requested to petition the legislature to exempt the White Plains property from taxation. Such expedition was, however, not in accordance with the conservative spirit of many of the governors. In March, 1887, the Asylum Committee was requested "to consider and report what in their opinion should be the future policy of this Board in reference to the Asylum as to the advisability of removal, the manner and time of such removal if in their opinion it is advisable, and such other matters as affect the future usefulness of this department." The committee made their report in April. They reviewed the present and prospective difficulties involved in remaining at Bloomingdale, and recommended removal of the asylum to another location. They also presented what they considered to be the views and policies of the governors at that time, as follows:

> The care and treatment of the mental invalids has become the most important and renowned part of the work of the Society of the New York Hospital, which is the only corporation of its character in New York which has a department for the insane. While its hospitals for the ordinary sick and injured enjoy a very high and well-deserved reputation, there are other institutions in this community which could, and in all probability would, supply their

places if the Society were compelled to discontinue these portions of its work, but its asylum for the insane meets in an especial manner the needs of the middle classes of the population in respect to means—the classes who are able to pay moderate rates in whole or in part for the treatment of those among them who are so unfortunate as to be afflicted by the most distressing of all human ailments, and whose sufferings would be aggravated by their surroundings if compelled to go to public pauper institutions for the insane. Among that class there is need for an almost unlimited expansion of our Asylum, while its advantages of comforts and treatment are known and sought for not only by the wealthy classes at home but by those of distant parts of the country, and to some extent by those of other countries on this continent. It is for the classes of this metropolitan district of only moderate means for whom the almost unlimited expansion of our Asylum is needed. For lack of sufficient accommodations we are almost daily turning from our doors patients who really can find nowhere else what our Asylum could give them if it had the room. To close such an institution or to diminish its means of usefulness would be a public calamity, but to enlarge and increase its usefulness is a duty because of the need and the opportunity.[4]

It was by such reaffirmations that the governors, on different occasions, reminded themselves and others that the main policy and purpose of the organization was, and must be, to provide treatment for the mentally ill of "the middle classes of the population in respect to means." The policy was well expressed by one of the governors during one of the public attacks on the character of the institution. In the New York *Tribune* of March 10, 1888, he stated: "We never refuse any deserving case of real destitution in an unfortunate person belonging originally to the better classes. We are charged with being an aristocratic institution. Well, if to take that class of patients is to be aristocratic, then we are aristocratic."

The Board of Governors, without further discussion, approved the proposal of the committee to use the White Plains property as a site for a branch, and, if removal of the entire institution from Bloomingdale should become necessary, to remove it there. This was shortly before the investigation of the asylum by a committee of the State Senate which was described in Chapter XXIV, and it seems remarkable that no reference was made in the testimony taken, nor in the report of that committee, to the active measures toward removal which had already been taken.

As not all of the governors had been members of the board when, after consideration of many other sites, the White Plains property was purchased in 1868, some of them, like their predecessors of that time, felt

[4] *Minutes of the Governors,* April 5, 1887.

that the advantages of beauty and of water carriage offered by the Hudson River valley should be obtained for the new asylum. In May, 1887, therefore, a committee was appointed and instructed to examine and report on any site that might be called to their attention by not less than three members of the board, and such other sites as the committee might deem suitable. This committee reported in October that they had looked particularly for sites with a water view, not more than forty minutes by railway from the city. They examined sites at Throgg's Neck on Long Island Sound, and at Garrison, Irvington, and Scarborough on the Hudson. They were particularly impressed by the Butler Wright estate at Scarborough, and recommended that the board examine it and other sites. For this purpose Mr. Elbridge T. Gerry, one of the governors, placed his yacht at their disposal. At the November meeting of the board, Dr. Nichols was requested to examine the sites and report. His report was presented in December and consisted largely of a comparison between the Scarborough and White Plains properties; he also mentioned some property at Oscawana on the Hudson. He made no specific recommendation, and used the opportunity again to emphasize the importance of adhering closely to the policy of the Society in regard to patients who could pay only moderate rates. He presumed, he said, that

> it is as certain as that there will not be any future demand upon this department of the hospital for the care of paupers, that you will continue to provide for the large class of respectable patients of moderate means, and for others of very restricted means, to the extent of your pecuniary ability. . . . The provisions of the charter, the annuity formerly granted by the Legislature, the exemption from taxation . . . . . the private donations you have received for the purpose and your own benevolent feelings would alike forbid any other change in this respect than an increase in the number of such patients provided for.

To this he added that

> the considerations now presented seem to indicate that, in removing this department to the country, the new grounds and buildings should embrace such an extent and variety of accommodations as the great and growing population and wealth of New York demand, whereby there may be such improvement in methods as will put the Institution abreast of all the true advances in practical psychological medicine; and that there is no occasion to make any change in the practice of the Institution for many past years with reference to the classes of patients received and cared for.

He also presented his views of what the plans of "a model institution of the corporate benevolent class should embrace"; namely, a systematic hospital for the acute, and all other active cases though chronic, of both sexes, to consist of a wing for each sex extending and retreating in echelon form, from a central administration building, that at a considerable distance right and left or to the rear of the wings of the hospital should be asylums or retreats less expensive in construction, appointments and administration than the hospital, for the quiet patients of moderate means, whether convalescent or chronic, and villas or cottages fronting, but at a suitable distance from, the wings of the hospital, with small parks and tree and shrubbery plantings between the villas and wings, for the use of quiet patients who have the means to live in small groups or separately, in as nearly a homelike way as mental invalids can live anywhere.

Dr. Nichols considered that provision should be made at the new institution for one thousand patients.[5]

When a vote was taken on the Scarborough site on December 22, six of the governors were in favor of accepting it, and nine were against it. The way now seemed to be clear for proceeding with plans for utilizing the White Plains property. On May 1, 1888, by a vote of thirteen to seven, the following resolution was adopted:

Resolved that the Farm at White Plains, in Westchester County, which is now owned by the Society of the New York Hospital, is adopted as the site of its Asylum for the Insane when it is removed from Bloomingdale.

In June, however, a resolution authorizing the Asylum Committee to employ an architect and prepare plans and estimates was laid on the table. In November another site was proposed by one of the governors. This was at Verplanck's Point. An examination with report by Dr. Nichols being unfavorable, the committee voted against giving it further consideration. In March, 1889, a bill for the exemption of taxation of the White Plains property having been introduced in the legislature, the governors authorized the commencement of building operations as soon as the bill should become a law. In the meantime Dr. Nichols had been proceeding with the preparation of plans, and in June he was given leave of absence for four months to examine recent institutional construction in Europe. He returned in October with much useful information and material.[6] He was, however, a very sick man, and on December 16 he died. This was an irreparable loss. He was succeeded by Dr. Samuel

[5] *Minutes of the Governors*, Oct. 4, 1887.

[6] Since the above was written it has been learned that Dr. Nichols with the help of his wife had placed his notes and sketches on foreign institutions in two large binders, and that they were in 1894 presented to the American Medico-Psychological Association. A search by the Secretary of the Association has been unsuccessful. See the *Transactions* of the Association, I (1894), 61.

B. Lyon, who had on Dr. Nichols's recommendation been appointed assistant medical superintendent in September, 1886. He had previously been employed at the United States Government Asylum in Washington, D.C., and it was considered that he was particularly qualified for the position as he "had not only a thorough practical knowledge of the care and treatment of the insane, but has had a business and architectural experience that specially qualifies him to assist in drawing plans of the contemplated buildings in the country and in overseeing their erection." [7]

In April, 1890, a plan prepared by the architect James Brown Lord was presented, and working plans and specifications were ordered. It was, however, not until December, 1891, that the governors, after reaffirming by resolution that "the Society's Farm at White Plains which was purchased for that purpose in January, 1868, is now finally adopted as a site for a new Asylum for the Insane," approved and adopted the plans reported by the Building Committee and directed them to proceed with the erection of the buildings. An appropriation of $1,250,000 was made. The governors also authorized the committee to enter into a contract with the Harlem Railroad Company for the construction of a branch from its station at White Plains to the asylum property, and to expend on the project not more than $35,000. This track, which was to have been laid in Martine Avenue, was, however, not provided. Four members of the board were still opposed to the White Plains site, and after voting against the resolution, three of them recorded the following objections:

(1) Great extra cost of construction and maintenance over places with shore front; (2) The costly and doubtful experiment (as it is yet unproved) of the proposed sewerage. (3) In the absence of water view an important factor in the cure of patients is left out.

The value attached to a water view in the cure of patients is noteworthy. Notwithstanding their objections, however, there was only one dissenting vote against the resolution which authorized the construction of the building. It was not until May, 1892, that a contract was entered into with Norcross Brothers and work was commenced. The amount of the contract was $1,131,144.45. It was estimated that electric lighting, kitchen and laundry equipment would add $22,282.

Delay was, to a considerable extent, due to uncertainty in regard to exemption from taxation. The law providing for exemption was passed

[7] Physician's Annual Report for 1885.

in June, 1889. In September, however, the property was assessed by the White Plains authorities and the governors appealed to the courts. An adverse decision against the Society at a special term of the state supreme court was recorded by the governors in August, 1890. This was reversed by the general term, but, in order to obtain a final settlement of the question, it was taken to the Court of Appeals, which in June, 1891, decided that the property was exempt.[8] Some delay was also occasioned by negotiations with White Plains in regard to sewage disposal. At first it was expected that a sewage disposal plant would be constructed on the property, and much study was given to this by a committee of the board. It was proposed, however, that the asylum join with White Plains in the construction of a trunk sewer through the Mamaroneck valley to the sound, and after much delay it was eventually arranged that the sewage from the property would be discharged into the White Plains system. It was ascertained that an abundant water supply could be obtained from wells on the property.

Building operations now proceeded steadily, with few noteworthy incidents. In November, 1893, Dr. Lyon proposed that villas be erected in addition to the main building, in accordance with the general scheme described by Dr. Nichols in 1887.[9] The building committee reported, however, that they were aware that "what is known as 'the Cottage System,' or the construction of separate buildings accommodating a limited number of patients, is more and more attracting the attention of Alienists at the present time, the McLean Asylum alone having on 176 Acres constructed some 18 buildings, and we might cite other instances on this point," but they considered it inexpedient to recommend a very extensive outlay in villas "in view of the present commitments and the large appropriations already made, and obligations incurred by the Society, and recognizing fully the indisposition of the Board towards further expenditures." They considered, however, that, in order to fulfill their obligations to the donor, it would be necessary to erect a new Macy Villa.[10]

In May, 1894, the title of Bloomingdale Asylum was, by order of the Board, changed to "Society of the New York Hospital, Bloomingdale, White Plains." This change was made, it was recorded, "to conform to the practice in the state of dropping the term Asylum from the titles of institutions for insane." The practice adopted by the state was, however,

[8] Letter from Dr. Lyon to Mr. Strong, a governor, June 18, 1891. New York Hospital, Westchester Division.

[9] P. 341.

[10] *Minutes of the Governors*, Dec. 5, 1893.

to substitute the title "Hospital" for "Asylum," and the title "Bloomingdale, White Plains" was never adopted in popular usage. It was not until 1910 that the title was officially changed to "Bloomingdale Hospital." [11]

In August the Asylum Committee reported to the board that the buildings were completed and ready for the reception of patients. The board thereupon authorized "the removal of the patients (by instalments) as soon as practicable; to be completed not later than October 1, 1894." The first transfer was made on August 12, when fifty-four women were taken to the new asylum and were reported to be "very much pleased." The remaining patients were transferred "by instalments," and the transfer was completed by September 18. The total number transferred was 284, of which 129 were men and 155 were women.[12]

On July 3, 1894, the Building Committee made a full report to the board of the expenditures for construction. The total amount was $1,444,839.95. It was estimated that the new Green Building cost $148,699 [13] and the Macy Villa $40,000. The buildings included the main building, the Macy Villa, the Green Building, the medical superintendent's residence, the greenhouse, and the stable. The expenditure included landscaping, grading, and road-making, much of which was done by Frederick Olmsted, who was the landscape architect of Central Park in New York. Funds for the project were taken from the general appropriation made by the governors, and $101,604.07 from "surplus income of the Asylum."

On September 1, 1894, the Asylum Committee held their last meeting in their relations with the old Bloomingdale. They recorded in their minutes that without one omission, the committee had held their regular monthly meetings from "May 5th, 1821 to September 1, 1894, a period of nearly 75 years."

The following notice was issued: [14]

BLOOMINGDALE

To the Medical Profession and Friends of the Institution:

The present expectation is that the medical work now carried on in the Bloomingdale Asylum at 117th Street, between Amsterdam Avenue and the Boulevard, will be transferred to the new BLOOMINGDALE, WHITE PLAINS, West-

[11] 1910 is the first year in which "Bloomingdale Hospital" appears as the official title in the annual report. Dr. Lyon had used it occasionally in his reports several years earlier.

[12] Physician's monthly report, September 1, 1894, in the *Minutes of the Asylum Committee.*

[13] *Minutes of the Governors,* Oct. 2, 1894.

[14] Annual report for 1893.

chester Co., N. Y., where for the last two years, an Institution of the most modern and liberal character has been in preparation, which is now nearly completed.

It is confidentially [*sic*] believed that the new BLOOMINGDALE will contain all essentials for the best care and treatment of the insane of the class among which the work of the Society has lain for so many years. The new buildings are of the Pavilion type, loosely grouped together, of a cheerful appearance, and are situated upon an elevation from which pleasant inland views are obtained on all sides. They are in the midst of extensive grounds, well adapted to the out-door enjoyments of the patients. The immediate surroundings of the Institution will be comfortable and attractive. Elevators, electric lighting, many single and connected rooms for the individualizing of cases, special departments for hydro-therapeutics, electro-therapeutics, massage, etc., are incorporated in the plan, and it is expected that these will be, in their proper places, essential features of the treatment.

No break will take place in the work of the hospital on account of its change of location.

The new Institution may be reached by the Harlem Railroad by some thirty daily trains, a dozen of which are express trains which make the trip in less than three-quarters of an hour. Public conveyances are always at the depot to convey passengers to the Institution, which is about twelve minutes further, and a special mode of transit may be provided, if the necessity seems to justify it.

The transfer of patients from New York to the new Institution will be made at the season of the year when such residents of cities as are able, are accustomed to go for some months to the country, and the new Institution is situated in a region which attracts many such summer residents, on account of its healthfulness, pleasant drives and ready accessibility from New York.

The Medical Superintendent may be seen on Mondays from three to four o'clock, and some Medical Officer on Wednesdays and Saturdays from twelve to one o'clock, holidays excepted, at the New York Hospital, 8 West 16th Street, New York City, by persons desiring to inquire about patients, or to obtain other information regarding the Institution.

After it was determined that the asylum would be removed, few expenditures for repairs and improvements were made at old Bloomingdale, except "such as were necessary to keep the Institution . . . . up to the highest standard of efficiency." [18] The only structural change made was the conversion of an "old unoccupied building" into a resort for patients, where they were provided with some simple gymnastic apparatus, a bowling alley, and a pool and card room. In 1889 a request was received for the use of the property for an International Exposition or World's Fair to be held in 1892. After consideration, however, it was found that the new institution would not be ready in time. Im-

[18] Physicians annual report for 1889.

provements in fire protection, plumbing, and in the wards for disturbed patients were made at various times on recommendation of the State Commission in Lunacy. Some concern was felt lest the provision in the Insanity Law of 1890 which restricted the legal confinement of an insane person to the state hospitals and to private institutions licensed by the state commission might be so interpreted as to exclude Bloomingdale, which operated under a charter.[16] The suggestion of the commission in regard to "establishing a uniformity in the status of all patients remaining . . . when the commission came into existence," some of whom had been admitted under earlier legal requirements, was, however, carried into effect, and copies of certificates and statistical and other information desired by the commission were furnished. In his annual report for 1889 the medical superintendent reported that requests and recommendations of the commission had been complied with, and "a harmony established with it." This has not been disturbed to the present day.

In 1891 negotiations for the sale of the property to Columbia University were entered into. An option was given the university for the purchase of four blocks extending from 116th to 120th streets and from Tenth Avenue to the Boulevard for $2,000,000, possession to be given on January 1, 1895; [17] and in 1892 an option for the purchase of the property west of the Boulevard and north of 116th Street was added, the price to be $650,000. A strip of land on 115th and 116th Streets was, in 1894, dedicated to the city, and also, with the consent of the university, forty feet along 120th Street from Amsterdam Avenue to the Boulevard. In September, 1894, after the patients had been transferred, permission was given to the Teachers College of the university to occupy the buildings, proper protection being provided in regard to legal possession on January 1, 1895, as agreed. Consideration had already been given to the disposition to be made of the proceeds from the sale of the property, and on February 7, 1893, the following resolution was adopted by the Board of Governors:

Resolved: That as the remaining real estate of the Hospital adjacent to or consisting of its Bloomingdale Asylum property shall be sold, the proceeds to the extent of one million five hundred thousand dollars shall be invested and held by the Hospital as an endowment fund for the purpose of providing for its annual expenses; and shall be invested by the Treasurer and the income only thereof used for such purpose; and the principal of such endowment fund shall not be diverted from this application except by a vote of a major-

[16] *Minutes of the Governors,* March 1, 1892.
[17] *Ibid.,* Dec. 1, 1891.

ity of all the elected Governors of the Board after notice of motion in writing signed by the Governor proposing it and duly entered in the minutes at a previous regular monthly meeting of the Board.[18]

[18] The total amount received for the property was $5,883,550, of which more than $5,000,000 was paid by Columbia and Barnard colleges. The last parcel was sold in 1909 for $11,000. *Minutes of the Governors*, Nov. 15, 1906, Jan. 5 and Feb. 2, 1909.

PART SEVEN

The Dawn of Modern Scientific Psychiatry at Bloomingdale 1894-1911

XXVII: "BLOOMINGDALE, WHITE PLAINS"

BLOOMINGDALE, with the term "Asylum" omitted from its title, was moved to White Plains at a time when rescuing the mentally ill from gross neglect and ill-treatment had been, in large measure, accomplished, and no longer absorbed most of the attention and effort of those engaged in the work. Intensive medical and psychiatric clinical study and treatment, and scientific investigation, were commencing to receive more attention and to be the object of provision made in the institutions. An editorial writer of the *American Journal of Insanity* considered the period to be one in which "upon the threshold of another era, the repetition of history brings again into prominence the requirements of the recent insane." He anticipated that in the hospitals for the mentally ill

> plans will be studied that quiet may be secured and unpleasant impressions removed; that acute cases may be seen frequently and conveniently by the senior medical officers; that a body of selected and trained nurses will provide the best care; that a *case* may be observed and studied by itself; that there may be reasonable and proper isolation during the critical stage; in short that the acute insane may be individualized. Upon the successful attainment of these requirements rests the distinctly professional character of the hospital. This, in brief, is the problem which now presents itself for solution.[1]

Such objectives had always had a large place in the service for the mentally ill of the New York Hospital, and it was expected that the new facilities would provide means for substantial advances.

When opened in 1894, the new Bloomingdale consisted of the main building and the Macy Villa for the accommodation of patients. There was also under construction the recreation building or gymnasium, which was completed the following year. The main building was considered to be of the "pavilion type." It consisted of a central building containing offices, the chapel, and living quarters for personnel, three service buildings, and six buildings for the accommodation of patients

1 *Am. J. Insanity*, L (1893), 316.

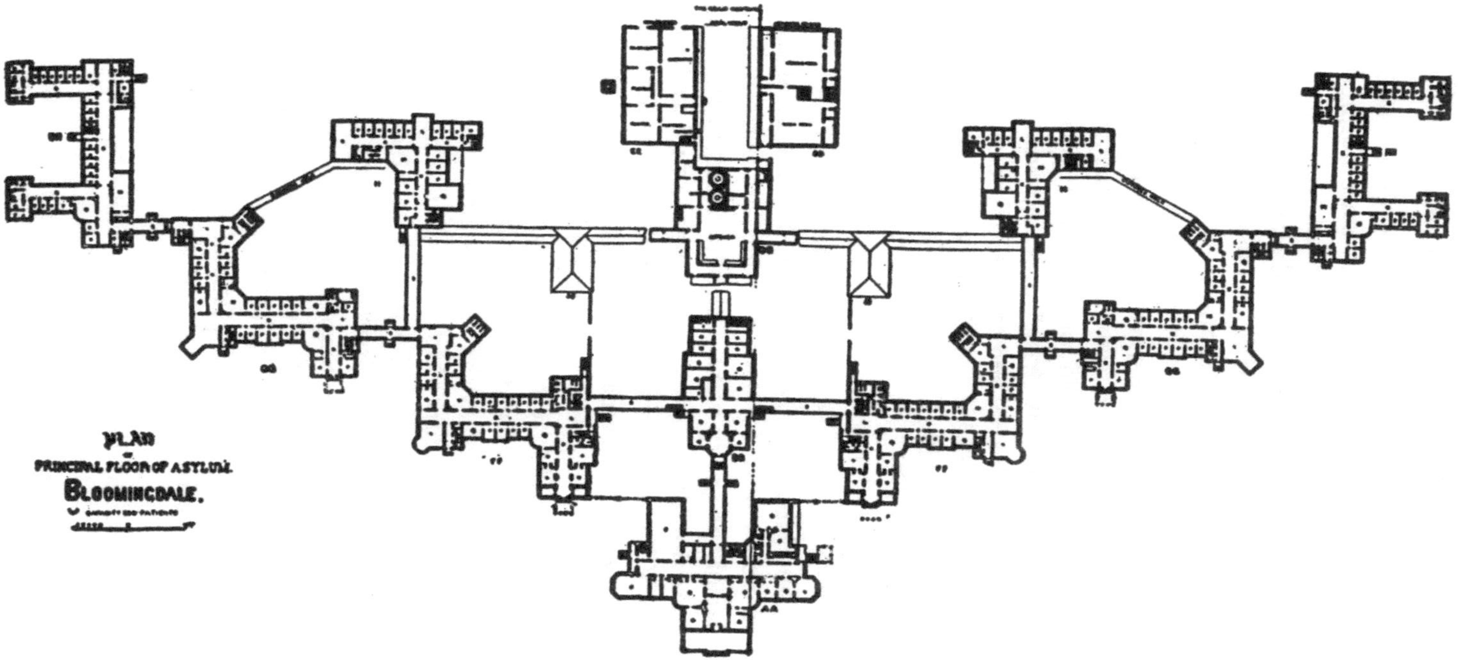

BLOOMINGDALE, WHITE PLAINS, 1894: FLOOR PLANS AS ORIGINALLY DESIGNED

(CENTRAL PAVILION FOR ADMINISTRATION AND DISTAL PAVILIONS FOR DISTURBED PATIENTS NOT CONSTRUCTED.)

and employees, all joined together by corridors of various lengths. The design was said to be similar to that of a new state hospital at Ogdensburg, New York. The pavilions of that hospital were, however, of two stories, with sleeping quarters on the second story, and day rooms only on the first. The Bloomingdale pavilions, on the other hand, were of three and four stories, the top stories, and in two instances a high basement, being occupied by employees. It was assumed that the pavilion plan was a means of combining the advantages of separate small buildings with those of convenient and economical supervision and administration. The original plan provided for three additional pavilions. One directly in front of the office and chapel building was designed for administration; two others, one attached to each of the terminal buildings erected, were designed for the accommodation of excited patients. These three pavilions were omitted, it was assumed temporarily, but actually they were never erected.

The proposed administration building was designed for reception rooms, a committee room, the medical superintendent's and the business offices, the library and laboratory, and social rooms for the patients. The second and third floors were for living rooms for personnel. The pavilions in the rear of the group were designed as an infirmary and hospital, and their use for disturbed patients was considered to be temporary. The Macy Villa was thought by physicians who visited it, some from foreign countries, to be remarkably satisfactory for the treatment of patients who paid the higher rates. It was contemplated that the completed institution would accommodate 500 patients, 400 in the main building and 100 in villas and cottages. Altogether the new Bloomingdale was generally regarded as the "high water mark of the close of the century . . . eminently adapted for the practical purposes for which it is intended." [2] The president of the American Medico-Psychological Association (now American Psychiatric Association) in his address in 1902 referred to it as one of four hospitals for the mentally ill which "have done magnificent work and stand to-day in the forefront of American psychiatry." [3] At the request of the New York State Commission in Lunacy, colored sketches and plans of the institution were exhibited at the Paris Exposition in 1900 and at the St. Louis Exposition in 1904.[4]

Little formality attended the inauguration of the new service. An

[2] *Ibid.*, LI (1895), 417.

[3] American Medico-Psychological Association, *Transactions*, 1902, p. 80.

[4] *Minutes of the Bloomingdale Committee*, Jan. 2, 1904. (The title of the Asylum Committee was changed to Bloomingdale Committee.)

invitation was extended to a group of physicians, journalists, and "prominent persons interested in general philanthropic measures," who on October 17, 1894, visited and inspected the institution and were served with supper in the chapel. An account of this appeared in the New-York *Tribune* on October 18. That paper had earlier (July 22) published a detailed description of the buildings, to which it was added that "the good work accomplished yearly by the New York Hospital and its branch the Bloomingdale Asylum is too well known to require comment here."

It will be recalled that Dr. Nichols considered that an institution for the mentally ill should consist of a central hospital and groups of villas and cottages. Unfortunately, his plans and descriptions have not been found, and the extent to which they were embodied in those followed cannot be ascertained. As has been mentioned, the Building Committee felt that economic considerations would prevent adherence to his views relating to detached buildings.[5] Soon after the opening, however, the wife of Mr. James M. Brown (who at the time of his death in 1890 was president of the Society) donated funds for the erection of a villa in his memory, to accommodate twelve or fifteen women. The building, known as the Brown Villa, was opened in 1896. Dr. Lyon was, perhaps, encouraged by this to suggest in the same year that an adjoining farm of fifty acres be purchased and used as a location for a group of cottages, "thus providing for the home and the hospital sides." This was not acceded to, however, and it was not until 1900 that the subject was again broached. In that year Dr. Lyon proposed that simple cottages of the "seashore type" be erected at a cost of five or six thousand dollars. He suggested that they would be "popular . . . for the insane of wealthy families." He was granted an appropriation of $6,000 for one cottage. Before it was erected, however, the father of one of the patients agreed to furnish the funds, and the cottage was completed in 1901 at a cost of $7,500. It was named "The Lucretia M. Dexter Memorial Cottage," and is now used for training school purposes. In 1900 also, a large skylight which had been discarded when some alterations were made at the New York Hospital was obtained by Bloomingdale and used in the construction of a recreation building for women; the second floor for the recreation room, and the first floor for the accommodation of nine slightly disturbed patients. This building was called "The Solarium." The recreation room was discarded in 1924 when the Taylor building was erected. No further addition to the accommodations for patients was made until 1904. In that year a legacy of $25,000 was received from James H. Banker, a

[5] See p. 343.

former governor, for the erection of a memorial villa. This building furnished accommodations for nine male patients. It was completed in 1905, and provided means for improving the classification of patients in relation with the Macy Villa. At this time the villas were restricted to the accommodation of patients who paid the higher rates. Later, medical considerations were of more weight than financial in determining accommodations.

In 1907, for the purpose of providing "additional rooms for our new scientific work" (which will be discussed fully in the next chapter) an extension attached to the rear of the office building was completed. This had been proposed by a member of the Bloomingdale Committee.[6] It contained on the first floor accommodations for a laboratory and a large room for occasional use by the governors and for informal social gatherings of the patients and personnel. The second story provided a few bedrooms. In the basement there were "a fine bathing suite" for hydrotherapy, and a mortuary and autopsy room. In 1911 a cottage for summer use was erected at Oakland Beach on Long Island Sound. For several years previously, rented cottages had been used with great advantage for day parties of patients, and for short periods of residence at the seashore. Permanent provision was, therefore, considered desirable; the property was purchased in 1910. In order to improve the milk supply of the hospital, a new barn was erected in 1907, and in 1909, following an extensive fire, the horse stable was enlarged and improved.

In 1910 Dr. Lyon again asked consideration of the question of cottages. He pointed to the increasing number of patients, occasioning detrimental crowding, and saw "no relief in sight except to use some of our receipts to add accommodations for a class of very remunerative patients of a somewhat disturbed or disorderly character." He recommended bungalows and also a villa for "women somewhat disturbed of the nice class . . . at a good price." In explanation of this he added that "while this is not a money making institution as such, all money received could be used very advantageously either here, or in New York in improvements and charitable assistance." [7] This proposal was approved by the Bloomingdale Committee but was apparently not considered by the board.

The governors were at that time much preoccupied with the question of again moving the New York Hospital to a different location. A site was, indeed, purchased and plans were prepared in which it was ex-

[6] *Minutes of the Bloomingdale Committee,* Dec. 2, 1905.
[7] *Ibid.,* Aug. 30 and Oct. 1, 1910.

pected that some provision would be made for mentally ill patients. It had long been felt that more extensive and adequate provision should be made not only at Bloomingdale but also at the New York Hospital for the reception of acutely ill mental cases. In one of his monthly reports in 1909, Dr. Lyon advised the governors that

there should be some more active supply of patients at Bloomingdale of the acute and hopeful class, so that the resources of Bloomingdale for the treatment of patients may be fully utilized, and that it may fulfill its mission of relief and cure of the insane, to a greater degree than it does at the present time. This month's census [343] emphasizes the need of reception halls in New York City for acute cases.

In December of that year he proposed that the houses at 16 and 18 West 16th Street should be used for the establishment of "an annex for nervous diseases." [8] The new site for the general hospital was, however, not used, and the project gave place to the negotiations with Cornell University which resulted eventually in the present development on East 68th Street.

Notwithstanding the consideration given to provision for patients who could pay the higher rates, there was never any intention of departing from the long established policy of devoting the service primarily to patients who could pay only the bare cost of maintenance or required assistance to finance their illness. As soon as the new institution was established it was considered that "in view of the probability of reduced expenditures for improvements, and the prospects of a good income from remunerative patients," the assistance to patients of limited means could be increased, "giving preference to those whose form of disease makes it probable that they may be restored to society after a few months' treatment at Bloomingdale." In fact, Dr. Lyon felt that "the ability of the Institution and its prospective ability to render assistance to a large number of indigent deserving cases is not contracted, nor is likely to be . . . it is confidently expected that a larger amount of such assistance can, from year to year, be rendered." [9] There was no diminution in the number of free patients during this period. In 1895 the number was 8 percent of the total number treated, and in 1910 it was over 9 percent. Many others paid rates that were less than the cost of treatment.

Because no outlay for repairs was needed on the new buildings and because the number of patients increased (many at the higher rate), for a number of years the income was greater than current expenses. In 1896 it was considered advisable to bring the Bloomingdale funds more

[8] See also pp. 471–472.

[9] Medical superintendent's report for 1895.

closely under the control of the treasurer, and it was directed that all balances not required for immediate expenditure should at the end of each quarter be transmitted to him. It was also decided that not more than $3,000 of any surplus income could be spent for improvements at Bloomingdale unless approved by the Board of Governors. The amount of petty cash in a White Plains bank subject to the order of the medical superintendent was fixed at $1,000. It was also required that a monthly statement of receipts and expenditures be made to the governors.[10]

The service was managed on very economical lines. A comparison with the similar hospitals of Butler, McLean, Hartford, and Pennsylvania revealed that the weekly per capita expenditure was less at Bloomingdale than at any of the others except Pennsylvania.[11] The number of patients treated at the Bloomingdale and Pennsylvania hospitals was, however, larger than at the others. The annual budget of Bloomingdale increased from $225,000 in 1888, when the average daily number of patients under treatment was 306, to $235,000 in 1903 when the average number was 336. The average weekly rate received in 1888 was $13.07 and in 1904 it had risen only $1. In 1910, however, it was $16.09. Quite substantial balances were transferred to the treasurer during this period; use of these funds for improvements and for the assistance of impecunious patients was not confined to the needs of the mentally ill.

When the new Bloomingdale was established it was assumed that no more buildings would be required "unless some new departure is made in convalescent homes or other special directions." [12] Apparently the question of utilizing a portion of the property for other classes of patients than the mentally ill was under consideration. In 1895 Dr. Lyon, in a letter to the president of the Society, pointed out the prospect presented by the southern portion of the property as a location for "a convalescent or incurable department" of the New York Hospital.[13] This project was proposed and fostered by the medical superintendent and the Bloomingdale Committee, and in 1897 they suggested that the farmhouse be utilized for convalescent women, and that a pavilion for men be built "slightly removed." Dr. Lyon suggested to the governors that this pavilion might be "utilized later for insane quiet laboring patients, perhaps, should you desire to establish a more distant and pretentious convalescent home for New York Hospital patients, somewhat further

10 *Minutes of the Governors*, April 7, 1896.

11 Report of the medical superintendent, *Minutes of the Bloomingdale Committee*, April 2, 1904.

12 *Ibid.*, for 1895.

13 Letter to Mr. Trimble, president, March 5, 1895, on file at Westchester Division.

from our present buildings." The proposal for a pavilion was adopted and in 1898 Dr. Lyon was requested to submit a plan for a building for ten men, as it was considered advisable to reserve the farmhouse for women. Later it was decided to reverse the order and to erect a pavilion for women. This was accomplished in 1900, and the new cottage, which was small and cheaply constructed, was named "The Orchard." At this time the daughters of Duncan Campbell (he had been one of the governors) became interested in the project, and contributed in all $30,000 for building purposes. The cottage, under the name of "The Campbell Convalescent Home," opened on May 1, 1901, and nine men and seven women were admitted. Before the close of the season it was decided to provide for the men in a cottage on an adjoining property which had recently been purchased. The service was found to be very useful; in October, 1904, in reviewing the work at the close of the season, Dr. Lyon reported that the homes "fill a very benevolent office towards convalescent people who have little or no means."

In 1906 the governors appointed a committee to inquire into the question of "Fresh Air Treatment." The committee report referred to one on "Cottage Hospitals" that had been made in 1876,[14] when the removal of the New York Hospital from its original site on Broadway was under consideration.[15] The committee also presented plans and specifications for a "Country Branch Hospital at White Plains." In November, 1907, they presented a supplementary report which contained an account of a conference on the subject with the medical board, and a number of letters from physicians. Among the letters favoring the project was one from Dr. John S. Billings, an authority on hospital planning, and one from Dr. Henry C. Burdett of London, author of *Hospitals and Asylums of the World* (1891–1893). The committee were evidently ardently in favor of the general plan, but did not approve of the architect's proposal of one large building instead of a group of small buildings. In their annual report the governors stated that "the Hospital is desirous of carrying out this most promising feature of hospital treatment." They estimated that the cost would be $150,000 or $200,000 and they appealed for funds.[16] Adequate funds were unavailable; the distance was great for the attending physicians to travel; and a full-time salaried staff would be required. For all these reasons the project was abandoned.

The Campbell Home was, however, enlarged by the addition of two

[14] Society of the New York Hospital, *Printed Reports, Addresses . . . , 1872–1909.*

[15] See p. 260.

[16] *Minutes of the Governors,* March 5, 1907.

cottages and an administration building; and, from 1907, under the able direction of Miss Alice E. Ellison until 1932, and thereafter of Miss Marie L. Troup, it was operated as the "Campbell Convalescent Cottages" for children and adolescent girls. In 1936, because of financial considerations, it was with great regret discontinued. Consideration of the establishment of a branch hospital on the Bloomingdale property again occurred in 1909, when removal of the New York Hospital to another location was pending. Again, however, it was objected that the distance was too great for the attending physicians and the project was dropped. This account of provision at Bloomingdale for New York Hospital convalescents, while not altogether pertinent in a history of the service for the mentally ill, is given because it was started, fostered, and supervised by the Bloomingdale Committee and the medical superintendent and was for a number of years financed entirely from the Bloomingdale income.

In 1904 the business administration was thoroughly investigated by the Committee on Finance of the Board of Governors, with the assistance of an expert accountant. Much testimony was taken and the business methods were carefully scrutinized. The report of the committee was printed. They recommended that the medical superintendent be relieved of the duties of general superintendent, purchasing agent, and manager. This would have been a reversion to the form of organization adopted when Bloomingdale Asylum was established in 1821 and maintained for many years, during which the authority of the physician was gradually extended until in 1877 he was given full control with the title of medical superintendent. The committee recommended the appointment of a purchasing agent to have charge of the purchasing for all branches of the Society's work. The report was referred to the Bloomingdale Committee for examination and report. That committee considered the report of the accountant to be "inaccurate, misleading, and erroneous in its deductions." They saw no advantage in a general purchasing agency, believing that the same result could be obtained by means of conferences and coöperation. They disapproved of divided authority and cited the experience and example of other institutions in regard to the position of medical superintendent. They believed that the majority of the recommendations "would result in injury, not benefit, to the Institution." [17] In a supplementary report the Finance Committee added that they did "not share in the admiration of that [Bloomingdale] committee for the business methods," and pointed out that the

[17] *Ibid.*, March 7, 1905.

medical superintendent and the farm steward had outside interests. They directed attention to improvements in the administration and economies made since the investigation, with consequent "better financial results." [18] The Board of Governors, a few days after the final report was presented, voted that "no further action in the matter is necessary."

It was anticipated, when Bloomingdale was removed to White Plains, that the facilities for outdoor activities as a means of treatment would be greatly increased. Much attention was, therefore, given to grading, planting, the construction of roads and walks, and provision for exercises and games. A glance at a view of the grounds in the vicinity of the buildings at the time of the removal will indicate the work involved in producing present-day conditions.[19] The buildings were, in most instances, located in the open fields. By May, 1896, however, it was noted that the grounds "now present a very attractive appearance, and the labor bestowed on them begins to show." A "tree expert" was employed in 1907. In 1901 the property had been extended by the purchase of fifty acres called the Onderdonk farm. It was on this property that Dr. Lyon proposed that a group of cottages for patients be erected. It is now the location of residences for physicians and nurses. Early in 1911 sixty acres of the extreme southern portion of the Bloomingdale property were sold to the Winifred Masterson Burke Relief Foundation as a site for a convalescent home. This furnished, perhaps, a substitute for the "convalescent or incurable department" proposed in 1895.

In 1897 an arrangement was made, in coöperation with other property owners, for the construction of a public road along the western margin of the property. After long negotiation, and the buying, selling, and exchanging of several parcels of property, the road was finally constructed and was dedicated to the city in 1916. It is now called Bloomingdale Road; the same as the name of the road to the original Bloomingdale site in New York. For the purpose of protecting the water supply, the governors provided for a sewer in the road. In 1897 the water supply was augmented by boring a well to the depth of about 500 feet. This provided about 12,000 gallons per day of an exceptionally pure water for drinking. In 1898 the lake was deepened, providing a supply of soft water for the boilers and laundry, an addition to the means of fire protection, an attractive feature to the landscape, and a means of exercise and pleasure for the patients during the winter. In 1902 an additional well was dug for the purpose of increasing the water supply from 45,000 to 50,000 gallons per day, which were considered adequate. In 1904 and

[18] *Ibid.*, April 4, 1905. [19] See illustration p. 334.

1905, on the recommendation of the fire underwriters and the State Commission in Lunacy, $13,000 were spent on water lines, pump, hydrants, and other equipment for fire protection. The iron gates and the iron fence which had stood at the main entrance to the Bloomingdale grounds in the city were, in 1895, placed at the entrance to the new Bloomingdale grounds. The gates were, some years later, transferred to the Mamaroneck Avenue entrance, in order to widen the main entrance for the passage of automobiles. The fence, however, which is the handiwork of the Bloomingdale blacksmith, still adjoins the main entrance. During the month of March each year this entrance is officially closed in order to avoid its becoming a legal thoroughfare for the public. The farm and garden were cultivated with advantage, and in some years all the potatoes and vegetables required were produced, besides much of the feed for the cattle and horses.

In entering upon the new service, it was announced that Bloomingdale was provided "with the necessary facilities for taking care of and treating by the most modern methods all the patients which it will accommodate." [20] Among these facilities, the equipment for hydrotherapy was considered to be of particular interest. Several rooms in the basement of the "infirmary building," occupied by disturbed women, were assigned for its accommodation. They contained a large electrical apparatus, hot-air and steam cabinets, a needle bath and a shower bath. Provision was also made for massage. In 1908 the department was thoroughly renovated and "brought up-to-date." In the annual report for that year it was stated that the hydrotherapy equipment was "among the first if not the very first of such installations in a hospital for the insane."

Carriages and wagons "not distinctly institutional" were provided for patients' drives. Those who had sufficient means were charged a small amount. In 1909 an automobile was provided in which patients were taken out without charge. An International Harvester Delivery Wagon chassis was also purchased, and a top and seats were made for it by the hospital mechanics. This was used to take patients to the beach cottage. Tennis courts and a baseball diamond were constructed, and the recreation building furnished facilities for bowling, handball, pool, billiards, and other games. "Vis-a-vis swings" placed on the lawn were considered to have a definite therapeutic value. A new organ was purchased in 1894 for $3,000.

In 1899 a start was made toward equipping a clinical laboratory. There

[20] Medical superintendent's report for 1895.

was "gathered into one place the apparatus and material for clinical laboratory work, which has formerly been done in the dispensary, or in the physicians' offices; and we now have a suitable place where examinations can be made without interfering with or being interrupted by other work." In 1907, as already mentioned, more adequate provision was made in the new extension to the office building. In a review of the ten years following the removal to White Plains, Dr. Lyon in his annual report for 1904 mentioned that there were "ample facilities for Physical Culture, Electric, Dental, Ophthalmic and Gynecological Departments, Clinical and Pathological Laboratory, Cabinetmaking and other manual training opportunities, salt water bathing, and a large variety of individual outings."

In 1908 "a small department for fancy manual occupation" for women was, at the suggestion of Dr. August Hoch, established under the direction of Mrs. Medora Amsden, wife of one of the physicians. She was actuated by purely benevolent motives, and for two years served without pecuniary compensation. She had, it was stated, had "experience in art culture and instruction in Massachusetts, and comes well equipped for this kind of work which she has undertaken with enthusiasm." Equipment was provided for weaving and basketry, at first in two rooms of the second floor of the Dexter Cottage and soon after in two rooms in Hall 1 for women. In his annual report, the medical superintendent referred to the project as "still in the nature of an experiment, but it is no doubt a small step toward the desirable condition of being able to afford manual occupation to persons whose minds are not in a condition to meet even the ordinary problems of life, but who are diverted by a new interest and by something which they can do themselves with their own hands." In the report of the following year the occupation department was called "valuable to the moral treatment"; and "owing to the good work which they have done, [it] has been less expensive than was expected. A considerable demand has existed for the fancy work, which has appealed to various women who visited the institution, so that there is every encouragement to pursue it." References relating to the work in the monthly reports during the year are to the effect that "the financial deficit is more than compensated by the beneficial results to the patients," half of the expense having been covered, and that "if the expenses can be minimized, it is a valuable adjunct to the means of treatment." This marked the rather halting beginning of what has since become a major resource in the treatment of both the women and the men patients. A corresponding department for men was not established until 1912. It will be described in a later chapter.[21]

Notwithstanding the increased distance to be traveled in visiting the institution, there was no diminution in the attendance of the governors, nor in their zeal for the interests of the service. In addition to the regular visits and meetings of the Bloomingdale Committee, and the inspections of the weekly and the inspecting committees, the officers and as many members of the Board of Governors as could attend held an annual meeting at Bloomingdale. For a number of years several of the attending physicians of the New York Hospital accompanied them on the visit. After the training school for attendants was established this annual inspection was made on graduation day.

There was at first some uncertainty concerning the title of the institution. In the revised by-laws in 1895 it is referred to as the "Society's department for the Insane, called Bloomingdale, White Plains." In 1910, the title was officially changed to "Bloomingdale Hospital," and by that name it was known until 1936, when it was changed to its present title of "New York Hospital—Westchester Division."

An innovation greatly appreciated by those who have occasion to consult the minutes of the Bloomingdale Committee was the adoption in 1894 of typewritten instead of handwritten entries. The thin, typewritten pages were pasted on the leaves of such books as were used when the minutes were handwritten, until, in 1899, the present loose-leaf volumes were introduced. In June, 1900, the medical superintendent's "summary" for the month began to contain more than a statistical statement and to take on the form of the report now presented at each monthly meeting. In 1909 the practice of spreading the full text of the annual reports on the minutes was discontinued.

In December, 1903, the service was first visited and inspected by the recently appointed medical inspector of the State Commission in Lunacy, and inspections by medical representatives of the state department have been made several times a year ever since. All patients admitted since the previous visit and still remaining, are interviewed by the medical inspector, and a complete inspection is made. For a number of years previously members of the commission had visited the institution once, and occasionally more times, each year. Much information in regard to the details of organization and administration of the service was re-

[21] Pp. 423–424.

quested by the commission during the first few years following its establishment. This was readily supplied, full understanding and confidence were obtained, and the cordial relations and coöperation which have ever since been maintained, were established.

XXVIII

EARLY TWENTIETH CENTURY MEDICINE AND PSYCHIATRY AT BLOOMINGDALE

As an aid in estimating the significance and character of some of the developments at Bloomingdale following the removal to White Plains in 1894 and up to 1911, a brief preliminary review of psychiatric progress in America during the period may be helpful. The removal occurred at a time when provision for the study and treatment of the mentally ill, and psychiatric thought and practice in America were subjected to much criticism and were entering upon a transition period. On the one hand, Dr. E. C. Spitzka, an eminent psychiatrist, was in July, 1894, writing in the *Journal of Nervous and Mental Diseases* that "the overwhelming majority of state and larger private asylums have attained the dignity of psychiatric clinics," and that "the main improvement has occurred within the ranks of those who are physicians to asylums." On the other hand, Dr. S. Weir Mitchell, an equally eminent neurologist, in the same year was deploring, in an address before the American Medico-Psychological Association, the "scientific unproductiveness" of the asylums, the torpor and unprogressiveness of boards of management, especially those of the endowed private institutions, the isolation and freedom of the asylum physicians from the critical observation of visiting and consulting colleagues, the inferior nursing service and lack of consideration of the individual patient.[1] In 1896 also Dr. Landon Carter Gray was declaring to the American Neurological Association that "we are startled to find that no new type of mental disease, no original pathological observation, no new departure in treatment, and not one text-book, has ever come from an American asylum, despite the millions of dollars and thousands of patients they have had at their command." [2] All these statements were evidently made without full knowledge and understanding, and the truth was somewhere in between. Progress was being made but was slow, irregular, and attended with many difficulties.

The change of title from asylum to hospital was more than a verbal gesture. Some of the improvements made in different hospitals in the state of New York were, in 1896, listed in the *American Journal of Insanity:* the establishment of laboratories (clinical, pathological, bacteriological), operating and treatment rooms, well-organized hospital and

1 American Medico-Psychological Association, *Transactions,* I (1895), 101.
2 *Am. J. Insanity,* LIII (1896), 324.

infirmary wards for physical treatment, special reception and intensive treatment departments, assembly halls and other facilities for recreation purposes, summer cottages, medical baths, workshops for patients, training schools for nurses. It was in 1896 that extensive industries in which patients were employed were established at the State Hospital, Utica, New York. Further improvements listed by the *Journal* in 1903 were an increase in the number of staff physicians, the employment of medical and surgical specialists, the adoption of a system of interneship, the segregation and treatment of tuberculous patients, the "open door" system and other facilities for "moral treatment." It was considered that mechanical restraint had been "practically abandoned." [3]

Apart from the special hospitals, a start was made towards provision for the treatment of mental illness at the general hospitals. A pavilion for the purpose was erected at the Albany (New York) Hospital in 1900. In 1901 a separate psychopathic hospital for treatment, research, and teaching was established at the University of Michigan Medical School. A similar institution, the Boston Psychopathic Hospital, was established in 1909, and the Phipps Psychiatric Clinic of the Johns Hopkins Medical School and Hospital was established in 1908. These developments marked an advancement in provision for psychiatric teaching in the medical schools, which, however, continued to be generally very inadequate.

In 1895 the New York State Commission in Lunacy (created in 1889) established in New York City a Pathological Institute, "the first time in the history of this hemisphere that a government has set to work to study insanity as it should be studied, viz., by an aggregation of discoverers in many fields, biology, anthropology, psychology, pathology, chemistry and the like." [4] Under the direction of Dr. Ira Van Giesen extensive scientific investigation was undertaken. In order to bring the work of the institute into closer relations with the hospitals it was, in 1902, moved to the Manhattan State Hospital and reorganized under the direction of Dr. Adolf Meyer. An educational and scientific program in collaboration with the hospitals was adopted. Courses of instruction for the hospital physicians were given at the institute and at the hospitals. Laboratories were established, libraries organized or expanded, and staff conferences reorganized. An orderly system of examination, classification, and case recording was introduced. In a remarkably short time a striking transformation occurred in the spirit and practice of the hospital physicians. A new type of psychiatric thought and practice was

[3] *Ibid.*, LIX (1903), 536.

[4] *Ibid.*, LVI (1899), 5: "Some of the Problems of the Alienist," by Frederick Peterson, M.D.

introduced which raised the standard of the whole service to a higher level and it has continued to operate with increasing excellence. It would have been fortunate if the Bloomingdale physicians had been given access to the advantages enjoyed by the state hospital physicians at that time.

A mark of advancement in attention to the mentally ill in New York communities was the provision made in 1902 for the transfer of the patients to the state hospitals by nurses instead of by deputy sheriffs or relatives. Another advance was the substitution in 1909 of medical health officers for poor-law authorities as the officials responsible for providing adequate care of the mentally ill pending their transfer to hospitals. Psychiatric out-patient service was established in different places. One of the first, and apparently the very first in New York, was that at the Cornell Medical College Clinic in 1904.[5] Provision for supervision and readjustment of patients after they left the hospitals began to be a subject of discussion about 1894, and a report relating to it was presented at a meeting of the American Neurological Association in 1898. In 1906 the State Charities Aid Association of New York appointed local committees for the purpose and was instrumental in establishing the social service which is now considered essential in every well-organized public hospital for the mentally ill.

Improvements which were made or contemplated in the provision and treatment of the mentally ill were subjects of papers and discussions at the meetings of the American Medico-Psychological Association and of the American Neurological Association. Many articles relating to them were published in the current psychiatric literature of which the *American Journal of Insanity* continued to be the principal, although no longer the only, medium. *The Journal of Nervous and Mental Diseases* also contained articles on psychiatric topics. The publications relating to staff organization and methods, laboratory and hospital equipment and their use, various forms of treatment, the training of nurses and attendants, and other details of hospital provision and treatment contributed greatly to raising standards throughout the country. The progress of psychiatric thought and clinical practice may also be traced in the discussions and publications of the period. The spread of knowledge relating to the role of microorganisms in disease led to the conception of infection from the intestines and other parts of the body as a

[5] 1904, according to a statement by Dr. Adolf Meyer, then professor of psychiatry at Cornell Medical College. It was first cited as the Department of Psychopathology of the Dispensary, at a Cornell University Medical College meeting held on April 21, 1906. Dr. Hoch was appointed chief of the clinic.

cause of mental illness. Autointoxication and its treatment received much attention in 1894 and later. In 1899 a study of more than a thousand cases of mental illness treated by thyroid extract was published by two physicians of New York state hospitals.[6] Several physicians, notably Dr. H. J. Berkley of Baltimore, practiced thyroidectomy in the treatment of dementia praecox, especially of the catatonic variety, and reported favorable results.[7] After surgeons were employed on the staffs of the hospitals for the mentally ill, articles relating to surgical treatment began to appear in the literature. Later surgery came to have a larger place—in some instances too large—in the practice of a limited number of physicians engaged in the treatment of the mentally ill. About 1895 and later much interest was manifested in constitutional factors in mental illness, in the form of "degeneracy" manifested by stigmata. Articles based on studies in the laboratories of the hospitals began to appear in the literature by the close of the nineteenth century. General paresis, cerebral arteriosclerosis, and hereditary chorea were frequent subjects of contributions. References to examination of the spinal fluid and cytodiagnosis began to appear in the psychiatric literature about 1903, and at the same time the role of bacteria and acute infectious disease in the production of mental illness was receiving much attention. In 1905 the possible bacterial origin of general paresis was a subject of interest. Alcoholism, particularly the Korsakow syndrome, was another subject of a number of communications. The blood pressure of the mentally ill began to be referred to in 1904, and metabolism tests in 1908. The term *dementia praecox* appeared in articles in the *Journal* in 1900, and the term *manic-depressive psychosis* in 1907, although Kraepelin's classification had been adopted in various American psychiatric services at an earlier date.

Medical thought and, to a large extent, medical practice in mental illness were, at the close of the nineteenth century, still dominated by the conception of structural and physiological disturbances as the basic factors in causation and as the main objects in treatment. About the time of the removal of Bloomingdale to White Plains, however, psychological considerations began with increasing frequency to receive attention in publications. Among significant titles may be mentioned *The Psychical Correlation of Religious Emotion and Sexual Desire* by James Weir, Jr., in 1897, "The Imagination in Relation to Mental Disease" by Robert H. Chase in 1899, and, in 1903, "Nature and Genesis of an Insane De-

[6] *Am. J. Insanity*, LVI (1899), 257.

[7] *Ibid.*, LXV (1908), 415. Dr. Berkley was also the author of a work on the *General Pathology of Mental Disease*, published in 1900.

lusion" by J. W. Wherry, in which the origin and formation of delusion were attributed to "subconscious cerebration." In 1908 articles relating to psychology in clinical and preventive medicine, to mental factors in psychiatry and to habit training as the "backbone of psychotherapy," [8] were becoming more frequent. In that year also an article by Dr. C. Macfie Campbell entitled "Psychological Mechanisms with Special Reference to Wish Fulfilment" was one of the earliest manifestations in America of the advent of psychoanalytic doctrine. In 1909 an article by Dr. Ernest Jones entitled "Psychoanalytic Notes on a Case of Hypomania," and a second article, "On the Nightmare," by the same author, brought psychoanalysis clearly into the purview of general psychiatric literature. Dr. A. A. Brill's translation of *Psychic Mechanisms of Hysterical Phenomena* and other papers of Freud were also published in that year. The subject of psychoneuroses in psychiatric hospital practice may perhaps be considered to have first received attention in Van Deusen's notable article in 1868.[9] Although an article on "Neurasthenia and Insanity" appeared in the *Journal* in 1900, it was not until about 1910 that the psychoneuroses began to have an established place in the psychiatric hospital literature of America. In 1910 Kent and Rosanoff's notable *Study in Association in Insanity* was published and found a useful place in psychiatric scientific investigation. The prevention of mental illness began to receive particular attention with the dawn of the twentieth century, and in 1909 the National Committee for Mental Hygiene was founded by Clifford W. Beers, who had himself experienced a severe mental illness with treatment in three types of hospitals and who wrote an account of it in *A Mind That Found Itself* (1908).

A considerable number of books on psychiatric subjects by American authors was published during this period. Among the principal were a *Text Book on Mental Diseases* by Theodore H. Kellogg, M.D., in 1897, Clevenger and Bowlby's *Medical Jurisprudence of Insanity* in 1898, Church and Peterson's *Nervous and Mental Diseases* in 1899, *Treatise on Mental Disease* by H. J. Berkley in 1900, Brower and Bannister's *Practical Manual of Insanity* in 1902. In 1902, also, Diefendorf's *Clinical Psychiatry* (an abstract of the sixth edition of Kraepelin's treatise) furnished to many American physicians a highly valued access to Kraepelin's teachings. In 1905 Stewart Paton's text book, *Psychiatry*, was published and was long a standard work for physicians and students. A number of

[8] Adolf Meyer, "Role of Mental Factors in Psychiatry," *Am. J. Insanity*, LXV (1908), 46.

[9] E. H. Van Deusen, "Observations on a Form of Nervous Prostration (Neurasthenia) Culminating in Insanity," *Am. J. Insanity*, XXV (1868), 445.

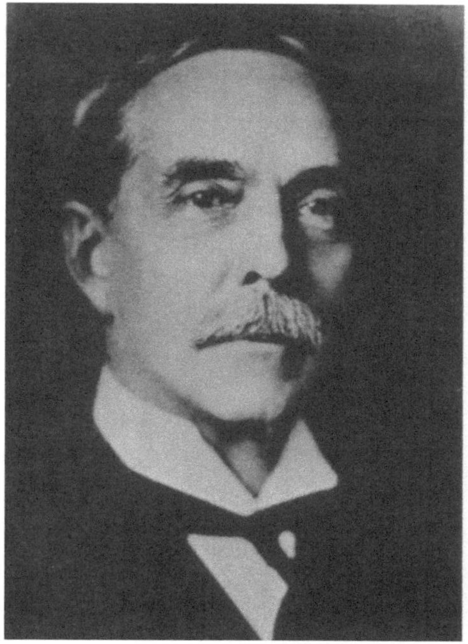

SAMUEL B. LYON, M.D.
MEDICAL SUPERINTENDENT, 1889-1911

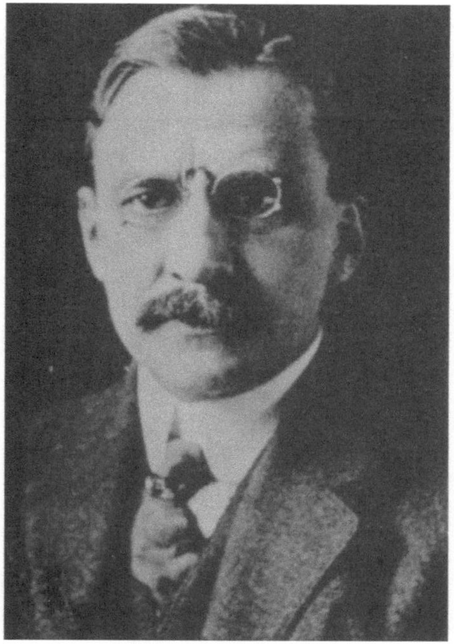

AUGUST HOCH, M.D.
FIRST ASSISTANT PHYSICIAN AND
SPECIAL PATHOLOGIST, 1905-1909

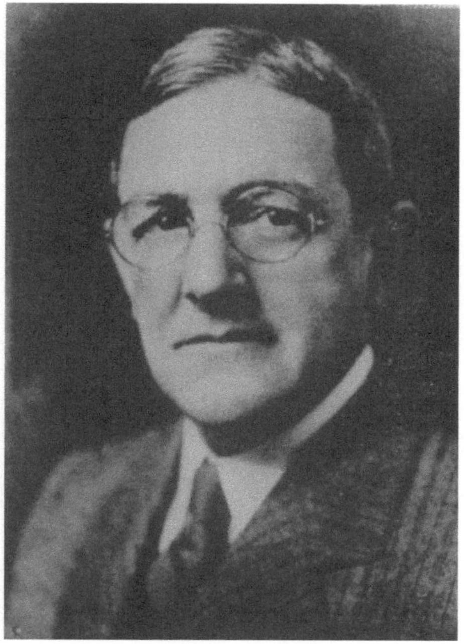

MORTIMER WILLIAMS RAYNOR, M.D.
MEDICAL DIRECTOR, 1926-1935

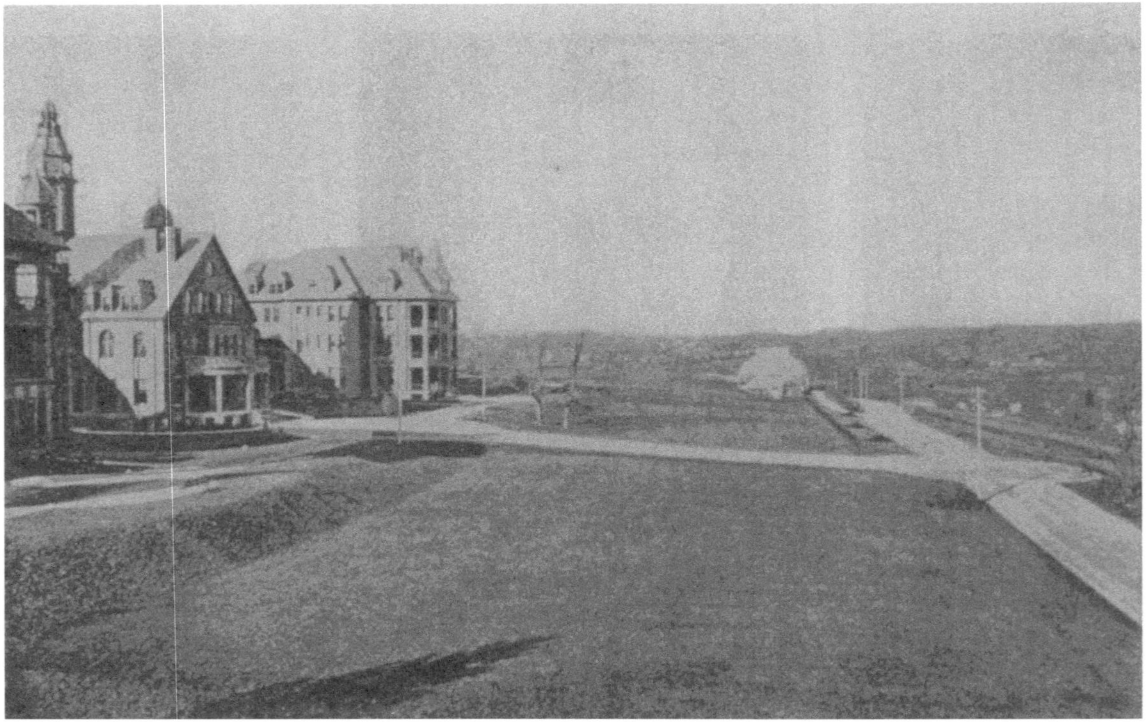

BLOOMINGDALE, WHITE PLAINS, 1894

other books on special psychiatric topics were published during this period. The first number of the *New York State Hospitals Bulletin* was issued in January, 1896. The neurologists in private practice manifested considerable interest in the public hospitals for the mentally ill, and were, on occasion, very helpful in promoting improvements. Much of the current literature on psychiatric topics consisted of articles which had been presented at meetings of national or local neurological societies.

It was anticipated that the removal of Bloomingdale to the new location at White Plains, with its better facilities, would enable it to take full advantage of these advances in medical study and treatment of the mentally ill. In 1896 it was reported that "the Hospital has made full use of all its facilities," and that the medical superintendent, after a visit to a number of hospitals in England and Scotland, found that "Bloomingdale is not behind any other Institution which he saw, in matters of comfort, convenience or medical efficiency." No change occurred in the relative number of physicians on the resident staff. In 1894 when the average daily number of patients was 294 the staff consisted of the medical superintendent, three assistant physicians, and one clinical assistant. In 1910 with a daily average of 352 patients, there were, besides the medical superintendent, three assistant physicians and two clinical assistants, one of whom was appointed for laboratory work. In 1895 Dr. Rose Pringle was appointed as a clinical assistant. Her particular duty, as described in the annual report, was "assisting in those matters of personal contact between the physician and the patient in which a woman can be more properly employed perhaps than a man." The New York law now specifies that the medical staff of every state hospital shall include a woman. In 1905 the first assistant physician was designated special pathologist also.[10] A dental service was introduced in 1896, and was gradually extended and systematized. The first dentist was Dr. D. Austin Sniffen. Specialists in surgery, ophthalmology, and other specialties were employed in a consulting capacity; the character and extent of service were, however, not clearly stated. A few gynecological operations and an operation for strangulated hernia were mentioned in the records. There was a sufficient number, however, to lead the governors, in 1905, to adopt a resolution that no dental or surgical operation should be performed without the consent of the Bloomingdale Committee, a relative, or a friend.

The case histories for fifteen years following the removal in 1894 continued to be recorded in the large volumes described in previous

10 *Minutes of the Bloomingdale Committee,* April 1, 1905.

chapters, in the handwriting of a physician or clerk. If notes were made by nurses, they have apparently not been preserved. The governors were evidently actively interested in the case histories, as it is sometimes mentioned in the notes of their visits that they had "found them in order" or that they "showed a careful, painstaking method of arrangement." The books were also brought to the committee meetings for inspection and their presence was sometimes mentioned in the monthly reports of the medical superintendent. Impelled, perhaps, by the adoption of the new form of case recording in the state and other hospitals, the president of the Society and the medical superintendent, in 1905, visited the Sheppard and Enoch Pratt Hospital, where they "found they had an elaborate system of keeping histories of patients, but not essentially superior to those of Bloomingdale." They also mentioned the laboratory, the good work of which they "hoped to duplicate." It was not until 1909 that Dr. Townsend, first assistant physician at Bloomingdale, who had previously been in the New York State service, introduced the typewritten loose-leaf system of case histories, together with the general plan of history adopted by the state service.

The publication of statistical tables in the annual report which, it will be recalled, was resumed in 1891,[11] was, with the exception of a single table showing the movement of population, again discontinued in 1907. The diagnostic terms used in the statistical tables and in the case histories during the period were acute mania, acute melancholia, melancholia, unclassified depression, manic depressive psychosis, dementia praecox and catatonia (after 1905). The statistical tables recommended for general adoption by the American Medico-Psychological Association were not accepted at Bloomingdale because, as explained in the annual report for 1897, it was considered that a "breach of continuity," and "difficulty in reconciling the various discrepancies" would result. The number of cases of general paresis which were treated at Bloomingdale was, as previously noted, quite large. In 1901 it was reported that of 1,230 admissions to the service during the previous ten years, 205 were cases of this disease. It was stated, however, that the number had decreased 6 percent.

The great advances in medicine during this period had, no doubt, an influence on the general medical study and treatment of the patients at Bloomingdale. Dentistry and the services of specialists contributed to greater efficiency in diagnosis and treatment. Medication did not change much except by the introduction of the synthetic hypnotics. The annual

11 See p. 325.

reports contained little relating to general medical treatment, the only reference being ordinarily such statements as "the physicians have been industrious and vigilant in their attention to the patients," or "all the customary forms of treatment have been followed with regularity and with a fair measure of success." Intercurrent illness of noteworthy importance occurred infrequently. An epidemic of influenza among patients and employees in 1898 was recounted in detail in the annual report. In 1904 "mild influenza and tonsillitis" reached noteworthy proportions, but in 1907 "head colds which it is fashionable to call the grip" were accorded brief mention only. A few cases of diphtheria were recorded in 1902 and in 1910, and in 1898 and in 1910 one case of scarlatina. None of these infections spread, which would seem to indicate good management.

Nothing in the treatment facilities provided in the new Bloomingdale seemed to be regarded with more hopeful anticipation than the physiotherapy equipment. This had been installed in 1894 under the supervision of Dr. Simon Baruch, "greatest authority on the subject in America," and the physician who was in charge of the treatment had received instruction from him and in Europe. An expert masseur was employed, and later "an operator familiar with the salt rub baths." In 1896 the medical superintendent reported that hydrotherapy was used more and more, in combination with massage, regulated exercise, enforced rest and supportive treatment. In the following year a statistical statement of the cases treated was given. Of 30 acute cases, 15 recovered, and 12 improved, some very much. Of 42 chronic cases, 11 were cases of general paresis, 5 of which improved and "the progress of the disease appeared to be retarded," 2 having been discharged from the hospital. Five cases of paranoia improved sufficiently to be discharged to the care of relatives and "have got along well at home." Half of the chronic female cases treated were grossly demented. Ten of these "showed material improvement in habits and in bodily condition, with more or less mental improvement." One circular manic case had received persistent treatment for ten months, after which she had been eleven months at home without active manifestation of her disease. The procedures that seemed most beneficial were, in acute excitable conditions, the vapor bath followed by tepid water spray, with gradual lowering of the temperature and increase in pressure. For rheumatism and neuritis the Scotch douche was found to be beneficial. Sphygmographic tracings made before and after treatment showed "improved tension and character of the pulse, with increased force and a firmer up-stroke." A static electrical machine was also "used in appropriate cases with gratifying results." The medical superintendent reported in 1898 that:

> These various forms of baths, while by no means a panacea for every ill, do an appreciable amount of good in two ways; one, by their actual application, and, in the other, by encouraging patients and their friends to feel that something active is being done for them which is likely to improve their condition, thus invoking suggestion as aid to cure.

It is interesting to note the estimate of the value of various forms of treatment at the time when they were first introduced. Even such commonplace articles as vis-a-vis lawn swings were, when introduced at Bloomingdale in 1898, found to have precise therapeutic value. The annual report noted that these swings

> proved to be especially soothing to a class of unstable patients, serving as an outlet for their nervousness and surplus energy. This is a class of patients inclined to be in constant motion, destructive or irritable and occasionally violent, and to several such people the swings seemed to act as a kind of moral restraint, and to reduce the confusion and discomforts of the disturbed halls to a very appreciable extent.

The term "moral treatment" was still used to designate the occupational, recreational, social, and other similar measures provided for the treatment of the mentally ill in hospitals. The new location and facilities at White Plains provided means of more fully utilizing and extending these measures. The annual report for 1895 listed as "diversions . . . to relieve the monotony" and promote patience and contentment "during the tedium of convalescence": regular Sunday services with good music; biweekly entertainments "of a nice character"; driving in carriages and wagons; frequent salt water bathing parties to the beach; abundance of current literature; and many games "at their own instance." The "Amusement Pavilion" was used every day except Sunday. In 1903 a shop was established for making mattresses and pillows "with the help of patients under the direction of an attendant." The hope was expressed that "it will be a useful enterprise both for the patients and the Hospital." Two patients worked at this occupation and it was reported at the end of a month that one hundred mattresses and eighty pillows had been made. There is, however, no further reference to this project. Among the new forms of exercise, the bicycle was, in 1896, considered of particular value. Twenty or thirty patients were taught to ride and took runs, "not only through the grounds, but over the adjoining country," in some instances unaccompanied. It was commented that "how far the wheel contributed to the cure of patients it is impossible to say; but the fact remains that quite a number of patients who went home cured . . . had become bicycle riders while here, and will have this additional outlet for their surplus energy, and, perhaps, diversion from morbid trains of thought." In 1897 a trained teacher of Dr. Sargent's method of physical culture was employed in the women's department, and in 1900 "on the women's division a professional entertainer comes to amuse, instruct, and divert patients on the various halls." Neither of these positions was given a place in the permanent organization during this period, but was filled only for temporary periods at varying intervals. A letter to an applicant for the post as entertainer stated that this was "not a recognized regular position."

In 1904 comment was made on the greater liberty accorded to the patients since the removal. Mechanical restraint, while still not completely discarded, was comparatively seldom resorted to. Eight patients succeeded in committing suicide during the period. It was reported that "the usual games, trolley rides, and individual visits to watering places, etc., and all available industries, varied the occupations of the summer and fall, while the winter was shortened by its appropriate indoor and outdoor recreations and sports." In 1899 it was noted that fifty patients had been taken on a sleigh ride, which they enjoyed greatly though the temperature was two degrees below zero. Tournaments of tennis, billiards, pool, and bowling, participated in by patients, officers, and employees were "a distinct object of interest." The rented cottage at Rye Beach was resorted to daily by parties of patients, and some were in residence there for varying periods. In August, 1903, trips in a naphtha launch were "greatly enjoyed." In 1909 it was reported that the cottage was "one of the most successful features of the Hospital during the past summer." The usual dancing parties were attended regularly. Dancing classes were also conducted. The music for the dances and for entertainments was furnished by an orchestra of sixteen employees under the direction of the bookkeeper, who was an accomplished musician. The Thanksgiving Dance was described as "a scene of cheerfulness and enjoyment." A Fancy Dress Ball and a play by amateur village and hospital talent gave "great enjoyment." In the words of the medical superintendent, "All these various attempts at supplying a motive and interest in life soon reach their limitations, and are by no means of universal application, but that they do a distinct amount of good, and that they are factors in the improvement and recovery of a certain number of patients, I think there can be no doubt." [12]

In the annual report for 1896 an account is given of a "Patients' School." Such a school was established at Bloomingdale by Dr. Earle in 1845, and was discontinued by his successor in 1849.[13] In 1886 the annual report contained a reference to a school for women patients conducted by a supervisor.[14] How long this was continued is not revealed by the records. A school had apparently been reëstablished in 1895, this time for men, and visiting governors in their notes recommended the purchase of equipment for it. It was attended by about thirty patients.

> "A competent teacher, with eight years' experience, and musical abilities conducts advanced pupils through the mysteries even of Euclid, Latin and Greek; but the object of the school is to awaken dormant energies by the actual participation of the patient in whatever study—the simplest being often of the greatest benefit—e. g. spelling and mental arithmetic, and reading of interesting portions of history.

The school was equipped with a blackboard, maps, charts, globe, and textbooks. The session of two hours each school day "affords change of surroundings, and . . . assists by substitution in breaking up the continuity of morbid ideas and mischievous acts." The results were described as "modest, but . . . good." Among the patients was a Spanish college student who learned English and, after being mentally ill for five years, "seems convalescent." He had appeared to be demented and was at first noisy and troublesome at the school, but became attentive, quiet, and interested. A case of chronic melancholia "finds life worth living since he attended the school." Three patients "who very rarely speak on other occasions, read aloud, and write on the blackboard. Two medical patients, and a former teacher construe the universal language, Latin, for their less proficient brethren, and introduce a vein of humor at times." One of these when in the halls "cannot be made to talk or assist others." Another "is extremely incoherent and noisy there." No other reference to the school has been found. Schools of this character were, when asylums for the mentally ill were first established, considered by many physicians a useful means of "group treatment." There must have been very few besides that at Bloomingdale in 1896. There was, however, one at the Willard (New York) State Hospital in 1897 and an interesting account of it was published in the *American Journal of Insanity*.[15]

[12] Medical superintendent's report for 1898.

[13] P. 237.

[14] P. 327.

[15] *Am. J. Insanity*, LVIII (1901), 141.

The occupation class for women, the establishment of which was described in the preceding chapter, was reported in 1909 to have continued to prove "valuable in the moral treatment of the patients." In 1910 employment was furnished 52 patients; the articles made were 270 reed baskets, 140 raffia knotted articles, 55 raffia sewed baskets, 5 woven rugs, 41 woven cushion covers, 69 woven draperies, bags, bureau and table scarfs, 5 hammered brass pieces, 2 bead decorated leather bags. Sales amounted to $431.58 and the materials cost $291.92. It was from this small beginning, at the initiative of an idealistic, generous woman, that the present extensive occupational department for women grew.

Previous to 1901 all the patients at Bloomingdale, with a few rare exceptions, were admitted by legal commitment. In that year, however, twenty-three patients were admitted on their own application. Since then voluntary patients have been admitted in increasing numbers.[16] In 1908 the medical superintendent reported that "a gratifying feature of this is that a number of former patients come back voluntarily." Writs of habeas corpus requiring the judicial determination of the propriety of the patient's further detention were occasionally issued and necessitated appearance in court with frequently prejudicial publicity. In the report for 1905 it was stated that there had been fourteen discharges by the courts during the twenty preceding years. In 1906 and 1907, at the instigation of two patients who had been discharged by the courts, several writs were served simultaneously or at short intervals with little time allowed for preparation. Evidently these occurrences produced considerable apprehensiveness as in January, 1906, the medical superintendent wrote to the chairman of the Bloomingdale Committee that there were several patients who could write a sufficiently intelligent letter to a judge, "and should they do so, with the present feeling, they might get us some more unpleasant criticism."

It was still the popular view that "lunatic asylums" were places of violence and close confinement and that sane persons were not infrequently confined in them. Some of the proceedings in White Plains were therefore attended by many demonstrative spectators and were highly sensational. At one time the governors appealed to the district attorney to attend hearings in the public interest lest dangerous patients be discharged. One patient who was discharged after a number of hearings had been in different hospitals for many years. She was discharged, however, and, although she had abundant means, she lived in penury and neglect and soon died. In another case, a man committed suicide

[16] See pp. 412, 455.

soon after his discharge by the courts. This incident was widely published and excited considerable comment in the newspapers in regard to the discharge of patients by the courts against the judgment of hospital physicians. It had a sobering effect on the local attorneys and judges and there has not been at Bloomingdale a repetition of this experience.

XXIX

NURSE TRAINING: ADVANCES IN SCIENTIFIC AND CLINICAL STUDY AND PRACTICE

FOLLOWING the removal to White Plains, the lecture course for attendants described in Chapter XXV,[1] was extended and in 1895 it was beginning to be regarded as a school. The course of instruction followed "the general model approved by the British Psychological Society." In 1897 the continued success of the course and an increase in the number of students was noted, and in 1898 the following communication was presented by the medical superintendent to the Bloomingdale Committee:

Bloomingdale, White Plains,
Aug. 30, 1898.

To the Bloomingdale Committee:

GENTLEMEN:—

I will state briefly regarding the training of attendants in our so-called school; that it was begun two years ago, and should, I think, have begun several years earlier, but that the greatly increased labor entailed upon the Hospital staff by the transfer of the work of the Hospital from New York, made it advisable not to enter on the matter until the Hospital was well established on its new basis at White Plains.

It has been recognized for some years that Hospitals for the Insane would secure a better class of attendants, and that the service they would render would be more efficient and reliable, if they were systematically taught the nature of their duties, and some general principles regarding sickness in general and insanity in particular. Bloomingdale was one of the latest of the prominent hospitals to start a training school. The Medico-Psychological Society of Great Britain, and the similar Society of the U. S. and Canada, both of which are largely made up of physicians in charge of hospitals for and taking special interest in insanity, not only endorse, but consider such special schools for training attendants essential to the proper care of the insane in hospitals.

Our brief experience of the results of the School at Bloomingdale, is that the nursing of the patients is more intelligently and faithfully performed. That the attendants use greater tact and judgment in managing troublesome cases, because, in realizing that they are dealing with sick, and not simply violent or irritating patients, they rely less on force and more on kindness and persuasion. The attendant who has diligently studied, and passed an examination, and has the evidence to show of his proficiency, has thereby increased his feeling of self-respect and responsibility, and with these qualities, he becomes a much safer reliance for the physician, who, however attentive he is

[1] See pp. 328–329.

personally to his patients, is nevertheless obliged to delegate the constant care of them to the attendant.

I will only add that I believe it is the general experience in hospitals for the insane in this country and in Europe, that where they specially train their attendants, they find in their servants the same increase of efficiency in their work as is found in general hospitals in the care of the sick and surgical cases, by their trained nurses.

I am, Very respectfully,

SAMUEL B. LYON, *Medical Supt.* [2]

In October of that year it was proposed by the Bloomingdale Committee that the by-laws be changed to read as follows:

OF THE TRAINING SCHOOLS

1. There shall be a Training School in the Hospital for the instruction of female nurses. . . .

2. There shall be also a training School for the Instruction of the male and female attendants at Bloomingdale, which shall be under the direction and management of the Bloomingdale Committee and such rules and regulations as that Committee may from time to time prescribe, subject to the approval of the Board.

At the same meeting the committee recommended the following rules for the government of the school, which were adopted by the governors in December, 1898:

(1). It shall be the policy of the Society of the New York Hospital to maintain a Training School for men and women attendants at Bloomingdale; but when the proportion of trained attendants there shall equal 50 per cent. of those employed on either side of the House, the School may be temporarily suspended, until the proportion again falls below 50 per cent. of those employed.

(2). The course of the Training School shall extend over a period of two years, and shall consist of one session each year, of about eight months' duration, commencing October 1st and terminating June 1st.

(3). The School will be divided according to sex, and the lectures will be given by the physicians of the respective departments, as they are assigned to that duty by the Medical Superintendent.

(4). There will be two terms each year, and one lecture per week throughout each term, with such special or extra lectures as may be considered necessary. It is expected that the course will be gone over four times during the two years.

(5). All time lost from their studies, due to sickness or other causes, must be made up before an attendant is eligible for final examination.

(6). The class will be composed of Junior and Senior members, and examinations will be held at the end of each term. The Juniors must pass satisfactory examinations before they can proceed with their senior work.

(7). The examinations will be conducted by some physician connected with

[2] Letter Book, "Executive Letters, Bloomingdale," at Westchester Division.

the Society of the New York Hospital, but not, as a rule, by one directly engaged in the instruction of the class, thus avoiding the appearance of favoritism.

(8). Attendants passing satisfactory examinations, at the expiration of two years, will receive a medal and a certificate of proficiency, to be issued by the Society of the New York Hospital.

(9). The course of instruction will consist of lectures and demonstrations, and will include anatomy, physiology, the first care to the injured or sick, the general care of the sick, the administration of medicines, hygiene, disinfection, bandaging and surgical dressings, theory and practice of massage, and the observation of mental symptoms and manifestations.

(10). Candidates joining the Training School, must be approved by the Medical Superintendent; must be between the ages of 20 and 35 years; must be of good moral character, and have a fair common school education; and they may be required to pass an examination (entrance) in primary English branches.

(11). Candidates will be admitted to the class on two months' probation, and they may be withdrawn at any time by the Medical Superintendent.

(12). Not more than 25 per cent. of the number of attendants employed on each side of the Hospital may belong to the class at one time.

This school was conducted without a nurse as director. The instruction was given by physicians and included, besides the lectures, some practical instruction in bandaging, first aid and a few other simple procedures, and in massage.

The committee had in June reported to the governors that fifteen attendants had completed the course and they were "authorized to examine said attendants and issue a certificate and inexpensive badge to those who had passed a satisfactory examination." The certificate was as follows:

THE SOCIETY OF THE NEW YORK HOSPITAL

BLOOMINGDALE

White Plains, New York

THIS IS TO CERTIFY THAT
has completed with credit a two years' course of instruction and practice in general nursing, and the care of the insane, at this Institution,
AND THAT
has passed a satisfactory examination, under the direction of the Bloomingdale Committee of the New York Hospital.

Medical Superintendent

Assistant Physicians

Dated White Plains, N. Y. *Chairman Bloomingdale Committee*

The badge was described as

> a silver badge, of the size and thickness of a half dollar, hung by three links from a bar of silver, with a pin. The name of the nurse appears on the bar; on the front of the medal "The Society of the New York Hospital, Bloomingdale" surrounds a wreath of gold, in the centre of which is a red cross. On the back of the medal is engraved "Graduate of the Attendants' training school, 1898."

Exercises were held on July 27, and two women and three men who had completed the course in 1897, and nine women and three men who had completed it in 1898 were given the certificates and badges. The governors, however, considered it inadvisable to adopt the red cross. The badges were, therefore, recalled and the cross was replaced by an enameled shield on which the words "Founded 1771" [3] were placed. At a meeting of the American Medico-Psychological Association in 1906, Dr. Lyon, medical superintendent of Bloomingdale, in a discussion of nursing gave his reasons for providing training for men as well as women:

> The majority [of male attendants] I have known were self-respecting, and up to the average intelligence. . . . Many of them have a fair education; some have failed perhaps in more active careers, but are fully capable of the duty we ask of them, and are more suitable than women as companions and associates for men patients.
>
> When we inaugurated our training school, it seemed to me it should be for the men, if for any one. We could get very good women, with a natural bent for nursing, but the men . . . need to be instructed. So we established a training school for men, as well as women . . . and I think the results have justified the effort, not only in better care for the insane, but in making better companions to the patients. We have many educated and refined patients, and it is not enough to put a spade in their hands, and tell them to work. They must be amused, and got out of their morbid conditions, and we find intelligent male nurses and companions a great assistance to us in restoring patients to their natural places in life. When the men patients want to go to the theatre, play ball, go to the city, etc., the competent male nurses can go with them, which women nurses could not do properly, and with manly companions, patients often brace up, and show a renewal of interest in manly pursuits, which is often a forerunner of their restoration to normal life. . . . Where good men can be obtained, and can be well instructed, I believe they should be the responsible caretakers of the majority of men patients, who are not sick in the ordinary meaning of that term, and who need the stimulating companionship of other men. If women are in responsible charge of the men, you can only get an inferior grade of men, who will be willing to take the irresponsible and degrading subordinate positions, such

[3] "Founded 1771" was later dropped.

men as are no proper companions for male patients of intelligence; and an important means of moral treatment is lost.[4]

From 1898 on, graduation exercises were held annually. The date was fixed to correspond with the annual visit of inspection of the board of governors, and the exercises were attended by the president and several others of the board, sometimes as many as ten in all, and also by some of the physicians of the New York Hospital. The proportion of graduates who remained in the Bloomingdale service diminished with the passing years. In 1904, 39 (12 men and 27 women) of 73 graduates were still in the service. In 1910, however, when the total number of graduates was 107, only 26 (7 men and 19 women) were still at Bloomingdale. In 1909 the medical superintendent noted that "as far as we know, all the graduates of the school have done well, and have been a credit to the Hospital, the service of which has been made more efficient by their help."

The school served a useful purpose and initiated at Bloomingdale a development in nursing education which, in common with similar developments elsewhere, made considerable progress. Adequate nursing for the mentally ill by well-educated, properly trained nurses remains, however, everywhere a provision which has not yet been securely established.

The year 1905 is notable in the history of the psychiatric service of the New York Hospital as that in which modern clinical and laboratory methods were introduced in the study and treatment of the patients. Previous to that year there was no properly equipped laboratory at Bloomingdale. In 1898 even the ordinary examination of urine, such as soon afterwards became a routine procedure, was considered important enough to be reported in detail in the annual report. The place in which, in 1899, the apparatus and material for laboratory work was gathered, was a small room in the basement under the administration offices. The equipment consisted only of that required for urinalysis, and the work was done by the clinical assistants. An indication of interest in scientific investigation was manifested in 1899 when Dr. R. J. E. Scott, who was not a member of the resident staff, was reported to have made a cell count of the blood of 35 paretics, and to have found a marked increase in the large mononuclear and transitional cells. He also made one examination for malaria, one for gonococcus, and four for tubercle bacilli. No other reference to laboratory work appeared in the annual report until 1905. A clinical study of the eyes of 196 patients was, however, made by Dr.

[4] American Medico-Psychological Association, *Transactions*, XIII (1906), 203.

R. G. Reese, the visiting ophthalmologist, in 1899, in order "to observe what relation if any existed between ophthalmic disease and mental disorder." He reported that 103 of the examinations gave negative results; that 14 cases, 9 of which were paretics, were found to have chorioretinitis; and that a high degree of insufficiency of the internal rectus muscle was observed in 55 of the 57 paretics examined, which was not apparent in patients with other forms of disease. At this time some of the ophthalmologists who had been added to the medical staff of different hospitals for the mentally ill considered that the relief of eye strain accomplished by their services contributed greatly to the recovery of many patients from their mental illness.

The governors, as well as the Bloomingdale physicians, were well aware that the mentally ill patients under their care should share in the benefits to be derived from the great advances in scientific and practical medicine which were elsewhere transforming the services for other classes of sick persons. In the past it had, more than once, been the governors who had initiated and accomplished the introduction of important advances in the service. There is ample evidence that, in the present instance, they, as well as the medical superintendent, were giving much consideration to ways and means of making progress. Dr. Lyon was disposed to place the emphasis on a department for the mentally ill in the city. In 1899 he presented at a meeting of the American Medico-Psychological Association a paper on "The Desirability of Close Connection between the Psychopathological Laboratories and Hospitals for the Acute Insane." [5] He pointed out the advantages of a city location, prompt service, and cooperation with educational institutions in teaching and scientific investigations. He brought the subject before the governors many times and made several definite recommendations, some of which have been referred to in previous chapters. The governors were entirely in accord with the object of his proposals, although many years passed before it was accomplished.

They were also, however, deeply concerned with the necessity of advancing the service at Bloomingdale. In 1903 Dr. Frederick Peterson, State Commissioner in Lunacy, and Dr. Pearce Bailey, an eminent neurologist of New York, suggested to Dr. Lyon that Dr. August Hoch, who had for ten years been engaged in laboratory and clinical work at McLean Hospital, and who had published some noteworthy articles, might be available for the Bloomingdale service. Thereupon, Dr. Lyon wrote to Dr. Hoch the following letters: [6]

[5] *Ibid.*, VI (1899), 364. See also pp. 353 and 471–472.
[6] Letter Book, "Executive Letters, Bloomingdale Asylum."

Dec. 5, 1903

DEAR DOCTOR HOCH,

Dr. Peterson who has been here today tells me that you had arranged to go to Michigan to carry on your work, but that something prevented the change and you are still at McLean—but he thinks that you have determined to sever your connection with that hospital, and that Doctor Cowles has or is about to secure your successor. If Dr. Peterson is correctly informed in all these particulars I will be glad to learn if your future arrangements are made or if perhaps we could arrange here for a temporary or possibly a permanent connection on your part with this hospital. I know Dr. Peterson is desirous of having you establish yourself near New York and we might see our way clear to assist in that very desirable result.

I am exceedingly anxious to treat other hospitals with perfect good faith and would not try for a moment to get you away from McLean—unless it is already determined that you are to leave there.

Yours very truly,
S. B. LYON

Dec. 19, 1903

DEAR DOCTOR HOCH,

Yours of the 11th inst. came duly. As I said in my letter to you, any negotiations are based on your having severed your connection with McLean—as I wish to observe to other institutions the same consideration I would expect from them. I note what you say about the clinical observations being under your charge. It would seem natural that the physician in charge of Laboratory work should have the largest facilities for observing the patients. I do not see how he could exercise any authority over other and senior physicians, like our First and second Assistants, both of whom are experienced alienists and one of them a neurologist connected with the Vanderbilt Clinic, but they would no doubt give their hearty support to any advanced clinical research.

Thanking you for your courteous reply, I am very truly,
SAMUEL B. LYON, *Med. Supt.*

Unfortunately, Dr. Hoch's replies have not been preserved; he did not join the staff until later. Apparently he wanted to be sure that his laboratory work would be attended with good clinical observations and with intelligent collaboration on the part of the clinical service.

Although no change was made at that time, consideration of advancement of the clinical and scientific work of the hospital continued to receive attention. Apparently the governors were proposing various expedients, as indicated by the following letter from the medical superintendent to the chairman of the Bloomingdale Committee in February, 1905:

MY DEAR MR. MORRIS,—

In view of our conversation today I think I may give you confidentially my idea of what would be for the best interests of Bloomingdale, and also might meet the sentiment which you say exists in the Board. I am as anxious as anyone can be to see Bloomingdale occupy the highest position possible. I have spent so much of my life in trying to build it up, that I cannot ever be indifferent to its reputation and its real usefulness.—

1. I may say first that no such hospital can prosper with two heads. It has been tried in New Jersey and at Norristown, Pa., for political reasons, the business head being the concession to politics. His independence of the Medical department and closer touch with the lay board, has made the medical side of the hospital virtually subordinate to the business and political side, to the great detriment of the institution. The head of a hospital for the insane, should be a medical head, for all departments are dependent on each other, and there should be no division of authority, and there can be none without the medical side suffering. Of the hundreds of such hospitals about which I have more or less knowledge in this country and abroad, I do not recall but one in Penn. and these two in N.J. organized with separate coordinate responsibility. And the general practice of having one medical head is not an accident, but the result of much discussion and experience.

2. In the second place, it is not necessary for the medical head to do everything, or even to be the most expert of all those connected with the service. He should have sufficient competent assistants, medical as well as business,—and he can have medical assistance with specialized and cultivated ability to carry on original research in various lines which promise to add to the knowledge of insanity, without either jealousy on his part of a subordinate who had gone further in some directions than the head of the institution might have done, or disloyalty on the part of such subordinate. In fact I believe it is generally the fact that physicians who incline to original lines of work, do not have much executive ability, nor inclination, but prefer the laboratory and speculative side of medicine. Indeed as a rule they prefer such work to the practice of the profession of medicine.

3. Last year I suggested to the Committee a departure in the direction of establishing a branch in the city, which should be more distinctly a school, hospital, and psychological institute of research than Bloomingdale, over twenty miles from town, can be,—and I had then a man in mind, who is now I believe doing original work in a hospital and who would be glad to get to this neighborhood.

4. The conclusion of the matter, as lead up to in the preceding, is this. Bloomingdale can well afford to employ a capable and well known man, an investigator but not a sensationalist, as the one I refer to is, I believe, to do other than routine work, as Special Pathologist and Clinician. It would help its reputation, and it might,—I do not feel confident that it would necessarily,—add something to its ability to relieve suffering and cure disease, the objects of its existence.

The arrangement could be proposed by the Committee and so be easily brought about, and the expense need not exceed perhaps $4,000 for the first year, during which it could be discovered if it was likely to be worth while. The number of the staff need not be increased, as with such a new member, the usual clinical assistant could be dispensed with. The salary would have to be at least $3,000 or $3,500,—but if you can get the value of the money that should not be allowed to prevent such an important departure. Laboratory appliances would cost something, but not a great sum. We have much already which would be applicable.

I am sure all concerned would rejoice to see the medical work at Bloomingdale extended in any really advantageous direction. The man I have in mind stands high among those interested in the scientific aspect of Psychiatry, and I can easily refer you to N.Y. physicians who know of him and his work. I may add that I think him conservative, and unlikely to attempt visionary departures.

This, as you know from its early response to your remarks, is not fully matured in my mind, but it is not entirely new either, and I am quite willing to cooperate in putting on foot such laboratory and original work here.

Yours very truly,
SAMUEL B. LYON

One proposal seemed to have been that responsibility for the medical work be separated entirely from responsibility for administration. This form of organization is frequently suggested by members of boards of management before they have learned by observation and experience the actual requirements of hospital treatment of the mentally ill. The "investigator" mentioned in the letter was evidently Dr. Hoch, and Dr. Lyon soon wrote to the medical superintendent and the first assistant physician of McLean Hospital in regard to his ability to manage the women's department at Bloomingdale. He also referred the governors to Dr. Peterson and Dr. Adolf Meyer for further information relating to Dr. Hoch's qualifications. A vacancy had occurred in the position of first assistant physician at Bloomingdale and, in April, 1905, Dr. Hoch was appointed with the title of First Assistant Physician and Special Pathologist. According to the medical superintendent, "his many valuable papers have given him a very high standing in the medical profession, and he will continue his scientific laboratory work at Bloomingdale, while also applying himself to executive and practical duties, an ideal combination of mental activities." [7]

Dr. Hoch entered upon his duties at Bloomingdale in July, having spent the intervening period in Europe. He recommended that Dr. George S. Amsden, who had been associated with him at McLean, be appointed as his assistant. Dr. Amsden was also recommended by Professors E. W. Taylor and Walter B. Cannon, with whom he had worked at the Harvard Medical School, and it was considered that his unusual experience in laboratory work would make him an "efficient assistant to Dr. Hoch in his development of such special work at this hospital." [8] He was appointed in June as a clinical and laboratory assistant.

[7] Medical superintendent's report for 1905.
[8] *Minutes of the Bloomingdale Committee,* June 28, 1905.

There was at Bloomingdale at that time nothing that could properly be considered a laboratory. A room on the office floor of the administration building was, however, taken over and in September the medical superintendent reported that "we are gradually getting our laboratory into convenient shape." The interest of the governors was manifested by visits to the new laboratory and talks with Dr. Hoch. In October he "explained details connected with his department" to Mr. Schuyler (president), who reported to the board that "examination of patients should not be conducted in the present room, which is practically the anatomical laboratory." In November it was reported that "the psychological laboratory is in good running shape. Some of the apparatus and books authorized have been procured, and more are on the way." The work extended beyond the laboratory, however; the medical superintendent reported that "the work of Dr. Hoch in perfecting a more minutely detailed record of the mental and physical condition of all the patients, both of longer residence here, and those who have come since the first of July, has gone on."

The annual report for 1905 quoted a communication from Dr. Hoch to the governors explaining the principles and plans which he proposed to follow.

> There are practical as well as scientific reasons why every attempt should be made to develop as much as possible the scientific medical work in a hospital. It is also obvious that in the centre of all attempts of this nature must stand a thorough observation of the patients. This implies a minute inquiry into the constitution of the individual to be treated and into the development of the disease, and a most careful analysis of the symptoms both physical and mental. The latter is done at the bedside, as it were, by carefully observing and questioning the patient and by studying the course and outcome of the disease. This bedside or clinical observation constitutes the largest and most important part of the scientific work in mental diseases. But in this study a need is often felt for special tests, be they of a chemical, microscopic, physiological or psychological nature; it is at this point that a clinical laboratory equipment becomes necessary. The laboratory is, therefore, only a tool which in a definite case may or may not be required and it forms a part of the general clinical work. The functions of a pathological anatomical laboratory are so well known that it is scarcely necessary to say much about them. The autopsies and the studies of the tissues will, of course, supplement the clinical studies and are therefore often of great value. But the idea that the chief scientific advance in the knowledge of mental diseases should come from a study of brain after death is erroneous, and this, we are glad to say, is an idea which is much less prevalent than it was ten years ago. The postmortem studies are only of real value when they are preceded by careful clinical observations.
>
> Of great importance, in addition to these various observations, is their full

recording, since this alone insures a possibility of summing up and attaining of accurate results from which more general conclusions may be drawn and new problems formulated which in turn will furnish the foundation of further work at the bedside and in the laboratory.

If the study of the patients and the recording of the observations is minute and accurate, the careful treatment follows as a necessary consequence, and all the legal questions, the other important issue in the care of the insane, are well looked after.

These are, in brief, the ideas which guide us in developing further the medical work of this Hospital. It has been shown in many places that even without such work a hospital may get along very well. But we hope to have made it sufficiently clear that the out-put of energy and expense required to do the best work will be sufficiently compensated and that the practical foundation of this development will show that it is necessary to adjust the entire activity of the hospital so that this work is possible to the fullest extent. No state of satisfaction should be reached before we can feel that all is done that can reasonably be expected.

Although the laboratory was developed and conducted with great efficiency by Dr. Hoch and Dr. Amsden, clinical studies formed a large part of their interests and activities. In February, 1906, Dr. Lyon reported that "much stress is being laid on the accurate observation of the patients, and recording their cases amply for the purpose of gaining more definite information for treatment, as well as for wider scientific reasons." In the annual report for that year the portion of Dr. Hoch's report which is quoted therein relates entirely to clinical studies:

The work has, during the past year, been conducted along the lines mentioned in the last annual report. Careful clinical studies in the manner indicated there, have been regarded as the essential part of the work, because we feel sure, and experience teaches us, that such studies have a very practical value, inasmuch as many important indications for treatment may be obtained which would be overlooked in a less careful analysis of the patients' conditions. This is a part of the general tendency towards greater individualization in mental treatment which makes itself felt in psychiatry and which indicates the line along which some of the progress in treatment will come. Much interest has been and will be, for a long time, centered upon a study of the development of certain diseases with an attempt at understanding the mental habits and reactions of the patients before the disease came on, and thus entering into the problems of their causation. This is possible to a much greater extent than is commonly supposed. It forms in our opinion one of the most important fields for research in mental pathology, since it is this, much more than anything else, which will eventually lead to that which we are all aiming at, a prophylaxis of certain forms of insanity.

The reference in the report to "understanding the mental habits and reactions of the patients before the disease came on," is, perhaps, the first indication in a publication of the particular and very productive attention given to this subject by Dr. Hoch and Dr. Amsden.

In 1907 the laboratory was established in the new quarters provided in the extension to the administration building described in a previous chapter.[9] The accommodations were now described as

a Psychological Laboratory containing two large rooms, one for examinations and various tests and reactions, and the other for microscopic and such work as is carried on in the most modern of these laboratories. This is in the immediate charge of the First Assistant, Dr. Hoch, and Dr. Amsden, who devote themselves more particularly to the work of investigation.

A further account of the work is given in the annual report:

The Laboratory in its new quarters, is now well equipped so that, so far as that is concerned, we have adequate facilities for work. The work which has been carried on during the year consists, not only in the study of the tissues from the nervous system and other organs, obtained at autopsy, but also in the study of lesions by means of serial sections through the brain as a whole. This work makes possible a proper co-ordination of clinical symptoms and anatomical changes in the nervous system. The additional facilities offered for the examination of the secretions and excretions of the body, as well as the blood and the cerebro-spinal fluid, are daily in use, and add efficiency to the clinical work.

A considerable amount of research has been devoted to the study of the causation of certain forms of insanity. The beginning of these studies was indicated in the report of last year. In this age of bacteriology the mental causes of insanity have been strikingly neglected, and only recently attention has again been directed towards them. Such studies teach us that what is at the bottom of certain—of course not all—mental disorders, are conflicts in the patient's life, usually of long standing, with which the patient has never been able to get square, and which owing to the lack of sufficient balancing factors and sound mental habits, give rise to a growing disharmony. That which we then call the mental disorder, is nothing more than the becoming dominant of such conflicts in various forms of peculiar abnormal reactions and faulty attempts at adjustment. These manifest themselves in delusions, hallucinations, peculiar acts, and the like. In each case, therefore, a careful psycho-analysis is necessary, not only for the purpose of research, but for the diagnosis as well. By diagnosis we no longer mean merely that which can be expressed in a single work, but we mean a thorough clearing up of the situation, that is, an understanding of the actual struggles and difficulties which the patient has, and which are hidden under the perplexing array of mental symptoms. It is becoming more and more evident that for a proper management and treatment of those forms of insanity which we have in mind, such a knowledge is indispensable, and that to be satisfied with anything less is a

[9] Pp. 352, 359.

procedure to be put on the same level as a treatment without any diagnosis at all, i. e., without adequate indications.

The advancement in the clinical laboratory work so as to provide for more extensive examinations, including the blood and spinal fluid, is noteworthy. The increasing emphasis on mental conflicts and life situations as the important problems in the study and treatment of the mentally ill is also significant of the lines of progress. Psychoanalysis is also mentioned for the first time in a Bloomingdale report, though probably not the Freudian pattern thereof. In April, 1907, the state medical inspector recorded at one of his visits that "a good start has been made in the better medical study and care of patients required by the progress of medicine and psychiatry."

In the annual report for 1908 Dr. Hoch's views on the place and importance of studies of the personality traits and habits of mind of mentally ill patients as they were manifested in their lives previous to their illness were explained more fully.

The general trend of the research work, of which the Report of 1907 spoke, and which has been continued during the past year, has logically led us to consider another side of the same problem, namely, the study of the personality before the outbreak of the psychosis. The question which here presents itself is this: Do the different types of mental disorder develop in different types of personality? To a certain extent this question is not new, and yet it has not received the attention which it deserves, and little aimful work has been done upon it. As a part of the general problem of the causation of insanity, it is, of course, very important to ascertain why the profound reactions of mental disorders can be produced in certain individuals by mental causes which in others do not produce such an effect; in other words, to ascertain where the weak spots in the personality are; or, to put it in still another way, what we desire to know is what are dangerous traits in a mental make-up, or dangerous habits of mind, which foreshadow a mental breakdown. If ever we are to develop a sound mental hygiene based upon a scientific foundation, and applicable to those who most need it, there would seem to be no better field upon which to gather data than this study of personality in individuals who have broken down. This, of course, is not the place to speak of the methods which we have adopted in this work; suffice it to say that the question has so far been studied partly in the patients who entered the Hospital during the year, partly in the clinical material collected during the last three years, and, finally, also in the large material collected by Dr. Hoch at the McLean Hospital. The results thus far obtained have been most interesting, but, of course, can only be regarded in the nature of a preliminary survey, since this is a study which will require years of painstaking and laborious work. In this connection, the special advantages which a private hospital offers, owing to the fact that the patients and their relatives and friends belong more particularly to the educated classes, are plain and make it directly a duty for hospitals of this sort to supply these facts which cannot be gathered as well in State Hospitals.

. . .

In the pathological laboratory the brains of two cases with focal lesions have been sectioned, studies of which are now being made. Considerable more material is now in progress of preparation. Aside from this and the daily routine examinations of the blood, excretions and secretions, furnished by the Hospital Ward, especial attention has been paid to the examination of the cerebro-spinal fluid of cases of long standing organic disease of the central nervous system.

In December of that year Dr. Hoch, in a paper read before the New York Psychiatrical Society entitled "A Study of Mental Make-up in the Functional Psychoses," presented a review of the work on this subject on which he and Dr. Amsden were engaged.

Although Dr. Hoch's attention was more and more devoted to clinical studies, autopsies and anatomical investigations were not neglected. The only publication of this work by Dr. Hoch during his Bloomingdale service was "A Report of Two Cases of General Paresis with Focal Symptoms," which appeared in the *Review of Neurology and Psychiatry* in 1906. This was a clinical as well as an anatomical study.

Dr. Hoch's position at Bloomingdale did not permit him to reorganize the whole medical service or to introduce, throughout, the methods of study and practice employed in his own work. The number of physicians was not increased, staff conferences were not held regularly, a systematic form of case recording was not adopted throughout the service, and the bound volumes of hand-written histories were continued. Nevertheless, the examination and treatment of patients were greatly improved. It was also the influence and work of Dr. Hoch, during his four years of service, which laid the foundation and started the superstructure of the advanced psychiatric clinical and scientific work that has been developed at Bloomingdale and the New York Hospital.

Dr. Hoch resigned his position at Bloomingdale in June, 1909, to succeed Dr. Meyer as director of the Pathological Institute of the New York State Hospital system, and as professor of psychiatry of Cornell University Medical College. Dr. Amsden remained, however, and continued the work of the laboratory. The position of First Assistant Physician in charge of the women's department was filled by the appointment of Dr. Theodore Townsend. He had previously been employed in the New York state hospitals, in which the medical service had been greatly advanced under the instruction and leadership of Dr. Meyer. Dr. Townsend remained at Bloomingdale for two years only, and his principal contribution to advancement of the service was the adoption of single-leaf typewritten histories and the systematic form of recording introduced into the state hospitals by Dr. Meyer.

Before assuming full responsibility for the laboratory work at Bloomingdale, Dr. Amsden spent six months in Europe pursuing studies at the laboratories and clinics of Professors Alzheimer, Jung, Plaut, Kraepelin, and others. He resumed his laboratory work in April, 1910. He had procured the equipment and mastered the technique of the Wassermann test, and until 1916 made this test for the New York Hospital as well as Bloomingdale. He continued the anatomical work, and, as the number of deaths and autopsies diminished at Bloomingdale, he obtained suitable material elsewhere. He had also been equally interested with Dr. Hoch in the study of personality traits with reference to their influence in the development and course of mental illness and with reference to prevention. In a report of his work during 1910 he stated:

> In addition we have continued the collection of data bearing upon the interrelation of psychosis and mental make-up or personality. The importance of this study, particularly in hospitals dealing with the better educated classes, should, we believe, be forcibly emphasized. It is more and more evident that consideration of this data not only makes it possible to handle cases with greater precision, but it indicates also in recoverable cases the direction in which training of the patient against subsequent difficulty may most efficiently be pushed. Moreover it appears hardly less than a duty to make this data, so easily accessible in hospitals in this class, generally available for whatever bearing it may have on the problems of limitation and prevention of mental deviation.[10]

These studies of Dr. Hoch and Dr. Amsden enabled them, in 1913, to publish for the use of practitioners and students a "Guide to the Descriptive Study of the Personality," [11] which was adopted extensively in psychiatric practice and scientific investigations, and was a useful contribution to psychiatric progress from the Bloomingdale service.

The increased interest and activity in the study and treatment of patients which followed Dr. Hoch's appointment may, perhaps, have led to particular consideration of the preponderance of chronic patients in the hospital. In 1905 a restatement of the policy relating to the patients was published in the annual report:

> Its policy has been to aid for a limited time as many hopeful cases as possible, but to retain chronic and hopeless cases only to a limited extent, and through these limitations to scatter its beneficence over as wide a field as possible.

10 Medical superintendent's report for 1910.

11 *State Hospital Bulletin,* New Series, VI (1913), No. 1.

Prospects of recovery were no doubt considered in the admission of patients. After admission, however, many were retained for long after their irrecoverability became evident. In 1910 the medical superintendent reported the "removal of certain chronic and non-paying patients to other Institutions, thus making room for new cases, as well as improving our financial position." [12] Many remained, however, for years, some at a rate below the cost and some entirely free. The effect of this preponderance of chronic patients had a tendency to give the service a static attitude and to limit the development of the organization and facilities, and the movement of population, required for active study and treatment and for scientific investigation. This was recognized and means were taken to correct it (see Chapter XXX).

Several papers, in addition to those already mentioned, were prepared by members of the Bloomingdale Medical Staff during this period, most of them by Dr. Hoch. A paper entitled "The Lesson Taught by a Few Hard Cases" by Dr. William E. Dold, first assistant physician, was published in the *Transactions* of the American Medico-Psychological Association in 1898. In 1897 a paper by Dr. Lyon on "The New Insanity Law and the Commitment of the Insane" was published in the *New York Medical Journal.* In 1906 he also read before the American Medico-Psychological Association a paper on "Miscarriage of Habeas Corpus Proceedings." In 1903 Dr. Charles Atwood published in the *New York Medical Journal* an article entitled "Do Our Present Ways of Living Tend to the Increase of Certain Forms of Nervous and Mental Disorder?" Dr. Hoch's other papers included, "A Study of Some Cases of Delirium Produced by Drugs," published in the *Review of Neurology and Psychiatry* in February, 1906; in 1907, "The Manageable Causes of Insanity," which was read before the New York Academy of Medicine; "The Psychogenesis in Paranoiac States," and "Psychogenesis in Dementia Praecox," both of which were read before the New York Psychiatric Society; "The Psychogenetic Factors in the Development of Psychoses," published in the *Psychological Bulletin;* and "On Psychotherapy in Psychiatry," read before the New York Neurological Society; and, at the meeting of the American Medico-Psychological Association in 1910, "Constitutional Factors in the Dementia Praecox Group," in which he used material gathered during his work at Bloomingdale.

The removal of the psychiatric department of the New York Hospital to White Plains tended to widen its separation from the other departments. Transportation was much slower than at present, and the service

[12] *Minutes of the Bloomingdale Committee,* July 26, 1910.

was deprived of the intimate relations with physicians and surgeons of the other departments which would have been mutually advantageous. The Bloomingdale physicians had, however, from an early period made visits to the New York Hospital with considerable regularity and were occasionally asked to see in consultation patients in the hospital. In December, 1898, this practice was made official when the Bloomingdale Committee directed that a representative from Bloomingdale should attend at the hospital every day except Sundays and holidays. This practice has been followed ever since.

PART EIGHT

Fulfillment of Some Long-cherished Aspirations

1911-1926

XXX: RENOVATIONS AND ADDITIONS

On July 1, 1911, Dr. Lyon retired from the position of medical superintendent of Bloomingdale Hospital. He had been connected with the hospital for twenty-five years, as medical superintendent for twenty-two. In accepting his resignation, the governors commended his term of office as especially notable for the removal to White Plains and the construction of the buildings there, "for whose design he was so largely responsible," [1] and felt that "the steady growth of the institution is the best evidence of the good repute and success of his administration." Dr. Lyon was an ardent and persistent advocate of resumption of service for the mentally ill at the general hospital in New York City.[2] On several occasions he submitted proposals and plans that were to be carried out in principle twenty years after his retirement and when he was no longer living.[3]

He was succeeded by Dr. William L. Russell, who assumed the duties of the position immediately following Dr. Lyon's retirement. Dr. Russell was, at the time of his appointment, medical superintendent of one of the New York State hospitals, and had previously been medical inspector for the State Hospital Commission. Before assuming his new duties, at the request of governors of the hospital he spend three months visiting hospitals and other institutions for the mentally ill in Europe. As state inspector he had frequently visited Bloomingdale Hospital and discussed the service with Dr. Lyon and Dr. Hoch. In 1909 he had, by request of Dr. Lyon, submitted an outline of his views relating to the further development of the work. In this he supported Dr. Lyon's proposal for a department in the city, and made a brief statement relating to its character and organization. He also proposed a program for the further development of the service at Bloomingdale. The communication was shown to the governors by Dr. Lyon, and Dr. Russell was invited to confer with the president and some other members of the board. The

1 *Minutes of the Bloomingdale Committee,* March 4, 1911.

2 See pp. 353, 380.

3 See Chapter XXXVI.

program then presented was essentially that undertaken two years later when Dr. Russell succeeded Dr. Lyon as medical superintendent.

Attention was directed to the unique position of the New York Hospital as the only "voluntary hospital" in the city which had always made provision for the mentally ill. It was pointed out that "for those able to pay a moderate rate, and for persons of refinement who, because of mental disease, have become indigent . . . the foundation and resources of the hospital are such as to enable it to furnish every case, without regard to the rate paid, with the kind of care and treatment actually needed," and there was no other hospital in the city which was equally prepared. The essentials of the program proposed were as follows:

(1) The policy of the hospital to be directed more exclusively than in the past to the treatment of curable cases; (2) To increase the activity of the service, and improve and extend the facilities and organization to this end, on the principle that "better facilities will help to bring cases" (Particular emphasis was placed on the necessity of ample clinical and laboratory service.); (3) The nursing service and the training of nurses and attendants to be "a special feature under a competent principal and assistants"; (4) Further development of provision for physiotherapy including prolonged baths, and for physical exercises, games, recreational, occupational and social therapy; (5) Provision for special reception services, nurses' residences, and for examination and treatment purposes; (6) A reception department in the city, adequately equipped and organized for in-patient and out-patient service.

In the period following the removal of Bloomingdale Asylum to White Plains, great progress had occurred in the general field of medicine and psychiatry, and in social and economic standards. Dr. Russell had participated in the advancements in the state service which had been made under the leadership of Dr. Frederick Peterson, commissioner, and Dr. Adolf Meyer, director of the State Psychiatric Institute, and he entered upon his duties at Bloomingdale with a hope of introducing into the service there the best of the spirit and methods of progress of which he had knowledge. The governors were aware that such a program was indicated and Dr. Russell's appointment was made with a view to its accomplishment. It was realized that it was a long-term program, which would necessitate a change in the character of the patient population, a more active admission and discharge rate, and many changes and additions to the buildings, to the facilities for service and scientific work, and to the organization. Many of the changes anticipated were not fully accomplished even at the close of the fifteen years to which this section of the history relates.

It was felt that first consideration should be given to increasing the activity of the service, and to improving and utilizing more effectively the resources for study and treatment. New construction at Bloomingdale had in the past been designed principally with a view to classification and to the fundamental requirements of living accommodations for an increasing number of patients. It was now thought advisable to give preference to facilities for the more efficient operation of the hospital as a place of active treatment. Although only seventeen years had elapsed since the removal to White Plains, progress in nearly every field of human endeavor had been so great that much that was fully abreast of the times when provided was rapidly becoming obsolete or inadequate for the advancing requirements. This was the case in regard to sanitary conditions. The property was infested with mosquitoes and the fairly recent realization of their connection with malaria called for action. Breeding places were treated, malarial cases were screened, and window and door screens were installed throughout the buildings. In a few years mosquitoes ceased to be a menace, and malaria was completely eliminated. The water supply was examined, further protection from possible contamination was provided for the wells and in 1912 the supply was supplemented by a connection with the White Plains system. A more extensive connection especially for fire protection was made in 1925. A separate distribution of the remarkably pure water of the deep driven well was provided in 1912. In that year also the hot-water system was improved by means of a circulating pump, and in 1926 an entirely separate system was installed by which the patients were never exposed to water at a dangerous temperature. The advancing dairy standards were adopted in the treatment of the hospital herd and in handling the milk. A milkhouse equipped with sterilizers was erected in 1912, and chemical and bacteriological examinations were made daily.

Toilets and bathrooms were made more sanitary by means of new fixtures and the substitution of tile and marble for wood and plaster. In 1921 a program was inaugurated for the replacement of all the plumbing and for renovation and extension of the toilet and bath sections throughout the buildings. The number of continuous flow baths was greatly increased. This extensive program in fully occupied buildings was not completed until 1926. The serving pantries were similarly treated, and, in some, equipment for light cooking was added, besides the sanitary sinks and food heaters with which all were provided. The main kitchen was enlarged and renovated. Most of the equipment was replaced and a sanitary floor was laid. Gas ranges were installed and a pipe line was laid to connect with the White Plains system. Food conveyers devised by the hospital mechanics produced great improvement in the service to the many dining rooms supplied from the central kitchen. A specially equipped diet kitchen was constructed, and, after the school of nursing reached its full activity, a suitable diet laboratory was provided.[4]

It was considered necessary to replace nearly all the laundry equipment, to enlarge the building, and extend the use of electric power for operating the machines. A sterilizer for mattresses and other large articles was installed. New and additional steam and hot-water boilers were provided. A filter was introduced to permit the use of the soft water of the lake in the boilers and laundry. The lake was also deepened and surrounded by a retaining wall. An incinerator for the disposal of refuse was constructed. The electric system was overhauled. A new engine and dynamo were obtained in 1912 and much of the electric wiring throughout the buildings was renewed. In order to obtain access to an alternating current, a connection was made with the White Plains system. In 1911 lights were installed in 105 of the patients' rooms, which had previously been without any.[5] The telephone system, which in 1911 had three instruments for outside calls, was extended throughout the buildings. Fire protection was made more secure by revision and extension of the water lines, and of the hydrants and standpipes. Automatic sprinklers in the basements, fireproof doors—some of them self-closing—and fire-fighting equipment furnished additional protection. To safeguard important medical, legal, and other records a basement room accessible only through the business office was equipped with a number of large fireproof safes.

Building operations during this period were directed especially to increasing efficiency. The Oakland Beach Cottage for summer use was completed in 1911. In 1913 a garage was built for the recently acquired automobiles, and a separate dining room for nurses was provided in accordance with the plans for improving the nursing service. In 1914 the basement barbershop used by the patients was replaced by an attractive little building attached to a corridor on the first floor of the main building. In 1916 the business management of the hospital was facilitated by the erection of a general store. The long-desired workshop for men patients was opened in the same year.

War conditions during the next few years delayed further building activity until 1921, when a dining room for the better accommodation of

[4] Annual report for 1926.

[5] *Minutes of the Bloomingdale Committee*, Oct. 24, 1911.

the male nursing service, with similar accommodations on a different floor for the mechanical and domestic service, was provided. Important construction in 1922 included an attractive and commodious occupational therapy building for women, donated by Mr. Frank K. Sturgis, chairman of the Bloomingdale Committee of the Board of Governors; and the first two of a series of cottages for married physicians, for which funds were provided by Mr. Payne Whitney, vice president of the Society. A medical-staff house containing additional accommodations for physicians was erected in 1924, also from funds donated by Mr. Whitney. In the same year a gymnasium or recreational building was added to the resources for the treatment of the women patients through the generosity of Mr. Henry R. Taylor of the Board of Governors, and also in that year a corresponding building for the men was provided by means of a legacy from a former patient. The Oakland Beach Cottage was in 1925 replaced by a much more extensive and attractive house and grounds on Orienta Point. The house was enlarged and facilities including a private bathing beach were provided for exercise and recreation. Also in 1925 the need for additional and more suitable accommodations for student and graduate nurses was supplied by provision for an attractive residence; this was a generous gift from the late Mr. Edwin Gould (who at the time requested that it be anonymous), augmented by a legacy from Mr. Taylor, who had died before the recreational building which he had donated was completed. In 1926 a third cottage for a physician's residence was erected by means of Mr. Whitney's donation and Mr. Taylor's legacy. In 1922 a comprehensive plan for the further extension of the hospital and its work was prepared, and to some extent furnished a guide to future developments.[6]

In addition to the erection of new buildings, much was done to improve the facilities of the hospital by means of alterations, and additions to equipment. The increasing medical and nursing activities necessitated the diversion of rooms designed as accommodations for patients to use as offices, examination and treatment rooms, bathrooms, pantries, utility and other service rooms. Small surgical operating rooms were provided for each service. A partition in the laboratory provided a room for psychological work. In 1912 a large room near the laboratory was equipped with shelving and suitable furniture and lighting and was taken over for the medical library. In 1922 when the Dexter Cottage was vacated by the occupational department and assigned to the school of nursing, the medical library was extended into the adjoining room,

[6] *Ibid.*, May 22, 1922.

which had previously been used as a lecture room for the nurses. In 1916 dentistry was assuming such magnitude that more space was required. The dentist was given a larger room, and in 1922 a suite of five rooms was provided by means of partitions in a large room in the administration building. In the same year a room adjoining the drug room was taken over for a new X-ray apparatus. About this time also the attention given to the health of employees was extended and organized, and a suitably equipped room for ambulatory cases was furnished near the laboratory. Infirmaries for sick employees were provided in the main building. In 1912 the balconies of the halls for disturbed patients were renovated and revised so as to be available enclosed or open throughout the year. In 1915 the assembly hall was remodeled and refurnished. In 1916 the general library which was used extensively by the patients was placed in a suitably equipped attractive room. The accommodations of attendants and domestics on the fourth floor of the main building and in other parts of the hospital, were thoroughly renovated and made more comfortable, sanitary, and attractive. The women's hydrotherapy department was renovated and extended. In 1914 the Dexter Cottage was remodeled and equipped for the accommodation of the expanding occupational therapy department. An extensive program of refurnishing the patients' halls and rooms was adopted and partly carried into effect. In 1916 a master clock with ten auxiliary clocks was installed, and in 1923 a call system for the physicians. Many useful but less noteworthy renovations, alterations and installations were made during the period. In March, 1925, a list of thirteen items of additional improvements was presented to the Bloomingdale Committee and approved, the estimated cost being $110,000.

Many improvements were also made in the patients' recreation grounds and other parts of the property. Several tennis courts and a nine-hole golf course were constructed, and fields were equipped for hockey, volley ball, and other games. Walks were renovated and extended. Outside lighting was increased and some of the wires were placed underground. The trees, shrubs and flowers were given much attention, and in 1917 a consulting arboriculturist was engaged to make regular examinations and advise treatment. A nursery for trees and shrubs was started in 1926.

The facilities thus provided contributed immeasurably to the advancement of the service to a higher level than had previously been possible. In undertaking improvements due consideration was given to the value of beauty in promoting contentment and wholesome adjustment.

The new residential and treatment buildings were architecturally designed with a view to adding an inviting domestic aspect to the hospital, and to contributing to the contentment of the patients, as well as disarming the aversion felt by many to entering an institution for the mentally ill even as visitors. It was sometimes remarked by visitors that on entering the grounds they had the impression of being in a private residential estate. A patient said that her fear of admission to the hospital was allayed when the beauty of the grounds met her vision on arrival. A European visitor who was in America to visit educational institutions remarked, after going through different departments and about the grounds where the patients, many quite young, were working or walking and playing games, that it seemed more like an educational institution than a hospital. The removal of the iron guards [7] from more than one hundred windows, in 1913 and 1922, contributed much to the general morale in relieving the impression of being "behind the bars." In 1913 the chairman of the Bloomingdale Committee recorded that "during the last two years . . . the entire tone has been raised and the efficiency increased."

The prediction in the program that "better facilities will help to bring cases" seemed to be fulfilled by the increasing activity of the service. In 1911 the number of patients treated was 498, and in 1926 it was 587. The number admitted in 1911 was 140, and in 1926 it was 278. In the years 1915 to 1919 the number admitted was 1,238, an average of 247 each year, while during the preceding five years only 772 had been admitted, an average of 154 each year. As already mentioned, however, the increasing activity necessitated the appropriation for clinical and administrative purposes of much space designed for accommodations for patients, and in consequence the average daily number under treatment fell from 351 in 1911 to 267 in 1926. In making room for incoming patients it became necessary to discharge many of the older patients whose outlook for further benefit was unfavorable. Only in this way could the expanding provision for an active curative service be adequately used. As the older cases were withdrawn and organically involved cases were refused, and as the medical and nursing services improved, the deaths fell from 22 in 1911 to 9 in 1926. Cases admitted on voluntary application increased from 66 (or 47 percent of all admissions) in 1911 to 176 (or 63 percent) in 1926; this may be attributed, in part at least, to an increasing confidence in the service by the medical profession and the public.

[7] A still more effective provision is described on p. 449.

The development of the facilities and service was, especially after World War I, much favored by the general prosperity of the country. The necessary expansion of the hospital organization and the operation of the new facilities required an increase in current income. This was secured principally through higher rates than previously obtainable from the patients admitted and from many of those already in the hospital. In 1911 the average weekly rate was $16.01; in 1926 it had risen to $59.08. The income from rates was $288,806.04 in 1911 and $819,417.08 in 1926. It was customary to transfer to the treasurer of the Society any credit balance that appeared on the Bloomingdale account at the end of each three months,[8] and in 1914 it was decided to place these balances in a separate fund to be used only for improvements at Bloomingdale.[9] From 1911 to 1925 the total amount obtained from patients and spent for improvements was $456,250. In the same period $245,900 were appropriated for this purpose from the general funds of the Society; $489,000 came from gifts as already described; $163,000 from a legacy; and $100,000 from the sale of property to the Burke Foundation. The total from all sources was $1,454,150. Although it was evident that, owing to the general increase in prosperity, patients could now pay higher rates, no change was made in the policy of admitting suitable cases at rates below the average cost of treatment or without charge. In 1911 the number of patients treated at less than cost constituted 41½ percent of the total number treated, and 45 were given free treatment. In 1925 the corresponding numbers were 48 percent and 34. The policy which had long been pursued was discussed in the annual report for 1912.

The income received from the patients who are fully paid for is of immense value in enabling the hospital to maintain a higher standard of treatment for all the patients than would otherwise be possible. In the application of its funds to the relief of those who are unable to pay the full cost or who must be cared for without charge, the highest good can be accomplished in the treatment of as large a number as possible of patients who are suffering from conditions in which cure or at least restoration to home and some measure of efficiency can be reasonably expected. This policy has been aimed at in carrying on the work of the hospital during the year. As room was required for new patients, the removal of many who were past the stage in which improvement could be expected was requested. In a number of instances the patients removed were transferred to the State Hospitals. The need of applying private benevolence to providing simply humane care for insane persons is not now as great as it was when the Society first undertook the treatment

[8] See pp. 353–354.
[9] *Minutes of the Bloomingdale Committee*, June 6, 1914.

of this class of sick persons. There were then and for years afterwards, no public institutions for the insane, and the only place in the State where hospital treatment for persons suffering from a mental disorder could be obtained was the New York Hospital and later Bloomingdale Asylum. Now, however, there are fourteen State Hospitals where free care and treatment can be obtained by any citizen of the State who may be in need of it. What private benevolence can still do to good purpose is, however, to provide for a high grade of treatment for many cases in which the circumstances are such that private rather than public care is clearly indicated irrespective of the ability of the patient to pay for it either entirely or in part. In providing for this class of cases, the hospital is performing an important social service. There is also great need for the application of private funds to the solution of the problems of cure and prevention of mental disorders, and private hospitals with liberal resources are needed to supplement the excellent work of the State Hospitals which is likely to be limited by the necessity of providing for mere numbers and by the changes and defects of public administration.

The economic and social status of those to whom this service was rendered may be judged by the fact that in 1913, 35 percent of the women admitted were self-supporting by gainful occupation; many of them were teachers.

In 1914, at the request of the Board of Trustees of the Village of White Plains, a committee of the State Legislature investigated the hospital with particular reference to the old question of exemption from taxation. The committee, like those which had previously explored the subject, and like the courts also, reported that the hospital was a department of a charitable institution and exempt from taxation. They also mentioned advantages derived by the village and the state from the operation of the hospital, and reported that the acreage of the property was no greater than required for the adequate treatment of the patients.[10] In 1918 a communication relating to the question of licensing the hospital was received from the State Hospital Commission.[11] This was referred to the attorney of the hospital and no further reference to it was found in the records.

10 Report of the Legislative Commission to Investigate into the Affairs of the Society of the New York Hospital and Bloomingdale Hospital, submitted to the Legislature Feb. 18, 1915.

11 *Minutes of the Bloomingdale Committee,* Aug. 27, 1918.

XXXI

CLINICAL AND LABORATORY SERVICES

In the period 1911 to 1926 the medical staff increased from five physicians besides the medical superintendent to twelve. One or more short-term appointments were also made from time to time in the position of clinical assistant, and after 1911 fourth-year medical students were usually taken on for work in the clinical and laboratory services during the summer. One of the staff physicians devoted himself entirely to the laboratory with occasionally a clinical problem included. In 1923, the position of Assistant Medical Director was created and Dr. Samuel W. Hamilton was appointed to it.

Much importance was attached to bringing to bear in the study and treatment of the patients the resources of advancing clinical medicine. In 1922 the medical service was augumented and quickened by the appointment of Dr. Joseph C. Roper and Dr. Edward Cussler, attending physicians at the New York Hospital, as visiting physicians at Bloomingdale. Thereafter regularly once a week the resident physicians' examinations of newly admitted patients were reviewed and supplemented by a visiting internist. Other patients concerning whom advice was desired were also examined. Urological service was similarly provided by the appointment, on the recommendation of Dr. Oswald S. Lowsley, consulting urologist at Bloomingdale from the New York Hospital, of Dr. Lisle B. Kingery as visiting urologist. The service thus obtained from the visiting staff was greatly valued by the resident physicians, and has ever since contributed substantially to the maintenance of the medical standards. The acquisition of a small X-ray apparatus in 1919 soon revealed as stated in the annual report, that "the amount of this work which is now required would justify the purchase of a complete equipment and the establishment of a department." This was accomplished in 1922 after the visiting physicians had strongly recommended it. The work of the laboratory was also, through their influence, quickened and additional equipment was obtained.

During this period the role of infected teeth and other focal infections in the production of mental illness was receiving much attention. Influenced by the published claims of remarkable results,[1] and by the understanding and interest of Dr. D. Austin Sniffen, who since 1896 had attended to dental needs of the patients as they were presented to him by the physicians, dentistry began to have a place of growing importance

1 Henry A. Cotton, *The Defective Delinquent and Insane* (Princeton and London, 1921).

in the treatment of the patients. The accommodations for this service were greatly increased. Additional and better equipment was furnished. In 1912 dental examination of all the patients at regular intervals was introduced as a routine procedure. In 1921 the practice was adopted of making a dental X-ray examination a part of the physical examination of all patients admitted. Dr. Sniffen gave increasingly more time to the work, and in 1922 he retired from private practice and has since confined his service to the mentally ill at Bloomingdale and at the psychiatric clinic of the New York Hospital. In 1921 a dental hygienist was appointed, and in 1923 a dental assistant. The constant attention given by this department to the mouths and teeth of the patients made a striking contribution to their comfort and health, and to the constructive plans of physical and mental treatment followed in the hospital service. The growth of the dental service is shown by the increase in the number of patients who received attention from 86 in 1911 to 607 in 1925, and in the number of examinations and treatments from 484 in 1911 to 2,874 in 1925. The dental hygienist also in 1925 gave 1,255 dental and oral treatments to 502 patients.

The small surgical operating rooms provided in 1919 facilitated surgical attention, although it was still considered advisable to send patients in need of major operations to the White Plains Hospital or to the New York Hospital. Most of the surgical service was given by Dr. J. Fielding Black of White Plains. With a view to sharpening interest and responsibility and to facilitating service, a consulting staff was appointed. It consisted of a surgeon, an ophthalmologist, two aurists and laryngologists, and a urologist, and facilities for their work were provided. An official anaesthetist was also appointed. In 1925, 189 visits to patients were made by the consulting and visiting physicians and specialists. Eighteen major surgical operations were performed and many others that were less serious.

In August, 1911, Dr. Charles Macfie Campbell was appointed first assistant physician. He had previously been for several years on the staff of the New York State Psychiatric Institute. He remained in the service for two years only and in 1913 left to become associate professor with Dr. Adolf Meyer at Johns Hopkins Medical School, and later professor of psychiatry at the Harvard Medical School. In 1912 he was placed in general charge of the clinical and scientific work at Bloomingdale, and made a notable contribution to the organization and advancement of the service. Regular biweekly staff conferences were established. At these all cases admitted to the hospital were presented; also other cases of special clinical interest, or whose parole or discharge was pending. Autopsies were reported and specimens presented. Questions relating to treatment and administration were discussed.

Much attention was given to the organization of the clinical and medical administrative services. Records and reports were adopted by which information from every service was readily transmitted and preserved and the work of the various diagnostic and treatment services were coördinated and made increasingly effective. Particular attention was given to obtaining as full and accurate accounts as possible of the history of the patient and his illness previous to admission. Following the methods introduced by Dr. Hoch and Dr. Amsden, a detailed description of the mental constitution or the personality of the patient previous to his illness was, perhaps for the first time in any hospital records, given a separate place in the case history. The single-leaf filing system adopted in 1909 for the case records facilitated the assembly in one binder of all the various records from several sources which made up the complete history. In consequence the histories increased in volume, in fullness, in precision, and in usefulness. As the patients were admitted each was assigned to a member of the staff as the patient of that physician. This contributed to establishing confidence and a sense of security for the patient. This physician made the physical and mental examinations, prescribed the physical treatment and the organized therapeutic measures, and gave the personal psychotherapeutic treatment required. The staff conference and the consultations with the medical director and the other physicians, however, brought the patient to the knowledge and interest of the other members of the staff, and were means of promoting orderly and thorough work with all the patients. Written reports relating to the various measures of treatment, to the organized activities and to any noteworthy incidents were made daily to the medical director. A brief outline of the general principles and methods of treatment followed at the hospital in this period was presented in the annual report for 1922.

Experience with the patients here does not permit us to subscribe to any exclusive theory concerning the nature of mental disorders, nor to believe that any specific or exclusive form of treatment is universally suitable or even properly applicable in all cases. It is considered necessary, therefore, in the study and treatment of the patients, to be prepared to deal on rather broad lines with the problems of the individual cases and of the various types and groups for which treatment is required. The treatment suitable in any case can, it is believed, be determined only by means of a good understanding of the case and of the principal factors involved. In the examination and treatment of the patients received at the Hospital, provision is, therefore, made for applying the best available resources of clinical medicine and of psychiatry. An effort is made to understand the patient with reference to the stock he belongs to and to inherited traits; the influence of parental and school training and of the contacts and experiences he was subjected to during his developmental period; the leading and significant traits in his personality which may have operated through his life in determining his emotional reactions, and in shaping his behavior; the adverse physical, emotional, domestic, economic, or social influences to which he may have been exposed and their effects; the immediate circumstances of his illness and the history of its onset and course. In the personal physical examination of the patient, the clinical and laboratory resources are fully utilized, the aid of specialists in the different departments of medicine and surgery being obtained whenever this seems to be necessary. The mental examination is made by the systematic methods generally in use in psychiatric practice. A full and orderly arranged record is made of all the significant information obtained in regard to the history of the patient and to his present physical and mental condition, and this is continued throughout his stay at the Hospital.

The knowledge of the patient thus obtained determines the treatment. The personal treatment administered by the physician consists in such measures as may be required by physical conditions which require attention, and in explaining to the patient, when he is in a condition to be accessible, the factors in his mental state which he should understand and endeavor to deal with himself. The physicians may also, by their understanding of the conditions from which the patients suffer, and by their intelligent sympathy, and firm and wise advice, be a support and guide to them in their distress and in their progress towards health and self understanding and management. The knowledge and advice thus conveyed is one of the most valuable contributions which the Hospital can make to the future welfare of the patients who leave the Hospital as it may enable them to exercise better self control and self direction than ever before, and to avoid or minimize further difficulties.

Under the direction of the physicians, certain organized treatment resources are also used with advantage. The patients present a variety of conditions, and the manner and extent to which these resources are applied are controlled by the physicians and vary in individual cases. Some require ordinary sick and surgical bedside nursing. Others require nursing attention because of mental and physical feebleness, emotional states, and behavior disorders. Measures such as hydrotherapy, massage, air, and sunshine, and dietary regulations are employed to promote vigor, sleep, relief of tension, and nutrition. Physical exercises, out-door and indoor games and sports, drives and walks, productive occupations, social entertainments, dances, and plays and reading are employed as invigorating measures, and as a means of promoting physical and mental application, objective interests, release from emotional tension and fanciful preoccupations and the production of easy, wholesome, enjoyable social relations. The ultimate object of treatment is, in all cases, the restoration of the normal functioning of the individual, not only in his own isolated life but as a member of a family, an industrial organization, and of society. The special measures of treatment referred to are, therefore, strongly reinforced by the orderly and systematic hospital regime, the regulated schedule of exercise and rest, work and play, the considerate and effective management of uncontrolled behavior, the attitude of the members of the Hospital organization, and even the beauty of the grounds and surrounding country. In the study and treatment of mental disorders the whole organism and personality of the individual must be considered. In a very few cases the removal of one outstanding disturbing factor, mental or physical, may accomplish the object. In most instances, however, the patient presents a problem which can only be solved by the most careful study, and the use of means directed to influencing his mentality as well as to repairing his body.

As the activity of the service increased, the average age of the patients under treatment diminished. Many were quite young: in some years a third of those admitted were under thirty; [2] many were under twenty, and some were sixteen or less; in 1916 three were under fourteen. Occasionally it was found advisable to decline to accept a child who was so young that association with mentally ill adults was considered too prejudicial. In 1913 a separate service was organized for a group of young girls who happened to be in the hospital. The results were satisfactory but as discharges occurred, the number of suitable applications for admission was too small to warrant maintenance of the service. The establishment of a special service for children and adolescents was for several years recommended in annual reports, and the need is still pressing.

As the number of physicians increased, and in accordance with the progress of psychiatry during the period, the practice of individual psychotherapy was gradually amplified and extended. Freudian psychoanalysis was exciting much interest and was permeating psychiatric thought and practice; it was therefore considered advisable in 1926 to give Dr. Thomas M. French of the medical staff a year's leave of absence with salary for the purpose of study in Europe with special reference to this subject. It was agreed that upon his return he would remain in the service of the hospital for not less than two years. This marked the advent of technical psychoanalysis at Bloomingdale in the study and treatment of a limited number of cases.

For the purpose of extending the usefulness of the hospital a few of the general practitioners of the vicinity who manifested interest were invited to the regular staff conferences. In 1912 a further step in the

[2] At the Asylum of the New York Hospital in 1817–1818, more than half the patients admitted were under 30 (p. 105).

same direction was taken by the establishment of open conferences to which a larger number of physicians were invited. A special program was prepared and members of the staff and specially qualified speakers from New York and elsewhere discussed topics relative to psychiatric conditions and problems which are met with in every branch of medical practice. These conferences have ever since had a permanent place in the activities of the hospital and have contributed substantially to spreading psychiatric knowledge and interest among the physicians of Westchester County. The County Medical Society was also invited to hold some of its meetings at the hospital, and eventually this became the practice for all its stated meetings. In 1926 a "Monday Evening Conference" was established, at first informally in the apartment of one of the physicians. This was soon made official and has been an extremely valuable means of keeping the staff abreast of psychiatric progress and of educating the new members. It will be referred to more fully in a later chapter.

A further extension of the service was made in 1914 by the establishment in connection with the public schools of White Plains of a clinic for the examination of atypical children. This was conducted by Dr. Charles I. Lambert, who after serving for nine years on the staff of the New York State Psychiatric Institute had succeeded Dr. Campbell at the hospital in 1913. He was assisted by Dr. Milton A. Harrington and Dr. Karl Bowman, members of the hospital staff. This work was continued until 1917, when the demands of war service interfered. With the creation of the position of county psychiatrist the need became less pressing. It was reported that the demonstration of the value of such work had enabled the school authorities to obtain an appropriation for the establishment of an ungraded class in the schools.

A similar undertaking of more significance and importance in the history of the hospital was the opening in 1924 of an outpatient psychiatric service at the New York Hospital on West 16th Street. Dr. George W. Henry of the Bloomingdale staff was placed in charge. Except for a long period of study in Europe, he continued to conduct the service until 1932 when it merged with the Cornell Medical College Clinic to form the outpatient department of the Payne Whitney Psychiatric Clinic of the new New York Hospital on East 68th Street. The growth of the service at 16th Street was limited by inadequate accommodations. Nearly half of the patients treated were referred from other services of the outpatient department and from the wards of the general hospital; a few were from the Probation Bureau of the city courts. About 30 percent came of their own initiative. In 1926 the number of patients treated was 416. A social worker was added in 1925. Dr. Henry had four assistants, two of whom were not connected with Bloomingdale. The out-patient service led to more frequent requests for psychiatric consultations in regard to ward patients, and eventually to a weekly round of all the wards by the psychiatrist. A quickening of interest and understanding of psychiatry at the general hospital was accomplished which helped in the further developments in psychiatric service, teaching, and scientific investigation which were undertaken later.[3]

Attention was also given to encouraging patients who were on visit or discharged from Bloomingdale, to return for consultation with the physicians either at the New York Hospital or at White Plains. This service was of advantage in aiding the patient to readjust to the requirements of life in the community and to avoid relapse. In 1926 the number who called for consultation was 91 at the city office and 191 at White Plains. It was possible, with the help in some instances of the social-service department of the New York Hospital, to aid patients to obtain suitable employment. Occasionally a patient visited his business from time to time while convalescing at the hospital, or went to and fro daily.[4] An increasing number of patients were permitted to return to their homes for visits of varying lengths, in many instances a prelude to discharge. In 1911 the average daily number on visit from the hospital was 16, all committed patients. In 1926 it was 49, of which 13 were voluntary patients. The need and value of a readjustment service for convalescent patients ready to leave the hospital, and for long-term cases who had regained some measure of capacity for productive employment and social relations, was discussed in the annual report for 1915 along with a proposal for the establishment of an "industrial colony." Such a colony, "managed as a partly self-supporting benevolence, the products of which would be marketed, would be a unique and remarkably useful addition to the present organized agencies for the relief of this most appealing and least understood class of sick persons." The project was not undertaken. Another form of extension of service was the interest and participation of members of the hospital staff in community mental hygiene work. At the first public mental hygiene conference, held in New York in 1912, three members of the medical staff and the director of nursing were among the speakers. Ever since mental hygiene organiza-

[3] G. W. Henry, *The Neuro-Psychiatric Out-Patient Clinic: a Clinical Report* (Society of the New York Hospital, General Bulletin, March, 1927).

[4] Compare with similar instances at the "medical asylum" of the New York Hospital in 1818 (see p. 115).

tions and community service were first established, members of the hospital organization have participated in local, state, and national activities.

In a previous chapter [5] an account was given of the origin and early development of the clinical and pathological laboratory. In 1911 Dr. Amsden was still in charge, and extension of the work and its coördination with the clinical service was continued. The following account of the introduction of the Wassermann test in 1910, and of the dwindling opportunities for neuropathological work was given by Dr. Amsden:

> Soon after returning from abroad I began collecting the equipment necessary for the Wassermann reaction. By the end of the summer our outfit was completed and since September the Wassermann test has been a part of the routine clinical work.
>
> We do this test according to the original method of Wassermann—the method employed also at the Munich clinic. In especial cases experience has shown the advisability of making use, in addition, of Noguchi's modification of this test. By this combination I believe that a maximum of accuracy is secured. Up to the present time we have done 193 reactions involving 78 cases, a part of which were in the New York Hospital and House of Relief. The results tally closely with those currently published. This test, together with the results obtained from examination of the spinal fluid, marks a distinct advance in precision of diagnosis and treatment.
>
> I have also given especial attention to the application of the more recent neuropathological methods to material from our autopsies. Although we have relatively few post-mortem examinations, this fact makes it possible to carry out a complete study of them. We are, as a means of control, employing the same methods on suitable material obtained elsewhere.

A history of the laboratory from its earliest inception to 1932,[6] written by Dr. George W. Henry, who was director of the laboratory and of the X-ray department from 1922 to 1932, was printed privately by the hospital. After reviewing the beginnings of laboratory work at the hospital and its development by Dr. Hoch and Dr. Amsden, Dr. Henry gave a chronological account of the additions to the equipment and organization and of the work engaged in. In 1911 a psychogalvanometer was obtained and a number of studies of reactions of the patients were undertaken by Dr. Campbell. From year to year new equipment was added, some of considerable importance. In 1919 the annual report indicated that "the laboratory is now well equipped for ordinary clinical work and

[5] P. 379 ff.

[6] George W. Henry, *Bloomingdale Hospital Laboratory: an Historical Survey* (Society of the New York Hospital, 1933); see p. 11 for above quotation from Dr. Amsden.

for some forms of research work." After 1918, however, anatomical work was no longer engaged in, and interest was confined principally to physiological and biochemical studies. When X-ray and ultraviolet and infra-red lights were added to the hospital equipment they were operated under the direction of the director of laboratories. In 1923 a special study of gastrointestinal conditions by means of X-ray examinations was made by Dr. Henry and a well-defined relationship between the motility, tone, and position of the gastrointestinal tract and the mood changes characteristic of some forms of mental illness was revealed. Communications on the subject were made by Dr. Henry to the American Psychiatric Association,[7] the New York Psychiatric Society, and other medical organizations.

Investigations of this character were pursued intermittently for several years. In 1925 Dr. Henry reported at a meeting of the Association for Research in Nervous and Mental Diseases [8] a study of 51 cases of schizophrenia in which it was observed that barium meals were retained in the colon for more than five days in 70 percent of cases in acute phases, and this did not occur in the chronic phases of this disorder. This seemed to indicate that the latter cases "had made a readjustment even at a vegetative level." Other scientific studies relating to disturbances of the ductless glands were engaged in by Dr. Norman Keith, now at the Mayo Clinic. Blood chemistry studies were, at various times, undertaken by Dr. Bowman, Dr. Henry, and others. In 1924 Dr. Henry endeavored to correlate the blood chemistry determination in routine examination with types of mental illness. It was found, however, that there were no abnormal deviations unless the patient had a complicating physical illness.

In 1927 Dr. Henry and Dr. Sniffen, the dentist, devised a technique which by eliminating mouth contaminations facilitated a study of the kinds of microorganisms found in the root canals of the teeth. These studies were made at both Bloomingdale and a public hospital. Bacterial invasion was found to be present in the teeth of psychotic and nonpsychotic patients with equal frequency, and there was four times as much infection in the teeth of public hospital patients as in the teeth of Bloomingdale patients. More than 50 percent contained streptococci, in 10 percent of the haemolytic variety. These percentages were noted in both psychotic and nonpsychotic patients, with no indication of re-

7 *Am. J. Psychiatry*, III (1924).

8 *Association for Research in Nervous and Mental Diseases. Schizophrenia*, V, 1928.

lationship to mental illness.[9] Studies of basal metabolic rates revealed that hypomanic and tense, agitated patients showed a higher rate than normal, and that depressed, underactive, or apathetic patients showed a rate lower than normal. Other laboratory work is described in Dr. Henry's history, as follows:

> During the year [1925] a study was made also of the calcium and phosphorus content of the blood with respect to personality disorders and of the effect of ultra-violet radiation on these constituents of the blood. These studies were made in addition to taking care of the full schedule of routine laboratory work. A special fund for research work was again recommended.
>
> During nine months in 1926, in the absence of Dr. Henry, the laboratories were in charge of Dr. S. Spafford Ackerly. Another Victor air-cooled ultra-violet lamp was added to the therapeutic equipment and the purchase of a Sanborn graphic metabolimeter, an electric thermostatic-controlled water bath, and a new chainomatic chemical balance, greatly facilitated the laboratory work.

Two technicians were added to the laboratory staff during the period, and medical students were frequently employed during the long summer vacation. The work of the laboratory advanced in five years by 300 percent, exclusive of steadily increasing X-ray work. Physicians who were in charge of the laboratory from 1916, when Dr. Amsden was transferred to the clinical service, to 1926 were Dr. Louise Frazee, Dr. Karl M. Bowman, Dr. Joseph P. Eidson, and Dr. George W. Henry.

Closely connected with the development of the laboratory and the clinical and scientific activities of the service was the medical library. In 1911 the medical books of the hospital were kept in a small room adjoining the office of the medical superintendent and in a room in the basement. Among them were valuable works of the eighteenth and early nineteenth centuries. Some of these had been purchased for the library of the New York Hospital before Bloomingdale was established. No catalogue has been found. In order to make better provision for the organization and use of the library, the books were removed to a prepared room near the laboratory. They were arranged and catalogued by Dr. Amsden. In 1915 a musician employed in the service gave some assistance. It was not, however, until 1918, when a trained librarian was appointed, that systematic skilled service was obtained. The first statistical statement relating to the library appeared in the annual report for 1915. In that year 66 volumes were added, and 43 in 1916. In 1919 the total

[9] G. W. Henry, and M. C. H. Doyle, "Focal Infection in the Teeth," *Am. J. Psychiatry*, VIII, Part 2; G. W. Henry, and D. A. Sniffen, "Root-Canal Infection," *Dental Cosmos*, Nov., 1930.

number of volumes was 1,115. The growth of the library was slow but by 1924 the number of volumes was 1,266, and in 1926 it was 1,646. The number of periodicals subscribed for in 1926 was forty-one, of which eight were foreign. From time to time members of the Board of Governors, notably Mr. Walter Jennings, made it possible by personal contributions to obtain books which were more expensive than could ordinarily be afforded from hospital funds.

The attention to illness and injury among the employed personnel of the hospital was also improved by the better facilities and organization provided. In 1924 efficiency was increased by means of an organized outpatient service. A suitably equipped room was provided at which a physician and nurse were in attendance at a regular hour. Employees were given a complete physical examination when first employed and a record was kept of their illnesses. In 1926, 514 persons made 1,361 visits to the clinic. Two hundred X-ray pictures were taken and 78 persons required bed treatment in the infirmaries which had been provided. Infectious diseases were quite infrequent in the hospital. Cases of malaria occurred in diminishing numbers until about 1918, when the mosquito pest and malaria ceased to require particular attention. In 1916 a male employee died of epidemic poliomyelitis of which there were a number of cases in the community. No other case occurred in the hospital. In 1918 the severe epidemic of influenza and pneumonia so generally prevalent sickened 17 patients and 52 employees. In a second outbreak in 1922 there were 78 cases, 42 of which were patients. In 1921 there were 12 cases of septic sore throat with one death. In 1911 it was decided that cases of active tuberculosis would no longer be accepted, and as soon as proper arrangements could be made those already in the hospital were discharged, in most instances by transfer to another hospital. The number of seriously involved organic and grossly deteriorated patients in the service was gradually reduced by discharge and by declining to admit them. The number of cases of general paresis, which in 1915 amounted to 21 percent of the male admissions, in 1925 was reduced to one case in a total of 290 admissions. Admissions were confined to cases in which the outlook for active treatment seemed to be favorable. The policy thus adopted brought about a great change in the social atmosphere of the hospital, to the great advantage of the patients in whose treatment social relations and activities have a large place.

The more enlightened and liberal attitude of the public toward the mentally ill contributed perceptibly to a better understanding and cooperation among patients, relatives, and officials. The laws and regulations governing admissions and discharges were liberalized. From the opening of Bloomingdale in 1821 to 1911, of 11,289 patients admitted only 307 were voluntary. Only 12 of these were admitted previous to 1901. From 1911 to 1926, however, of 3,777 patients admitted 2,492 were voluntary. The effect of this freedom from court procedures and commitment on the morale of patients, their relatives, and of the hospital personnel can hardly be overestimated. In the annual report for 1923 the views then held relating to voluntary admissions were presented. It seems appropriate to quote them in full.

Of the patients admitted, one hundred and ninety-two, constituting nearly seventy-two per cent. of the admissions, signed their own applications and were brought under treatment without certification or court orders. The number of patients who have been admitted to the Hospital by this method now amounts to about 2000, of which 1600 were received during the ten years last past. The experience thus obtained would appear to be a sufficient demonstration of the propriety and practicality, in a large proportion of the cases, of dispensing with legal encumbrances in the way of obtaining access to hospital treatment for persons afflicted with illnesses which affect the mind. In not a single instance has any serious embarrassment or any disadvantage to the patient or to the Hospital been occasioned by the operation of the voluntary system. In the large majority of instances the issues are purely medical and personal, and it requires only ordinary judgment and discretion for the physician to determine when application to the courts becomes necessary. The present system of State supervision furnishes all the precautions needed for safeguarding every interest concerned, and it would be extremely unfortunate if, as sometimes seems imminent, there should be a reversion to the more rigid and technical legal systems which, without discrimination, were formerly employed in the admission of every case. Patients who present extremely gross manifestations of mental disorder are so obviously unfit to take care of themselves that no formal procedure is required to furnish to the most uninformed in such matters convincing evidence of the propriety and need of hospital treatment. Such cases may, in an interval of relative clearness, even though they may not fully grasp the true state of affairs, accept the judgment of their friends and medical advisers and willingly enter the Hospital. In cases which are quite incapable of cooperation, application may be made by some legally authorized person, and the patient admitted under certification by one physician. This procedure was followed in eighteen instances during the year. The large majority of patients who sign their own applications fully realize, however, that they are in need of help and they are glad to seek it at the Hospital. Those who decline to cooperate, or who after admission on their own application, serve the agreed upon notice of their intention to leave, or persistently request to be discharged even though they refrain from presenting the written notice, cannot, of course, be received or detained unless a court order is obtained. The system of indiscriminate and ruthless commitment as a necessary preliminary to obtaining hospital treatment for a person whose mind is disordered, belongs, however, to a period when mental disorders were not as well understood as they are today, and when the well organized means of dealing with them, which are now available, had not been developed. It is being gradually superseded by more enlightened methods which are flexible enough to meet the varying needs of individual cases and situations, and at the same time provide all the protection which is necessary. Soon it should be possible, in a state like New York with its remarkably well organized system of management and supervision, for the large majority of persons in need of treatment for disorders which affect the mind to find access to public and private hospitals without much if any greater formality than is required in procuring relief in any other form of illness. An organized effort to educate the public to this end would seem to be desirable. At present, in order to escape the legal encumbrances, hundreds of patients are every year placed in nursing homes and other institutions which are quite free from official supervision, or they are sent to institutions in adjoining states where the laws are more liberal or are laxly enforced.

Inebriates and drug habitués were admitted in limited numbers under the provisions of a special law passed in 1913 which provided for their commitment for a period of not more than one year. The discharge of patients by means of writs of habeas corpus was occasionally undertaken, and at times succeeded, frequently with unfortunate results. Thirteen patients (six were women) committed suicide at the hospital during the period.

The publication in the annual report of statistical tables of various facts relating to the patients, which had been discontinued in 1907, was not resumed. Statistical statements in regard to age, occupation, duration of illness previous to admission and other data were, however, incorporated in the text. A tabulated statement in regard to movement of the patient population was contained in each report. In 1916, for the first time, the table of diagnoses requested by the State Hospital Commission was published. The hospital also participated in the system of statistical data furnished by all the hospitals for the mentally ill as a means of compiling nation-wide, uniform statistics in coöperation with the National Committee for Mental Hygiene and the United States Bureau of the Census. In the same year a tabulated statement of the laboratory work was published. Beginning in 1921 the X-ray examinations were similarly tabulated, and in 1922 and after, the dental statistics were presented in tabular form. In that year and thereafter statistical tables of the work in the occupational, physical education, and physiotherapy departments were published in the annual report. In 1925 statistics of the outpatient service at the New York Hospital were published.

It has long been considered that the type of psychiatric service conducted by the hospital is of particular benefit to society in that "the patients received . . . belong principally to the more productive classes, and their restoration to usefulness is a distinct contribution to the public good." [10] The annual report for 1914 stated that of the patients admitted there were among the men 6 physicians, 3 lawyers, 6 teachers, 2 chemists, 3 engineers, 5 manufacturers, 2 writers, 6 merchants, 9 salesmen, 3 clerks, 3 farmers, 3 mechanics, 3 tradesmen, 12 students in school or college, and one each, musician, dock-master, dyer, gardener, restauranteur. Among the women were 2 physicians, 9 teachers, 5 social workers, 4 writers, 5 nurses, 4 stenographers, 4 saleswomen, and one each, librarian, designer, art critic, actress. milliner; 6 were students in school or college. Another report noted that only one of the men and two of the women were supported from invested funds, and that "practically all the men had been overtaken by the misfortune of mental disease while engaged actively in productive pursuits, and thirty-two percent of the women had been similarly engaged." [11] In another year, 22 of the patients admitted were students in schools or colleges, 19 were teachers, 6 were physicians, and 6 were lawyers. Thirteen of the women were in business positions and 8 were nurses. Over half the women were married and supported by their husbands, who were either business or professional men.[12] Ordinarily 30 to 40 percent of the women admitted were self supporting by gainful occupations.

The use of prolonged baths, improvements in the nursing service, and advances in the general medical service of the hospital made it possible to discard almost entirely the use of sedative and hypnotic medication. In fact medication of every kind was considerably reduced. The treatment of general paresis by salvarsanized serum was the only new remedy of noteworthy importance to be employed during the period. The method was abandoned when fever treatment was introduced. The advances made in the general medical service were accomplished by improved facilities and organization by means of which more complete and precise examinations were made, and treatment was more vigorously and accurately directed. Physical therapy, which had long been employed at the hospital, was greatly extended. Previous to 1911 a masseur and a masseuse who also administered hydrotherapy were employed. In

[10] Annual report for 1914.

[11] *Ibid.*, 1922.

[12] *Ibid.*, 1926.

1926 three women and two men were engaged in this service. Two hundred and forty-nine patients received 6,787 massage treatments in that year, and 290 received 8,274 hydrotherapeutic treatments. This was exclusive of 12,003 prolonged baths for 192 patients, and 3,659 packs for 120 patients, which were given by the nurses. Sea bathing and sun baths were also provided for at the cottage on Long Island Sound, and 1,747 treatments by ultraviolet ray were given at the hospital.

A considerable change was made in the management of the dietary of the hospital. Knowledge and standards in dietetics were advancing, and in medical practice scientific and therapeutic considerations were replacing mere appeals to the patient's appetite. The transition was slow and attended with difficulties. All the cooking at Bloomingdale is done in a central kitchen and distributed to more than twenty dining rooms. In 1911 the kitchen was governed by a head cook or matron, who, with the help of her husband, who was storekeeper, determined from day to day what the regular meals should consist of. Special consideration was given to patients who paid the higher rates. Most of these patients were in the villas, and the more liberal menu was called "Villa Diet." In 1908 an attempt had been made to prepare in the steward's office a menu to be followed. This occasioned dissatisfaction in the kitchen, however, and was abandoned. In 1911 the attempt was renewed and thereafter the menu was coördinated with the inventories and purchases. The following is a sample of the dietary at that time:

FEMALE DEPARTMENT

BREAKFAST *(for all halls except 3 and 4)*

Cantaloupe, Force & Cream, Steak, Baked Potatoes, Bread, Coffee. (On Hall 4, boiled eggs were substituted for steak, and on Hall 3 both were omitted.)

Villa Diet: Cantaloupe, Cream of Wheat, Bacon & Eggs, Baked Potatoes, Muffins, Toast, Cocoa, Tea, Coffee.

DINNER

Halls 1, 2, 4, 5: Soup, Roast Beef, Spinach, Cucumbers, Potatoes, Cottage Pudding.

Halls 3, 6, 7, 8: Soup, Beef Stew, Spinach, Potatoes, Lettuce, Cottage Pudding, Milk.

Villa Diet: Same as Hall 1 except that creamed squash and lettuce were substituted for spinach and cucumbers, and coffee, milk, and tea added.

SUPPER

Halls 1–5: Tea, Milk, Bread, Butter, Toast, Tomatoes, Huckleberries, Cake.

Halls 6–8: Milk toast substituted for milk and toast.

Villa Diet: Cocoa, Tea, Coffee, Milk, Broiled Chicken, Boiled Eggs, Baked Potatoes, Huckleberries, Cake.

Ice cream was served once a week.[13]

A supplementary "sick diet" consisted of milk toast, broth, eggs, custards and junkets, which was ordinarily ordered by the physician for any patient unable to eat the regular meals. There was also much ordering of special dishes for patients who expressed dissatisfaction with the regular dietary or who were suffering from diabetes or other conditions in which dietary treatment was imperative. All special diet orders required the signature of the medical superintendent. The distribution of food was by ordinary serving dishes on open trucks. Eggs were boiled and tea and coffee were made in the kitchen, and in distant dining rooms might not be served until an hour later. There were no warming tables nor cabinets in the dining-room pantries.

In 1913 and thereafter the position of dietitian was listed in the annual report. It was not filled, however, until 1917. Some improvements were made in the dietary, and instruction in dietetics was given to the student nurses by a part-time instructor engaged during the teaching sessions for the purpose. In 1914 the need of a special diet kitchen for the preparation of sick diet as well as for teaching was mentioned in the annual report. It was provided in 1916, but was not organized for food service, and contributed little to the dietary of the patients. The first full-time dietitian was employed in 1917 and soon after an assistant was added. Some difficulty was experienced in reorganizing the kitchen and it was not until the firmly established cook had resigned in 1919 that a new dietitian was placed in complete charge and progress in advancing the dietary service was greatly facilitated. Even then, however, it was a long time before scientific and therapeutic considerations entirely superseded catering as the controlling principle and practice. Steam tables and cabinets and tea and coffee urns were placed in the dining-room pantries in 1917, and it was made possible to boil eggs and do other light cooking there. The special diet kitchen was manned for service in 1919. In 1922 food containers were provided for keeping the food warm and covered during transportation from the kitchen. In 1924 a committee consisting of the assistant medical director, the steward, and the dietitian was established to have charge of the dietary. Several standardized special dietaries were provided, and extra dishes were, as before, ordered on occasion. In 1926 the dietary staff consisted of the dietitian, her assistant, and two student dietitians.

[13] This dietary may with interest be compared with that of an earlier period, p. 156.

A notable event of this period was the celebration of the hundredth anniversary of the opening of Bloomingdale Hospital in 1821, held on May 26, 1921. Addresses were made by Mr. Edward W. Sheldon, president of the Society of the New York Hospital, Dr. Adolf Meyer and Dr. Lewellys F. Barker of Johns Hopkins University, Dr. Pierre Janet of Paris, Dr. Richard Rows of London, Dr. George D. Stewart, president of the New York Academy of Medicine, and the medical superintendent of the hospital. The audience of over three hundred consisted principally of distinguished psychiatrists from many places. A tableau-pageant was presented on the lawn, in which dramatic scenes representative of the early history and present work of the hospital were portrayed by a large company of patients, physicians, nurses, instructors, and others of the hospital organization. A full account of the proceedings was published in a volume entitled *A Psychiatric Milestone.*[14]

Between July 1, 1911, and September 1, 1926, forty-five physicians besides the medical director were, for varying periods, members of the Bloomingdale staff. Some of these were medical internes with a short service. Only one of those in the service in 1911 remained in 1926. Several who obtained their early training and experience in psychiatry at Bloomingdale in that period have since become distinguished in psychiatric education and practice. Among these, Dr. C. Macfie Campbell (1911–1913) became professor of psychiatry at Harvard University Medical School. His successor at Bloomingdale, Dr. Charles I. Lambert (1913-1922), and Dr. Howard W. Potter (1916–1920), Dr. Robert B. McGraw (1921 and 1924–1925), and Dr. George E. Daniels (1925–1927) became professors of clinical psychiatry at the Columbia University Medical School and eminent psychiatric practitioners. Dr. Milton A. Harrington (1911–1915) became the medical hygiene adviser and teacher of mental hygiene at Dartmouth College and the author of two books.[15] Dr. Sanger Brown II (1912–1917) became assistant commissioner in the New York State Department of Mental Hygiene and the author of two books.[16] Dr. Karl M. Bowman (1915–1917 and 1919–1921) is (1944) professor of psychiatry of the University of California, and author of a book [17] and many scientific articles. Dr. George W. Henry (1917–), associate professor of clinical psychiatry of Cornell University Medical College, has distinguished himself in research and as the author of three

[14] Published privately by the Society of the New York Hospital, 1921.

[15] He wrote *Wish Hunting in the Unconscious* (New York, 1934); *A Biological Approach to the Problem of Abnormal Behavior*, (Philadelphia, 1938).

[16] *Sex Worship and Symbolism* (Boston, 1922); with Howard W. Potter, *The Psychiatric Study of Problem Children* (New York, 1930).

[17] *Personal Problems for Men and Women* (New York, 1931).

books [18] and many articles. Dr. Thomas M. French (1924–1929) became associate director of the Chicago Institute of Psychoanalysis and a professor at the University of Chicago. Dr. Herbert E. Chamberlain (1921–1925) is consulting psychiatrist of the California State Department of Social Welfare. Dr. Samuel W. Hamilton (1923–1936) is director of surveys of mental hospitals and state mental hygiene for the United States Public Health Service. Dr. George S. Amsden (1905–1924) became professor of psychiatry at the Albany Medical College and later (1931–1936) held the corresponding position at Cornell University Medical College. Dr. S. Spafford Ackerly (1925–1926) is professor of psychiatry at the University of Louisville School of Medicine. In November, 1913, Dr. Albert Durham resigned after serving as a faithful, earnest member of the staff since 1898.

More than twenty-six communications relating to the mentally ill were published by members of the medical staff during this period. A number of these were read before psychiatric and other medical societies. Many other articles which were not published were presented at medical society meetings or at the open and Monday evening conferences at the hospital. Contributions to psychiatric literature were made by other members of the organization, including Mr. Louis J. Haas, director of occupational therapy, who published a book [19] and many articles in current literature.

At this period progress in psychiatry and mental hygiene in America was becoming so prolific in facilities for service and contributions to the literature that it will no longer be practicable in this history to present even a scanty review. It seems appropriate to mention, however, the monumental work on *The Institutional Care of the Insane in the United States and Canada,* edited by Henry M. Hurd and published in four volumes by the American Medico-Psychological Association in 1916–1917. Publications relating to psychoanalysis and to mental hygiene began during this period to take on considerable proportions. A number of psychiatric periodicals were established, among the more important of which were the *Archives of Neurology and Psychiatry* of the American Medical Association, and *Mental Hygiene,* the quarterly of the National Committee for Mental Hygiene. *The Psychoanalytic Review,* edited by Dr. W. A. White and Dr. S. E. Jelliffe, was established in 1913.

[18] *Essentials of Psychiatry* (Baltimore, 1925); *Essentials of Psychopathology* (Baltimore, 1935); *Sex Variants* (New York and London, 1941).

[19] *Occupational Therapy* (Milwaukee, 1925).

XXXII

NURSING SERVICE AND THE ORGANIZED THERAPIES

DURING this period advances of considerable importance were made in the nursing service. In 1911 the training course for attendants[1] had been accompanied by little change in the nursing organization, in the conditions of work and living, and in the position of the nurse in the hospital. The average daily number employed in that year was 128, of whom 62 were men and 66 women. The hours of duty were twelve and fifteen on alternate days, and eleven and a half on night service. As only three maids and two men were employed for domestic work in the patients' quarters, much of this work devolved upon the attendants, with such help as they could obtain from the patients. The advantage of the esprit de corps to be derived from separating those engaged in the personal care of patients from other groups in the hospital organization had not yet been fully recognized. Domestics and attendants, with the exception of those in charge of halls who had their meals with the patients, were treated with little or no discrimination in arrangements for living quarters and meals.

The appointment of a superintendent of nurses in 1912 marked the inauguration of a new type of nursing service. The courses of instruction, the graduates and students engaging in the work, and the better nursing facilities were of particular value in the treatment of physical conditions. The better nursing of severe illnesses frequently restored to health patients who would otherwise have died. The nursing records relating to both mental and physical conditions took on a more complete and useful form. The hours of work were in 1912 reduced to an average of ten for day duty, and in 1919 an eight-hour day was adopted for graduate and student nurses. In 1915 the average daily number in the nursing service had increased to 183,[2] of whom 86 were men and 97 women. By increasing the number of domestics, the nurses and attendants were enabled to devote their services more exclusively to the patients. Salaries and wages were increased, more liberal provision was made for time off duty, and in 1914 a pension system for all employees was adopted. The separate dining room for the women erected in 1912, the corresponding provision for the men made in 1919, and improvements in living quarters also contributed to the stability and character

[1] P. 329.

[2] Thirty-three of these were domestics employed in the ward service.

of the service. Separate residences for those employed in the nursing service were long desired, but it was not until 1925 that the first of these residences was provided. The liberal provision made for entertainments and for recreational and social activities, and the advances in clinical medicine in the treatment of the patients and employees were also means of promoting health and contentment for all. Notwithstanding, however, the thought, effort, and expense devoted to the problem and the great advances that were accomplished, difficulty in maintaining a satis-

Nursing Service

1911

Men

1 supervisor
1 night supervisor
10 charge attendants
49 attendants
—
61 (Total)

Women

1 supervisor
1 assistant supervisor
1 chief night attendant
10 charge attendants
53 attendants
—
66 (Total)

1926

1 Assistant Director of Nursing and Nurse Education
2 supervisors (1 for night service)
1 relief supervisor
9 charge nurses
1 charge attendant
10 assistant charge nurses and attendants
2 relief night nurses
3 floor nurses
25 attendants
8 student nurses (men)
—
62 (Total)

1 Director of Nursing and Nurse Education
3 supervisors
10 charge nurses (1 for operating room and employees' clinic)
3 night charge nurses
11 floor nurses
15 attendants
28 student nurses
6 graduate students
—
77 (Total)

In the men's service, some of the attendants were graduates of the two-year course. Two domestics were employed in 1911, and 18 in 1926.

In the women's service also there were graduates of the two-year course; the advent of graduate nurses and students is noteworthy. Three domestics were employed in 1911, and 21 in 1926. The daily average number of patients in the hospital was 351 in 1911, and 267 in 1926.

factory service was of frequent occurrence. The turnover was large, and there were never enough candidates for training. The advance that was made in the organization during the period is indicated by the table on page 420.

When in 1821 the mentally ill patients were removed from the "medical asylum" at the New York Hospital to Bloomingdale, it was believed that by kindly, considerate management, and adequate facilities for directed work and recreation, the readjustment of the patient to normal life and pursuits would be more frequently and certainly accomplished. Particular attention had long been given to the mitigation, reduction, or abandonment of mechanical restraint and seclusion. The means employed and the varying degrees of success obtained during different administrations have already been described. In 1911 the only form of mechanical appliance used was the closed sleeve canvas jacket called a camisole. Resort to it was infrequent. Patients were still placed alone in rooms with the doors closed. A large panel of glass, however, provided for constant observation. State regulations governing restraint and seclusion required frequent relief for the patient and that records be kept for inspection. After the use of prolonged baths and packs had been more extensively introduced, and the medical and nursing services had been enlarged and activated, restraint by mechanical appliances was practically dispensed with. A graduate of the Bloomingdale School of Nursing, who some years later was appointed director of a psychiatric service at a general hospital, was, when asked to instruct the student nurses in the use of mechanical restraint, unable to comply because she had never seen the appliances used and did not know how to apply them.[3]

In the plan of "moral treatment" much importance was attached to engaging the patient in useful employment. It was found that the women, who were accustomed to sewing, knitting, and household work in their homes, could be more adequately employed than the men. While the number of women thus employed was considerable, the range of employment was narrow and without the charm and incentive of novelty and variety; only those with sufficient initiative to be volunteers took any interest or part in it. Dr. Nichols had in 1850 suggested that competent instructors should be employed to instruct and engage the patients in occupations.[4] It is doubtful if at that time competent instructors, especially for the men, could have been found. In 1911, however, the growth of interest and the provision for education in art and handicrafts which

[3] Personal communication.

[4] See p. 244.

had occurred in America seemed to have provided means of adopting directed employment as a positive method of treatment of the mentally ill. The development in the women's service, proposed by Dr. Hoch and undertaken by a voluntary instructor in 1908, has already been described.[5] This was gradually being expanded. In addition to their voluntary work in the halls, the patients were given instruction in weaving, basketry, knitting, crochet and needlework. In 1911 two attendants who had been given some instruction spent part time in assisting the instructor. The number of patients who received instruction that year was 70, and 886 articles were made. In 1912 a full-time capable assistant was appointed. After more space had been obtained by transfer to the Dexter Cottage in 1914, the number of crafts was increased and more of the patients attended. In that year 216 patients were treated and 18,222 articles were made or repaired. Two additional assistants were soon engaged and the work steadily progressed. Again in 1923, after Sturgis Hall was in operation, the number of patients employed had increased to 263, and the number of articles made and repaired was 14,255. At the end of the period, in 1926, the staff consisted of the director and seven assistants, besides a porter. Crafts engaged in were metal and jewelry, basketry, bookbinding, block printing, cardboard construction, crochet and tatting, cooking, drawing and designing, dressmaking, embroidery, fancy needlework, gesso and clay modeling, jigsaw toys and wood construction, knitting, leather tooling, printing, plain sewing and machine stitching, painting in water colors and oil, winding skeins and warps, typewriting, and weaving. Gardening was also engaged in, for a time under a special instructor. It was not attended with great success, however, except for a very few patients ordinarily and for many in wartime. Patients who were too disturbed, resistive, or feeble to attend the shops, were given instruction where they resided in the halls. After Sturgis Hall[6] was opened, however, a class for difficult patients was formed there. It was amazing to see the calming effect on these patients of work in the shops. Some of the show pieces on exhibition in the building were made by them.

Sturgis Hall was a remarkably valuable acquisition. It is an attractive building located in picturesque surroundings. The views from the windows are an incentive to contentment and joy in producing beautiful articles. The building was designed by Mr. Grosvenor Atterbury, architect, with the assistance of Miss Pauline G. Gundersen, who had succeeded Mrs. Amsden as director of the department in 1914. It contained

[5] Pp. 359–373.

[6] See p. 424.

eight work rooms on the main floor, and four on the sunlit side of a lower floor (part of which was underground because of the slope of the land). Entrance was made through a large lobby with beamed ceiling, leaded windows containing craft designs, and a variegated slate floor. So much charm was there in the building, with its air of activity, suggestive equipment and finished products, that patients who were too apathetic or resistive to accept invitations to work, and who nevertheless were brought to the building with the other patients, would sometimes be so attracted that they would ask permission to repeat the visit, and eventually after a period of idle observation would follow the example of those about them and engage in some interesting craft.

In the early reports of the Bloomingdale Asylum Committee it was stated with regret that it was "difficult to contrive suitable work for the Male Lunatics." [7] The governors expected that the removal to Bloomingdale and again to White Plains would supply means of overcoming this difficulty. The women had their own original resources. The men, however, were in most instances without interest or practice in such manual employment as could be provided in the routine operation of the hospital and nothing else was available. Some degree of success had attended the attempts at solving the problem. At times it was reported that 40 percent of the men and over 50 percent of the women engaged in some manual employment, that "both sexes render much voluntary assistance in the care of the halls, in the making of beds, washing of dishes etc.," and that a few men did a little work on the farm, in the mechanical shops, and in the kitchen and laundry. For the women it was found "easy to provide a certain amount of sewing and divide it around so that all may do a little and none be made weary with long hours of labor." [8] The idea of employing instructors had been entertained, and for a short time a sewing instructor was engaged.

It was not, however, until the success of the measures adopted for the women in 1908 had been demonstrated that an attempt to make similar provision for the men was undertaken. In 1912 an instructor was procured from an educational institution, two rooms in the old gymnasium were furnished with equipment, and twenty-five of the male patients were employed in joinery, basketry, rug making, brass hammering and piercing, leather work, jig sawing, broom making and chair caning. It was explained to one of the governors, who observed that the brooms were better than he found in the stores, that these brooms were

[7] *Minutes of the Governors*, Dec. 4, 1821.

[8] Annual report for 1890.

made by college graduates. It was evident that the undertaking was promising and after another year, during which 69 were employed, the governors made an appropriation for an occupational building. While this was under construction the department was expanding. In 1914 a room in the main hospital building was taken over as a printing shop; in 1915 the output of this shop was 201,112 pieces of printed matter and the binding of 1,175 books, magazines, and pads. Garden plots were provided for some of the men, and an assistant was appointed to engage the patients in gardening and a number of other kinds of outdoor work, mostly of a very practical character. The number of patients who were treated in the department in that year was 93. The new building was occupied in May, 1916, realizing at long last a recommendation that had been repeatedly made by the asylum physicians since 1835. The building was located on a prominent site in the men's recreation grounds. It contained nine workshops, besides service rooms and an entrance lobby which was also used as an exhibit room. Much interest was shown by the patients in the construction of the new building and they made the benches, stands, cabinets, and other pieces of equipment.

Three appointments were made in the position of director during the first three years of operation of the department. Sometimes a vacancy extended over a considerable period. Assistants were at first provided by attendants who gave part-time service, and they were able to keep the department operating during the vacancies. In October, 1915, Mr. Louis J. Haas was appointed director. During his long service the department was brought to its present high state of efficiency. Mr. Haas also, by his inventions, his many publications, and his active participation in organizations, exhibits, and other means of promoting occupational therapy, made a notable contribution to the introduction and advancement of this form of treatment in America. At the time of his appointment four full-time assistants had been added to the department. One of these was a printer and bookbinder for whom a power press and other necessary equipment had been provided. Other shops in the new building were a fully equipped carpenter shop, a smithy, shops for small metalwork, basketry, caning, weaving, and other crafts. Many articles of use and beauty were made for the hospital or to be taken home by the patients. The outdoor party aided in the construction of tennis courts and the golf course. They made benches and other articles of cement and wood for the lawns and the beach cottage. In 1918, after the new shops had been well established, the number of patients treated in the department was 197 and 1,476 pieces of shop work were finished. The printing shop produced 245,526 pieces of printing, and bound 3,600 books, pamphlets, and pads. At the close of the period, in 1926, the staff consisted of the director and five assistants, 8,458 articles were made and 523 were repaired. Fifteen different crafts were engaged in. The department had contributed to the development of occupational therapy in other places much instruction and advice, and also samples of devices and products. Sample baskets and brush blocks, model chairs and drilling jigs were made for the New York State Commission for the Blind, with instructions printed in Braille. Models of small looms designed for use by patients in their rooms were furnished to the superintendents of hospitals in Sweden and China.

Closely allied to productive occupation in the plan of "moral" treatment were activities that had formerly been designated "amusements." These embraced physical exercises and sports, parlor games, social parties, reading, and assembly-hall entertainments. The value of this form of treatment had always been recognized, and on several occasions a qualified person had been employed as instructor and supervisor. This service had, however, never gained a permanent place in the system of treatment. In 1911 the patients were dependent upon the physicians and attendants for any assistance needed in utilizing the available means of recreation. Much was accomplished. It seemed advisable, however, as in occupational therapy, to endeavor to develop more fully and permanently a form of treatment that had been highly valued ever since medical treatment of the mentally ill had received attention. A start was made in 1911 by a class of men patients under the leadership of one of the supervisors. In 1912 Miss Gratia Eldridge, a graduate in physical education of Columbia University, was engaged to work with the women. She had remarkable personal as well as professional qualifications for the undertaking. She remained for eight years and made a valuable contribution in establishing a department, and making it an indispensable and permanent part of the treatment resources of the hospital. An article published by her in 1921 [9] gives an account of her experiences and of the problems with which she was confronted and her ways of meeting them. In 1914 an assistant to Miss Eldridge was appointed. In 1920 she had four assistants and the service of two students from a school of physical education during the summer. The activities

[9] Gratia Eldridge, "Recreational Activities in the Treatment of Mental Disorders," *Am. Phys. Educ. Rev.*, June, 1921.

were at first only such as could be engaged in by means of the available facilities. There was a gymnasium with little equipment, a grass tennis court, a golf putting green and a bowling alley in the men's gymnasium, to which the women had access. There were also the recreation grounds, the walks and woods on the hospital property, the cottage on Long Island Sound, and the assembly hall for social parties and entertainments. Formal gymnastics, folk dancing, a few simple games, and bowling were the first activities undertaken by the instructor. By 1920, however, when Miss Eldridge retired, provision had been made for field hockey, basketball, baseball, and volley ball; the number of tennis courts had been increased, and a nine-hole golf course constructed.

The department had assumed responsibility for the social activities and for the assembly-hall entertainments. The regular dancing parties which had, for many years, been a highly appreciated form of entertainment, were reorganized on a less formal plan. The alteration and redecoration and furnishing of the assembly hall added much to the attractiveness of the dancing parties. There was also a change in the patients themselves; under the new policy of admission they were now younger and less frequently affected with long-standing disorders. On special evenings such as Thanksgiving a costume party was given, for which the patients, in some instances with the assistance of the occupational therapy department, made their own costumes. At an afternoon Christmas party the patients had an opportunity to invite their visiting friends. Dancing classes were formed and some who had never danced or who had refrained for years were induced to take lessons. Parlor games, dramatics (five plays in one year), music, informal dances, beach parties with swimming, picnics, cross-country tramps, skating, coasting and skiing in winter, and many other similar activities were pursued with a continuity and vigor that could not have been maintained without the skilled and persistent attention of the physical instructors.

Throughout the summer season, day parties of patients drove to the beach cottage for a meal and a swim. In the new cottage at Orienta Point, which was, however, not available until 1926, provision was also made for tennis, golf putting, croquet, and indoor games. Overnight accommodations were provided, so that a few patients at a time could remain for varying periods. The homelike conditions, the relaxation of institutional regimentation and the greater liberty were a source of encouragement to many patients, whose recovery, in many instances, received a noticeable impetus. The number of day parties in a season was usually about seventy, in which six hundred or more participated;

and the number of patients who remained for several days was usually about forty-five. Among the pleasures at the beach were, for several years, trips on a forty-foot launch which was generously placed at the disposal of the hospital by Dr. Lyon, who had been the medical superintendent. The launch was unfortunately wrecked in a severe storm in August, 1915.

The work continued to advance under other leadership after Miss Eldridge retired in 1920. It was greatly implemented in 1925 when a fully equipped gymnasium of liberal dimensions and beautiful design was opened, a donation from Mr. Henry R. Taylor, one of the governors of the hospital. In appearance the building without and within is more like an old English hall than a conventional gymnasium. It is conveniently and attractively located in the women's recreation grounds. It contains, besides a main hall 90 by 50 feet, a number of smaller rooms for pool, billiards, ping-pong, bowling, and individual correctional treatment, and also a kitchen, showers and lockers, an office and service rooms, and two galleries, one of which contains a mechanical pipe organ. An attractive and useful feature of the interior is a clock dial harmonizing with the design of the room and made by the men's occupational department. Not infrequently, even before a patient could be induced to engage in constructive occupation, the impact of a medicine ball or ever so listless participation in bean bags or some other simple exercise would penetrate her inactivity and start her on the way to wholesome interests and pursuits. At the close of the period, in 1926, the staff of the department consisted of the director and four assistants, besides for varying periods one or more students. Fifteen forms of games, sports, social and other activities, in addition to general entertainments, were engaged in under the management of the department, and 257 different patients participated.

Greater difficulty was experienced in establishing a department for the men. It was hard to find an instructor who was professionally well qualified and had also the personal qualities and attitude required for the management and treatment of the mentally ill. A retired Danish army officer, who was appointed in 1912, succeeded fairly well after a start had been made by one of the supervisors in 1911. In 1913 attention was received from the instructor by 146 patients. In the annual report for 1914 the following activities were listed as though they had been engaged in by both men and women: calisthenics with and without dumbbells, striking-bag, medicine ball, Indian clubs, chest weights, ring and bar stalls; basketball, baseball and tennis, indoor and outdoor;

handball, bowling, golf, field hockey, roque, croquet, quoits, skating, coasting, skiing, country walks, picnics, social parties and dances. The loss of the bowling alley by fire occurred in 1914. Bowling on the green was added to the games for men in 1917. Tennis, golf, and billiard tournaments excited much interest, and fans of both sexes attended these and the baseball and other match games. A moving-picture machine was obtained in 1914 and thereafter furnished one of the scheduled entertainments. The men also had the use of the beach cottage, resorting there alternately with the women.

Provision was made for an assistant to the director in 1914, but for several years this position was either vacant or unsatisfactorily filled. In 1918, after a year of temporizing, Mr. Michael Collins, a graduate of the Bloomingdale Training School for attendants, who had during several years of nursing service shown exceptional ability in understanding and caring for patients, was appointed director of the department. By taking some short courses and by visiting various departments of physical education and gymnasiums, Mr. Collins acquired adequate facility in the various exercises and games considered most efficacious in the treatment of the mentally ill. Experience had demonstrated that, in this position, superior educational and technical qualifications could be better spared than understanding and skill in work with patients. With this appointment the work was established on a permanent footing and under Mr. Collins' direction made steady progress. In 1918, 108 patients were enrolled with an average daily attendance of 52; this rose in 1919 to 207 enrolled and an average daily attendance of 66.3. The number of activities engaged in had doubled. The increase in facilities, especially the golf course constructed in 1915, did much to add to the interest and furnish incentives to participation by the patients. By 1917 there were six tennis courts on the property, in the construction of some of which the patients had participated. A legacy from a former patient gave another impetus to the work in 1924 by furnishing a new gymnasium. The building is of more conventional design than the women's gymnasium. It is equally commodious, and in addition to the provision similar to that made for the women it contains a squash court, an attractive, nicely furnished lounge, and a larger number of bowling alleys. In 1926 the staff consisted of the director and two assistants. Students of schools of physical education were when available added to the summer staff. The staff were not as fully responsible for social activities and entertainments as that of the women's department, though they frequently participated.

The number of patients who came under their attention in 1926 was 202, with an average daily attendance of 85.5. Much of the work of both departments cannot be exhibited statistically.

The placing of directed employment and recreation on a well-organized and permanent footing was, perhaps, one of the most important accomplishments at Bloomingdale Hospital during this period. Reports of the program were probably in some instances exaggerated, but apparently were not without influence in promoting similar advancements elsewhere. An English psychiatrist, who, when visiting the hospital, was first shown the laboratory, X-ray and dental departments, and other facilities for scientific examinations and treatment, expressed great surprise, saying that he had been informed that Bloomingdale was a "work cure."

Employment was at first considered "diversional," and was so designated in reports and published papers. Recreational activities, while perhaps no longer regarded as mere amusements, were probably seldom thought to have much if any different purpose in a hospital for the mentally ill than in any ordinary community. But, through practice, the true place and value of directed employment and recreation in a constructive plan of treatment were revealed more clearly. The employment of educated and observant men and women as instructors or therapists, and their understanding and the results of their observations and relations with individual patients, contributed much to an appreciation of the positive medical value of these measures. When intelligently directed they afford valuable means of promoting healthy adjustments to social relations and responsibilities, which is the ultimate aim of treatment of the mentally ill. How well this is understood and turned to account by capable therapists may be gathered from such articles as that of Miss Eldridge and others. Many patients at Bloomingdale and no doubt at other hospitals, become extremely helpful to other patients. Some of them act as valuable assistants, in some instances with knowledge and skill in some art or pursuit in which they are professionals. Some have been permitted to prolong their stay at the hospital or to return in order to learn more thoroughly one or more of the crafts for the purpose of utilizing them in the community as a means of support. Three of the women patients discharged during this period received appointments as occupational therapists in other institutions; one at a state hospital where she contributed substantially in the establishment of a department, another in a private hospital where she established and conducted for years the occupational treatment of the patients. The third introduced occupational therapy in an institution for delinquent girls and has ever since conducted it with very beneficial results. In many instances patients have, after returning home, found in some craft learned at the hospital a health-promoting hobby and even a means of revenue, and more than a few men and women, who had never realized the value of recreation and play in the maintenance of health and capacity for social relations and work, have returned home conditioned to give them a larger place in their lives. The attractive exhibits which were displayed by the departments at meetings of the American Psychiatric Association and at other places year after year for several years, were a means of promoting the widespread introduction of occupational therapy in the treatment of the mentally and physically ill.

Although religious services, which have been regularly conducted at Bloomingdale since 1819,[10] were in this period—perhaps not without loss—no longer given the important place in "moral treatment" which they held in earlier periods, they were conducted regularly and were well attended. Good music was provided, and on special occasions such as Easter and Christmas the floral display from the greenhouse was of more than ordinary beauty. For many patients the services contributed to their normal interests and gave them comfort and encouragement. Perhaps when clergymen have better learned the nature of man and his needs, especially when he is mentally ill, these services may have some of the positive medical value in treatment attributed to them by former governors and physicians.

A library for the use of the patients was established in 1822. That it had value as a means of treatment was early recognized. Much attention was given to reading and the use of the library and the establishment of a reading room by Dr. James Macdonald in 1827.[11] At first a patient acted as librarian and later an attendant received extra compensation for attending to the library. In 1911, however, no special library service was provided and the books were scattered in bookcases on different halls. In 1914 the musician who acted as librarian of the medical library gave some service to the patients' library also and the books were assembled in one room. In that year it was stated in the annual report that 44 books had been added, some of which were gifts of the authors. In 1915 it was reported that 136 books had been added. In 1916, through a

10 P. 192.

11 Pp. 187–188.

bequest from Catharine Jane Pryor, 264 books were added. In that year also the room in which the books were assembled was completely transformed into a handsome paneled library lined with built-in bookcases. A generous fireplace and comfortable library furniture made it an inviting resort for such patients as were in condition to come to it. The librarian was also provided with a cart by which she conveyed books about the patients' halls, and by means of catalogues and descriptions of other books endeavored to interest the patients in suitable reading. Care was exercised in the selection of books, all of which were examined by the librarian and usually by one of the physicians before they were accepted. The librarian conferred with the physicians with regard to particular patients. She learned much about them in her visits through the house, and she also attended conferences and lectures at which the problems presented by the mentally ill were discussed. It was not until the trained librarian was appointed in 1918, however, that the effective use of reading as a treatment measure began to be understood and employed. The librarian gave talks to the nurses on the use of reading in the treatment of the patients. The library has now come to be accepted for what it was called by one of the governors in 1827—"one of the essentials of moral treatment." The Board of Governors provided that a definite amount might be expended for books from the budget each month. In 1917, of 586 books added, 200 were a personal donation from Mr. A. J. Smith, one of the governors. In 1919 the president of the board, Mr. E. W. Sheldon, donated 100 volumes. In 1925 another of the governors, Mr. Walter Jennings, gave $250 for the purchase of books. The first report of circulation from the library was made in 1916, when 3,787 books were distributed. In 1919, after a trained librarian had been employed, the circulation rose to 7,800, and 380 books were added to the collection. In 1921 it was reported that the library contained 3,966 volumes. In 1926 it contained 5,021 volumes, and the circulation during the year was 10,435, of which 5,482 were distributed to patients and 4,953 to employees. The hospital at that time also subscribed for 65 popular magazines.[12]

In this period much progress was made in adding to the efficiency of the psychiatric service of the New York Hospital as an organized means of accomplishing the main purpose for which it was established. The measures which the governors had hoped to provide when they designed Bloomingdale were at last developed and amplified into a fine

12 W. L. Russell, "The Library in the Modern Hospital," *Library J.*, Dec. 15, 1924.

medical instrumentality to work with the physicians in their personal therapy. In fact, occasionally when personal psychotherapy seemed to have reached an impasse, the discouraged physician would be advised by the staff conference to "leave him to the organization" for a while. This sometimes worked very well, and after a period of directed exercise in social adjustment by means of the organized therapies and the constant influence of wholesome relationship, personal therapy could be resumed with happy results.

XXXIII

EDUCATIONAL WORK AND WAR SERVICE

One of the principal motives actuating the physicians instrumental in the establishment of the New York Hospital in 1771 was to make provision for medical education. In this they had the full support of the governors. Medical teaching was engaged in at the hospital from its opening for the reception of patients, and even before.[1] References in Alexander Anderson's diary indicate that, at least while mentally ill patients were treated in the general service, medical students had opportunities to observe and study them. Some of the attending physicians, notably Dr. Hosack, Dr. Mitchill, and Dr. Hammersley, wrote and lectured on mental illness or related subjects.[2] Whether the patients in the "medical asylum" operated at the hospital from 1808 to 1821 were subjects for clinical teaching, cannot now be determined with certainty. It seems probable, however, that they were. It is also indicated in Dr. Handy's report to the governors in 1818 that the house physicians of the general hospital assisted in the study and treatment of the patients in the asylum.[3]

There can be no doubt that the removal of the service to Bloomingdale in 1821 and to White Plains in 1894 not only separated it from the other medical services, but from the medical schools and easy access for teaching as well. Consequently, collaboration with medical schools and formal medical courses were not undertaken at Bloomingdale. The physicians learned their psychiatry by observation and experience, by reading, and from their more experienced colleagues. Some took special courses in New York or went to Europe for observation and study. Several gained well-deserved reputations as specialists.

The establishment of the laboratory in 1905, and the precise and thorough clinical methods employed by Dr. Hoch and Dr. Amsden, may be considered the beginning of developments at Bloomingdale which enhanced the value of the service as a means of medical and psychiatric education. Since 1911 daily morning conferences have been held, at which the physicians, supervisors, and directors of organized therapies discussed the state of their services and their observations and experiences with the patients. These conferences, together with the clinical staff conferences four times a week, the open conferences, and the Monday evening conferences,[4] the advance in the general clinical stand-

1 P. 27.

2 See Chapter V.

3 Pp. 103–104.

4 See p. 406.

ards, and the organization and use of the library furnished an atmosphere and means of learning that were an incentive to study and to proficiency in practice. Senior members of the staff instructed new members and supervised their work. Special studies and the preparation of articles for presentation at the hospital conferences and at medical societies, or for publication, were encouraged. In 1919 the governors authorized the expenditure of $500 annually for traveling and other expenses in attending meetings and presenting papers. In proposing an increase in the number of physicians the medical director suggested that "in accomplishing this the educational resources which the Hospital possesses might perhaps be better organized and utilized as a means of securing and training physicians for the field of psychiatry." [5] In 1924 the Council on Medical Education and Hospitals of the American Medical Association proposed a plan of systematic work and instruction for physicians, to be approved by the council as a definite course for qualifying physicians as psychiatrists; the plan was not undertaken at the time. Time from duty was allowed for special courses and for gaining broader experience and greater proficiency in psychiatry. Student internes were appointed in the clinical and laboratory services during the summer vacation. Recent graduates awaiting entrance upon their service as internes in general hospitals were appointed medical internes at Bloomingdale for varying periods; some of them, after completing their general hospital service, accepted positions at Bloomingdale. Near the close of the period a member of the staff was given a year's leave of absence with salary to study in Europe. The subsequent careers of a number of physicians who obtained at Bloomingdale most or all of their first practical instruction and experience in psychiatry are living evidence of the educational value of the service.

The New York Hospital School of Nursing, established in 1877, was one of the earliest in America. The first school in America for the training of nurses for the mentally ill was established in 1882 at McLean Hospital. That training would improve the character of the nursing at Bloomingdale had long been anticipated. In 1845 Dr. Pliny Earle "hoped that the time would come when persons would be especially educated to be attendants." He had in the preceding year prepared as a means of instruction a "Guide for Attendants." [6] In 1883 Dr. Nichols went a step farther in proposing that nurses from the New York Hospital be given a course of three to six months of "training and service" at Bloomingdale. It was, however, not until 1891 that a preliminary move was made towards

[5] Annual report for 1919.

[6] Pp. 232, 233.

the introduction of an organized system of instruction and training. This, and the developments which followed up to 1911, have been described in previous chapters. At the close of 1910 the number of attendants who had received certificates of graduation from the school established in 1895 was 107, of whom 26 (7 men and 19 women) were still in the service. In 1911 there were under training in the school 6 men and 8 women. Seven of these were in the first year of the course, and 20 others who had been admitted had dropped out. One of the great difficulties in maintaining a satisfactory nursing service was the constant turnover: the annual report for 1911 noted that, with an average of 62 men in the service, 148 had been engaged during the year and 143 had left; and with an average of 66 women, 77 had entered and 69 had left.

A special report to the governors in November, 1911, recommended that the instruction of attendants be continued, and that a teaching organization be formed for the purpose of improving the character of the course and, by means of additional training at a general hospital, of graduating as trained nurses those who could qualify. This had been accomplished at other hospitals, notably at McLean in Massachusetts. It was recommended that a capable nursing superintendent be appointed and that psychiatrically trained supervisors and charge nurses be obtained as soon as possible to form an educational organization. It was realized that this would be a comparatively slow process, owing particularly to the difficulty both in obtaining adequately qualified graduates as teachers and supervisors and in obtaining candidates qualified for the extended course contemplated. The report also took note of a number of other difficulties:

The nursing of mental cases is not generally looked upon as an attractive field of work. The traditional views of insanity and the insane still have great influence, and few who have not seen for themselves have any true conception of the nature of the work. . . . Nurses who have been trained only in general hospital work are rarely qualified for important positions in which the first essential is knowledge of mental diseases and of the insane and their needs. . . . The main object must be to improve the work of those already employed in the nursing service, and to furnish opportunities and training for those among them who may be qualified to become thoroughly trained nurses. All the attendants should, therefore, be given some systematic instruction, not only a few who may be selected with a view to graduating them as nurses. The school organization and work are not to be looked upon as something apart from the present system, but simply as an elaboration with a view to better service, and better standards of training for those who are to be in the future entrusted with the delicate and difficult work of nursing cases of mental disease, not only in special institutions but wherever these cases are met with. Bloomingdale should eventually furnish much needed leaders in this field of nursing.[7]

It was recommended that courses be established "which might be attractive to graduates of general hospital training schools who might be led to take these courses after graduation." Attention was directed to the necessity of "improvements in the conditions under which the members of the nursing force live and work," specifically, shorter hours and better living quarters, including a separate Nurses Home. The recommendations were approved by the governors and steps were taken towards carrying out the program.

Nurse training and practice had for many years been conducted without state regulation. The physicians and governors of the hospitals for the mentally ill had, therefore, been free to undertake any plan or system of instruction and training which, in their judgment, would best meet their needs. Now, however, laws had been enacted for the regulation of all nursing education and practice. The law and its administration were shaped and controlled by nursing organizations composed of graduates of general hospital schools in which no provision was at that time made for instruction and training in the nursing of the mentally ill. It was evidently not understood that laws, regulations, schedules, and syllabi appropriate in the regulation of nursing and nurse training in the well-established schools of general hospitals might not only not contribute to the advancement of nursing and nurse training in the hospitals for the mentally ill but might actually prove prejudicial to developments which had been established and maintained under the most difficult circumstances and had accomplished remarkable improvements in the treatment of the patients. In fact, considerable apprehension was occasioned by the inclusion of the hospitals for the mentally ill among those for narrow specialties such as orthopedics, eye, ear and throat, and skin diseases; these were considered suitable only for short courses in undergraduate nurse training in affiliation with general hospital schools and for post-graduate training.

Nearly all the hospitals for the mentally ill in America encountered the same problems in endeavoring to establish and conduct a school of nursing; therefore a fuller account of the Bloomingdale experience than would otherwise seem necessary may serve a useful purpose. The position of director of nursing, established in 1912, was filled by the appointment of Miss Adele S. Poston, who had previously held a corresponding position in the state hospital service of Illinois. In order to prepare the men's

[7] *Minutes of the Bloomingdale Committee,* Nov. 13, 1911.

service for the educational work contemplated, Mr. W. C. Roden, a graduate from the Butler Hospital School, Providence, Rhode Island, was appointed assistant supervisor. In 1913 a graduate of the New York Hospital School was appointed instructor in general nursing; she remained for a year. The instruction in the two-year course was extended and improved, and a thirteen weeks' course was established for all new attendants, irrespective of their qualifications for the longer courses which they might or might not enter. A three-year course, including one year at the New York Hospital and a maternity hospital, was established, and the school was registered by the State Department of Education. In 1911 there were 35 students in the two-year course, and 2 men and 2 women finished and were given certificates. In order to increase the number of well-qualified graduate nurses in the service to aid in the educational work, two graduates, one from McLean Hospital and the other from Butler Hospital, were in 1914 engaged as supervisors. Five other graduate nurses from hospitals for the mentally ill were added. Miss Gertrude Trefry, a graduate of the White Plains Hospital School, was engaged as instructor in general nursing. She remained in the position for sixteen years and made an important contribution to the establishment and development of the educational work, especially in the three-year course.

Many candidates were enrolled in the two-year course, but only a small proportion remained through to graduation. The largest number to graduate in any year was thirteen in 1916 and again in 1918, when twelve of the thirteen were women. Eight women and twelve men entered the course that year. In the following years the number received and the number graduated fluctuated greatly, and in 1920 the course received its death blow. In August of that year the medical director of the hospital reported to the governors that "recent legislation which has practically abolished the two-year course has added to our difficulties." In the annual report for the year it was explained that

Some of the most valuable nurses in the service are graduates of this course and many of them hold excellent positions elsewhere. Under an amendment to the Nurse Practice Act which has recently become operative graduates of this course will be entitled to the designation of trained attendant (T. A.). As, however, the law specifies that a training of nine months qualifies for this form of certificate, it is unlikely that candidates for the two years' course can be obtained, and nine months is much too short a period of training for the responsibilities of the nursing of persons suffering from mental disorder. The way in which this amendment will affect the training schools and the nursing service of the hospitals for this class of illness can scarcely as yet be estimated. Nothing has, however, done so much to improve the character of the hospitals, especially the State hospitals, as the courses of training . . . and it would be nothing less than a calamity affecting the welfare of thousands of the most helpless of sick persons, if anything were permitted to impair the standards of these courses or reduce the number and quality of the candidates.

During three years following the passage of this act attendants were encouraged to enter the course, and a large number did so, most of them men. Few, however, finished. No women entered after 1923. Two men were given certificates in 1925, and in 1926 none was admitted and the course was discontinued.

According to a short review of the history of the course (issued in 1923), all the instruction was at first given by the physicians, "especially Dr. Pringle [8] who . . . has reason to feel gratified that some members of the nursing service who are to-day depended upon to perform the most difficult and delicate tasks, are graduates of this course." Candidates "were selected from the untrained attendants then employed, by reason of their demonstrated practical fitness for the work, and as a result of an entrance examination." Furthermore, the state department of education stipulated that candidates be selected with reference to their formal schooling in particular subjects as shown by credentials or "counts" from their teachers, and that the former method of selection by examination and observation of practical suitability was no longer acceptable.[9] The brief account added that those who entered "have, after varying periods, been dropping out, and for two years none has finished." This was the valedictory. The total number of graduates of this course from its establishment in 1895 to its close was 171, of whom 114 were women and 57 were men. In the words of Dr. Lyon in 1909, the nursing service "has been made more efficient by their help."

The future of the nursing service was now believed to depend upon the development of the three-year course, and of courses of six months or more for graduates of general hospital schools. In 1914 six students had entered the three-year course. In the following year there were eleven, three of whom went to the New York Hospital for the part of the course given there and to the Manhattan Maternity Hospital. At the close of 1917 sixteen students were enrolled in the course, one of whom was a man. The first graduates, two women, finished the course that year; and the first annual report of the director of nursing to be pub-

8 Dr. Rose Pringle, assistant physician, 1895–1927.

9 A request to admit by the former procedure in special instances was refused.

lished appeared the same year. Letters were addressed to high school principals, physicians, clergymen, and others who might be interested in referring candidates. Hundreds of inquiries were received but the number who applied was disappointingly small. Physicians and nurses whose knowledge of mental illness and of the resources of Bloomingdale for nursing education was meager, and who were influenced by traditional views and prejudices, usually advised against applying for admission to the school. Moreover, the nursing organizations and periodicals were opposed to separate schools in specialized hospitals, irrespective of their size or character. Neither they nor the state authorities proposed any policy or program by which, in the advancement of nursing education, the nursing needs of the thousands of patients in the hospitals for the mentally ill, nearly all public, might be adequately supplied; and they opposed or gave only halfhearted support to proposals made by physicians and others who sought to maintain and further develop the provision for training already established. In order to retain registration it was necessary to conform to technical forms and procedures in the admission of students, to follow prescribed schedules and syllabi prepared primarily for general hospital schools, to employ charge nurses who met certain academic requirements, and to make what was considered a necessary distinction socially and officially between registered nurses and students on the one hand and unregistered nurses and attendants on the other. It was, however, realized that the object of the state department was to advance general nursing education and practice, and every effort was made to work in harmony with it and to promote its general aims.

The work of the school was carried on in a hopeful, coöperative spirit and a measure of success was achieved. Notwithstanding the small number of graduates, an alumni association was organized with the hope that, in time, it would aid in building up the school. In 1919 the nursing organization was further strengthened by the employment of more well-qualified graduates, and the working hours of nurses were reduced. The number of students continued, however, to be far too small. Six entered in 1919 and three in 1920. In her annual report for 1920 Miss Poston admitted some discouragement, and offered the consolation that "our School is one year older and has gained in experience and in a degree of prestige among other schools." In 1921 Miss Poston resigned and was succeeded by Miss Katherine Hearn, who had been for many years in the service as supervisor and assistant director of nursing. A vigorous campaign of information was again instituted and again hundreds of letters were received. The number admitted in 1922 was, however, only six.

In 1923 the school entered into an arrangement with four of the general hospital schools in the vicinity, by which a highly qualified teacher was employed to give academic instruction to junior students at a central school, for which accommodations and equipment were provided at Bloomingdale. This course absorbed four months of the first year, during which there was little time for practical service with patients. Seven students entered the hospital school that year and one graduated. With a view to advancing educational work in the men's department, a woman supervisor was placed there. In 1924, after thirteen students had entered, Miss Hearn reported that "if this number can be maintained for the next few classes, the school will have arrived upon a secure footing." In 1926 this optimistic view seemed to be confirmed by the admission of 28 students, 8 of whom were men. There were in the school that year 93 students—48 in the hospital school, 35 from affiliated hospitals, and 10 graduate students. In the meantime, in 1925, the working and living arrangements for male students were improved, and supervision and practical instruction were delegated to Mr. Roden, who was advanced to the position of assistant director of nursing. An affiliation was made with the Mills School for Male Nurses at Bellevue Hospital for a year's instruction and training in general nursing for the Bloomingdale students. At the close of this period it did seem that the school had "arrived upon a secure footing." (See Chapter XXXV.)

The course for graduates of general hospital schools may be said to have received its first candidates when, in 1913, three nurses from the Johns Hopkins Hospital were given a short course of instruction and training to prepare them for service in the new Phipps Psychiatric Clinic. In 1914 two nurses were given a four months course. The course was later extended to six months, and an additional three months were required in order to obtain a certificate. During the period from 1913 to 1926 there were students in the course in all except three years. The total number was 42, all women.

Short courses for senior students of general hospital schools were first provided in 1914, when three students were received from the Mt. Sinai School, each for three months. The number of affiliated hospitals was gradually increased until the limit of residential accommodations was reached. The United States Army School sent groups of twenty students for periods of three months during one year. The total number of students from affiliated hospitals in that year (1921) was 98; the highest number in any other year was 55. In 1919 the New York Hospital School joined the affiliation and sent five students. In 1923 the course for Bloomingdale students at the New York Hospital was, at the request of the state department of education, extended to one year, with three additional months at the Manhattan Maternity Hospital. The annual report of the medical director of the hospital for 1921 noted that 170 students had thus far been received from the affiliated general hospital schools for the three months' course, and added that

> the experience thus obtained has demonstrated that, while relatively short courses in psychiatric nursing . . . can be given with advantage to the students and the Hospital, a system of this kind, which some have thought might provide all that could be furnished in the field of education by the special hospitals, is quite inadequate for maintaining the highly qualified nursing service required for the Hospital and for supplying nurses for the general field of psychiatric nursing in which there is a growing demand. The maintenance and further development of the full three-year course is, therefore, of paramount importance.

The report of the following year repeated that "affiliations will not, however, solve the problem of maintaining our own service at a high level by means of graduates who have had a thorough training and experience in the work. Nor, without these, could those who entered for short courses be given adequate instruction and training." The same note is sounded again in the report for 1924:

> It would seem advisable for a hospital of the size and type of Bloomingdale, with its close relationship with a general medical and surgical hospital, to devote its educational resources in the field of nursing to producing graduates who are highly trained and experienced in psychiatric nursing, and to furnishing courses for the graduates of other schools who wish to enter this field.

In view of the further history of the Bloomingdale school, and of what occurred in many of the other hospitals for the mentally ill at which schools were conducted, these excerpts from the annual reports are noteworthy.

As a means of encouraging professional reading, a special library for nurses was established in 1912; several of those in the nursing courses later contributed books to it. The library was located in the Dexter Cottage, where facilities for study were also provided. The appointment of a librarian supplied the service needed for the maintenance and use of this library. In 1926 the number of volumes was 293. The nurses and students had access also to the medical and the general libraries. Lectures were given by the librarian, together with advice in regard to the use and value of reading in the treatment of the patients, and the selection of books for different types of patients.

Ample means of recreation were provided for the nurses and students. A social club was organized and the recreational facilities of the hospital were placed at their disposal. Although patients, visitors, and others who were interested in the nurses were requested not to offer money or gifts to them, contributions were accepted for the general entertainment fund which was used for picnics, theaters, and other forms of entertainment, many of which, such as dances, theatricals, and sport tournaments, were conducted by the nurses themselves. In 1920 an entertainment of special interest was a pageant commemorating the hundredth anniversary of the birth of Florence Nightingale, founder of the mother school in England from which our American schools were derived. Provision was made for the further education of the graduates through a scholarship supported by the income from a donation made by Mr. Edward Floyd-Jones in 1918. The first recipient of the scholarship was a graduate of the three-year course who was given an opportunity to take a course in dental hygiene, after which she was given a position as the first dental hygienist at the hospital.

The various departments of organized therapy also engaged in educational work. The students in all the nursing courses received instruction in physiotherapy, occupational therapy, recreational therapy, and, except the affiliates, in dietetics. Occupational instructors from other hospitals were received for varying periods of observation and training every year from 1915 on. In 1922 the total number of students and craft workers who received instruction was 70. In 1924 a six months' course for training qualified craft workers in the practice of occupational therapy was established. Graduates of occupational therapy schools were accepted for a three months' practice course. In 1926, 9 students were given the six months' course, 8 were given shorter courses, and 43 student nurses were given instruction.

Students, nurses, and some attendants were given instruction in physical exercises and games from 1912, when a recreational director was appointed. Corrective exercise classes were organized for the benefit of the nurses in 1917. In order to enable them to participate effectively in the dancing classes for patients, many of the nurses were also given lessons. Patients not infrequently aided in the work of the department and in one year it was reported that four of them had been "quite competent assistants." During one summer a former patient who was a schoolteacher returned to serve as an assistant. Students of schools of physiotherapy were employed during the summer, especially to assist in the extensive outdoor activities. The instruction and practice in recreational therapy extended to many members of the nursing service contributed much to creating an atmosphere and a quality of social and recreational activity throughout the hospital that was of inestimable therapeutic value.

In the department of physiotherapy, all nurse students were given instruction in hydrotherapy and light therapy. Some lessons in light massage were also given, but it was considered that much more extensive instruction and practice than could be provided in the time available was required for proficiency.

Beginning in 1913 all student nurses were given instruction in dietetics. A special diet kitchen was provided in 1916. Until a full time dietitian was appointed in 1918, however, part-time teachers were employed to give a scheduled course. After 1918 much more thorough instruction and practice courses were given and in 1926 a well-equipped diet kitchen or laboratory for teaching was provided. In 1919 courses for student dietitians from domestic science schools were introduced, and by the end of 1926 thirty-one such students had received instruction. The interest and intelligence in dietetic treatment produced by the educational work of the department were of great advantage to the dietary service of the hospital, which, especially for patients who required special dietary treatment, was completely transformed.

During World War I, the educational as well as the clinical resources of Bloomingdale were utilized for the benefit of the military forces. An account of the services rendered was published in the annual reports of 1918 and 1919. Fifty-three of the men and women employed at the hospital left to enter military service. Three were Belgians who went home in 1914 to help defend their native land, three joined the Canadian army and the others served under the Stars and Stripes. Five were physicians, four of whom entered the United States Army Medical Corps, and one the Canadian army. The director of nursing and fifteen graduate nurses, of whom three were supervisors and four were male nurses, joined the United States Army Nurse Corps. Three attendants also entered the army medical service, one as an occupational therapist, the other two as attendants for mentally ill soldiers. Ten male attendants and nineteen other employees joined the combatant or other nonmedical military services. Two of the men were killed, both of whom had been faithful, efficient, and well-liked employees. One of the physicians, Dr. Sanger Brown, Major, M.C., had charge of the neuropsychiatric service of the base hospital at Saveney, the French port at which disabled soldiers embarked for return to America. Miss Poston, director of nursing, in 1917 undertook the task of assembling for the National Committee for Mental Hygiene the nursing staff for the first neuropsychiatric unit to go overseas. In March, 1918, she accompanied the unit to France as chief nurse of United States Army Base Hospital No. 117 at La Fouche. After a notable service for which she was awarded the distinguished service medal, she resumed her position at Bloomingdale in March, 1919.

After a study of the hospitals for disabled soldiers in Canada by the medical director, the governors of the hospital offered the Surgeon General of the Army fifty beds for the treatment of commissioned officers. It had already been suggested that a special hospital for military use be established on the hospital property or that the present buildings be appropriated. The offer of fifty beds was, however, accepted and the first patient was admitted on May 2, 1918. The service was continued until October 14, 1919, when the last officer under treatment was discharged. The officers were classified and treated in exactly the same way as the civilian patients, with whom they mingled freely. For official purposes the hospital was considered by the army as a department of United States Army General Hospital No. 1 in New York City. A medical officer from this hospital visited the military patients daily and during part of the time he resided at Bloomingdale and worked with the other physicians. Treatment, however, and administrative control by the medical director of the hospital remained undisturbed. Patients were transferred to and from Hospital No. 1 with little formality, and relations with the administration there and with the Surgeon General's office were in every respect entirely harmonious. The total number of officers treated was 90 (of 91 admissions, one was admitted twice). An army nurse was also admitted for treatment. Sixty-five, nearly three fourths, of the officers had been overseas. Thirty-one belonged to the combatant services, 30 were physicians or dentists, 6 were engineers, and 8 belonged to the quartermaster's department. Sixty-eight were lieutenants, 14 captains, 4 majors, and 2 lieutenant colonels. Many were extremely ill, excited or suicidal. The disorders from which they suffered were classified as follows:

Manic Depressive, Depression	38
Manic Depressive, Excitement	9
Delirium (Exhaustion)	5
Psychoneuroses	2
Constitutional Psychopathic Inferiority	7
Traumatic Psychoses	2
Alcoholic Psychoses	2
Dementia Praecox (Paranoid 5, Catatonic 1)	6
Paranoid Condition	9
General Paresis	3
Luetic Meningitis	2
Drug Delirium (Bromide)	1
Not insane (Alcoholism)	1
Unclassified	3

The large proportion of manic depressive cases, 52 percent, most of them depressed, is noteworthy. One was a case of amnesia, which was precipitated by a collision at sea and lasted until the officer was in hospital. The average duration of the illness previous to admission was, so far as could be ascertained, about 2.78 months, and the average period under treatment at Bloomingdale was 3.09 months. Fifty-six of the cases (62 percent) left the hospital entirely recovered or very greatly improved. Twenty-two had improved, and 12 had not improved. There were no deaths.

At the request of the Surgeon General, an army nurse was received for a short course of training in the treatment of the mentally ill, including some instruction and practice in occupational therapy. A three months' course for occupational therapists was approved by the Surgeon General, and twelve students were admitted. They were already trained in crafts at a school which had been established in New York for training for army service by Mrs. Helen C. Mansfield. Living accommodations for those in the course were provided in a cottage on the hospital property which was renovated and furnished for the purpose by the governors. No charge was made for tuition, and a reimbursing rate for board and lodging was accepted only from those able to afford it. Two of those who entered the course were given army appointments before they finished. Of the ten who finished, five went overseas, some of them to Base Hospital No. 117, four went to army hospitals in the United States, and one became a teacher of occupational therapy in a Western college in which therapists were being trained for the army. The men's department of occupational therapy, besides participating in the instruction of students, was much interested in devising equipment for the use of army-hospital patients who were confined to bed or were incapable of leaving the wards. In the women's department the patients made for the army and navy 674 knitted sweaters and socks and 50 attractive scrapbooks. Some of the latter were sent to the New York Hospital unit in France. The patients were also greatly interested in raising vegetables during this period. Both men and women cultivated their own gardens. There were many visitors to the occupational departments during the war and rehabilitation periods. Notably among them were representatives of the Surgeon General's office, of the Federal Bureau of Vocational Education, and of the Canadian Department of Soldiers' Civil Reestablishment. Visits were also received from the National Society for the Promotion of Occupational Therapy, from teachers and students of classes for army reconstruction aides, and from many others who were interested in occupational therapy.

Other war services engaged in were Red Cross work, in which patients and employees and members of the families of physicians and others who lived on the hospital property participated. Over 40,000 articles were made. Liberal contributions were made to Red Cross and other funds for war relief. The physicians served on various boards engaged in the examination of recruits and in other services. The service of former patients in the armed forces is also worthy of mention. Some of them corresponded with us, and evidently served well without developing serious nervous symptoms. One psychoneurotic woman was a canteen worker near the front; for her courage and resourcefulness in attending to soldiers and the civil population under bombardment she received great praise in the report of Marshal Pétain and was awarded the Croix de Guerre.

The appreciation and thanks of the Surgeon General of the Army for the service rendered, especially in the treatment of the officers, were expressed in a letter received by the governors in April, 1920.

PART NINE

A Complete Organization for Service, Education, and Research

1926-1936

XXXIV: ADVANCEMENT OF MEDICAL AND EDUCATIONAL RESOURCES

In September, 1926, Dr. Russell was appointed general psychiatric director of the Society with special reference to extending the service in connection with contemplated developments in New York City. He was succeeded at Bloomingdale by Dr. Mortimer W. Raynor, who for a number of years had served with distinction in various positions in the New York State hospitals, and also in the medical corps of the American Expeditionary Force during the first World War. At the time of his appointment he was medical superintendent of the King's Park State Hospital. His interests were intensely clinical and educational and he entered upon his new duties with great understanding and ardent zeal for the advancement of the service. The facilities and the organization of Bloomingdale were developed to a point at which they were equal, and perhaps in some respects superior, to those of most other hospitals for the mentally ill. Dr. Paul Schilder, Professor of Psychiatry of Vienna, who spent a month teaching at the hospital, considered that "nowhere in the world, and certainly not in Europe, is there an institution having the facilities and doing work equal to that done at Bloomingdale Hospital." [1] Dr. Raynor's sound interests and ideals and his dynamic executive ability peculiarly qualified him to utilize the facilities more effectively and to press on to further developments.

By means of generous gifts and the favorable condition of the Society, further measures were taken to carry forward the building program. As the work progressed, Dr. Raynor advised the governors that the facilities recently provided and others proposed "may be looked upon as those which are required to modernize both the accommodations and the equipment; to round out the facilities which have not yet been fully provided for; to provide for continued development to meet the needs of the community; and to continue the scientific and educational work

1 *Minutes of the Bloomingdale Committee,* March 2, 1929.

of the Hospital." [2] Although Mr. Whitney died in 1927, his beneficent interest in the service continued to be manifested by means of appropriations from funds administered by the trustees of his estate. In 1930 a fund of $1,250,000 was appropriated for use at Bloomingdale. Plans were thereupon adopted for the erection of three cottages for married physicians, two for women patients, two extensions to the main building for medical and surgical purposes, and a building for acutely excited women. Construction of all but the last mentioned was at once proceeded with. The cottages for patients were named "Bard House" and "Bruce House," in commemoration of Dr. Samuel Bard, one of the founders of the New York Hospital, and of Dr. Archibald Bruce, who was the first physician of the asylum when it was established in 1808. In accordance with the plan proposed by Dr. Nichols in 1887,[3] these houses were designed for patients no longer in need of the intensive study and treatment measures provided in the main hospital building. It was also intended to compensate for the demolition of the "solarium," in order to provide a site for the proposed building for the acutely excited. Unfortunately, before the plans for this building were adopted, the general financial depression had set in, and the project was deferred. (A building for the same purpose but on a different plan was designed by Dr. Raynor's successor and was opened as "The Nichols Memorial" in 1941.) The medical and surgical wings attached to the central corridors of the main building were a particularly valuable addition to the facilities for clinical and scientific work. They contained a surgical suite adequate for major operations, offices equipped for the medical and surgical specialties, a greatly enlarged X-ray department, a spacious dental suite, and rooms for psychological examinations and studies. The employees' clinic was also provided with liberal accommodations in one of these wings.

Besides the new construction, extensive renovations, renewals, alterations, refurnishing, and additions in equipment were accomplished. The Rogers and Taylor recreational buildings and the student nurses' residence were completed. The shore cottage at Orienta Point, named "York Lodge," was enlarged, and equipped with facilities for recreational treatment. Many of the halls in the main building were transformed by means of new furniture, rewiring, and more attractive and efficient lighting fixtures. The renovation of the toilet and bath sections and electric wiring, which had been progressing as funds were provided, was continued, and added steadily to the sanitation of the accommodations

[2] Annual report for 1931. [3] See p. 341.

and to the convenience and comfort of the patients and their nurses. Rooms originally designed for the accommodation of patients were in some instances converted into utility rooms, bathrooms, and offices for the physicians and nurses. Eventually every physician was provided with a separate office. The privacy thus obtained was of advantage in conducting interviews and in facilitating the work of the physicians. The medical, nursing, and laboratory services were furnished with additional equipment. The safety of the patients was made more secure by the installation of nonshatterable glass in many of the windows. Quietness was promoted by means of absorbent material on the ceilings of rooms occupied by disturbed patients. The removal of iron guards from many more of the windows relieved the patients of some of their apprehensions and resentment and reduced the prisonlike aspect of the exterior of the building. In 1933, Dr. Raynor, encouraged and supported by Mr. and Mrs. Barklie Henry, experimented with various forms of screening material with a view to replacing all the iron window guards by a screen identical in appearance to an ordinary fly screen and at the same time secure enough to resist attempts at breakage or removal. In 1935 the problem had been solved and an appropriation was made for installations in several of the patients' halls and rooms. The transformation was striking, and it may be anticipated that in a few years all hospitals for the mentally ill will dispense with the forbidding iron bars and grilles that are so reminiscent of former crudities. The governors authorized the manufacturer to use the name "Bloomingdale Hospital Screening." (It was discovered later that this screen could be cut. A different unobtrusive screen devised under the direction of Dr. Raynor's successor was, after thorough testing, adopted in 1936 and installed in many of the windows.) The removal or alteration of some of the porches afforded freer access of light into the buildings, especially at the Brown Villa, which after renovation and refurnishing was taken over for convalescent women. The improvement that followed the transfer of these patients from the main building was reported to be remarkable, and led Dr. Raynor to comment that "the treatment value of small units and an environment approaching normal living conditions is of great importance in the treatment of psychiatric disorders." [4] Various improvements were also made in the dietary and other service departments. The diet kitchen was much enlarged and additional equipment installed. A self-operated passenger elevator in the women's department added greatly to ease and

[4] *Minutes of the Bloomingdale Committee,* June 1, 1929.

convenience. Many other structural improvements were anticipated and in 1934 extensive sketches were made of alterations of the main building to adapt it more fully to advancing ideas of requirements.

It had long been anticipated that, as the population of the vicinity increased, the further development of the property to provide more fully for the outdoor activities of the patients would be necessary. As long as open country was available (and before the advent of the automobile), the patients could safely walk, ride, bicycle, and picnic beyond the hospital grounds. This was, however, found to be no longer practicable and a program of further development of the property was adopted. In 1928 the dairy was discontinued. The cows were indeed of interest to the patients and provided a picturesque feature in the meadows. Nevertheless, there seemed to be little economic advantage in conducting a dairy, since excellent milk could be purchased, and the attention required could be better directed to medical purposes. The vegetable garden was also dispensed with. The cow stable was converted into a group of garages for employees who lived on the property, and the garden into a lovely summer flower garden and nursery which added to the beauty of the grounds and was a source of interest and pleasure to the patients. The stone farm fences were gradually removed and used for building purposes.

The old question of public streets through the property again became a problem. Streets indicated in the White Plains maps would, if opened, pass in such close proximity to the buildings occupied by patients that it seemed as though another removal might have to be considered. Negotiations were entered into, and it was agreed that, if the hospital would donate the land and finance the opening of one wide street, legislation would be obtained to enable the city forever to refrain from cutting streets through or taking any part of the property for any use whatever during its occupancy by the hospital. It was also agreed that the zoning ordinance which permitted the use and development of the property for hospital purposes would be maintained. A contract was thereupon entered into and a strip of land 120 feet wide, situated at a considerable distance from the hospital buildings, was donated and funds furnished for opening the street through the property. This separated about twenty acres from the rest of the property and an approach was made by a tunnel under the road. A strip of land 50 feet wide was also donated to provide for widening Bloomingdale Road, and a strip of 20 feet for widening North Street.

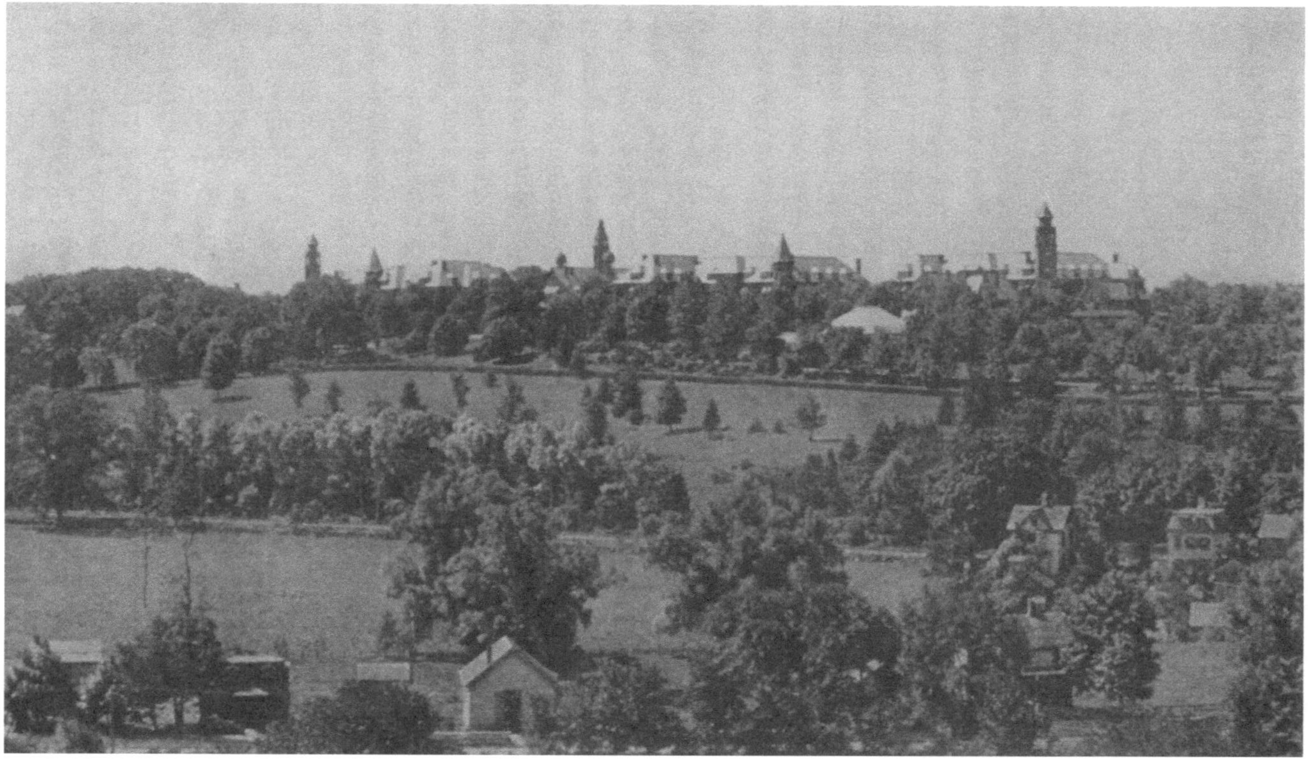

BLOOMINGDALE HOSPITAL, 1936

The separated property had been included in the building program as a location for additional buildings. In 1928, therefore, a landscape architect was engaged to survey the whole property and prepare a plan of roads and attractive walks through the woods and to suitable building sites, and a beginning was made toward construction. A pavilion for the convenience of the patients, a golf putting green and a driving range were constructed south of the new street. Picnic grounds supplied with conveniences were also provided at different points. It was expected that by such means a spacious hospital park would be developed where the outdoor recreational facilities, which are as indispensable as the buildings in the hospital treatment of the mentally ill, would be adequately provided. Much attention was also given to the trees and shrubbery, especially about the new buildings and in providing a screen around the borders of the property. Additional tennis courts and other facilities for exercise and games were constructed. A new fence, and along the southern boundary a wall, encompassed the whole property. The main approach to the hospital was improved by a hard surface on the drive and by new electric lanterns with underground wires. Several additional wells were dug and a water supply sufficient for general purposes was obtained on the property. The fire lines, were, however, connected directly with the White Plains system and could be operated separately. The opening of the Mamaroneck Valley sewer facilitated the disposal of the hospital sewage.

The operation of the hospital was considerably embarrassed by the general financial depression, the effect of which began to be manifested in 1930. The number of applications for admission diminished, rates were lower and collections difficult. It was necessary to close some of the halls and dining rooms. Repairs which were not considered vital were deferred. Salaries and wages were reduced. Notwithstanding the difficulties, however, the essentials of good service were maintained. In endeavoring to maintain the established policy relating to the admission of patients, Dr. Raynor, in his annual report for 1931, made a plea for additional special funds for this purpose and reminded the governors of "the tradition of the Hospital for more than a century of its existence that no person, otherwise suitable, be refused admission because of temporary lack of funds." Even in periods of financial difficulty this tradition and policy have been faithfully adhered to. The opening of the Payne Whitney Psychiatric Clinic at the New York Hospital in 1932 was thought by some to have diverted a few patients who would ordinarily have applied to Bloomingdale. This was, however, temporary only, and, as was expected, the Clinic has augmented applications to Bloomingdale.

More important than the possession of facilities are the manner and extent of their use. A considerable advance in this respect was made at Bloomingdale during this period. The number of resident physicians was increased; and also the number of visiting physicians, from three in 1926 to seven in 1935 (their title was changed from visiting to attending staff). These physicians visited the patients regularly at stated intervals. They examined all admitted since the last previous visit, and treated any in the hospital who were in need of their special service. The consulting staff was also increased from five in 1926 to eight in 1936. What these changes accomplished in medical service may be gathered from the increase in the number of visits by attending and consulting physicians from 189 in 1925 to 1,468 in 1935. The advantage of improved facilities for medical examinations and treatment at the hospital is indicated in the decrease in visits made by hospital patients to the private offices of these physicians from 82 in 1925 to one in 1935. It was no longer necessary to transfer acute operative cases to general hospitals. In 1932 medical administration was advanced by relieving the assistant medical director of ward service and providing him with a central office. Similarly in 1933, "for the purpose of assisting the medical Director in further advancing the medical work of the Hospital, broadening its scope and maintaining present standards," the position of director of clinical psychiatry was established.[5] The first to be appointed was Dr. Gerald R. Jameison, afterwards medical director of the Payne Whitney Psychiatric Clinic and Assistant Professor of Psychiatry of Cornell University Medical College. In 1932 the physician in charge of the laboratory was given the additional title of "Resident Internist." He was placed in charge of the medical examination and treatment of employees, and their outpatient clinic in its new accommodations was more fully organized. The activity of this clinic was increased from 1,145 visits by 458 persons in 1927 to 1,705 visits by 760 persons in 1935. The number of employees sick in bed also increased. Nevertheless it was noted that the total time lost from illness was diminished. The resident internist also accompanied the visiting physicians on their visits to patients, noted their findings and recommendations and saw that these received proper attention. He also saw that clinical conditions found by laboratory tests and X-ray examinations were attended to, and he himself made electrocardio-

[5] *Ibid.*, Nov. 4, 1933.

grams, electroencephalograms, basal metabolism and other technical examinations. In this way another advance was made in the practice of internal medicine at the hospital. In 1933 the title of assistant physician was changed to resident physician. That year, in order to lend special distinction to one of the positions and to honor a former physician of the hospital who was considered one of the most distinguished psychiatrists of his time, one of the positions was designated "Pliny Earle Resident in Psychiatry."

As already indicated, the medical service was during this period considerably advanced. The general plan of organization and the methods of examination, recording, and treatment were not materially changed but the organization was expanded and the work was done more thoroughly. The attending internists, in 1928, after a careful survey of the facilities and general medical work during the preceding year, reported that internal medicine at the hospital was equal to similar work in the best general hospitals.[6] The work of the resident medical staff was supplemented by that of the attending specialists, and the improved medical and surgical facilities were utilized with great advantage in the general medical and surgical work. The number of dental visits increased from 2,834 in 1926 to 3,646 in 1935. X-ray examinations increased from 650 to 873, and examinations in the clinical laboratory from 6,614 to 15,218. In the psychiatric work individual psychotherapy was pursued more intensively. It was probably quickened by the introduction of psychoanalysis by Dr. French after his return in 1927 from a study period in Europe. Other members of the staff were also given an opportunity to obtain instruction and training in this system of study and treatment. In 1929 a course of lectures was given at the hospital daily for a month by Dr. Paul Schilder, psychoanalyst from Vienna. He also attended the staff conferences and examined and discussed their patients with the physicians as they made their rounds, and he gave some lectures to the nurses. In 1930 further lectures and conferences were obtained from Dr. Franz Alexander of the Berlin Psychoanalytic Institute (he later became director of the Psychoanalytic Institute in Chicago), who spent a week at the hospital. Dr. Alfred Adler also visited the hospital and discussed patients and their problems with the physicians. In this way some degree of understanding of psychoanalytic doctrine and practice was obtained by the whole hospital organization, and found a place in the study and treatment of the patients. The established policy of the hospital of maintaining a well-balanced attitude toward any new method

[6] *Ibid.*, March, 1928.

of treatment and avoiding exclusive specialization in the treatment of the complex and various conditions met with in psychiatric practice, was, however, adhered to, and experience has shown that, even in the treatment of the psychoneuroses, equally good results have been obtained by means of other measures long employed at the hospital.[7]

The treatment of favorable cases of general paresis by malaria was continued to a limited extent. The increasing number of active conditions among the admissions augmented the danger of suicide. Dr. Raynor, in November, 1933, reported to the governors that of 2,609 patients who had been treated at the hospital since January, 1925, eleven (0.42 percent) had committed suicide there. Of the 229 patients in the hospital when the report was made, 115 had displayed suicidal tendencies, and 24 percent had made overt attempts. Thirty-six had made in all 109 attempts and one man had, during two years, made 125. The large majority of the patients who committed suicide were women, and the means chosen was, in most instances, hanging. Dr. Raynor noted that fewer attempts were made in spring and summer.[8]

The facilities for the measures formerly designated "moral treatment" were used to their fullest capacity. The Taylor and Rogers recreational buildings, the extended sport and play fields, and the new shore cottage were of inestimable value in implementing these measures. The variety of activities was increased and the work was conducted with growing understanding and precision. It is an inspiring sight when patients who for weeks or months have been in the depths of physical and mental depression, or in such a state of excitement as to be incapable of normal social relations, begin to show interest and to take part in wholesome activities with gradually increasing capability and, eventually, all the qualities of healthy, useful persons. Some of the patients in their convalescence acted as voluntary assistants in various activities. One supervised cooking in the occupational department, another furnished skilled assistance in preparing for an amateur theatrical performance. Patients, instructors, physicians, and nurses participated in dramatic and musical entertainments, and in sport tournaments, exhibition games, costume dances, and social activities. The earnest spirit in which sports were engaged in was manifested in the occasional minor injuries which were reported. Occupational therapy claimed increasing attention: the number of articles made and repaired in the departments rose from 23,604

[7] D. M. Hamilton and J. H. Wall, "Hospital Treatment of Patients with Psychoneurotic Disorders," *Am. J. Psychiatry*, XCVIII (Jan., 1942), and XCIX (Sept., 1942).

[8] *Minutes of the Bloomingdale Committee*, April 28, 1934.

in 1927 to 37,752 in 1935. These departments had already been supplied with adequate facilities and were at the beginning of the period well developed. The way in which Dr. Raynor endeavored to bring all these measures under thoughtful consideration with a view to increasing their effectiveness is referred to later in this chapter.[9] Cigarette smoking had become so general among the patients that in April, 1933, arrangements were made—after long hesitation and with great regret—permitting women to smoke.

The number of continuous flow tubs was increased, and prolonged baths and wet packs were used extensively. A similar increase took place in the use of massage, hydro and light therapy (in which the number of treatments was 18,217 in 1927 and 27,093 in 1935). The library as a means of treatment was fully utilized; circulation increased from 10,537 volumes in 1927 to 17,974 in 1935. This increase occurred solely in the distribution to patients, although the employees had also access to the library.

The admission of patients voluntarily accepting treatment without resort to court proceedings continued to be of inestimable value to the morale of the patients themselves, to their relatives and friends, and to the physicians, nurses and the whole of the hospital community. This enlightened advance has also contributed to promoting public confidence in the management of the institutions for the mentally ill. It seems hardly credible now that although before 1842 not even medical certificates were required, and before 1874 no court approval or order of commitment, during the many years of operation of the hospital previous to 1900 only twelve patients were recorded as voluntary. In contrast, at the close of 1935, 72 percent of the patients in the hospital were again without court orders and 81 percent of those admitted during the year entered on the same terms. And during the whole period from 1926 to 1935 it was necessary to produce only one patient in court on a writ of habeas corpus. In his annual report for 1928 Dr. Raynor stated that the policy was "to resort to legal restriction only when it was clearly required to protect the patient and to furnish legal authority for detention." The excellent laws and administrative system which, in the course of years, have been adopted by the state of New York, furnish ample protection from improper treatment or abuses.

As a further means of maintaining confidence and coöperation, patients who were on visit or were discharged from the hospital were kept under observation and treatment for a period through consultation

[9] Pp. 458–459.

with the physicians either at the Bloomingdale office at the New York Hospital or at White Plains. The average daily number of patients away from the hospital on visit increased from 39 in 1925 to 57 in 1935. In 1927 former hospital patients consulted the Bloomingdale physicians 134 times at the New York office, and 241 times at White Plains. In 1935 the number had increased to 256 in New York, with no increase at White Plains. The increase in New York may perhaps be attributed, in part at least, to the more satisfactory office provision made in 1932 at the new psychiatric department of the New York Hospital.

From time to time Dr. Raynor directed attention to the question of establishing a service for children and adolescents. It was suggested that some of the property south of the new street would be a suitable location for this development. It was also suggested that a department on this property for the study and treatment of protracted physical disease would provide much needed service for a class of sick persons who became dependent because of discouragement and lack of adequate treatment. The question of extending the treatment for alcoholism was raised when the publication by a former patient of an embellished account of his experience at the hospital precipitated a flood of applications from alcoholics. It was considered inadvisable, however, to admit more than a limited number of such patients.

In the first two or three years of general postwar prosperity the nursing service suffered from difficulty in filling vacancies, especially in the men's service. The number of women graduates employed was increased, however, and special nurses were on occasion engaged for individual patients. Additional women were employed in the men's nursing service. With the onset of the financial depression the number of graduates available for employment or as applicants for the graduate courses increased. By 1935 there was a large number in the service and the standards were high. The character of the nursing service was inextricably linked with nursing education (see Chapter XXXV). The hospital nursing service and school had gained a wide reputation and during this period was visited by many nurse directors and other prominent nurses from foreign countries as well as from different parts of America. Many occupational therapists and officials interested in occupational therapy, some from foreign countries, also visited the hospital; among distinguished psychiatrists, some came from as far away as China, Japan, and Latin America, and a considerable number came from Europe. Professor Eugen Bleuler of Switzerland remained for several days. His son, Dr. Manfred Bleuler, who later succeeded to the position long held by his father at the university and the psychiatric hospital at Zurich, was at the time a member of the Bloomingdale staff. At a Monday evening conference he made a valuable contribution by interpreting to the members of the staff his eminent father's views on schizophrenia.[10] In May, 1934, 85 members of the American Psychiatric Association, of which three former physicians of the hospital had been president, were entertained at the hospital.

Although in 1928 two positions on the medical staff were established as residencies in which special provision would be made for study and training, it was not until 1934 that the educational work of the hospital in qualifying physicians as specialists in psychiatry received the official approval of the Council on Medical Education and Hospitals of the American Medical Association, a representative of the Council having visited the hospital in that year. The periods of training designated were from two to five years. In addition to the plan followed at the hospital, members of the staff were enabled to obtain special courses and instruction and experience in laboratories and clinics in New York. Three of the hospital physicians were given a year's leave of absence with salary for study in Europe. Of educational value to the physicians and all others engaged in the personal care and treatment of the patients was an undertaking to submit to a systematic study at the Monday evening conferences "everything we do for patients in the hospital, why we do it, and what is accomplished." [11] Examples of the particular subjects discussed were suicide with special reference to prevention, individual psychotherapy, various other forms of treatment, accidents to patients, and the therapeutic value of a dental department. The studies of prevention of suicide made at the hospital led to observations of much value in anticipating attempts.[12] In 1933 a thorough consideration was given to the different forms of organized treatment such as occupational, physical and recreational therapy, and dietetics, as practiced in the hospital. These were accepted as established routine without sufficient scientific consideration. The communications in the symposium were made by the heads of departments and by the physicians in charge of services, who described their services and gave their views and estimates of the various treatment measures employed. The symposium was then summarized by the director of clinical psychiatry, who described it as a discussion of "various

10 Later published as "Schizophrenia: Review of the Work of Prof. Eugen Bleuler," *Arch. Neur. and Psych.*, Sept. 1931.

11 Personal statement of Dr. Raynor.

12 G. R. Jameison and J. H. Wall. "Some Psychiatric Aspects of Suicide," *Psychiatric Q.*, VII (April, 1933), 211; G. R. Jameison, "Suicide and Mental Disease," *Arch. Neur. and Psych.*, XXXVI (July, 1936).

resources, which, when combined, make for a complete therapeutic organization." This discussion of the organized therapeutic resources had a noticeable influence in quickening the interest of the physicians to utilize them with greater understanding and precision. The proceedings of this and other Monday evening conferences were bound and are preserved in the hospital library. They contain much of value relating to psychiatric hospital practice. Nothing is perhaps more distinctive of Bloomingdale than the character of its therapeutic departments and the intensive way in which they are operated separately and also so as to constitute "a complete therapeutic organization" exercising a constant pressure towards the rehabilitation of the patient physically, mentally, and socially.

The medical library was, during this period, used assiduously. Much attention was given to its management, use, and expansion by Dr. Raynor. In this he was aided by some of the governors who gave of their personal funds for the purchase of specially expensive books. The number of volumes was increased from 1,646 in 1926 to 5,296 in 1935. During the interval the nurses' library, which contained a few hundred volumes, was merged with the medical library. Among the books a group of twenty-four, the authors of which were former patients, are noteworthy. They were presented by the authors and some of them carry inscriptions such as: "This is my first testimonial to the best alma mater I ever had." "With the kindest regards of one who enjoyed its marvellous ministrations for many months and recalls them with gratitude." The reviews of books and periodicals presented regularly at the Monday conferences kept the staff informed. Assistance was given by the trained librarian, and for a time an additional research librarian was employed. Dr. Raynor encouraged research and advised the governors that special funds should be provided for this purpose. He referred to Dr. Schilder's opinion, expressed when he lectured at the hospital in 1929, that "he knew of no clinic or hospital, because of the type of patients and the facilities available, where the opportunities to carry on research would be greater." [13] Dr. Manfred Bleuler, who made a study of heredity [14] while at the hospital, expressed a similar opinion.

The increasing number of articles prepared by the hospital physicians for presentation at medical meetings and for publication is an indication of the advancement in the qualifications, interest, and activity of the

[13] *Minutes of the Bloomingdale Committee*, March 2, 1929.

[14] M. Bleuler, "A Contribution to the Problem of Heredity among Schizophrenics," *J. Nerv. and Mental Dis.*, LXXIV, Oct., 1931.

staff. From 1911 to 1926 there were about 70 articles published or read at meetings by members of the medical staff, and 5 by a member of the occupational therapy department; also three books were published.[15] From 1926 to 1936 the number of articles by physicians was increased to 120, and there were also 18 from the occupational therapy department, and 2 from the nursing staff. In the latter period also 11 articles, not included above, were published by the general psychiatric director, and one book by a member of the medical staff.[16] It was a time of increasing activity in psychiatric service, teaching, and research, and there were many publications on the subject. Notable accessions to the facilities in New York City were the greatly enlarged and reorganized psychopathic department of Bellevue Hospital, opened in 1933, and the State Psychiatric Institute and Hospital at the Columbia-Presbyterian Center, opened in 1929.

The closing three years of the period were saddened by the death of five of the governors, all of whom had been strong and active supporters of the service for the mentally ill. Three had been presidents of the Society, and one chairman of the Bloomingdale Committee and a generous benefactor for many years. Finally in October, 1935, Dr. Raynor, who, though his interest and efforts seemed undiminished, had been failing in health, died after a few days of acute illness. His contribution to the advancement of the service was of inestimable value, and he was personally much respected and beloved. In a memorial spread upon the minutes of the Bloomingdale Committee, he was characterized as "wise, just, kindly, tactful and forceful, endures as an integral part of the whole organization," and as "most helpful in shaping the psychiatric developments undertaken."

On June 1, 1936, Dr. Clarence O. Cheney assumed office as his successor, the duties of the position having in the interval been capably performed by the assistant medical director, Dr. Samuel W. Hamilton. Dr. Cheney, like his two immediate predecessors, had previously been employed in the New York State Hospital service. At the time of his appointment he was director of the New York State Psychiatric Institute and Hospital and Professor of Psychiatry of Columbia University. He had previously had a distinguished career in various positions in the state hospitals, among them that of medical superintendent, and just

15 Sanger Brown, II, *Sex Worship and Symbolism of Primitive Races* (Boston, 1916); G. W. Henry, *Essentials of Psychiatry* (Baltimore, 1925); Louis J. Haas, *Occupational Therapy* (Milwaukee, 1925).

16 G. W. Henry, *Essentials of Psychopathology* (Baltimore, 1935).

previous to his appointment he had been president of the American Psychiatric Association. His appointment maintained the understanding and relationship with the aims and policies of the public system of study, treatment, and prevention of mental illness which had greatly influenced the character and administration of Bloomingdale during the previous wenty-five years.

XXXV

PROGRESS AND DECLINE OF NURSING EDUCATION AT BLOOMINGDALE

In providing for the mentally ill, adequate nursing attention has always been regarded of paramount importance, and much difficulty has been experienced in furnishing it. Some of the difficulty can be understood only by realizing that prejudicial views and practices which once prevailed in the treatment of the insane still exercise an influence in shaping public opinion and the lines of progress which can be followed. When, in the course of time, it was clearly perceived that training was the means by which properly qualified persons for nursing the sick must be provided, it was hoped by those concerned with the welfare of the mentally ill that the day of their deliverance had arrived. The "Nightingale Movement," however, which in the middle of the last century represented the good Samaritan bringing to the medical and surgical hospitals highly qualified candidates for nurse training and nursing, passed the insane traveler by "on the other side." Nurse training in the hospitals for the mentally ill was introduced by their governors and physicians without help from outside. No special means of support were available and no particularly qualified candidates. They took upon themselves, therefore, the necessary instruction and training of attendants in the service.

The course was for two years, but even before there was governing legislation, many of the graduates voluntarily entered upon another year of instruction and training at a medical and surgical hospital. After various preliminary stages, schools were established in most of the principal hospitals throughout the country. There was, at first, no provision for a teaching organization and no qualified instructors and directors from which to form it. Here and there, however, a medical superintendent of a hospital managed to obtain a salary for someone to head the school. The position of superintendent of nursing was established by law in the New York State hospitals in 1908, and, as has been related, the position was established at Bloomingdale in 1912. Because the physical as well as the mental functions are disturbed in mental illness, it was at first considered advisable to engage as superintendents of the schools nurses with medical and surgical training. No others were in fact available. That they were without understanding of the mentally ill and of what was required in adequately nursing them had to be accepted as a temporary handicap. Their remoteness from an understanding of the problem was illustrated by a capable medical and surgical nurse, who, soon after she was appointed superintendent of a school, reported that there were so few patients confined to bed in the hospital that she would have to limit greatly the number of students admitted. When asked what would be done about the other patients, her reply was, "You don't call that nursing, do you?" Many such superintendents were, however, interested, energetic, and progressive. They learned by observation, study, and experience and made a substantial contribution in the establishment and development of the schools. Many of their students progressed to important positions, and eventually candidates well qualified in both psychiatric and medical and surgical nursing became available as superintendents and instructors.

An account has already been given of the early steps in nursing education at Bloomingdale, and of the development of the courses established up to 1926. The two-year course was, it will be recalled, abolished that year, and the three-year course, organized in 1912, was considered to be securely established. Twenty-eight students entered the course in 1926, eight of whom were men. The educational requirements for admission had been gradually advanced, and the nursing standards, especially in the men's department, were noticeably higher. In 1929 the nurse inspector of the State Department reported that "there has been outstanding improvement in the standard of nursing care." Dr. Raynor also reported to the governors that "the appointment of Mr. Roden as Assistant Director of Nursing has proved to be of distinct advantage to the Training School and the nursing service in the Men's Department." [1] Experience at other hospitals had demonstrated that nurse training of men could be successfully conducted only when directed by a properly qualified male nurse. In 1925 an affiliation was made with Bellevue Hospital by which Bloomingdale students were admitted for a year's instruction and training in medical and surgical nursing at the Mills School for Male Nurses there. This was continued until 1931 when the Grasslands Hospital School in Westchester County was substituted. Eventually the number of male students exceeded the number of women. Of twenty-eight students admitted in 1928, fifteen were men. In 1930 both the medical director and the director of nursing referred in their annual reports to the advancement of the standards in the men's department, and to the fact that it had been found advantageous to give

[1] Annual report for 1926.

the women students a period of instruction and practice there. The requirements for admission to the school were advanced to four years of high school with an average rating of 85 percent. The men admitted were as well qualified educationally as the women. In 1932 six of the students admitted had from two to four years of college education. Three full-time instructors were employed. The number of graduates in the service was increased as they could be obtained, and the nursing organization steadily advanced as an effective medium of education. At the close of 1932 there were 54 students in the course, of whom 28 were men and 26 were women, and 65 were given instruction in 1933. The three-year course was demonstrating its supreme usefulness as a means of solving the age-old problem of adequate nursing of the mentally ill. After a long period of slow growth it seemed at last to be favorably regarded by well-educated candidates for nursing education. Notwithstanding this apparent prosperity, however, it was really on the verge of dissolution.

In November, 1932, the state nursing inspector made a report on the school. After referring to the time spent by the students at the affiliated hospitals she asked: "Would it not be more profitable from an economic standpoint and as satisfactory from the standpoint of nursing service if postgraduates and affiliating students only were received?" She considered that "it would be very desirable also to have the affiliating course open to more students and to decrease the size of or discontinue the regular school." The six-month postgraduate course to which graduates of schools at medical and surgical hospitals were admitted, should, she stated, "help prepare more nurses for supervising and executive positions and supply the qualified nurses needed in charge of departments in psychiatric hospitals." This report reveals the lack of understanding of the time and practice required to qualify for adequate nursing of the mentally ill, and especially for the higher positions in organized psychiatric service. Evidently even the most intelligent and influential leaders in nursing education had little conception of what nursing the mentally ill consisted of. At a conference on "Whether mental hospitals should maintain schools of nursing" it was stated that as "the student in a mental hospital is learning the application of nursing procedures to a special type of patient," she should first learn the procedures in a medical and surgical hospital. (As though this was all.) No wonder the short courses in a psychiatric hospital are even by leaders in nursing education considered adequate and that a widely distributed and influential report of a study of nursing education refers to an undergraduate course of two months as a "thorough training in the specialty." [2]

In December, 1932, Dr. Raynor discussed the situation with the governors and advised them that "sooner or later definite provision would have to be made for the School of Nursing other than for its being financed from the funds received for the care of patients, if we were to meet all the requirements of the State Department and be able to continue the School." [3] The requirements which were most difficult to comply with were evidently those relating to theoretical instruction. In 1933 the director of nursing reported [4] that the New York Hospital School, with which Bloomingdale was affiliated for fifteen months' instruction and training in medical, surgical, and obstetrical nursing, was being reorganized "in keeping with modern progressive educational theories, the chief consideration of which is a greater accent on theory with enough correlated practice to achieve proficiency," and that at Bloomingdale the students "are a very important part of the actual nursing service and we cannot make any further changes in the curriculum in 1934 without endangering the patients' care." The preliminary course for first-year students was given at the Westchester Central School, which had also been required to change the schedule from four months to seven and a half, during which little time was available for practice in the care of patients. The director of nursing advised in regard to the Bloomingdale School that "in any reorganization for this school, the question of a school entirely independent of the hospital budget and nursing care of the patients should be considered." It is doubtful, however, if financial provision alone would have been sufficient to sustain the school at that time. It was becoming difficult to provide means of training the students in procedures employed in nursing patients in bed, and some reorganization in relations with the New York Hospital school seemed to be necessary. The director of nursing drew attention in her report to the large number of unemployed nurses in the community, although at the same time there was an unfilled demand for nurses with qualifications in psychiatric nursing. The question was raised as to whether the schools of the hospitals for the mentally ill might not advantageously devote their facilities to preparing undergraduates and graduates of the general hospital schools for psychiatric practice instead of conducting separate schools. In 1933 also, some of

[2] *Nursing and Nursing Education in the United States* (Rockefeller Foundation: Report of the Committee for the Study of Nursing Education, New York, 1923).

[3] *Minutes of the Bloomingdale Committee*, Nov., 1932.

[4] Director of nurses annual report, 1933 (on file at the Westchester Division).

the schools which participated in the operation of the Central School withdrew, leaving only one beside Bloomingdale, and it was soon after closed.

The situation was frequently discussed at the meetings of the governors. In March, 1934, Dr. Raynor again reviewed it with them and reported that "because of the increasing demands for more theoretical instruction by the State Department of Education the students are now spending at the Hospital in the care of patients only 13½ months of the three years' course"; he recommended that no students be admitted for the ensuing year and that the postgraduate course be extended from six to twelve months. The governors thereupon adopted the following:

Resolved that the Medical Director be authorized to reorganize the School of Nursing by omitting the entering class and extending the postgraduate course from six to twelve months.

This was done ostensibly with a view to further consideration, but it marked the end of the three-year course. The course had furnished 147 well-qualified graduates to the nursing of the mentally ill, 101 of whom were women and 46 were men. All were usefully employed; some advanced to important positions. An estimate of the value of the school was given by Miss Poston, its first director.

One of the first registered schools, high academic standards, proof is evidenced in the demand for its graduates to fill important positions as teachers, administrators and last but not least as Private Duty Nurses, to care for patients in their homes. The school has not only met standards but has set them. Its reputation has been enviable among other Mental Hospitals and the schools in close affiliation with general hospitals. Its being represented at National and Local meetings, has done much toward establishing respect and interest, as well as knowledge of the needs and problems in the field of Mental Nursing.[5]

What was occurring at Bloomingdale was much more than a local experience. The school had come within the scope of a widespread educational movement; nursing education was being related to activities other than nursing care of the sick as well as to the basic sciences of medicine and public health. The general scheme was to provide basic training for all nurses in schools conducted by general medical and surgical hospitals only; hospitals devoted to the study and treatment of some special form of disease were to train in their specialty students and graduates of the basic schools. By means of laws and regulations the

[5] Personal letter from Miss Poston, Sept., 1939.

schools at the hospitals for the mentally ill were subjected to state supervision and control in a program designed to implement that conception which took little account of the real nature of mental illness and the long period of training and experience required to qualify for its nursing. Schools could be operated only if licensed by the state, and were consequently obliged to conform to the views and regulations of the educational authorities. The experience at many of the hospitals for the mentally ill throughout the country was similar to that at Bloomingdale. Many felt compelled to close their schools, or to restrict the number of students to a point where they could intensively follow the requirements of the educational authorities. This was, however, incommensurate with the number of graduates needed for adequate nursing of the mentally ill. Many schools restricted their educational work to conforming with the general scheme of nursing education by furnishing short courses, in most instances three months, for students of general hospital schools.

At the time the three-year course was discontinued, the economic depression had occasioned so much unemployment that many general nurses sought positions at Bloomingdale or applied for admission to postgraduate courses. Dr. Raynor reported that he felt "confident that there will be a sufficient number of applicants for the course to take the place of a new class," which would ordinarily have been admitted to the three-year course. In 1933 a postgraduate course was given to twenty-one nurses. The course as adopted by the governors was in 1935 changed from "a twelve months' basic course, to an eight months' basic and a four months' advanced course. . . . Those students who demonstrate executive ability and an unusual adaptation to psychiatric nursing will be admitted to the advanced course." [6] Additional subjects were general and educational psychology, psychobiology, psychopathology, sociology, and mental hygiene. Two weeks of outpatient and social service instruction and practice were also provided at the psychiatric clinic of the New York Hospital. Ten students were enrolled in September, 1935. In usefulness to the hospitals, the graduate students were expected to be more valuable than the three-year students were for a considerable time after admission. They were more mature and were already qualified in general medical and surgical nursing. There was some advantage in this. It could not be expected, however, that, unless after finishing the course they remained for a longer period of training and practice at Bloomingdale or some other psychiatric hospital, they would be as

[6] Director of nurses annual report, 1935.

capable as the graduates of the three-year course as this was originally planned. The understanding of the mentally ill and the adjustment of one's own personality necessary for successful psychiatric nursing require the observation and practice obtainable only by means of prolonged association and experience. However, even if it had been certain that this plan of educating nurses for psychiatric service would best solve the problem, there was no assurance that a sufficient number of candidates could be obtained. There was reason to suspect that when the general economic depression was over and avenues of employment reopened, candidates for postgraduate courses in psychiatry would diminish in number or disappear altogether. Later experience confirmed this suspicion. As long as some of the other hospitals for the mentally ill succeeded in conducting schools there remained a possibility that Bloomingdale would be able to obtain sufficient nurses from that source. Dr. Raynor, however, evidently felt some misgivings; in 1935 he reported to the governors that though it was possible at that time to staff with graduates "under current economic conditions" and that there were many in the service, "this fortunate condition may not much longer be easy to maintain especially in the men's department." Nevertheless, some from this source continued to be available and, by providing training for graduates of general hospital schools who were appointed to salaried positions in the service, the standards of nursing were with some difficulty maintained.

The abandonment of the course for men when it was contributing so greatly to the standard of service was especially unfortunate. Few candidates for positions and none for postgraduate courses could be obtained from among the graduates of the few medical and surgical hospitals which conducted schools for male nurses. These hospitals had their own psychiatric services. The graduates of the Bloomingdale School found prompt and continuous employment in hospitals, industrial organizations, and private practice. Even during the economic depression not one of them was unemployed. It was anticipated that after the New York Hospital was established in its new location Bloomingdale would furnish male nurses for the psychiatric service there. It was also anticipated that the male students would be given additional training at the New York Hospital and that their service in the care of the medical and surgical patients there would replace the clumsy attentions of untrained orderlies. Special accommodations for male nurse students and graduates were provided at the new buildings. Dr. Raynor reported to the governors in 1932 that "in all probability the men student nurses would be received for their period of affiliation but this would have to be deferred probably for another year." [7] Why it was deferred was not made clear, but before another year the school at Bloomingdale for men as well as women had been discontinued.

Thus, unfortunately, was interrupted the plan of nurse training which had been independently adopted and which, with remarkable effectiveness, was providing in the hospitals for the mentally ill in America a trained personnel comprising in some instances half or more of those engaged in the care of such patients. Three-month training courses for students of affiliated schools at medical and surgical hospitals and postgraduate courses of a few months for graduates of these schools are of acknowledged value; they will not, however, maintain an adequate supply of trained nurses for the hospitals for the mentally ill. The importance and magnitude of the problem—and public interest in it—will, no doubt, eventually compel the powerful interests now concerned primarily with nursing as an educational problem to adopt a more adequate policy and system. It may be not too much to expect that the Society of the New York Hospital, with its long experience in providing for the mentally and physically ill and its superior facilities and organization for the training of men and women in the work, may lead off in this undertaking as it did many years ago in introducing the training of nurses in many of the medical and surgical hospitals of the country.

The three months' courses provide a valuable service to the advancement of psychiatry in the field of medical and surgical nursing. The students are seniors who have acquired some proficiency in general nursing and are also able to participate in the recreational and social treatment of the patients. It can hardly be considered, however, that they constitute a substantial part of the dependable nursing resources of the hospital or that the maintenance and advancement of the nursing service can be accomplished by this system of education.[8] Ten schools were affiliated for these courses for various periods, most of them from the beginning. From six coöperating schools in 1933, 63 students received instruction. In 1935 the total number of students since 1914 was 809. A very few of these returned for the postgraduate course. It was learned that the effect of the courses, in some instances, was to produce a noticeable change in consideration and treatment of personality reactions and problems in the affiliated hospitals. The students who had been at Bloomingdale, and more particularly the Bloomingdale stu-

[7] *Minutes of the Bloomingdale Committee*, April 2, 1932.
[8] See Chapter XXXIII.

dents who were in medical and surgical hospitals for part of their training, were enabled sometimes to aid in the medical understanding of a case. Some years ago a surgeon at one of these hospitals who was sceptical of the usefulness of psychiatry in medical and surgical practice, was puzzled by the slow recovery of a patient after operation and by her mental confusion and mild delirium during the night. Finally he asked the nurse if she could offer any suggestion as to the cause of the condition. He was startled when she replied, "She seems to me to have a mild post-operative infective exhaustive psychosis."

After the three-year course was discontinued it was possible to give more attention to the affiliated as well as the postgraduate students. The organization for nursing education was maintained as before. The instruction in occupational and recreational therapy was continued and a large number of students received instruction in these departments. The courses for students from schools of occupational therapy and physical education were also continued, and instructors from other institutions were accepted for periods of observation and instruction. For five years a head-nurse course was conducted in coöperation with Teachers College of Columbia University, two students enrolling each year. The number was too small to warrant the expense, and the course was discontinued by the college in 1933. Bloomingdale graduate nurses were on occasion given an opportunity, by means of the Floyd Jones scholarship,[9] to pursue advanced studies in nursing and related subjects, and some of them were enabled to obtain degrees. The thirteen weeks' elementary courses of instruction for all attendants as they entered employment at the hospital, which were established in 1912, were maintained as a routine practice. It may be considered that, in principle, they were first introduced by Dr. Pliny Earle in 1844. The Westchester Central School for first-year students, in the operation of which the schools of several hospitals participated, and which was established in 1923, was also discontinued in 1934. Ten schools had in all been associated, and the number of students who attended daily was ordinarily more than a hundred.

In 1936 the writer retired from active participation in the psychiatric service of the New York Hospital. It seems appropriate, therefore, to end at this point the story of nearly one hundred and fifty years of its development and activity. Inspiration and encouragement may be derived from contemplating the noble sentiments, sound judgment, and earnest endeavors of those by whom the service has been developed from

[9] See p. 442.

humble beginnings to its present high distinction and usefulness. Notwithstanding many disheartening difficulties and delays it is manifest that constant pressure towards progress has never ceased to operate. That this will ever be maintained by their successors there can be no doubt. Reaching toward the future is the resumption of psychiatric service in close relations with the other services of the New York Hospital, which, after a separation of over one hundred and ten years, was accomplished by the establishment of the Payne Whitney Clinic in 1932. This will be described in the next and last chapter.

XXXVI

THE PAYNE WHITNEY PSYCHIATRIC CLINIC OF THE NEW YORK HOSPITAL

When, on October 1, 1932, the Payne Whitney Psychiatric Clinic was opened at the New York Hospital, more than a century had elapsed since the service for the mentally ill at the hospital was removed to Bloomingdale. This occurred in 1821, and in 1894 a second removal was made to White Plains. The first removal separated psychiatry from the other services of the hospital. The removal to White Plains, however, not only widened this separation, but rendered the service less accessible to the community from which most of its patients were received. The only emergency hospital provision for the mentally ill that remained in the city was the public service for temporary care at Bellevue Hospital. Acutely ill and otherwise difficult patients who would previously have been brought directly to Bloomingdale were now received by transfer from Bellevue. Many favorable cases were taken to proprietary institutions which were more accessible,[1] and, not infrequently, after their financial resources had been depleted or exhausted, application was made for transfer to Bloomingdale. This may in some measure account for an accumulation of long-term and unfavorable cases there.

When the situation became sufficiently clear, it was realized that in order to furnish the kind of psychiatric service that the Society of the New York Hospital had always aimed at maintaining, it would be advisable to reëstablish a service in the city, preferably at the New York Hospital. For many years this was a deeply cherished wish, frequently considered but denied fulfillment. In 1899, Dr. Lyon, medical superintendent, advocated the establishment in New York City of an institution for the treatment of acute mental disease, "in close touch with our noble psychopathic institute." [2] In 1904 he proposed "a new centre for investigating all the questions connected with the causes, treatment, and care" of the insane, "and a teaching hospital for students." He suggested that, in order to be near the College of Physicians and Surgeons, then on West 59th Street, an arrangement for space might be made with Roosevelt Hospital. He recommended that, although the institution could be

1 Communication from Dr. Lyon to the governors, April 22, 1909.

2 S. B. Lyon, "The Desirability of Close Connection between the Psychopathological Laboratories and Hospitals for the Acute Insane," American Medico-Psychological Association, *Transactions*, VI (1899), 369.

affiliated with the "chair of nervous and mental diseases" of the college, "it could and should be under the direction of the New York Hospital through the Bloomingdale Committee and under the direct charge of a paid Resident Physician of the investigating type." He knew a suitable man whose services could be secured. (This was about the time that Dr. Hoch came to Bloomingdale.) Dr. Lyon believed that to this institution "a class of patients with nervous prostration and early or very mild phases of insanity might be attracted. None should stay long," and that "generally only patients not excited or violent beyond comfortable control should be admitted and committed, and voluntary admission should be by arrangement only. No ambulance cases should be rushed into it." Conditions have, of course, greatly changed since then and it is no longer considered advisable to provide for committed patients in this kind of a service. In regard to teaching Dr. Lyon recommended that

> the patients or some of them should be available, under proper restrictions, for observation and study by medical graduates and students, and a relation for this purpose could probably be established with the Department of Mental Diseases at the College of Physicians and Surgeons, which should exercise no control over the wards, but might advise as to treatment.

He proposed that this project be financed from the current income of Bloomingdale and, if necessary, from the proceeds of the sale of the Bloomingdale property in New York City.[3]

Again, in 1905, he advised the governors that the establishment of a reception hospital in the city would be "a progressive step, which is being taken in other cities and countries"; as for the Society of New York Hospital, it was "not only its opportunity, but its duty to add this feature to its many beneficent operations." [4] He brought up the subject again in 1909, advising that "the New York Hospital should again get a foothold in New York, for the immediate treatment of the increasing number of insane persons, whose attack may begin suddenly, and without warning." He urged the governors "to try the experiment in an economical and efficient way" by using two or three private houses adjoining the hospital, and, if this temporary provision proved a success, to provide more liberal and appropriate quarters later.[5] On this occasion he was supported by the medical inspector of the State Commission in Lunacy (see Chapter XXX). The governors seemed favorably disposed, but the

[3] Communication from Dr. Lyon, June 1, 1904. See also his annual report for 1905.
[4] Communication from Dr. Lyon, June 2, 1905.
[5] *Ibid.*, April 22, 1909; also, Dec., 1909.

question of the removal of the New York Hospital shortly began to engage their attention.[6]

After Mr. Payne Whitney became a member of the Board of Governors in 1912, the association with Cornell Medical College probably assumed greater significance, and consideration of provision for the mentally ill at the New York Hospital was thereafter governed by the prospect of a development in which hospital and college would be brought into close organic relations. It had, however, long been established in the policy and plan of development of the psychiatric department that provision at the New York Hospital would eventually be made, and when at last the way opened what was needed for the long-contemplated extension of the service was well understood.

From year to year the subject continued to be considered in the annual reports, particularly in those for 1921 and 1922. In 1925 Dr. Russell, who was about to retire from the position of director of the Bloomingdale service, prepared, at the request of Mr. Sheldon, president, and Mr. Whitney, vice president of the Society, a "plan for extending the work into the field of early recognition and treatment, prevention, education and research." In this plan further developments at Bloomingdale were proposed and described briefly, as it was considered that they had already been "pretty well defined in the Annual Reports and in special communications to the Bloomingdale Committee, notably that of April 1922." The views held in regard to a psychiatric service at the New York Hospital were explained pretty fully, and served as a guide in shaping the development that was later undertaken.[7] At this time the association with Cornell University had not been established. It was understood, however, that negotiations were proceeding and that, sooner or later, close relations would be formed. With a view to advancing psychiatric developments at the hospital (and doubtless those that were contemplated in association with the college, although this was not announced), Dr. Russell was, in 1926, appointed general director of the psychiatric work of the Society.

In May, 1927, Mr. Whitney died and, by the terms of his will, the governors found themselves in a position to realize, far beyond their most sanguine expectations, their long-cherished wish to resume at the New York Hospital the service for the mentally ill which had been one

[6] A site was, in fact, purchased, and plans in course of preparation in 1911 contained provision for forty mentally ill patients. This project was, however, soon supplanted by other considerations and prospects.

[7] This communication was printed and is in the Archives of the Society.

of its earliest activities. Mr. Whitney had been particularly interested in the psychiatric service. He referred to it as the most important work the Society was engaged in. He used in his will the phrase "neurological or psychiatric work" only because he was not clear concerning the relation of the one to the other. This was confirmed by a letter, in July, 1927, from Mr. Frank K. Sturgis, chairman of the Bloomingdale Committee, in which he gave an account of a conference with Mr. Lewis Cass Ledyard, who drew the will and was one of the executors.[8] It was accepted, therefore, that Mr. Whitney's intention was to provide funds for the development of psychiatric work at the New York Hospital, presumably along the lines of the plan prepared at his and Mr. Sheldon's request in 1925.

The New York Hospital–Cornell Medical College Association was established in June, 1927. Dr. G. Canby Robinson was appointed director, and plans for buildings to accommodate both the hospital and the college were at once undertaken. The medical supervision of the designing and construction of the building for the mentally ill was delegated to the department of psychiatry of which Dr. Russell was general director. Relations with the medical college were established when, in 1928, Dr. Russell was appointed professor of psychiatry, and Dr. Henry, director of the psychiatric outpatient service, was appointed instructor. Thereafter, until the hospital was moved to its new location, Cornell medical students received instruction in psychiatry in both the outpatient and inpatient services of the hospital on Sixteenth Street. In the preparation of the plans, the advantage of having available the advice and practical aid of the capable and experienced Bloomingdale organization can hardly be overestimated. Much in the construction, equipment, and furnishings of the building that is most effective in facilitating administration and in promoting the comfort, security, and successful treatment of the patients was obtained by means of the interest and skillful assistance of this highly qualified group. The hammock frame for the continuous flow bath tubs, the direct connected seamless irrigation table, the comprehensive lock system, the noiseless door latches, and many other specially adapted devices were of their design. It was assumed, in planning the development, that the policy and form of service which for many years had governed the operation of Bloomingdale Hospital, would be the primary consideration, and that the plan outlined in 1925 would be followed in its principal provisions. According to this plan, "a development in the city that would provide adequate facilities for the

[8] Letter on file in the Archives of the Society.

study and treatment of patients in the hospital and at the out-patient department, for teaching and for research, would assume almost, if not entirely, the proportions of a complete hospital unit." Reference was made to the character of the "special construction, equipment, organization, and management" required in the operation of a psychiatric service, and also to the prevailing ignorance on all these matters among general hospital administrators and physicians. It was recommended, therefore, that the building be located "adjacent to the other departments of the general hospital, and to the medical school." The site

should permit of sufficient separation from adjacent buildings to prevent overlooking, disturbing noises etc. An elevation overlooking the river or a park would best secure the quiet, air, light, and pleasant outlook that are so beneficial in the treatment of nervous patients. Provision, separate from that for patients, should be made for physicians, nurses, and other employed persons, and for teaching and laboratory purposes. The need of outdoor exercise, recreation, and of employment should also be provided for.

These recommendations were made without any knowledge whatever of the location of the new hospital and college. It was rather remarkable, therefore, that a site on the property conformed fairly closely with these recommendations. The building stands on a bluff and commands a wide view of the river and of Welfare Island. It is well removed from the streets and from residential and industrial buildings, but is adjacent to the other buildings of the hospital group with which it is connected by corridors, which, however, are not visible in the front of the building. It is near the main entrance to the hospital premises, and presents no indication of isolation or confinement. The windows are of the safety casement type, and require no guards. The land slopes away, at the rear of the building, toward the river; here two stories, which in the front are below grade, are provided with ample windows on three sides. In the upper of these stories provision was made for the outpatient service and the dental department; in the lower were placed the kitchen and other domestic service rooms, the physiotherapy department, and the large lecture room. The first of the eight floors above grade was designed for administration, reception lobby and consultation rooms, library, and a few living rooms for physicians. A reception room and two offices were provided for the use of the Bloomingdale physicians. The second-floor plan contained the laboratories and some examining rooms. The third was designed for children, and the fourth, fifth, sixth, and seventh for adult patients. Each floor for patients was divided into two sections so as to provide for separation of the men and women. The equipment and furnishings were, however, sufficiently uniform to permit of occupation by either sex. It was assumed that the policy pursued at Bloomingdale in regard to the class of patients would be followed at the new service, and the only differences in the accommodations throughout the

Out-patient Service

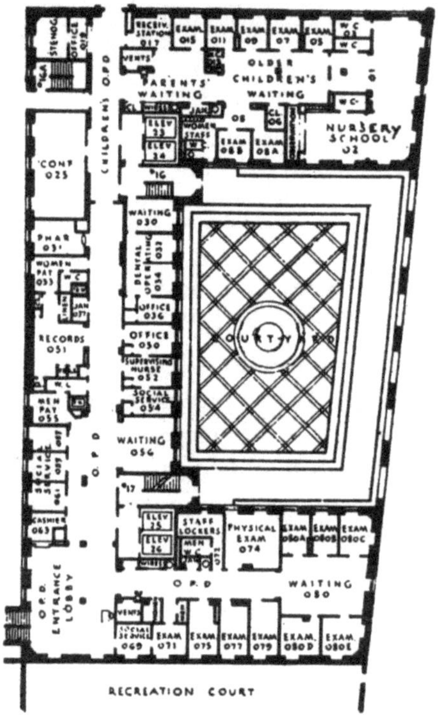

Laboratories

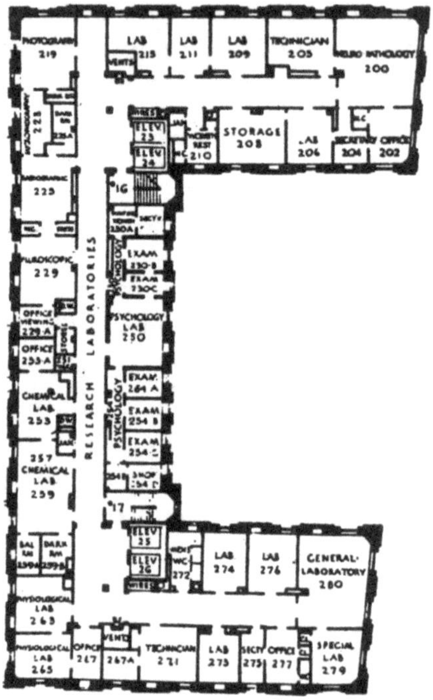

PAYNE WHITNEY PSYCHIATRIC CLINIC: FLOOR PLANS

building were those required by the condition of the patients. The accommodations for the more demonstrative patients were placed on the seventh floor. The eighth floor was designed for occupational and recreational therapy, and class rooms for children. A penthouse on the roof was designed for animals. The roofs of the wings were protected so as to be suitable for outdoor exercise. The space between the wings, and between the building and an adjacent building, was also designed for patients' exercise, and a yard for squash and other games was provided. Liberal provision was made for every form of study and treatment that could be anticipated. Many offices for physicians and others were provided in convenient locations, and conference and lecture rooms for teaching and scientific purposes. It was expected that the building would accommodate 88 adult patients and 23 children.[9] It was named the Payne Whitney Psychiatric Clinic.

As construction progressed, consideration was given to the form of organization and administration. In the plan prepared in 1925 the form

Children *Orderly Patients*

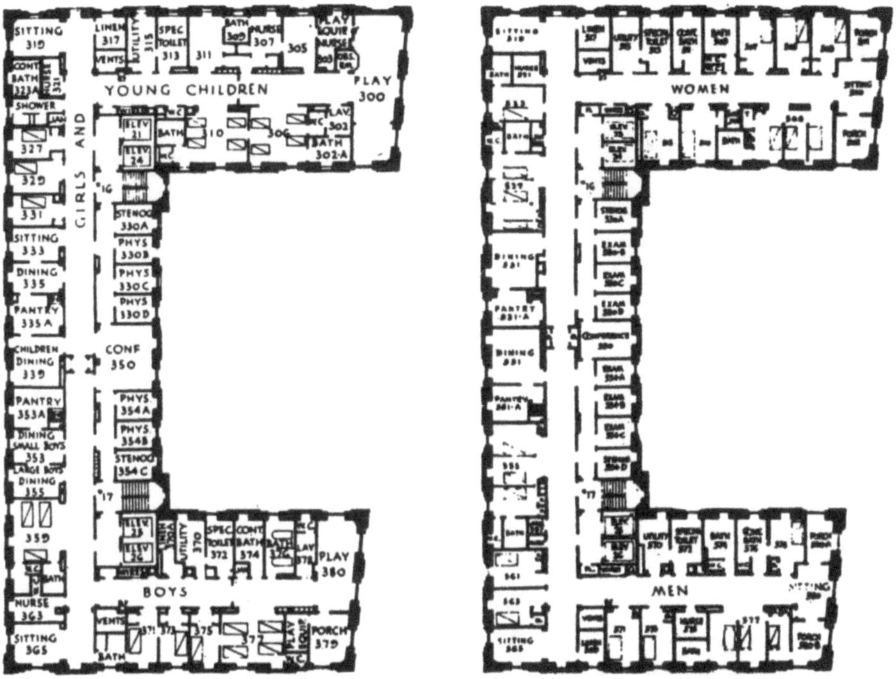

PAYNE WHITNEY PSYCHIATRIC CLINIC: FLOOR PLANS

proposed was patterned after that of Bloomingdale, which is universally considered most satisfactory for a psychiatric hospital. It was recommended, therefore, that the

> director . . . should be a psychiatrist and scientific investigator of superior qualifications. The relations with the medical school would be best adjusted if he were also the professor of psychiatry. He should be appointed and be removable by the Governors of the Society of the New York Hospital. All assistants and other employed persons should be appointed and removable by the director. One of the assistants should be an executive officer who would relieve the director of the details of the administration.

The organic relation with the medical school which was established later was not, at that time, anticipated. It was assumed that the governors

[9] A full description may be found in the *Journal of Nervous and Mental Diseases*, LXXVIII (Aug., 1933), and *Modern Hospital*, XL (June, 1933).

of the hospital would administer the service as an extension of the established psychiatric department, and that working relations with the college would be entered into in somewhat the same fashion as at the New York State Psychiatric Institute and Hospital, Bellevue, the Boston Psy-

Disturbed Patients

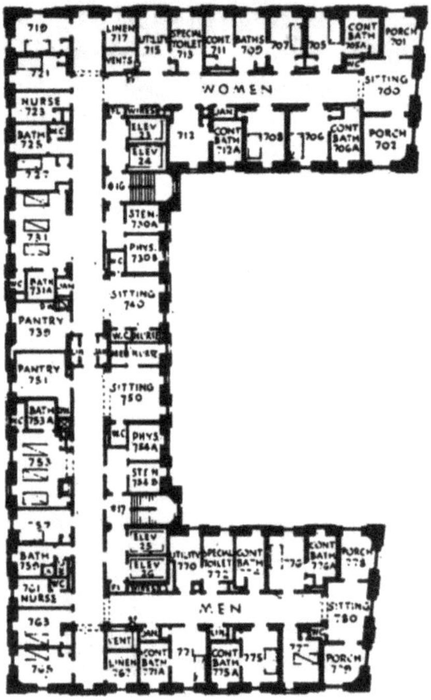

Occupational and Recreational Therapy

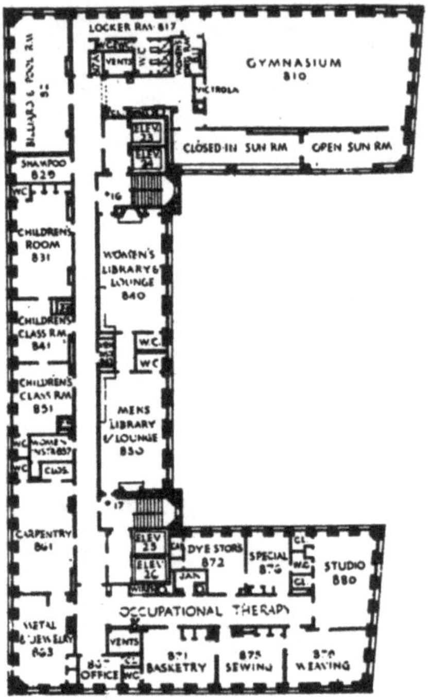

PAYNE WHITNEY PSYCHIATRIC CLINIC: FLOOR PLANS

chopathic Hospital, and many other educational institutions at which the psychiatric service and the college are separately administered. It will be recalled that in previous communications, notably that in 1904, the advisability of hospital control of the service was emphasized.[10]

In considering the appointment of a director, primary importance was attached to obtaining a psychiatrist who could be depended upon to maintain the Society's policy and standards of service to patients and their friends and to the community. If possible, the candidate should possess the qualifications of educator and scientific investigator as required by the university. It was difficult to find such a person. After a thorough search had been made in America and Europe, the appointment was given to Dr. George S. Amsden, who had for five years been

[10] Pp. 471–472.

professor of psychiatry and director of the psychiatric service at the Albany Medical College and Hospital, and had previously been for several years a member of the Bloomingdale staff. He was accepted by the college, and, in conformity with the general plan of organization of hospital and college, he was given the title of psychiatrist-in-chief and professor of psychiatry.

Some apprehension was felt lest the standards and methods of the psychiatric service of the hospital, which had been "shaped principally with reference to furnishing superior treatment to the individual patients" [11] might be too greatly subordinated to the interests and demands of education and scientific investigation. In the past it had been necessary for the governors to remind the physicians of tendencies in this direction.[12] In organizing the service, it was considered advisable to follow the plan adopted in 1808 by which a special committee of governors was appointed to have charge. For the organization of the service it was therefore proposed that "the Committee on Bloomingdale Hospital is, by reason of its special knowledge, experience, and interest, best qualified to undertake the task." The governors, however, decided to appoint a separate committee with the title of the The Payne Whitney Psychiatric Committee. The following departments were established: 1) Medical and Administrative; 2) Nursing; 3) Occupational Therapy; 4) Physical and Recreational Therapy; 5) Laboratories; 6) Social Service; 7) Dietary; 8) Domestic; 9) Clerical; 10) Miscellaneous. Provision was made for an executive business assistant to relieve the director of the Clinic of non-medical administrative details. He was to aid in the economics of administration, keep the director informed of the state of the finances, and aid in the financial relations with patients and their relatives which, in psychiatric practice, have not infrequently an important place in treatment.

In filling positions much advantage was derived from the relations with the long-established psychiatric department of the hospital. The unselfish and helpful coöperation of Dr. Raynor, its director, was of inestimable service. From the Bloomingdale staff Dr. George W. Henry was appointed attending physician at the Clinic, and Dr. Charles Diller Ryan, chief resident and Clinic executive. Miss Carolyn Sprogell, assistant director of nursing at Bloomingdale, became the director of nursing at the Clinic, and Mrs. Alma Rose, assistant housekeeper, became housekeeper. Dr. Harry M. Tiebout, who had previously been a member of the Bloomingdale staff, was appointed chief of the children's

[11] Plan of 1925, pp. 5–6.

[12] See p. 266, above.

service at the Clinic, and Dr. Joseph P. Eidson, chief of the Cornell outpatient service was transferred to the Clinic to have charge of its outpatient service. Dr. Eidson had also been on the Bloomingdale staff, and so had his chief assistant, Dr. William H. Dunn. Nearly all the nurses —men as well as women—had received their psychiatric training at Bloomingdale. Miss Pauline Gundersen, who was appointed director of occupational therapy, had for several years occupied the corresponding position at Bloomingdale. As the psychiatrist-in-chief had also a long service at Bloomingdale, the organization was thus, in large part, composed of members who were well schooled in the policies, standards, and practices of the psychiatric department and could be expected to integrate them firmly in the extended service. It was necessary, however, to look to other organizations in filling several important positions. Dr. Adolf Meyer, director of the Phipps Psychiatric Clinic of Johns Hopkins Hospital, generously released three of his senior medical assistants to accept similar positions at the Clinic. Two who had been in the service of other hospitals were appointed junior assistant physicians. In the organization of the outpatient department several members of the Bloomingdale staff were given appointments for part-time service. Dr. Raynor was appointed consulting psychiatrist of the Clinic, and Dr. George H. Kirby, who had just retired from the position of director of the State Psychiatric Institute and Hospital and professor of psychiatry of Columbia University, was appointed attending psychiatrist on a part-time schedule of psychiatric service in the medical and surgical departments of the hospital. He had formerly been professor of psychiatry at the Cornell Medical College.

In a previous chapter an account was given of the psychiatric outpatient and the consulting inpatient services which were established at the New York Hospital in 1924.[13] A similar outpatient service had been conducted at Cornell Medical College since 1904. These services were now merged and the outpatient service of the Payne Whitney Clinic became the largest in the city in which provision was made for thorough treatment. Appointments to the medical staff were limited to psychiatrists whose qualifications included at least a year in a psychiatric hospital. Special training in child psychiatry was required for appointment in the service for children. Salaries were provided for the director, the assistant director, and some of the attending physicians, and a modest stipend for psychiatrists in private practice or engaged in other psychiatric or mental hygiene employment, who were available for one or more

[13] Pp. 406–407.

afternoons a week at the Clinic. Patients were admitted on an hourly appointment system. The number of psychiatrists available was sufficient for half-day sessions only. It was anticipated, however, that when the number increased, morning and evening sessions would be held. Consideration was also given to specialization, as psychiatrists who were sufficiently interested and qualified became available for psychoanalysis, mental deficiency, alcoholism, convulsive disorders, speech defects, and so on. Much importance was attached to social service. A director of superior qualifications was appointed, with several assistants, all of whom were especially trained in psychiatric social work. Coöperative relations with physicians in private practice and with welfare organizations were established, and arrangements were instituted for the introduction of practice courses for student social workers. Special provision was made for coöperation with the other departments of the hospital. The department was connected by corridor with the department of pediatrics and relations of mutual advantage were established.[14] A nursery school for the study of the personality, development and training of young children was provided.[15] It was anticipated that, when the projected city Health Center was established in the vicinity of the hospital, an opportunity would be afforded for mental hygiene work and teaching.

The 1925 plan of organization noted that

> the more latitude and independence that can be given the better. This is especially the case in regard to a psychiatric hospital, as the requirements are not well understood by physicians and hospital administrators engaged in other fields. For economic purposes, however, purchasing, storage and distribution of supplies, accounting, repairs, laundry, transportation, heating, lighting, and other similar service might be furnished by a central administrative office for all the hospital departments.

It was also recommended that provision be made for independent support and for this purpose Mr. Whitney provided a separate fund.

The plan proposed was, however, not in accordance with the general scheme of administration adopted for other departments of the hospital. In the latter case, those engaged in introducing the scheme were unable to perceive that there were any problems peculiar to the administration of a psychiatric service; they proposed that in the operation of the outpatient service and of the nursing, domestic, dietary, physio-

14 Substantial aid in developing psychiatry in pediatric service and education was obtained from the Commonwealth Fund.

15 This was accomplished by the encouragement and support of Mr. and Mrs. Barklie Henry.

therapy and all the other departments of the Payne Whitney Clinic, "the heads of these departments be centralized, with such assistants in each unit as are required, and the services geared to meet fluctuating requirements." [16] It was assumed that to meet these requirements, nurses, social workers, physiotherapists, stenographers, domestics, and practically all others in the psychiatric organization except the physicians and their immediate assistants would be liable to transfer in and out of the service by central heads of departments, who in all probability, would be quite inexperienced in psychiatric service. The governors, however, to whom this proposal was submitted, having themselves had much psychiatric experience in their relation with Bloomingdale, found it advisable to adopt the recommendations of the psychiatrist in organizing the service. It was decided, therefore, that in the administration of the Payne Whitney Clinic there would be

> (1) A separate budget in which items for corresponding positions may differ from those of other departments, (2) Separate funds and accounting (Whitney fund and earnings), (3) Freedom from control by centralized heads of departments who are not trained and experienced in psychiatric administration. . . .
>
> Pro rata charges would apply only to general administrative offices (director, assistant director, superintendent, accounting) and all other charges would be unitary for supplies and services rendered, the charge made to include overhead.

In the estimates, this plan was much less expensive than that proposed for central administration. In pursuance of the plan, all heads of the various departments of the Clinic and all other persons employed in the service were appointed by the director and responsible directly to him. In the general scheme of organization and administration it was provided that the funds for psychiatry, except those required for a budget for educational and research work, should be budgeted with the general funds of the Society and administered by the central administrative officers. It was considered advisable, however, to keep the funds for support of psychiatry separate, to adopt a separate annual budget, and to report to the Payne Whitney Psychiatric Committee at each of their monthly meetings a statement of income and expenditures, rates charged to patients, and a report of any noteworthy occurrences. The plan of administration was, to a considerable extent, patterned after that which had been found satisfactory in the operation of Bloomingdale in its relation with the Campbell Convalescent Cottage. It was considered

[16] Communication to Dr. Robinson from the superintendent of the hospital.

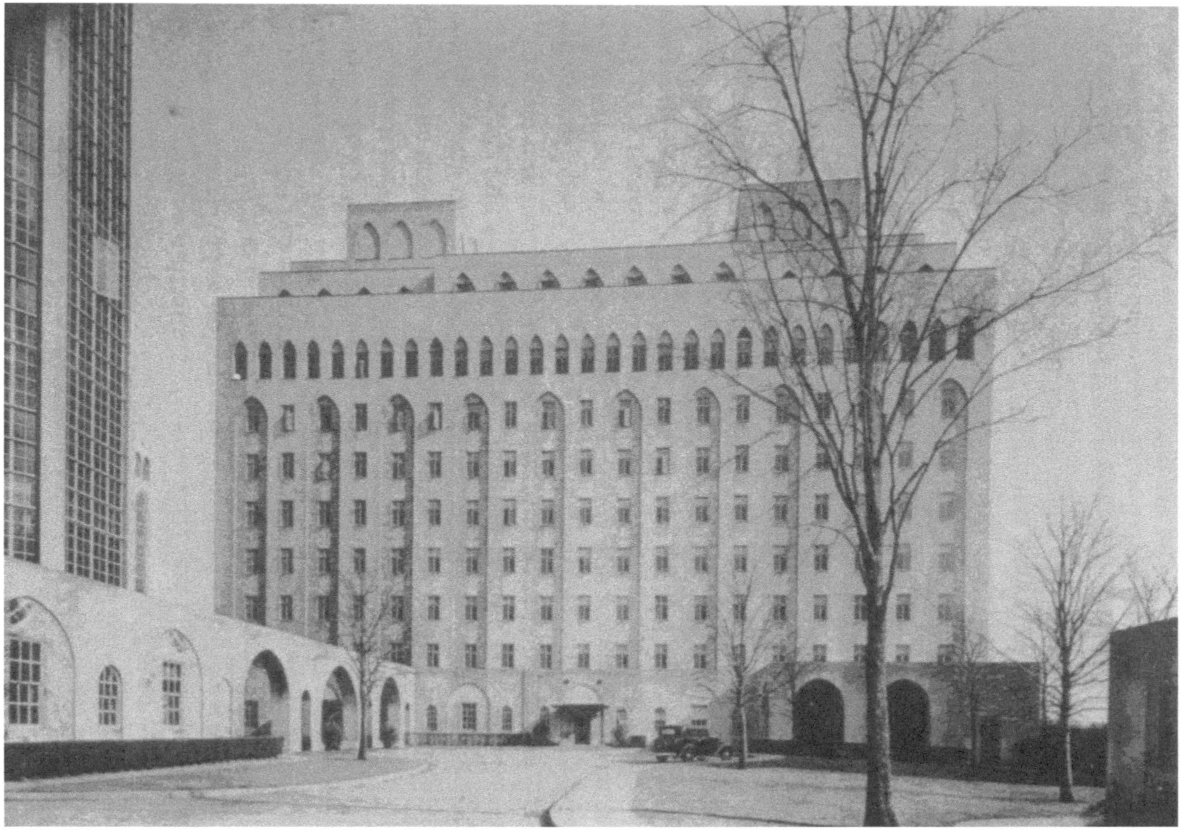

PAYNE WHITNEY PSYCHIATRIC CLINIC, 1932

that, as had for many years been anticipated, the resumption of psychiatric service at the New York Hospital would be treated as an extension of the long-established psychiatric department and that, in organizing and operating it, the well-tried policies and methods and the knowledge and experience gained would be the principal guides.

It will be recalled that the advantages for educational and research work were considered in every proposal made for resuming psychiatric service at the New York Hospital. The plan prepared in 1925 proposed "the establishment in New York City, in connection with the New York Hospital and a medical school, of an institution to be devoted principally to educational and research work in nervous and mental disorders, and to early treatment and prevention." It apparently did not occur to anyone in previous consideration of a development in the city nor during the planning and construction of the Payne Whitney Clinic, that the policy in regard to the admission, classification, and treatment of patients would be an obstacle in the operation of a teaching and research program. The space provided for laboratories, lecture and conference rooms, library, and animal house in the Clinic indicates the consideration that was given to these interests. It was expected that a large outpatient service, and the psychiatric conditions that are found frequently in patients of the medical and surgical services, would also be available. It was assumed that the teaching privileges at the Manhattan State Hospital, which for many years had been extended to the Cornell Medical College, would be retained. Hopes were also cherished that an arrangement might be made for a Cornell service at the State Hospital similar to that of the State Psychiatric Institute when it was located on Ward's Island. It was considered, therefore, that the facilities for psychiatric education and research would be extensive and of superior character. As in the classification of patients in the psychiatric department of the New York Hospital no sharp differentiation is made on financial considerations, it was expected that many of the patients would be utilized in clinical teaching. That this view was held in other organizations is indicated by the following statement by a teacher in psychiatric work who was consulted in the planning of the Clinic:

> The question of a sharp differentiation of private and ward patients might be considered. Although variation in accommodations and therefore of cost of hospital care seems to be desirable, could not all patients be used for teaching and research purposes, to a greater or lesser degree, relative to suitability and cooperation rather than relative to the amount they are paying?

A little more than ordinary tact, patience, and consideration of the sensibilities of the patients and their relatives, is nothing more than what all medical students, young physicians, nurses and others in training for psychiatric, and in fact for any branch of medical practice, should be schooled in.

It was thought that a large part of the educational work of the department of psychiatry of the New York Hospital would be in preparing physicians for private psychiatric practice, institutional service, and mental hygiene work, as well as for teaching and scientific investigation. Much had already been done at Bloomingdale, and it was expected that by means of staff appointments and fellowships this form of educational service would be much extended at the new Clinic. It was considered also that the need for provision for the training in child guidance and mental hygiene created by the closing of the Child Guidance Institute would be to some extent supplied by the New York Hospital.

In planning the teaching program, arrangements were made for utilizing all the resources mentioned. The time allotted to psychiatry in the college curriculum was more than doubled. Besides the professor and associate and assistant professors, selected members of the resident and attending staffs were added to the teaching staff. Dr. Raynor, who was appointed professor of clinical psychiatry, arranged for the members of the senior class to visit Bloomingdale in groups, in order that they might observe and have explained to them the character of the patients and the facilities and methods employed in their treatment. Several members of the Bloomingdale staff who were attending psychiatrists in the outpatient service of the Clinic were appointed instructors by the college and engaged in teaching. It was anticipated in the plan prepared in 1925 that psychiatric education of a somewhat elementary character but of considerable social value would be provided by means of lectures for parents, teachers, clergymen, judges, lawyers, probation officers, and others who engage in child training, religious, public health, medico-legal, vocational training, and other educational work.

The arrangement for a three months' course in psychiatric nursing which the New York Hospital School of Nursing had made for its students with Bloomingdale was, with the opening of the Clinic, discontinued, and a four months' course at the Clinic was substituted. A period of study and practice in the outpatient service was added to the course. An eight months' course for graduates was also established. These courses have proved to be quite successful and have brought into psychiatric nursing a number of much needed capable nurses, some of whom have advanced to important positions. In the considerations relating to educational work at Bloomingdale and at the Clinic much importance was attached to the necessity of maintaining a high standard of psychiatric administration and treatment of the patients. It was realized that the principles and the quality of practice which the physicians and nurses trained in psychiatry would follow in their future work would be to a great extent those which they had observed and participated in when students, rather than those they had heard about in lectures or learned from books.

The organization of the Payne Whitney Clinic when it was opened for the reception of patients on October 1, 1932, consisted of 171 persons, as follows: 42 physicians (28 in the outpatient service), 1 dentist, 53 nurses (all graduates), 3 occupational therapists, 3 physical and recreational therapists, 6 social workers, 3 laboratory technicians, 13 stenographers and clerks, 5 schoolteachers, 29 domestics, 9 in dietary service, 4 miscellaneous. Positions were filled as needed, and were added to with the growth of the service. Two of the floors for patients were all that were at first opened. Nineteen patients were admitted in October, and the total admitted by the end of the year was 67. It is an interesting coincidence that these figures correspond closely to admissions to the first building for the mentally ill at the New York Hospital, which was opened in 1808. It was reported that 19 patients were admitted at that opening and that the total admissions by the end of the year was 67.[17]

In planning the Clinic service it was considered that it would be advisable to operate it in such a way that the admission and treatment of patients would be as free from legal formalities as in the other departments of the hospital. It was believed that many mentally ill persons and their relatives who were unwilling to resort to court procedures or even to apply voluntarily for admission to institutions which were known as places for "the insane," and in consequence failed to receive needed treatment, would readily accept admission to a department of a well-known general hospital. It seemed probable too that, as had been anticipated in Dr. Lyon's proposal in 1904, many persons suffering from forms and degrees of mental illness which had not in the past been recognized as conditions in which hospital service was needed, would apply for admission to the Clinic. Such cases, in greater numbers than ever before, were applying to psychiatrists in private practice and to psychiatric out-

[17] *An Account of the New York Hospital* (New York, 1820), p. 6; see also p. 72, above.

patient services. The treatment of the mentally ill, all of whom in the law are designated "the insane," is, however, governed by state laws and regulations administered by the Department of Mental Hygiene. These laws and regulations were adopted when practically all mentally ill patients under hospital treatment were committed by court order. They had been gradually modified, however, so as to permit the admission of patients who signed voluntary applications or whose condition was so extreme that admission for a limited period without court order was imperative. Under the law, the Payne Whitney Clinic is governed by the section of the Mental Hygiene Law which relates to psychiatric departments of general hospitals. Such departments were at first established only at public hospitals, and were designed merely for the protection and observation of mentally ill persons who seemed to be proper subjects for commitment to a state hospital or private institution authorized under state license to treat committed patients. The period of detention permitted was only a few days. With the advancement of psychiatry, and the diffusion of knowledge relating to its character and to the treatment required, the psychiatric departments of general hospitals were organized and equipped to furnish adequate medical service, and the period of detention permitted was extended to thirty days. Many of the patients admitted soon recovered under treatment and it was unnecessary to transfer them to state or licensed institutions. The law governing psychiatric departments was also amended so as to authorize hospitals operated by privately supported hospital corporations to exercise the same powers as the public hospitals in the admission and treatment of the mentally ill. By virtue of this authority the Payne Whitney Clinic is enabled, without resort to judicial formalities, to admit for treatment any suitable case of mental illness.

The development of psychiatry in relation with the other departments of the New York Hospital, and with general medical progress might, perhaps, have been different if the service had not been separated in 1821. Possibly, however, the present understanding, organization, and highly developed facilities for personality study and treatment at Bloomingdale may be due to the independence and extreme specialization with which the service has been operated. The main interest and all the resources of the institution have been concentrated on the immediate problems presented by the patients under treatment. The extent to which every person employed in the organization, irrespective of his position, is aware that the welfare of the patients is the first consideration is remarkable. In reviewing the history of the service, progress seems at times to have been regrettably slow, even when what was needed was obvious to all concerned. Coincident, however, with the general progress in provision for the mentally ill in America, the main task at Bloomingdale for many years was to obtain accommodations suitable for the different types of patients, and the extensive facilities required for their physical and mental treatment. This task has now been practically accomplished. The advancement at Bloomingdale and the excellent provision for resumption of service at the New York Hospital have prepared the Society as never before to enlarge and extend, with increased efficiency, its service to patients, to psychiatric education and research, and to the community. In carrying forward the work the advice of an eminent physician, who was consulted in the planning of the Clinic, may sometimes be considered with advantage.

> Such an institute, whatever its scientific achievements may be, fails or succeeds in proportion as it serves the community. . . . Coordinate [therefore] the activities of research, teaching and care of the sick, and mental hygiene, in such a way that the community in which it is situated may feel constantly the pressure of its service.

The resumption at the New York Hospital of service for the mentally ill completed a cycle and restored the service to its original relations with the other departments. When the separation occurred in 1821, the disadvantages to the mentally ill were evidently recognized and an unsuccessful attempt was made to provide an attending medical and surgical service.[18] Probably at that time, no one considered that the removal was anything but an advantage to the other departments. The great advancement since then in understanding of the place of psychiatry in general medicine is now strikingly manifested in the genuine appreciation of the opportunity for mutual coöperation shown by all the departments. Psychiatry, on equal terms with the other branches of medicine, has now assumed its proper place among the resources for service, teaching, and research of the New York Hospital.

18 See p. 135.

APPENDICES

I: REPORT OF DR. ARCHIBALD BRUCE ON ALCOHOL

June 7, 1814 *

The Physician to the Lunatic Asylum, in compliance with the desire expressed by the Asylum Committee, in relation to Cases of insanity arising from Intemperence in the use of Ardent Spirits, begs leave respectfully to state,

That since the opening of the Asylum 572 patients have been received. 65 of these Cases from the best information which could be obtained are to be attributed to the immoderate Use of ardent Spirits,—of these 49 were Males, & 16 Females—of whom 4 died. (Two in a few hours after admission.) 3 were discharged at the request of their friends—4 relieved. 1 Eloped, 53 Cured.

In addition to the above may be mentioned 17 other Cases, which might be ascribed to the use of Ardent Spirits,—but who on inquiry were found to have been temperate, & the disease arising from other causes, but who after the symptoms of derangement had taken place, drank to excess. In these instances the intemperance is to be consider'd an effect, rather than the cause of Insanity—of these 11 were Males, & 6 Females—4 died. 1 Eloped. 2 discharged by request of friends—2 reliev'd, & 8 Cured.

By the inordinate Use of Ardent Spirits, the Memory is destroyed, the judgment becomes impaired, the Coats of the Stomach corroded, and diseases of the most miserable kind induced, as Gout, Dropsy, Fevers, Apoplexy, palsy, and not unfrequently Mania.

Where the fondness for Ardent Spirits has not been too long established it frequently yields to Medical and Moral treatment—where however it is of long standing, the habit is with the greatest difficulty removed; and indeed in many instances, notwithstanding the most rigorous treatment, and the greatest privations, the propensity is altogether insurmountable.

A Man of respectable standing in Society, who in consequence of repeated intoxication had rendered himself obnoxious to his Connections, in a fit of remorse attempted Suicide by cutting his throat, which he so far effected as nearly to terminate his existence; in this State he was brought into the Asylum—& recovered. Every Argument was made use of, to dissuade him from Intemperance—he left the House with a full determination of Amendment. After adhering to his resolution a few Months, he again relapsed into his former habit, and from symptoms of incipient Mania, would probably have become a second time an object of the Asylum, had he not have fallen a victim to Typhus fever.

A Woman far advanced in life, who had for many Years been Maniacal from the immoderate Use of Spirits, was admitted into the Asylum—in a

* From the *Minutes of the Governors*. Throughout these Appendices the spelling and punctuation of the originals have been retained, with minor exceptions in the interest of clarity.

few months She fell into a state of Atrophy, and died—during the time She was in the Asylum, She constantly expressed her desire for Rum; even to within a few moments of her death.

A middle aged Woman, whose fondness for ardent Spirits was such as to induce a derangement of mind, so as to render her dangerous to her friends, was placed in the Asylum. One Night unperceived by her Keeper, she attempted an escape, by tying her Blankets and Sheets together, and letting herself down, from a third Story Window. As soon as She began to descend, the rope broke near the Upper part, when she was precipitated to the bottom; by which She was materially injured. This accident could not deter her from drinking. No sooner had She recovered, than She again returned to her former habits of intemperance.

Altho' the prevention of this Cause of Mania falls within the province of the Legislator, the Undersigned trusts he will be excused for suggesting the following, as a means of lessening the Evil.

1st. By Confinement—Intoxication to be consider'd a punishable offence. Persons who are in the habit of using Ardent Spirits to an excess, so as to render themselves Nuisances to Society, on a proper representation to a Magistrate, to be subjected to Confinement for a longer or shorter period, according to circumstances, in an Establishment expressly for the purpose—during Confinement to be occupied in some useful pursuit, & when discharg'd to find Security for good behaviour.

A Country Merchant for Several years past, had been occasionally addicted to the immoderate Use of Ardent Spirits—every fit of intoxication was followed by Mania, which continued from a few days to several Months, during which he was highly dangerous to Society. When in a deranged State he was placed in the Asylum, where he was soon relieved by copious bleeding, blistering, and low regimen. He returned to his friends, and conducted himself with propriety for several Months, when he again relapsed, and during a fit of intoxication he fractured his leg. His Maniacal symptoms and propensity to drink continuing, he was a second time admitted into the Asylum, and [by] the same Means was again restored. Being fully sensible of his infirmity, and having frequently expressed a great fondness for Money, he was easily induced to enter into a Bond with two respectable Sureties to forfeit $1000. the first time he should drink to intoxication. This expedient had the desired effect—he has continued from the time of his discharge (Feby. 26, 1811) to the present, perfectly temperate.

2. Discouraging the Consumption of Ardent Spirits by substituting the use of light Wines—Cider, Malt liquors—&c.

It may be urged that strong liquors, as rum, Brandy, Whiskey &c, are necessary in hot Climates. To this it may be observed, that in the Southern parts of Europe, Intoxication is seldom known to occur. It is held in the greatest detestation. This arises from the constant Use of light Wines, which contain but a small portion of Spirit. Ice in Italy is consider'd a luxury, and by the labouring poor, esteemed almost a necessary of life. The price of this Article at Naples is regulated by the Government. The Italian considers a glass of iced Water preferable to the best of vinous Liquors. The Beggars pittance is frequently expended in obtaining a Drought of this wholesome beverage.

With the View of encouraging the Use of light Wines, might not the duties on Wines, be in proportion to the quantity of Ardent Spirit which they contain, and this in a ratio that would render the price of Ardent Spirit too expensive for the laboring Class of the Community.

The great facility of obtaining Ardent Spirits afforded to the poorer Class of people by the numerous small Shops, under the denomination of Groceries, renders it desirable that their number should be limited to the smallest possible. The Licence to be heavy, particularly for those who retail Ardent Spirits under the form of Drams. Whereas in order to encourage the Consumption, to have the Licence for the vending of small Wines, Malt liquors, & Cyder, proportionably low.

No Debt contracted for Drams, to be recoverable by Law.

A. Bruce

New York
5th April 1814

II: MEMORIAL TO THE NEW YORK STATE LEGISLATURE

February 6, 1816

Appeal for Funds for Establishment of Bloomingdale Asylum *

To the Representatives of the People of the State of New York in Senate & Assembly convened—

The Memorial of the Governors of the New York Hospital

Respectfully Sheweth

That by their annual report to the Legislature, it will appear that about 1500 poor and distressed sick persons, from the City and from different parts of the state, and from various parts of the world, without distinction of Country, or regard to the causes of their Maladies, have been admitted into the hospital, during the last year. As no institution is productive of greater goods to those whose sufferings entitle them to our commiseration and assistance, so nothing can be more honourable than the liberal and continued patronage afforded to this public charity by the Legislature.

The attention of your memorialists has been early excited towards that unhappy description of persons who had by various causes been deprived of reason, and for whom no public assylum was provided. After affording them the partial and imperfect aid of the Hospital, your memorialists ventured, under the incouragement of the Legislature to erect a suitable and convenient building, on the same ground with the Hospital, exclusively appropriated to the reception of lunatics, and in the plan of which particular care was taken to provide whatever was thought conducive to their comfort and convenience, as well as the mitigation and cure of the disease.

This edifice however is not capable of accommodating more than seventy five patients, and it being the only institution of the kind in the state, the number of applications for admission during the three last years, has greatly increased, so that your memorialists are under the painful necessity of almost daily refusing admittance to new patients, for want of room. A large number of insane persons are consequently at this moment unprovided for, many of whom remain a great burthen on their relatives and friends, and some of them highly dangerous to the community.

The increased experience of your memorialists, and a more attentive observation of the insane under their charge, have induced them to believe that many advantageous improvements may be made in the treatment of this class of diseased persons, but which, for want of adequate space in the present establishment, are now impracticable. It appears to your memorialists, that the indiscriminate mixture unavoidable in the narrow limits of the present institution, of persons of different characters, of various and opposite religious sentiments, the serious and profane, the profligate and virtuous, is rather calculated to check the progress of returning reason, than to awaken it from its morbid slumber, to depress the mind and to fix its unhappy bias, than to correct the wild wanderings of disordered intellect, or to break that chain of melancholy and misanthropic ideas, which precede, in most instances, the approach of madness.

* From the *Minutes of the Governors.*

Impressed with this belief your memorialists supposed they could not better discharge their duty towards this afflicted portion of our fellow beings, or more effectually promote the desirable object of an approved and extended plan for the management & cure of lunatics, than by obtaining, within a proper and convenient distance from the City, an area of ground sufficiently large for the accommodation of all the insane, and affording ample room for the best possible modes of treatment. The execution of such a plan your memorialists conceive would not only relieve the several towns and counties, as well as the near relatives of these unhappy persons from a serious charge and great responsibility, but tend greatly to improve the health of the patients and increase the means of their recovery.

A more extended space than they now occupy, where during lucid intervals or in a state of convalescence, patients may enjoy more rational and congenial society, a freer and purer air, innocent amusement, agreeable employment, or salutary exercise seems indispensably necessary to the compleat establishment of a judicious and enlightened plan of medical and moral treatment of the insane.

Your memorialists are confirmed in their opinion of the importance of combining a course of moral treatment towards insane persons, with the usual medical aid, by the experience of institutions for the insane in other countries, and more particularly of the one near *York* in *England* in which the number of these under its care, restored to society and their friends has far exceeded that afforded by any other establishment in which the ordinary mode of treatment has been pursued.

This course of moral treatment consists chiefly in regarding the patient, as far as his state of mind will allow, as a rational being, and in withdrawing his attention from that train of thought connected with the cause of his unhappy state of mind; and for that purpose to provide him with regular employment, as gardening or the various agricultural pursuits, innocent and agreeable sports and exercises, as the care and management of domestic birds and animals, riding, walking, conversation and whatever may tend to sooth his feelings, promote his comfort improve his health, and rouze the dormant energies of his mind.

With a view to such an enlarged scheme of treatment of the insane, your memorialists have lately purchased at a reasonable price in a very eligible situation, about six miles from the City, thirty eight acres of land; but their present means do not enable them to carry the plan into execution by erecting the necessary buildings. Your memorialists feeling the strong claims on public sympathy of that miserable and unfortunate portion of our fellow citizens, in whose behalf they now appeal to the fathers of the state, for assistance and support, and relying on their well known liberality earnestly & with confidence sollicit the Legislature to grant such pecuniary aid, by an annual sum or otherwise, as may enable your memorialists to compleat an establishment on the plan here suggested which must not only conduce to the relief of suffering humanity, but redound to the lasting honour of the state.

All which is Respectfully submitted

III: RULES AND REGULATIONS TO BE OBSERVED BY THE KEEPERS OF THE PATIENTS AT THE BLOOMINGDALE ASYLUM, 1821 *

Of the Men Keepers

1. They shall take the greatest care to preserve cleanliness and good order in the patients rooms and in the Halls of which they have respectively the charge.

Every patients room, and Halls No. 1 and 3 are to be swept daily—and in Winter each Hall throughout the house is to be swept every day.

2. Each patient is to be obliged to wash his face and hands and to comb his hair immediately after rising in the morning. The Keepers are to see this regulation strictly enforced, unless in cases where the malady of the patients will prevent its being executed—and each patient shall be shaved twice a week by their respective keepers.

3. Every patient in sufficient corporal health must be obliged to rise about sun-rise every morning, and must go to bed not later than at 9 o Clock in the Summer & half past seven in the Evening in winter.

4. Immediately after the patients are washed and combed in the morning, those whose health & condition will admit of it, must in good weather be taken to the yards. As soon as they are out, the rooms & Halls must be swept, spitting boxes and all filth and dirt must be removed and the apartments must be made perfectly clean and be put in good order before the patients are called in to breakfast.

5. Breakfast must be on the table, and the patients be called in to eat by the ringing of the Bell at 7 o Clock in the morning. The dinner must be served and the patients called to it, in the like manner at noon—And supper is to be given to them & they called to it in the same way at 4 o Clock in the evening in the Winter & at seven o Clock in Summer.

6. The patients must be brought in from the yards at sunset throughout the year.

7. The Keepers must use their utmost endeavours to preserve order and decency when they are at their meals. They must be restrained as far as practicable from entering into any loud conversation and from using angry, violent or indecent expressions. They must be taught that no one is to begin to eat until all are seated and the keeper has given them a signal to commence.

8. Any keeper or person employed by the Asylum, who shall be intoxicated, or introduce any Spirituous Liquors into the House or any part of the premises, or shall be known once to enter a Tavern or place where liquors are sold (except on express lawful business) shall be discharged the moment such offence shall be known to have been committed.

9. At 10 o Clock each keeper shall employ and superintend two men attached to their respective Halls in removing dirt, straw &c proper to be removed around the Asylum, which shall be placed in a Box provided for

* From the *Bloomingdale Asylum Committee Minutes*, Sept. 29, 1821.

the purpose, & to be emptied every day—and in hoeing up the grass near the House, that may have grown up in the different walks.

10. No keeper shall go off the premises without the knowledge of the superintendent.

IV: REPORT BY DR. MACDONALD ON HIS TRIP TO EUROPE, 1832 *

To the Bloomingdale Asylum Committee

GENTLEMEN:

Honoured by your choice as physician to the Bloomingdale Asylum and directed to spend a portion of time abroad in search of information relative to the treatment of insanity, the undersigned has endeavoured to dispose of his time in the most profitable manner.

He feels he would be wanting in respect to the Board of Governors did he not on this occasion acknowledge his sense of the high and important trust confided in him; and in candour towards himself, did he not confess how slender he thinks his abilities for so responsible a station. But however conscious of deficiencies in this respect, he can speak with more assurance of those qualifications depending on the will.

In pursuance of the general plan marked out by the Committee, he has visited those countries whose institutions promised the greatest advantages. These countries were England, Ireland, Scotland, France and the Italian States. The progress of civilization and the increase of disease seem to have been followed in different countries, though often times slowly, by the establishment of Public Hospitals and other means of relief. But till the latter part of the last century did philanthropy overlook the unfortunate Lunatic. His treatment in former times is involved in mystery, he seems to have been shut up in prisons; to have been burnt as a demon or allowed to run at large a subject of ridicule, pity or veneration according to his condition or the peculiarity of his countrymen. Before the above named period, however, it is true that in France the eloquence and zeal of Vincent de Paul had procured an amelioration; in England Bedlam was known, while in Italy and other European countries the Insane were placed under the care of religious orders.

At the close of the past and beginning of the present century an almost simultaneous wish for improving the condition of Lunatics and Lunatic Asylums manifested itself. The two great rival nations of Europe in particular, England and France, seem to have commenced a rivalship in this respect. But reforms of abuses, however gross, are slow when these abuses have been sanctioned by time.

Great Britain, France, the Italian States, Germany &c now turned their attention towards providing proper receptacles for the Insane and succeeded according to the wealth, genius, or wants of each particular people. In England, Scotland and Ireland wealth has not been wanting to erect numerous new and commodious buildings; in France old buildings have been altered and additions made; in Italy Convents have been converted into Lunatic Asylums and the dormitories of monks have been most rationally changed into cells for Lunatics; while in Germany in one instance, at least, an ancient fortress has been made subservient to humanity, and is now one of the best Asylums in the North of Europe.

* From the *Bloomingdale Asylum Committee Minutes*, Nov. 3, 1832.

Although the credit of having broken the chains of the Lunatic and of having proclaimed to the world the feasibility of treating him with kindness is partly due to France, the stability of the British government and the wealth of the nation have enabled the latter to outstrip the former in the construction of proper buildings.

In England there are three sorts of establishments for the Insane, viz

1. Private mad-houses
2. District Asylums for the poor
3. Public Asylums built by voluntary subscription or established by large legacies.

The first are, in the metropolis, under the surveillance of a board of special commissioners appointed by the Secretary of State, and in other parts of England under that of the Justices of Peace who also appoint from their numbers commissioners and visitors. These commissioners are empowered to grant licenses to keepers of mad-houses and to visit and inspect such establishments four times a year. The licenses granted, are for keeping "two or more insane persons," so that any individual may keep one Lunatic. It is necessary that in every licensed House containing one hundred patients there shall be a Resident Medical Officer. Besides many not licensed, because they contain only single patients, there are 128 licensed private mad-houses in England; 30 of which are the property of and are kept by Females—in these both sexes are admitted. Females are also employed as Superintendents of private houses not belonging to them. While in London the writer visited a private establishment belonging to one of the most respectable physicians of the place—it was for male patients only and under the entire superintendence of an unmarried Female; the physician himself residing some miles distant. The rich are generally found in this class of houses, but in the great metropolis itself Lunatic Paupers are sufficiently numerous to excite the cupidity of dealers in human misery, and hundreds are still kept in what are called the "Red and White Houses" for six and eight shillings a week by the father of a member of Parliament and that too with profit to the keeper. Consequently private houses, notwithstanding all the enactments and amendments that have been made, are still deservedly unpopular.

2. *District Asylums for the poor.* Previous to the memorable investigation before a Committee of the House of Commons into the condition of Lunatics and Lunatic Asylums, there was no provision for the Pauper Lunatic except in miserable workhouses and ill regulated prisons. One of the results of that investigation was the empowering the magistrates of the several counties of England and Wales to erect suitable buildings. Many of the counties taking advantage of this law have constructed and organized Hospitals that will do everlasting credit to the nation. They are modern, and are consequently built with all the improvements of the present era. Some of them, indeed, are models and in many respects undoubtedly excel any similar establishments. They are under the control of county magistrates.

3. *Public Asylums built by voluntary subscription or established by large*

legacies. These Asylums in their organization, method of inspection &c. are like the public Hospitals of our own country and generally receive Pay-patients; though Paupers are admitted into some of them on certain conditions;—indeed until District Asylums were established these were the only institutions in which the poor were regularly treated. Under this head may be ranked the notorious Bedlam or Bethlehem where Lunatic Convicts also are kept.

In Scotland, from a dread of poor-rates, there are no District National Asylums, but in most of the large towns there are public institutions erected by the voluntary subscription of benevolent individuals and supported by the pay of patients, many of whom are Paupers and maintained by their respective parishes. From the high respectability of these establishments, Private-Houses are not patronized; consequently there are but few of them in the country. There are no commissioners nor visiting justices as in England for inspecting these establishments. Besides the inspection of the ordinary Directors or Governors, the Sheriff of each county is authorized to visit both public and private Houses, to correct abuses &c.

Until within a few years, Ireland with the exception of the cities of Cork and Dublin, was destitute of public institutions for the Insane. Acts were passed under George IV appointing commissioners to investigate the wants of the country in this matter and to superintend the construction of suitable buildings. Besides Richmond Lunatic Asylum at Dublin, which, converted into a District Asylum, answers the demands of four counties, and that of Cork which is sufficient for the city and county of Cork, it was found expedient to divide the remaining part of Ireland into Eight distinct districts and to erect an Asylum in each large enough to accommodate from 120 to 150 patients. Four of the establishments under the above mentioned acts viz; those located at Londonderry, Belfast, Armagh and Limerick are in full operation. Three more are now building, and an eighth proposed, which will complete the original design. They are all on the same general plan, and under the same system of government. The commissioners at Dublin have control over all, appoint their officers and local Directors, investigate their fiscal concerns and if necessary, appropriate money for their maintenance. It is thought that the present system when in general operation will answer the wants of the country—if not, it is proposed to attach a distinct House to each institution, for incurables.

Private Asylums are not numerous in Ireland, and the only one of note established by individual beneficence or voluntary subscription besides those already named at Dublin and Cork is St. Patrick's founded by the eccentric Swift. And this is one of the worst constructed and worst regulated establishments in the United Kingdom.

All Lunatic Asylums in Ireland are inspected by two Officers named by Government and styled "Inspectors General." These persons also inspect and report annually on prisons, houses of industry &c.

Although in the different parts of the United Kingdom, the system of Lunatic Asylums differs in some respects, yet in England and Ireland, those establishments devoted to the Insane Poor and denominated "District

Asylums," are conducted on similar principles and are probably superior in construction and management to any similar institutions extant.

But as a system the Irish is more complete than the English. The latter authorises, but does not compel every county or district to erect new buildings. Consequently its operation is partial, being yet confined to a few counties; the former is compulsory and general and it will not be long before every district will be provided for.

The Hospitals of this class in both countries have been erected with an eye to all improvements made and to be made in this species of architecture. Classification, considered now in all countries of the first importance, has been amply provided for.

The public institutions established in these countries by voluntary subscription or by private beneficence, though in general managed with skill under the auspices of the most philanthropic individuals, are mostly deficient in construction not because they do not belong to the District or it may be said to Government itself but because the Houses were erected without the advantages of modern experience.

The "private madhouses" in England intended for the rich, and this comprises the most of them, are fitted up with all the comforts and frequently with many of the luxuries and superfluities of life. Old buildings, such as Gentlemen's seats in the environs of large towns generally serve for this purpose.

The establishments for the Insane in Scotland instituted as above mentioned by private charity, are of the very first order, and although they do not answer the demands of the whole country, yet they dispense a vast amount of good to the poor as well as to the rich. Indeed it may be said of the one at Perth, if there be anything on a small scale like an approach to perfection, it is here.

The number of Lunatics in England by a calculation was 16,222—proportion to the whole number of inhabitants as 1 to 783. The number in Wales 896, proportion to the population 1 to 911. The whole number in Scotland 3652, proportion to the population as 1 to 573.

From the assimilation in language, laws and customs which has of late taken place between the different parts of the United Kingdom of Great Britain and Ireland we are not surprised to find their charitable institutions similar; but we are scarcely prepared to observe so striking a difference as those of England and France, countries separated by an arm of the sea which requires at most but a few hours to traverse, present.

In England, Asylums established by voluntary subscription are numerous; in France, so national in public sentiment, they are not known, on the contrary Hospitals for the Insane are all mediately or immediately under the national government; in the metropolis of the former country a thousand formalities are necessary for a medical man whether foreigner or resident to gain admittance—in that of the latter to be a stranger or physician is a passport that opens all doors; in England the buildings are three or four stories high, in France a single story (Rez-de-Chaussée) is deemed sufficient, and all recent improvements have been made on this plan; in England convalescents have separate chambers, in France where society is so necessary to the enjoyment of life, that to be deprived of it is to be deprived of much that renders existence agreeable, many are placed in large halls or wards and with advantage. This to any other people than to one so much accustomed to live in public would be injurious.

In England during winter it is necessary to keep up a temperature of 60 and upwards, in France a large proportion of patients is without artificial heat.

To mention no other points of difference the diet of the one is as different from that of the other as the food of distinct species of animals.

In France there are three kinds of establishments for the Insane, viz.

1. Private Institutions (Maisons de santé des alienés)
2. General Hospitals (Hospices et Hopitaux generaux)
3. Special Hospitals, in which none but Insane are admitted

Private Institutions for the reception of the Insane are not so numerous as those of England—they are in general remarkably well kept and have not been guilty of those abuses which have disgraced the private "Mad-houses" of England. They are all under the surveillance of the Police and it is obligatory on each one even if there be but a single patient under its care to have a Resident physician. The private establishment of the celebrated Esquirol at Ivry near Paris is a model of this kind.

General Hospitals. Most of the Insane confined in France are found in the general Hospitals. These Hospitals are usually for the reception of the *aged,* the *infirm,* the *Insane* and the *old "employes"* of these and other establishments of Charity. The latter Class in consideration of former services is well provided for and has many privileges.

Apart and entirely distinct from the rest is the division for the Insane, and although it would be desirable to have these in buildings independent of every other establishment, yet so systematic are the French in the minute details of these matters that order and good management are visible in all the numerous subdivisions.

These general Hospitals with the other establishments of Charity in Paris are under the charge of a *general council* (Conseil général des Hopitaux et des Hospices) and of a distinct *administrative Commission,* both appointed by the King and subject to the control of the minister of the Interior.

In all the provincial towns and Communes where there exist institutions of charity, there are distinct administrative commissions which are either nominated by the Prefects of the respective Departments or directly appointed by the King.

The celebrated establishments of Bicêtre, Salpêtrière, and Saintyou at Rouen come under the head of general Hospitals.

The construction, distribution &c. or to use a comprehensive French term, the "materiel" of these establishments is more imperfect than that of the most modern English Asylums. The reason is obvious—the former are more ancient, and but few of them have been expressly built for the Insane; some, indeed, having been abbeys and convents. So excellent however are the additions made to many of them that in some respects they vie with or excel those of modern origin.

Special Hospitals. The number of special Hospitals in France destined for the reception of the Insane solely, does not exceed a dozen. Each one is under the authority of the Prefect of the department to which it belongs, and of a commission of surveillance; except that of Charenton which being the principal establishment of the kind in France, is directly under the jurisdiction of the minister of the Interior who appoints a commission of five to aid him in its superintendence. None but *Pay patients* are taken into this great Hospital, and the amount received for their board is sufficient to support it.

The same remark may be made of this as of the last mentioned class of establishments. For want of means to erect entire new buildings in other localities, the greatest skill has been displayed in altering and working up old materials.

The whole number of Lunatics in France is reckoned at 30,000—the number in Lunatic-establishments, not more than 7 or 8000.

The proportion of the Insane to the whole population is as 1 to 1000.

Proceeding from England and France to other European countries, Lunatic Asylums are generally observed to be inferior both in construction and management.

In Italy they are numerous and of the best and worst character. But as far as construction and internal arrangement are concerned, they may be pronounced to be without a single exception defective. This is not surprising when it is considered that they were erected for other purposes, mostly for convents. As in the general Hospitals of France, Lunatics are frequently placed in the same establishment with invalids &c &c. All the Public Hospitals are either directly or indirectly under the respective governments to which they belong, and Private Asylums, it is thought, are not known. Their internal administration was formerly, and is yet in some instances, in the hands of religious orders; but in this as in other temporal affairs the influence of the Roman Church is daily diminishing. Although Religious orders have lost their control over Hospitals yet the sisters of Charity are still preserved to nurse Female patients. In the dominion of the Pope Priests are generally if not universally at the head of all Hospitals.

As far as the writer has been able to learn from observation and enquiry the number of Lunatics in the different Italian Hospitals amounts to between 3 and 4000. The actual number in the whole of Italy is not known.

In Switzerland the number of Lunatics in public establishments is small. This is chiefly owing to the paucity of insanity in this as in other mountainous districts where Idiots are much more numerous. The latter being harmless, are not necessarily subjected to the more rigorous treatment of maniacs.

In Belgium and Holland, Lunatic Asylums are numerous but exceedingly defective both in their "material" and "personnel." The whole number of Lunatics by a census taken shortly before the late separation was 5591—

that is 1 to Eleven hundred inhabitants. The number of necessitous poor in public establishments was 1867 besides 1112 boarded with Private individuals.

In Austria and Prussia there are several well regulated Asylums—in the smaller German states there are said to be many miserable and some excellent establishments (particularly one in Saxony and another in Bavaria).

For the rest of Europe excepting Norway, a country on the very confines of Civilization, but little can be said.

In the north the Insane are usually confined in the same Hospitals with the poor, the aged and with venereal patients—in the South as in Spain and Portugal, chains and stripes are still too much in vogue. While in the East, the Turks regarding insanity as a special mark of divine favour, never undertake its cure. The harmless are allowed to run at large both in town and country, and are treated with great respect by pious mussulmen who on meeting them prostrate themselves and religiously kiss the hems of their garments. The furious are confined and *chained* in *magnificent* houses.

The Norwegian government has recently published a complete Statistical account of the Insane and has proposed a general national system for their care. The number of Insane in Norway is 1909—making one Lunatic for every 551 Inhabitants; the largest ratio known. As in other mountainous districts a large portion, one third, are Idiots.

Such is a rapid and imperfect outline of the different kinds of establishments for the Insane in many parts of Europe.

It may not be uninteresting to speak of some of the more important points of their internal economy. Although as already mentioned these buildings vary in construction according to the views of each people, yet in one thing all nations who have given the subject their attention, agree, it is [as follows:]

The Classification of the Insane

With this object constantly in view England has erected her only good Asylums—to attain this end France has altered and is still making additions to her old establishments. These divisions are not founded according to the distinct forms; such as Mania, Monomania &c that Insanity assumes, but according as the patient is quiet or noisy, cleanly or filthy, convalescent or incurable, paralytic, epileptic &c. In some of the New Hospitals of England there are no less than six Classes of each sex. An equally minute division is observed in the best Hospitals of France.

European Hospitals for the Insane have generally what American Asylums are destitute of.

Infirmaries—At the Royal Lunatic Asylum of Charenton in France those are no less than three distinct kinds of infirmaries:

1st. For the sick generally
2nd. For the Epileptic and Paralytic
3rd. For those disposed to suicide

Objections have been made to the last mentioned method of associating numbers of melancholics on the ground that they might assist each other in the execution of their sad designs; or at least, in suggesting various methods of self destruction, but it is well known by those conversant with the subject that melancholics, and above all, those disposed to suicide have but little sympathy for others, confine themselves within the narrow limits of their own sombre ideas and seldom or never act in concert with their fellows. This method of bringing together this class of the Insane was once abandoned, but was soon resumed because it offered too many advantages of safety by concentrating several keepers, where so much and so untiring vigilance is necessary.

As there is perhaps nothing in which people of different countries differ more than they do in their notions of comfort, so the Hospitals of distinct countries vary exceedingly in those arrangements that conduce to comfort. According to an American's or an Englishman's views, French and Italian Hospitals are faulty in many particulars; but in nothing more than in a deficiency, it might almost be said, in some instances, a destitution of those comforts afforded during Winter by artificial heat. In England great attention has been recently directed to this subject. The various methods of Stoves, open grates, air furnaces, hot water and steam have been employed, and decided preference has been given to the latter. The last district Asylum built, that of Middlesex, is warmed in this manner. Among its advantages it is said to be perfectly manageable, economical and salutary for those who breathe the atmosphere heated by it, while on the contrary, air heated in furnaces is pronounced deleterious to all individuals disposed to pulmonary diseases.

Warm bathing has now become an object of so general importance that in the Asylums lately erected in England there are conveniences for giving all the patients baths on the same day. For this purpose there are large tubs containing 1500 gallons each, in which several patients are put at the same time.

In this Country as well as America baths are chiefly used for cleanliness, but in France they are extensively employed as medicinal agents. As a general rule all patients under treatment, and this comprises all that are curable, take warm baths—some once a day, some every second day and others again twice a day—the time spent in the bath varying from half an hour to three hours. At the Hospital at Rouen this is carried to a very great extent. In some instances strong and violent patients are bathed three times a day and remain in the bath three hours each time. Of all the agents in the hands of the French physician this is the most powerful and if it does not deserve absolute imitation, is at least worthy of consideration.

In England great attention has been paid and much money expended in constructing water closets—they are in general all within doors, one belonging to each class. They are washed with water and so arranged in some buildings as to be entirely inoffensive. At Florence and Sienna in Italy, there is one in every room, the seat of marble. The act of sitting on them fills the vessels—to a certain height with water—the act of rising empties them. The personnel or administrative department of Hospitals in Europe is in many respects different from ours. Division of labour is much greater and there are more persons employed in each division than in America.

In France generally, one nurse or keeper is allowed to ten patients. M. Esquirol thinks this insufficient. At his own private establishment each patient has at least one attendant and in some instances more.

At Charenton the proportion is much greater than 1 to 10. In this establishment where there are usually 500 patients there are no less than 196 "employés." The following is a list of some of them.

Medical department and those attached to it

1 Physician in chief
1 " adjunct
1 " inspecting
2 " elèves (Students of medicine)
1 Surgeon in chief
1 " elève in surgery
1 Apothecary in chief
1 " elève
1 Surveillant (Superintendent) who executes the orders of the physician
1 Surveillant (matron) with duties similar to the last
1 Infirmier en chef (Head keeper or sub-superintendent)
1 Infirmiere (Sub-matron)

Non medical department

1 Director
1 Secretary in chief
Many Clerks
1 Econome (Steward)
1 Sous Econome (under Steward)
Many Clerks
1 "Receveur."
1 Bookkeeper
Several Clerks
1 Architect
1 Master-mason
1 Chaplain

As the government committee visits this establishment but four times a year, the ordinary duties of inspection fall on the physicians. This, consequently renders the number of medical officers greater, but it is scarcely necessary to add that the persons employed in both departments are more numerous than necessary.

In the Pay-Hospitals of England the proportion of keepers is about as great as it is at Charenton—but in the strictly Pauper Asylums where the patients are used to labour, the proportion is much less than that allowed by the French administration, (1 to 10). It is in some Houses but 1 to 25.

In the new Pauper Lunatic Asylums of Ireland there is 1 keeper to 7 and 8 patients.

In Italy there is 1 to from 10 to 20.

The deficiency of keepers both in numbers and character is a general subject of complaint and is considered one of the most difficult things in the management of Lunatic Asylums.

In the course of this tour of observation the writer has been impressed with the importance every where attached to moral treatment; not however to moral management exclusively, but to a judicious combination of moral and medical treatment—so closely indeed are they allied that it is difficult to say where the one ends and the other begins; it is difficult to put one into successful operation without bringing in the other. Active exercises and amusements are called moral agents, yet is not their operation on the physical as well as on the moral part of man?

On the other hand the very exhibition of a dose of medicine whether by persuasion or force may exert a powerful (good or bad) effect on the patient and in this way may be viewed as a moral agent.

In the early period of insanity when disorders in the physical functions are palpably manifest, medical is equally as important as moral treatment. It is for this reason that recent are so much more curable than old cases of insanity; though at the same time it must be admitted that the habit of wrong-thinking like inveteracy in vice gains force with time and adds to the incurableness of insanity. As moral agents then, and those kinds of agents that combine a moral and physical influence, are the remedies chiefly employed in the treatment of chronic insanity, and as by far the largest proportion of cases in Lunatic Asylums is old, it becomes important to give this part of treatment the highest consideration.

Moral treatment which in general terms is so comprehensive and includes the various kinds of employment and recreation, the personal influence of physician, attendants &c. in a word every agent brought to bear directly on the *"moral"* of the patient begins with *Classification.*

The injury that a raving maniac or disgusting idiot would do to a sensitive convalescent is too evident to require any argument in favor of such an arrangement.

It is now generally considered that after classification, the most important of all considerations in the management of the insane is employment. In the strictly Pauper Asylums of England, Ireland and Scotland a large proportion of patients has of late been employed and with advantage both to themselves and to the institutions to which they belong; thus in the Middlesex Co. Asylum two Fifths are employed—the men as Shoemakers, tailors, carpenters, brick layers, gardeners, bakers, brewers, labourers &c.

The Women in knitting, washing, sewing, cleaning house, feeding poultry, working in the garden, making baskets, straw hats &c.

At Wakefield nearly the same proportion is employed.

In the Dundee Asylum, a still larger proportion; more than one half, is employed.

Accidents from trusting patients with tools are unheard of.

It has been doubted if religious exercises could be introduced into Asylums for the Insane. From numerous experiments made in England and Scotland the question is now at rest. At least it is the opinion of the majority of persons connected with public establishments, that the precepts and consolations of religion may be made most useful in the moral management of the Insane. Chaplains are now attached to most of the large county

Asylums in England which they visit at least once a week when service is performed. In Catholic Countries Chapels seem to form an essential part of all Hospitals where such patients as are in a proper condition, attend mass once a week. A priest is usually attached to each House where he permanently lives. At the Asylum of Aversa near Naples, besides performing mass once a week and confessing patients individually, he pronounces a general benediction every day.

At Wakefield nearly one third, at York nearly one half, at Glasgow one half and at Dundee two thirds of the patients have been found well enough to join in the services of the chapel.

In the preceding remarks from a desire to make this communication as brief as possible, the description of particular institutions has been avoided —as brief as it is the subscriber fears that it is already too long and begs leave most respectfully to submit it in its crude form to the inspection of the Committee.

JAS MACDONALD

V: REPORT BY DR. MACDONALD ON ORGANIZATION

July 1, 1837 *

To the Bloomingdale Asylum Committee

GENTLEMEN:

In conformity with the resolution that Dr. Macdonald be requested to furnish the committee, as soon as his convenience will permit, with a more full and detailed account of the best method of conducting an Asylum for the insane and to point out the action of the whole plan; I beg leave to submit the following remarks.

The chief defects in the present administration of the Asylum are want of unity of action. Want of system and want of employment.

Unity of Action. The first endeavour should be to establish this which can only be done by making one individual generally responsible not only for the ordinary management of the patients, but for carrying into effect all schemes of manual labor whether on the Farm or in Work Shops and also for the cleanliness of the different Houses and pleasure grounds. The individual thus responsible must necessarily have authority to hire and discharge all subordinate persons in the employ of the institution, excepting perhaps those under the immediate direction of the Farmer.

The functions of the head of an establishment like this should be to plan, direct and supervise, as from him must originate all methods of treatment whether Medical or Moral, so in him should be concentrated sufficient power to carry his plans into effect, all superior officers should be so far under his control as to receive instructions from him. A system like this will prevent a division of interests and keep one part of the Household from arraying itself against the other. It will harmonise the action of the whole machine and if properly used will make every thing tend to one point: the comfort and restoration of the insane; if this plan confer upon one individual increased power it imposes additional obligations, his direct responsibility for the welfare of the institution and the conduct of its officers must check him in making wrong use of his power.

The functions of a physician to a Lunatic Asylum should not end with the performance of his daily duties. He has also professional duties to discharge, placed in an extended field of observation he can collect facts which may be of immense service to his medical brethren. But this he cannot do satisfactorily without a professional assistant, in this department as well as in every other he must have some one to attend to Minutiae, to do the drudgery. Otherwise he cannot take those large and impartial views which are so necessary for a person at the head of a great philanthropic institution. If obliged to attend to all the necessary details in the application of medicinal remedies, such is the tendency of the Human mind that he may assign to these an undue importance and prescribe them where labour or mental diversion might be much more efficacious. Or fatigued by mechanical drudgery he may take a partial and superficial view of every case

* From the *Bloomingdale Asylum Committee Minutes.*

presented to his observation. Though in the various Professions of Life great advantages undoubtedly are to be derived from the practice of selecting particular branches and subjects for study and observation yet this may be so exclusively done as to warp and contract the mind. Acting under this apprehension while cut off from general practice and believing there is no branch of his profession which may not afford some aid in the treatment of mental diseases, the writer has taken great pains to make Medicine generally his study. It has been his opinion therefore that a physician exclusively devoted to mental diseases cannot treat them medically so well as he might do with his mind enlarged by the observation of other diseases.

The above remarks relative to the performance of the details of the medical service by an assistant apply with equal force to the details in the other departments of the establishment.

Want of System. This being the result of a want of unity of action, System will naturally follow the establishment of the latter.

Want of Employment. Though the Patients of the Bloomingdale Asylum have been employed in different ways, their occupations have not been sufficiently varied and systematic nor conducted on right principles. The undersigned would remind the Committee that he has always been of this opinion and refers them to his various reports in which the subject has been introduced. Employment has not always been urged on right principles. The Patients have too often been asked to labor as a duty or as a matter of course. This would answer very well for a certain description of Lunatics; for those who are imbecile, who have neither wants nor desires, and whom motives do not influence, but there is another class who as much require motives to action as persons of sound mind. Few reasonable persons would work day after day for the mere pleasure of working. So it is with the insane, something must be associated with their labor: either the idea of benevolence, of aiding the destitute or the expectation of reward. Reward in one shape or another, let it be some delicacy of diet or article of clothing or money or other inducement, must be the motive of the great mass of patients. Thus if a carpenters shop should be established and boxes made for sale, let a regular account of the disbursements be kept and the surplus distributed among the patients who do the work. Let those patients who are above receiving a compensation for their work give their labor for some benevolent object, such as clothing the destitute, many of whom may daily fall under their notice. The cultivation in this manner of the higher sentiments cannot fail while it improves the Moral character to draw off the attention from those subjects that oppress the mind. To point out the action of the place it will be well perhaps to give a brief sketch of the operations of a single day. The whole Household to rise at a certain Hour at the ringing of a Bell. The cooks to repair to the Kitchen to prepare breakfast, the nurses and attendants to put their rooms in order for the use of patients—to call up the patients and see that they are washed and dressed; on the ringing of the Second Bell as many of the patients as are well enough and as many of the attendants and servants as can be spared to assemble in the room used as a chapel for morning Prayers. On the ringing of the third bell breakfast to be served throughout the House. After breakfast the ordinary attendants to put the bed rooms and Halls in order and to have the immediate care of those patients taking medicines and necessarily confined to the House, the other attendants, those engaged to amuse and employ the patients, to proceed in the execution of their various duties, some to walk with, others to ride with, others to work in the garden and fields with, others to sew, knit &c, with them until the hour of dinner, when preparation will be made for this meal: the patients in ordinary to dine at noon, the better class at 1 or 2 o'clock. After dinner useful exercises and amusements both in and out of doors until tea time. The evening to be spent according to the taste and condition of Patients: Needle work &c for females, Society, music, Games, reading to be the general amusement of the House. On the ringing of a Bell at a fixed Hour the whole Household to retire to rest and one or more of the superior officers to visit every part of the Establishment to see that the last order of the day is strictly enforced, that fires are secure and lights extinguished. According to the method above proposed, exercise, amusement, and employment will not be left to general directions but each person having charge of patients for these different purposes will be obliged to render a daily or weekly account of all that has been done: of the number of patients walking and the extent of their walks, of the number at work, the kind of work and of the work accomplished. Such is an outline of the general movement of the House. The following will be the daily duties of the different officers. The Physician accompanied by his assistant will as soon as the House is settled visit and inspect every part of it, see all the patients, examine strictly every one under treatment, make prescriptions and give directions for their management, cause their cases to be written down and regularly continued. After completing his indoor duties he will inspect the premises generally, look after the patients employed out of doors and supervise the operations of farming & gardening. The assistant Physicians duties will be confined to the House and Patients. Besides accompanying the Physician and making minutes of his observations and directions in each particular case he will see that the latter is carried into effect, and that medicines are properly administered and what are their effects. He will perform all the minor operations and visit the patients under treatment as often during the day as necessary. He will also make an evening visit to all patients under treatment and assist generally in carrying out the curative plans, Moral as well as medical of the principal.

The first duty of the Matron or Sub-matron after rising in the morning will be to visit the Kitchen and see that things are going on properly there, to visit the Female wing and Lodge, to see that the patients are dressed and washed for breakfast and that those who may be sick are not suffering. The first of these officers with the Steward will preside at the table where all the best patients will assemble for their meals. After breakfast the matron will proceed in her duties in supervising the domestic affairs of the House, of watching over the interests of the Female patients, that they are kindly treated and suitably employed and amused, that the nurses administer the medicines and diet prescribed by the Physician and in general perform their duties; in fine that she will do all she can in her power to carry into effect the general plan of treatment.

The *Physician* in treating Females deprived of reason finds it a delicate and difficult matter to arrive at a knowledge of all their ailments without the co-operation of an intelligent person of the same sex who will so interest herself in their behalf as to get into their confidence and to be able to point out all their secret suffering whether of mind or body. To be accompanied by such a person in his daily visits would give the Physician an advantage which nothing else could offer—besides the importance of this the necessity of having a superior Female constantly in the wing or in the new building just erected will render it almost imperative on the Committee to appoint an assistant Matron.

The *Steward* besides attending to the fiscal concerns of the institution should have some duty to perform that will bring him in contact with the patients and create a personal interest in their welfare. Let him daily make an early visit to the male wing and Lodge and see that the attendants are beginning the day properly by setting the House in order and attending to the cleanliness of their respective patients and as it will be his duty to supply their ward robes and examine their clothing.

As it has been suggested by some of the Committee that a single individual cannot perform all the duties of Steward, it may be deemed advisable to appoint a person to take all the Stores under his special charge to distribute provisions to the cooks, and to see that nothing is wasted or improperly taken away. As it may be the duty of this officer to watch over the economy of the House: in order to keep his peculiar functions constantly in view, let him be called the Economist.

The *Gardener & Farmer,* under this plan of making the Asylum an establishment of practical industry, will become a person of great importance. Having the farm and garden under his care, all the Labor on them must necessarily be under his direction. Let him be hired with the express understanding that much of his labor must be got from the patients and he will find means to induce them to work. One or more of the ordinary attendants might be always with them when employed.

The *Carpenter's* services may also under this plan be made highly advantageous, as many have been accustomed to work with joiners tools. He will furnish occupation for such patients as have a taste for this kind of Employment. Of the former ——— are now in the establishment and of the latter there are no doubt many who would be pleased with this kind of exercise.

All these Schemes for the more Systematic employment of the Insane may by some be deemed visionary. But when we recollect that useful Occupation has been successfully introduced into many European institutions for the insane and that is there no longer considered as an experiment the plan must be deemed practicable—and where we reflect that the great majority of patients in the Bloomingdale Asylum are old cases (beyond the reach of medical aid) and that if abandoned to their own inclinations they will almost surely degenerate, we cannot but think that a project that offers a reasonable promise of benefit should be adopted. The method of conducting the financial affairs of this institution I leave to the better Judgment of the committee. The Physician unfit by education and habit would of course wish to have little or nothing to do with them.

With much Respect your
most obedient Servant
JAS MACDONALD

VI: REPORT BY DR. NICHOLS ON THE CONDITION AND ENLARGEMENT OF THE WOMEN'S LODGE

June 28, 1851 *

To the Bloomingdale Asylum Committee

GENTLEMEN:

I beg leave to call your attention to the subject of an enlargement of the building occupied by the more excited, noisy and violent class of females, known as the "women's lodge," and an increase of facilities for their comfort and cure.

A majority, at least, of the members of your Committee are already quite familiar with this subject, and I have been most happy to find, in my conversations with you respecting the improvements and additions to which I refer, such a full appreciation of their very great and pressing importance. It would not seem necessary, therefore, that I should treat you to an essay in bringing this matter formally before you, and I will content myself with merely a succinct recapitulation of the present defects to be remedied and of the remedial measures I propose.

1. Classification. Perhaps the most crying defect in the architecture of the present building is the entire absence of any arrangements whereby the noise of excited and vociferous patients can be shut off from those who are quiet or would be but for the noise of others, and are greatly molested and injured by loss of sleep by night and unquiet by day.

Vociferation or other great noise in any one room in the building can readily be heard in all the other rooms. The three single rooms on the east side are usually occupied by the most noisy patients, because noise made in them disturbs the patients in the main house and in the men's lodge less than when made in the west rooms, tho we are always obliged to have patients more or less noisy in the latter rooms, but it will be readily seen that those east rooms being placed *in* at a distance from the east outer wall of the building, are nearly a central point from which the noise made in them radiates in every direction. Indeed, the noise made in that building not only radiates all over and through it, but, six of the nine single rooms on each floor being on the west side next to the men's lodge and main house, the noise made there radiates over and through the whole establishment and premises, and I do not a whit exaggerate the serious evils of the present state of things there and here when I say that during the warm season when patients are most excited and noisy, no individual can sleep there for on an average of as many as five nights out of seven who could not, with weariness and custom, sleep in as perfect a pandemonium as was ever witnessed on the earth. There were three nights in succession this present week in which not one wink of sleep was enjoyed by any patient on those Halls, except by a small proportion of demented, oblivious persons who could sleep any where. During some part of every night this week I have while lying in my bed in the main centre building, not only heard the noise

* From the Physician's Reports, Westchester Division.

but distinguished words and whole sentences vociferated by one or more of the patients in the women's Lodge. As I now write a patient leaves us, who has prevailed upon her husband to remove her, chiefly on account of the suffering she has experienced from loss of sleep and from hearing almost constantly by day and by night blasphemous, vulgar and invective declamation.

Patients and their friends generally have an unconquerable prejudice against the "lodge," and it is on account of the incessant annoyances to which I have alluded, and the absence of comforts and conveniences to which I will allude.

2. *Bathing and other uses and facilities for the use of Water.* The only convenience for bathing for both Halls in the female lodge is a tub situated in the basement beneath them. The bath room is always of the temperature of the external atmosphere and there are not and cannot well be any safe means of heating it, and the consequence is that in winter, in addition to the difficulty at all seasons of taking excited, feeble or filthy patients up and down a narrow, crooked flight of stairs, it is wholly improper to take such patients into a cold room and strip and wash them there—that room being often at the temperature of freezing, and sometimes lower. I have often been under the absolute necessity of administering stimulants to patients either before or after a bath on account of the coldness of the bath-room and the distance to reach it.

Every ounce of the great quantity of water that is or should be used on the Halls in keeping them clean and in the ordinary washing of the patients' faces and hands, and in cleansing them from their hourly accidents of nature, is carried by hand up one or two flights of stairs and used in little half effectual slops at any point about the Halls where a stove with a basin upon it can be set down in temporary safety. During at least three days of every week all the hot water used is brought by hand in pails all the way from the main centre building—a burden which should not be unnecessarily imposed upon the attendants whose duties are at best of the most severe and trying nature.

The consequence of the absence of conveniences for the use of water just spoken of, is, that nearly half of our female patients enjoy only its most ordinary comforts and benefits—such as are enjoyed in all the shanties which line the ungraded avenues and dot over the commons in our neighborhood.

3. *Heating and Ventilation.* The heat supplied to both Halls of the women's lodge is insufficient in quantity and of a bad quality. A single furnace only is used and the air chamber is only just as large as will suffice to contain it. The consequence is that a single stream of scorching hot air issues into each Hall, the privilege of being baked by which every patient struggles to monopolize and the monopoly is oftenest enjoyed by those who least need it, while the rest shiver with cold or growl with envy at a distance.

The draft of the furnace is so poor that every morning and evening when the fire is replenished and during the long time which, on account of the bad draft, is required for the coal to become thoroughly ignited and the combustion of it free, such a quantity of Carbonic Acid is thrown into the corridors as almost to suffocate those confined in them and to operate most injuriously on their general health. I have often entered those Halls when the gas has at once excited coughing and induced a very unpleasant sense of fullness in the head, and I have been obliged to throw up all the windows and then retreat till the atmosphere had become changed and purified, and, of course, as cold as the external air. Indeed, the custom has been throughout the season of fires, to throw open the windows morning and evening, and let the patients shiver through a couple of hours, in preference to their breathing such an unpleasant and deleterious atmosphere as they would necessarily have done had the windows been kept closed and the temperature maintained at a suitable elevation.

Again, in the case of patients (and there are always several such in every Institution) who, on account of excitement or dementia, will not attend to keeping themselves covered with their bed-clothes at night or whose beds become wet and otherwise defiled, there is no provision whatever in the women's lodge (nor in any other part of the establishment) to elevate the temperature of the rooms they occupy except in the slight degree occasioned by the passage of a very little heat from the corridor through the unglazed sash over the door. The consequence is that during the coldest months many of our patients suffer exceedingly, particularly at night, and, in order to make them as comfortable as possible, we are obliged to tie the worst in their habits and feeblest into bed at night, and tie their clothes upon them —a species of restraint which is calculated to induce filthy bodily habits and to confirm those already existing. It may, I think, be laid down as an axiomatic truth, that feeble and excited insane patients cannot be made even safely comfortable unless their sleeping as well as day rooms can if necessary be maintained at a temperature of from 60° to 70° of Fah. at all times, and the air changed often by a system of active ventilation.

4. Supervision of the Patients by the Attendants at night. There are no arrangements by which an attendant may exercise a supervision over the associated dormitory at night or over a feeble or suicidal patient occupying a single room unless she sits up and keeps wholly awake. Such a thing as an associated dormitory in the Hall occupied by the worst class of patients is, under the best arrangements, wholly wrong—I never saw one so situated in any other Institution—but ours, in my opinion, admits of no defense. Into it from four to six of the worst class of patients are locked at night and the attendant is out of sight and hearing (accustomed as she is to sleep, unless the noise be very near or very extraordinary) and whatever accidents occur among them, no one is wiser for it till morning. The attendant's room should be adjacent to the associated dormitory and separated from it only by a lattice door, through which all disturbances could be readily heard and seen.

5. There is no Water Closet in the women's lodge. The privy, which is placed at a little distance in the rear, is reached by a covered walk or passage with lattice sides. This arrangement answers tolerably well in summer, though it is then objectionable in affording patients frequent opportunities to get out of the view of their attendants, and to injure themselves or each other by violence, or to indulge in filthy or indolent habits. In the winter season the quite feeble cannot go to the privy at all, and the frequent use of *pots de chambre* in the house tends to render the air foul and unpleasant. The much demented, tho in fair bodily health, will not in cold weather go to the privy unless accompanied on every occasion by an attendant, but if alone will almost invariably defile the passage before reaching it.

By an examination of the two following plans a general idea of the improvements I would respectfully suggest, will readily be gained. The plan marked *A* represents either of the Halls in the women's lodge as they at present exist, both being precisely alike in all their arrangements. The plan marked *B* would represent the lower Hall (that occupied by the most excited class) after the proposed additions and alteration are made. The upper Hall would differ from the lower merely in having the new floor beyond the bathroom divided into only three instead of six rooms, as below. These three upper rooms are much needed to isolate a few highly excited patients of the higher class socially, whose friends are willing to remunerate the Institution liberally for their care and do not want them thrown in with from fifteen to twenty others, comprising persons of every grade of character and of every disgusting form of disease and habit.

The basement of the addition I would propose to occupy by a room in which to deposit the dead, by a large air chamber with its furnace, and by another compartment with water closet etc. in it for the accommodation of the wash-people, so that the present highly improper inter-communication between patients and their attendants and the wash-people might be altogether avoided.

From such rough estimates as I have been able to make I conclude that such an additional building as I propose, erected in the most thorough and substantial, but plain manner, together with water closets, baths etc. and the slight alterations proposed in the present building, would cost about five thousand dollars. Nearly an additional thousand dollars would be required to paint the present building throughout thoroughly and to purchase furniture for the new building and additional furniture for the present halls.

I respectfully but earnestly commend this subject to your favorable consideration.

C. H. Nichols

VII: REPORT BY DOROTHEA L. DIX ON THE ASYLUM

October 7, 1851

General and Concise Summary *

DEFECTS, WANTS, CONSEQUENCES

1. Inconvenience resulting from architectural defects.
2. Crowded Lodging Rooms.
3. Wholly unsuitable accommodations for highest class of patients.
4. Insufficient and ineffective modes of heating wings of the main building and the lodges.
5. Imperfect ventilation in all.
6. Contiguity of strong rooms in main building to the common dormitories.
7. Want of dumb waiters in the main building and proper means of carrying food to the Lodge buildings:
   - 1st Occasionally unsuitable congregation of nurses and attendants and often of patients in the passages leading from the kitchens in the basement.
   - 2nd Transportation of heavy trays over several flights of stairs—confusion and discomfort in serving—intercommunication of patients and nurses in different halls, etc., etc.
   - 3rd Exposure in reaching the Lodges in severe or inclement weather, etc.
   - 4th Delays, Temptations, Neglects, Confusion.
8. The Lodges: insufficiently warmed; insufficiently ventilated; insufficiently
   - 1st Protected—inspection and uniform oversight on the part of the officers entirely insufficient and infrequent comparatively.
   - 2nd Danger from fire; from lights.
   - 3rd In Females' lodge—from explosion of Boiler in the wash room beneath the Lodging rooms.
   - 4th Offensive nuisance and unhealthful vicinity of laundry to patients' rooms.
   - 5th Communication of servants in the same with the nurses and patients.
   - 6th No bathing rooms, wash sinks, and other requisite accommodations for invalids and excited patients in either lodge.
   - 7th No supervisor, no night watch in either.
   - 8th Noise of steam engine disturbs the quiet and stimulates the violence of the excited patients.
9. No seats nor shelter in the airing courts for excited patients attached to the Women's Lodge.
10. Excited patients left unguarded and the more quiet unprotected in the absence of nurses and attendants, while bringing food at meal hours from the basement kitchens in main building.—

etc. etc.

* Full report not found.

WANTS, ABSOLUTE

1. Competent supervisors in every department—either steward and matron required to serve in these departments, as in some institutions, or additional officers as in others.
2. It is a positive obligation and acknowledged necessity that no institution for the insane shall be left at any hour at any season without a physician within its walls; consequently that there should be an assistant physician; in an asylum having but few patients, the second medical officer might act as supervisor on most occasions in the Men's Wing and Lodge.

11. Material arrangements of the Institution at Bloomingdale defective and *must* for the most part remain defective under the present defective organization.

Three commanders in chief leading an army; three captains commanding a ship; three magistrates ruling a city; three presidents governing the union, might well lead respectively to defeat, to loss, to contest, to confusion, to anarchy and overthrow.

12. Buildings defective; extension necessary
   1st for improved internal arrangements;
   2nd the comfort and advantage of patients;
   3rd the admission of a larger number of patients;
   4th for the reputation of the institution;
   5th for the greatest possible usefulness.
13. Consequences of present position
   1st inefficiency in its operation.
   2nd Distrust throughout the community
   3rd Disapprobation of medical men—well informed and experienced in the treatment of the Insane
   4th Disadvantage through frequent change of physician

(Facts) The Bloomingdale Asylum has been established (I think) about 30 (thirty) years, and has had already 8 (eight) or *more* resident physicians; since 1830 there have been 6 different physicians in charge of the institution, the average duration of whose professional connection has been about 3 years and

14. No physician has ever entered upon his duties at the Bloomingdale Asylum approving its organization.
   2nd No physician (so far as I have knowledge) has retired from his charge without great dissatisfaction; without having
   3d made efforts for improving its condition;
   4th without a conviction of the impossibility of carrying out the greatest good under the existing organization.
   5th No physician, respecting his own reputation, strictly conscientious, respecting the rights and claims of his patients, and his obligation to their friends and to the community at large will ever long hold the office under the present system.

Finally the Institution should accomplish good it does not accomplish;

should take a rank it does not now hold; should reflect honor, not ask reproach on its Officers and Governors, tho all have done too much that is well, not to advance to that which is greatly better. The Institution they direct should do honor to their City, to their State, to their Country:—it now does neither.

Excuse me Gentlemen, if I seem severe; I am only truthful.

Very respectfully,
D. L. Dix

Highwood, Hoboken
October 7th, 1851

VIII: REPORT BY THE BLOOMINGDALE ASYLUM COMMITTEE ON THE SUBJECT OF MISS DIX'S REPORT

December 2, 1851 *

To the Board of Governors of the New York Hospital

GENTLEMEN:

The Asylum Committee to whom you referred the memorial of Miss D. L. Dix have with much deliberation considered the statements therein, and feel constrained to say that in their judgment the defects of the Institution are materially magnified and its many merits overlooked.

In the summary of Miss Dix the first thing called to notice is architectural defects. If the buildings were now to be erected doubtless improvements would be made. The Main Building the committee consider in its general arrangement, convenient and comfortable, the wings are warmed by two of Beebe's furnaces placed in each basement, the flues from which open on the several halls; if the flues were separate to each hall, a more equal distribution of heat would be made. In addition to the warmth derived from the furnaces, each hall has a large sitting room with open fire in grate; the committee believe the occasions very few if any in which a sufficiency of heat is not obtained both for health and comfort.

The dormitories can not well be otherwise than comfortable, provided a sufficiency of bed clothing is furnished, and a proper care observed in closing windows.

The water arrangements are certainly, both as regards bathing tubs and water closets, very complete.

Dumb waiters for the purpose of conveying food from the basements to the several halls, would doubtless be a convenience, but are not essential, nor does the want of them affect the convenience or comfort of the patients.

The communication of male and female attendants in procuring food, can doubtless be prevented by proper directions from the Physician, or so regulated as to avoid any evil growing therefrom. The same care on the part of the Physician will prevent all other intercourse between them which he deems improper or injurious.

As regards patients having intercourse with each other on the stair ways leading to the several halls, there is no necessity for it whatever; and proper care on the part of those whose duty it is to direct attendants and patients can effectually prevent it.

It would be pleasant to the committee, if they were able to present the condition and arrangement of the Lodges in as favorable a light as they have the wings of the main building, but candor will lead them to name many defects.

The female Lodge has one of Beebe's furnaces in the basement, a flue from it opening on each hall. Gas from it is frequently unpleasant, particularly when fires are renewed by fresh coal. It is believed this may and will be remedied; each hall has a sitting room, on one floor it is warmed by

* From the *Minutes of the Governors.*

a drum, on the other by open fire in grate—this building is believed to be comfortable as regards warmth. The bathing tub is in the basement, which is inconvenient, and in cold weather uncomfortable; water can only be obtained by being carried in pails.

Water closets there are none in the building, the passage ways to the privy are under cover—the engine which supplies the main house with croton water is in the basement of this building; the man in charge of it has expressed the opinion that should there be an explosion, the halls above would not be injured. The committee do not learn that the noise of the engine is heard in the halls, or in any way disturbs the patients.

The men's Lodge is also heated by a furnace, the flues of which open on three halls; in the basement, the opening is some feet from the floor; on the others very near the floor—the basement is not what it should be, or what the Committee desire to see it, either as regards warmth or purity of air—complaints have not reached the ears of the committee of want of comfort on the other halls; the bathing tub in this, as in the Female Lodge is in the basement, consequently in cold weather uncomfortable—it is supplied through pipes with both warm and cold water.

This Lodge is also without a water closet, and there is more exposure in reaching the privy than from the other lodge. When the condition of most patients in this building is considered, generally men of fair bodily health, but little suffering need be experienced, if attendants are watchful in their going out and coming in—close stools are used when occasions call for them.

The remarks of Miss Dix as to this building and its inmates, that "should enquiry be made of the Physician and other officers and attendants, facts would be revealed showing censurable circumstances too numerous to detail, and too unpleasant or offensive to record" has reference mainly, as Miss Dix states, to the want of proper arrangements for bathing and water closets—the Board will judge as to the propriety of such strong language in relation to it.

Classification could doubtless be much improved if accommodations were provided for the violent patients separate from others; this has long been considered by the committee a deficiency in the arrangements, and they have been anxious to remedy it,—the erection of additional accommodations has been under consideration for some months past.

In relation to Night Watcher, Dr. Earle soon after he took charge of the Asylum employed a watch in the male department whose duty it was to pass through the mens hall and Lodge once in each hour of the night. Dr. Nichols has dispensed with a watch during the summer, but employed one in the winter; a man is now in the house engaged for that duty.

The recommendation of Miss Dix, that a well educated intelligent female should be employed whose duty it shall be to visit from hall to hall with the endeavor by reading and otherwise to sooth, comfort, and counsel the afflicted, also to assist nurses in extreme cases, is worthy of consideration. If such a person can be obtained, the committee think the experiment should be made. Appointment and dismissal to rest with the Committee.

The principal defects and difficulties presented by Miss Dix, have now been considered, except that of Government.

The several members of the Board who in former years have served on the Asylum Committees, and are familiar with its management, are as capable of forming a sound judgment on this head as those now on duty—the committee however will say, they are not in favor of enlarged power in the hands of the Physician.

Miss Dix's statement that no Physician has ever entered upon his duties at the Asylum approving of its organization is believed to be a mistake—the rules of government now existing were drawn up by the late Dr. Mcdonald after his visit to European Asylums and it is believed was in entire accordance with his judgment as to what was wise. Dr. Earle when commencing his duties at Bloomingdale expressed his satisfaction in being relieved from responsibility of duties to be performed by the Warden.

The Committee in conclusion cannot refrain from expressing their conviction that the Institution possesses merits which entitles it to the confidence of the community.

Respectfully submitted
STEPHEN ALLEN, *Chairman*
STACY B. COLLINS, *Secy.*

IX: REPORT OF THE COMMISSION APPOINTED BY GOVERNOR HOFFMAN TO INVESTIGATE CHARGES AGAINST BLOOMINGDALE, 1872 *

To His Excellency John A. Dix, Governor:

SIR.—On August 20th, 1872, his excellency, Governor Hoffman, addressed to the undersigned the following communication:

STATE OF NEW YORK
EXECUTIVE CHAMBER,
Albany, August 20, 1872.

GENTLEMEN.—Charges of abuse in the Bloomingdale Lunatic Asylum have lately been made in the public prints, by parties who give their names, and avow their ability to prove their allegations. This asylum is, in common with others of less note, a purely private establishment, subject to no supervision of the public authorities. Our laws permit the confinement of alleged lunatics as well in these private institutions as in the public asylums of the State, upon the order of magistrates of the grade of justice of the peace, issued upon the certificate of any two physicians. This condition of the law giving opportunity for abuses, I have, more than once, asked the Legistature to correct. At the last session, two bills passed the Assembly, furnishing better safeguards in connection with the commitment and care of lunatics; one of these provided (very properly,) that no person or institution should undertake the care of lunatics, except when licensed by the State Commissioners of Charities, and thus subject to their inspection; this bill failed to pass the Senate. It was publicly asserted (and not denied,) that the failure of the bill in the Senate was due chiefly to the personal efforts at Albany, of the chief physician of the Bloomingdale Asylum. An aversion, thus manifested, to proper supervision of the public authorities, makes it the more important, as well to the repute of the institution itself, as to the public interests, that the charges now made should be investigated.

I therefore appoint you as a commission for the purpose of investigating these charges, and others that may be laid before you against this or any other asylum for lunatics, whether under public or private management, and of visiting and inspecting the several asylums for the insane, with or without charges being made against them, with a view of discovering abuses wherever they exist, requesting that you report the result of your inquiries to me as soon as possible.

The duty which I impose upon you is, I know, onerous. At the present time there is no provision of law enabling me to compensate you for your labors or your expenses. I feel warranted, however, in assuring you that the Legislature, at its next session, will not fail to provide a just and liberal compensation.

Knowing that the people will have the same confidence that I have in your fitness for this very important trust, I make an earnest request that you will, out of regard for the general good, accept the duty.

Very truly yours,
JOHN T. HOFFMAN

To Hon. Francis C. Barlow, Attorney-General, M. B. Anderson, LL.D., President Rochester University, Thomas Hun, M.D., Albany, N.Y.

In accordance with this request we have visited and examined the Bloomingdale Lunatic Asylum, and several other of the asylums of the

* *Journal of Insanity,* XXIX (April, 1873), p. 591.

State, to wit, the establishments known as Sandford Hall, at Flushing, Brigham Hall, at Canandaigua, the establishment of Dr. Kittredge, at Fishkill, and the State Lunatic Asylum at Utica, and we have heard the statements of those who, after public notice of our meetings, chose to come before us, including those by whom the charges against the Bloomingdale Asylum, mentioned in the letter of Governor Hoffman, were made.

The inquiries made by us have been limited by what we conceived to be the object and motives of our appointment.

Complaints and charges in the public prints had created a fear in the public mind that the several insane asylums of the State were made instruments of oppression, by the incarceration of persons who were not of unsound mind, and stories of abuses in the treatment of patients had excited apprehension in those whose friends were necessarily committed to the care of these institutions.

We conceive that the information of the public on these two points was the object of our appointment.

It would serve no good purpose for us to publish the mass of evidence taken by us, or to go into all the details of our investigations, or to set forth a variety of minor points in regard to which we might feel inclined to criticise the management of these institutions. We could only say in conclusion, what we now say, that, in our opinion, there should be some system of public supervision.

Having early come to the conclusion that the *possibility* of abuses in these institutions, without reference to their actual existence at the present time, is such that some system of supervision and inspection by the public authorities is desirable, we have not considered it necessary to continue our investigation further than we have above stated; and we therefore submit our general conclusions upon the points indicated, and we unite in recommending the passage of some law providing for a system of visitation and inspection.

First. We are of opinion that there is no just foundation for the apprehension that persons not insane are improperly confined in these institutions.

There will always be some cases in which there may be doubt as to the degree of the unsoundness of mind, and as to the danger to himself and others which would result from the going at large of the patient.

Not being experts on this subject, we obviously could not attempt to pass upon these doubtful cases; but as long as the persons in charge of these institutions are believed to be upright and skillful, the decision of these questions is more properly left to them with their large experience and opportunities of examination.

We would not be understood as intimating that we have doubts as to the propriety of the confinement of any of the persons who came under our observations, for we have not.

Having recommended the passage of a law for a supervision of asylums by persons skilled in the treatment of the insane, we do not feel it to be our duty to do more than express our opinion that these institutions, so far as we have visited them, are not knowingly and designedly made instruments for the incarceration of sane persons.

We do not hesitate to say that, in our opinion, the public anxiety on that point is wholly unfounded.

Second. As to the treatment and discipline of the insane, and the internal management and regulation of asylums, we do not consider it within our province to make any extended criticism of the methods of treatment and discipline pursued, or to point out any improvements which we might think could be made in the details of management.

A proper system of licensing and supervision will result in the laying down such rules and regulations as science and experience shall approve.

We only think it necessary to inform the public whether we find any gross abuses in the treatment of these unfortunate persons.

The great difficulty to be met with in these institutions is to protect the patients from the harsh and impatient treatment of the attendants. It is very difficult to find persons of kindness, patience and consideration, who are willing to spend their time in the care of the insane; and the difficulty of ascertaining, among the numerous complaints of persons of disordered minds, whether any particular ones are well founded, must be obvious.

Instances of abuse occur in all asylums, and attendants are not unfrequently discharged for that reason.

The utmost vigilance can not entirely prevent it, and all that can be required of the managers of such institutions is an active and vigilant scrutiny into all cases of complaint.

We have no doubt that any such conduct on the part of attendants would be promptly punished in the asylums above named whenever brought to the knowledge of the officers; but it is obvious that such officers do not properly discharge their duty unless they are ever wakeful and vigorous in detecting such abuses, and in maintaining a most thorough supervision over all subordinates.

In regard to the charge made against Bloomingdale Asylum in the public prints, we think that in order to do justice, both to the institution and the public, we may fairly say this: That the gross cases of mismanagement and misconduct charged against it have not been substantiated, and that great injustice has been done to the institution in representing it as the scene of outrages and habitual maltreatment of patients.

At the same time we are compelled to say that some instances of the improper treatment of patients by attendants have been fairly proven before us, and that we do not think that the utmost vigilance in detecting and guarding against this kind of abuse has prevailed in this asylum during the past summer.

Nothing but the sternest discipline, and the most careful watching over attendants, and the most searching and prompt investigations into [any] suggestions or suspicions of harsh treatment by them, should be tolerated in an institution of this kind, and we think there has been some laxity in this respect.

It is proper to say that one of the attendants, charged with improper treatment of the patients, had been discharged before our visit to the asylum, and that any relaxation of discipline during the past summer may have been the result of the absence of the superintendent for a considerable period by reason of the illness of himself and his family, and of the illness and death of one of the assistant physicians. We are bound to state the facts as we found them.

We have also visited the insane asylums at Ward's Island and Blackwell's Island, but as controversies were going on between the Commissioners of Charities and Correction and some of their physicians in regard to the management of these asylums, and the subject of the conduct of some of the attendants was then before the courts, it became clear to us that any investigation by those who, like ourselves, had no power of examining witnesses under oath, would be of little value, and we, therefore, did not press the examination.

In regard to the legislation needed to place insane asylums under supervision, we differ among ourselves.

Dr. Anderson is of the opinion that authority should be given to State Board of Public Charities to appoint a superintendent of lunatic Asylums, whose duties and powers should be defined by law, and who shall be associated in the discharge and exercise of those duties and powers with the members of that board.

General Barlow and Dr. Hun believe that such commissioner should be appointed by the Governor and Senate, and that he should be an officer separate and distinct from the Board of State Charities, and they submit a bill herewith creating such officer and defining his powers.

It is, perhaps, not of much consequence who has the appointment of such an officer, but it is the opinion of General Barlow and Dr. Hun that when appointed he should have the powers indicated in the accompanying bill, and that the various asylums should be put under the strict supervision provided for therein.

While differing as to the method of supervision, we all agree that in some way the public authorities should have control over this large class of helpless citizens.

We do this, not because we distrust the management of the various asylums and institutions which we have visited, for we believe that, subject to the criticism hereinbefore made, they are conducted and managed by skillful and humane men; but because we believe that a proper system of supervision would relieve the public anxiety in relation to these institutions, and at the same time be a protection to the asylums themselves from unjust suspicions and aspersions.

We have found the managers and officers of the several asylums and institutions heartily in favor of some system of public supervision.

Very Respectfully,
Francis C. Barlow
M. B. Anderson
Albany, Feb. 13th, 1873. Thomas Hun

X

A: ADMISSIONS, 1792–1936

Decades	Voluntary Admissions			Number Treated			Number Admitted		
	M	*W*	*Total*	*M*	*W*	*Total*	*M*	*W*	*Total*
New York Hospital General Service									
1792–1807 [a]	...	...	...	...	...	444	...	...	444
New York Hospital Special Dept.									
1808–1821 [b]	...	...	...	...	...	1,148	...	...	1,148
Bloomingdale Asylum (Hospital)									
1821–1830 [c]	...	...	...	...	...	1,268	...	...	1,268
1831–1840	...	...	...	...	...	1,320	...	...	1,228
1841–1850	...	...	...	...	...	1,254	...	...	1,123
1851–1860	...	...	...	...	...	1,335	636	589	1,225
1861–1870	...	...	...	...	...	1,495	650	690	1,340
1871–1880	...	...	...	...	...	1,246	518	563	1,081
1881–1890	...	...	2	913	885	1,798	811	773	1,584
1891–1900	...	...	10	...	...	1,592	674	613	1,287
1901–1910	...	...	295	768	725	1,493	610	543	1,153
1911–1920	615	698	1,313	1,210	1,270	2,480	1,041	1,081	2,122
1921–1930	831	1,035	1,866	1,375	1,640	3,015	1,219	1,470	2,689
1931–1936 [d]	490	746	1,236	752	1,058	1,810	627	897	1,524

[a] Records incomplete. See pp. 50–51.
[b] See p. 93.
[c] See p. 163.
[d] Five years only.

X

B: DISCHARGES, 1792–1936

Decades	Recovered			Improved and Much Improved			Unimproved and Transferred			Died			Total Discharged
	M	W	Total	M	W	Total	M	W	Total	M	W	Total	
New York Hospital General Service													
1792–1807 [a]	...	...	206	...	...	58	...	...	111	...	...	40	415
New York Hospital Special Dept.													
1808–1821 [b]	...	...	503	...	...	174	...	...	...	...	...	111	788
Bloomingdale Asylum (Hospital)													
1821–1830 [c]	...	...	541	...	...	264	...	...	296	...	...	75	1,176
1831–1840	...	...	604	...	...	202	...	...	235	...	...	147	1,188
1841–1850	...	...	529	...	...	290	...	...	171	...	...	153	1,143
1851–1860	249	233	482	140	148	288	121	101	222	105	83	188	1,180
1861–1870	261	290	551	186	197	383	79	83	162	109	115	224	1,320
1871–1880	140	187	327	148	209	357	102	65	167	97	84	181	1,032
1881–1890	190	276	466	258	233	491	133	134	267	187	80	267	1,491
1891–1900	159	192	351	212	239	451	98	70	168	192	93	285	1,255
1901–1910	164	165	329	217	178	395	71	100	171	146	94	240	1,135
1911–1920	204	259	463	437	414	851	226	305	531	122	74	196	2,041
1921–1930	210	373	583	506	622	1,128	295	301	596	68	46	114	2,421
1931–1936 [d]	123	186	309	261	466	727	153	179	332	12	18	30	1,398

[a] Records incomplete. See pp. 50–51. [b] See p. 93. [c] See p. 163. [d] Five years only.

Not included in this table are 205 patients listed in the annual reports from 1911 to 1936 under *Discharges* as "Not insane" or "Without psychosis," which include alcoholics, drug habitués, etc. Such listing does not appear before 1911, although occasionally in the earlier periods may be found "Improper Objects" (very few), also "Eloped" and "By Request," which have been included here under "Unimproved and Transferred."

XI: NEW YORK STATE LEGISLATION, 1785–1905, RELATING TO THE CARE OF THE MENTALLY ILL BY THE NEW YORK HOSPITAL

In the colony of New York idiocy and lunacy were civil disqualifications as in the English common law.

1785. Order of Common Council of the city of New York: Not more than five rooms in almshouse to be used for insane. (Until the New York City Lunatic Asylum was established in 1839, there was no other special provision except the New York Hospital.)

Laws of 1788, Chap. 31. All persons "furiously mad," etc., must be apprehended and confined by order of two or more justices of the peace. For text, see p. 73, this volume. (English Statute 17, Chap. 5, Sec. 6.)

1801. Act depriving insane of power to devise personal or real estate. Chancellor to see to maintenance and care of lunatics and their estates.

Laws of 1809, Chap. 90. Overseers of the poor authorized to contract with the governors of the New York Hospital for the care of lunatics.

March 23, 1810. Grant of $3500 a year for ten years. (Stopped by Act of April 15, 1817, Sec. 5.)

April 17, 1816. Grant of annuity of $10,000 until 1857, thereby permitting erection of new building for insane patients (Bloomingdale).

Laws of 1822, Chap. 257, Sec. 4. No property of the Society of the New York Hospital to be subject to taxes by any law of New York State.

Laws of 1827, Chap. 294. "An Act Concerning Lunatics." Insane persons should not be confined in prison, jail, etc., but should be sent to "the asylum in New York" or other place provided for reception of the insane.

April 17, 1830. Committee appointed by Legislature to investigate the use of funds by New York Hospital and Bloomingdale, and the need for a state institution.

March 10, 1831. Assembly Doc. 263, 1831. Report of above committee. (See pp. 158–160, this volume.)

Laws of 1842, Chap. 20. State Asylum organized. Certificates by two physicians required for admission to asylums. Patient may appeal to judge of the county against confinement, and judge may call a jury "to decide upon the fact of lunacy."

1857. Grant of $10,000 extended for two more years.

Aug. 20, 1872. Governor appointed commission to investigate charges against Bloomingdale and condition of asylums.

Feb. 13, 1873. Report of above commission. (See Appendix IX, above.)

Laws of 1873, Chap. 571. Creates office of Commissioner of Lunacy, responsible to State Board of Charities. Provides for licensing and inspection of asylums.

Laws of 1874, Chap. 446. Revision of lunacy law; no person to be confined except on certificate of two physicians and with approval by judge within five days. Jury may be called.

Laws of 1875, Chap. 446. "The portion of the property real and personal of the Society of the New York Hospital, a charitable corporation located in the City and County of New York, from which no income is derived, shall be exempted from taxation so long as the same shall be used exclusively for the purposes for which said Society was chartered."

April 18, 1879. Opinion of Attorney-General as requested by State Commissioner, no obligation on part of Bloomingdale to receive pauper insane. (See p. 311, this volume.)

Laws of 1884, Chap. 17. City prohibited from opening streets from 115th to 119th through Bloomingdale property.

May 4, 1888. State Senate Docs. No. 61 and 62. Report of Committee on Taxation etc., in the matter of the memorial of the Morningside Park Association. (See pp. 315–316, above.)

Laws of 1889, Chap. 283. Three Commissioners in Lunacy instead of one, directly responsible to the Governor.

June 12, 1889. Bill passed for laying out 116th Street from 10th Avenue to Broadway, to take effect Jan. 1, 1894.

June 13, 1889. Bill passed exempting property of New York Hospital "Wherever situated, from which no income is derived," from taxation.

April, 1890. State Care Act.

June, 1891. White Plains property judged not taxable by Court of Appeals.

1905. Medical inspector appointed by Commission in Lunacy to visit public and private institutions.

New-York, *30* day of *June* — 18*51*

Admit *Mary E* a **Patient into the**

Asylum. *at the rate of $4- per week for Board - the requisition of the Law being first complied with -*

To the superintendent of the Bloomingdale Asylum.

M. A. [illegible]

N. B. Security for Board, &c. must be given by the friends of the Patient immediately on admission, and the Board paid in full when, or before the Patient is removed.

A written statement of the circumstances of the case, and the causes, (as far as can be ascertained) of insanity, drawn up by the Physician, or some friend of the Patient, is expected at the time of admission.

B

1st R. S. p. 638. § 4, 5, 8, 10.

STATE OF NEW-YORK,
CITY AND COUNTY OF NEW-YORK, } ss.

To the Constables and Overseers of the Poor of the City of New-York.

Greeting:

WHEREAS, Complaint on Oath has been made to us, *John W. Wyman & Oliver M. Lowndes* Esquires, Special Justices for preserving the Peace in the said city, by *Benj. L. Swan*

That *John S* by reason of Lunacy or otherwise, is so far disordered in his senses as to endanger his own person, or the person or property of others, if permitted to go at large, and being satisfied upon examination, that it would be dangerous to permit the said *John Saidler* to go at large:

These are therefore in the name of the People of the State of New-York, to command you, the said Constables and Overseers, and every of you, to cause to be apprehended the body of the said *John Saidler* and him safely to be locked up and confined in such secure place as may be provided by you the said Overseers, within the said city of New-York, and to be dealt with as the law directs.

Given under our hands and seals, this *18* day of *July* in the year of our Lord, 183*1*

John W. Wyman

O. M. Lowndes

XII: FACSIMILES OF DOCUMENTS RELATING TO ADMISSION OF PATIENTS

A. Permit for Admission of Patients, 1821

B. Order for Commitment, 1831

C. Physician's Certificate, 1869

C

2d R. S. 5 Ed. part 1. Chap. xx. Title 3. Art. 1. Sec. 4 & 5.—Laws of 1860, Ch. 506, § 6.

Police Court—Third District.

STATE OF NEW YORK,
City and County of New York, } ss. Charles R Gill

of No. 244 Union Street, in the City of ~~New York~~ Brooklyn, *Physician*,

and Thos Ponce de Leon

of No. 214 East 13th. Street, in said City, *Physician*, being duly sworn, severally say. That Richard De L[illegible] is **Insane**, and is so far disordered in his senses, as to endanger his own person, and the persons and property of others, if permitted to go at large.

That they have personally examined said Richard and are satisfied that he is afflicted with such a vitiated understanding, and alienation of mind, as disables him from judging correctly between good and evil, and of the consequences of his acts, amounting to an absolute dispossession of the free and natural agency of the human mind.

Sworn before me, this 24th *day* of Jan 1869

[illegible] *Police Justice*

Chas. R Gill M.D.

Thos Ponce de Leon M.D.

XIII: THE ASYLUM COMMITTEE OF THE BOARD OF GOVERNORS OF THE NEW YORK HOSPITAL, 1808–1821

Gilbert Aspinwall	June 7, 1808–June 6, 1809
	June 4, 1811–Oct. 10, 1812
	June 6, 1815–June 4, 1816
John R. Murray	June 7, 1808–June 5, 1810
	June 1, 1819–June 5, 1821
Thomas Eddy	June 7, 1808–June 5, 1810
	June 7, 1814–Jan. 7, 1817
Thomas Franklin	June 7, 1808–June 5, 1821
William Johnson	June 7, 1808–June 6, 1809
Valentine Hicks	June 5, 1810–June 4, 1811
Benjamin D. Perkins	June 5, 1810–Oct. 1810
Matthew Franklin	Nov. 6, 1810–June 2, 1812
	Nov. 3, 1812–June 1, 1813
Jacob Sherred	June 2, 1812–June 6, 1815
	Jan. 7, 1817–June 1, 1819
Cadwallader D. Colden	June 1, 1813–June 7, 1814
Cornelius Dubois	June 4, 1816–June 2, 1818
John McComb	June 2, 1818–June 5, 1821

XIV: ORGANIZATION OF NEW YORK HOSPITAL, WESTCHESTER DIVISION, 1936

Board of Governors of Society of the New York Hospital

Westchester Division Committee

Medical Director

Assistant Medical Director

usiness Administration

1 Steward
4 Clerks and Stenographers
2 Storekeeper and Assistant
1 Barber
3 Watchmen
2 Ushers
3 Chauffeurs

Medical Staff

12 Resident Physicians
7 Visiting Physicians
9 Consulting Physicians
1 Dentist
1 Apothecary

Nursing Staff

1 Director
2 Assistant Directors
2 Instructors
6 Supervisors
66 Nurses
41 Student Nurses
34 Attendants

Plant Maintenance

6 Engineer and Assistants
6 Firemen
3 Plumbers
2 Blacksmith and Assistant
3 Carpenters
9 Painters
2 Tinsmith and Roofer
1 Plasterer

Laboratories and X-ray

1 Director
2 Technicians

Therapies

6 Directors
21 Assistants
1 Chaplain
5 Choir and Organist
1 Librarian

Dietary Service

3 Dietitians
3 Student Dietitians
1 Butcher
34 Cooks and helpers

Farm and Grounds

1 Supervisor
2 Florists
20 Laborers

Domestic Service

4 Housekeepers and Assistants
2 Laundry Overseer and Assistant
101 Maids and Porters
24 Laundry workers
2 Upholsterers
3 Dressmakers and Seamstresses
2 Clothing and Linen Clerks

Summary

Medical Staff	32
Nursing Staff	152
Laboratories	3
Therapies	34
Business Administration	26
Dietary Service	41
Domestic Service	138
Plant Maintenance	32
Grounds	23
	481

NOTE: 587 patients treated in 1936; average daily number 264. (From the Annual Report for 1936.)

INDEX

MENTAL ILLNESS AND SOCIAL POLICY

THE AMERICAN EXPERIENCE

AN ARNO PRESS COLLECTION

Barr, Martin W. Mental Defectives: Their History, Treatment and Training. 1904.

The Beginnings of American Psychiatric Thought and Practice: Five Accounts, 1811-1830. 1973

The Beginnings of Mental Hygiene in America: Three Selected Essays, 1833-1850. 1973

Briggs, L. Vernon, et al. History of the Psychopathic Hospital, Boston, Massachusetts. 1922

Briggs, L. Vernon. Occupation as a Substitute for Restraint in the Treatment of the Mentally Ill. 1923

Brigham, Amariah. An Inquiry Concerning the Diseases and Functions of the Brain, the Spinal Cord, and the Nerves. 1840

Brigham, Amariah. Observations on the Influence of Religion upon the Health and Physical Welfare of Mankind. 1835

Brill, A. A. Fundamental Conceptions of Psychoanalysis. 1921

Bucknill, John Charles. Notes on Asylums for the Insane in America. 1876

Conolly, John. The Treatment of the Insane Without Mechanical Restraints. 1856

Coriat, Isador H. What is Psychoanalysis? 1917

Deutsch, Albert. The Shame of the States. 1948

Dewey, Richard. Recollections of Richard Dewey: Pioneer in American Psychiatry. 1936

Earle, Pliny. Memoirs of Pliny Earle, M. D. with Extracts from his Diary and Letters (1830-1892) and Selections from his Professional Writings (1839-1891). 1898

Galt, John M. **The Treatment of Insanity.** 1846

Goddard, Henry Herbert. **Feeble-mindedness**: Its Causes and Consequences. 1926

Hammond, William A. **A Treatise on Insanity in Its Medical Relations.** 1883

Hazard, Thomas R. **Report on the Poor and Insane in Rhode-Island.** 1851

Hurd, Henry M., editor. **The Institutional Care of the Insane in the United States and Canada.** 1916/1917. Four volumes.

Kirkbride, Thomas S. **On the Construction, Organization, and General Arrangements of Hospitals for the Insane.** 1880

Meyer, Adolf. **The Commonsense Psychiatry of Dr. Adolf Meyer**: Fifty-two Selected Papers. 1948

Mitchell, S. Weir. **Wear and Tear, or Hints for the Overworked.** 1887

Morton, Thomas G. **The History of the Pennsylvania Hospital, 1751-1895.** 1895

Ordronaux, John. **Jurisprudence in Medicine in Relation to the Law.** 1869

The Origins of the State Mental Hospital in America: Six Documentary Studies, 1837-1856. 1973

Packard, Mrs. E. P. W. **Modern Persecution,** or Insane Asylums Unveiled, As Demonstrated by the Report of the Investigating Committee of the Legislature of Illinois. 1875. Two volumes in one

Prichard, James C. **A Treatise on Insanity and Other Disorders Affecting the Mind.** 1837

Prince, Morton. **The Unconscious**: The Fundamentals of Human Personality Normal and Abnormal. 1921

Putnam, James Jackson. **Human Motives.** 1915

Russell, William Logie. **The New York Hospital**: A History of the Psychiatric Service, 1771-1936. 1945

Sidis, Boris. **The Psychology of Suggestion**: A Research into the Subconscious Nature of Man and Society. 1899

Southard, Elmer E. **Shell-Shock and Other Neuropsychiatric Problems** Presented in Five Hundred and Eighty-Nine Case Histories from the War Literature, 1914-1918. 1919

Southard, E[lmer] E. and Mary C. Jarrett. The Kingdom of Evils. 1922

Southard, E[lmer] E. and H[arry] C. Solomon. Neurosyphilis: Modern Systematic Diagnosis and Treatment Presented in One Hundred and Thirty-seven Case Histories. 1917

Spitzka, E[dward] C. Insanity: Its Classification, Diagnosis and Treatment. 1887

Supreme Court Holding a Criminal Term, No. 14056. The United States vs. Charles J. Guiteau. 1881/1882. Two volumes

Trezevant, Daniel H. Letters to his Excellency Governor Manning on the Lunatic Asylum. 1854

Tuke, D[aniel] Hack. The Insane in the United States and Canada. 1885

Upham, Thomas C. Outlines of Imperfect and Disordered Mental Action. 1868

White, William A[lanson]. Twentieth Century Psychiatry: Its Contribution to Man's Knowledge of Himself. 1936

Willard, Sylvester D. Report on the Condition of the Insane Poor in the County Poor Houses of New York. 1865

Bei Fragen zur Produktsicherheit wenden Sie sich bitte an:
If you have any questions regarding product safety,
please contact:

Walter de Gruyter GmbH
Genthiner Straße 13
10785 Berlin
productsafety@degruyterbrill.com